PATHO

SECRS

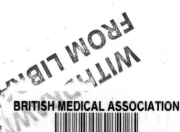

PATHOLOGY

SECRETS

Third Edition

Ivan Damjanov, MD, PhD
Professor of Pathology
Department of Pathology and Laboratory Medicine
Univerisity of Kansas School of Medicine
Kansas City, Kansas

MOSBY

ELSEVIER

MOSBY
ELSEVIER

1600 John F. Kennedy Blvd.
Ste 1800
Philadelphia, PA 19103-2899

PATHOLOGY SECRETS, THIRD EDITION   ISBN: 978-0-323-05594-9

Copyright © 2009 by Mosby, Inc., an affiliate of Elsevier Inc.

NOTICE

Knowledge and best practice in this field are constantly changing. As new research and experience broaden our knowledge, changes in practice, treatment and drug therapy may become necessary or appropriate. Readers are advised to check the most current information provided (i) on procedures featured or (ii) by the manufacturer of each product to be administered, to verify the recommended dose or formula, the method and duration of administration, and contraindications. It is the responsibility of the practitioner, relying on their own experience and knowledge of the patient, to make diagnoses, to determine dosages and the best treatment for each individual patient, and to take all appropriate safety precautions. To the fullest extent of the law, neither the Publisher nor the Editor assumes any liability for any injury and/or damage to persons or property arising out of or related to any use of the material contained in this book.

The Publisher

Library of Congress Cataloging-in-Publication Data

Damjanov, Ivan.
    Pathology secrets / Ivan Damjanov. – 3rd ed.
        p. ; cm.
    Includes bibliographical references and index.
    ISBN 978-0-323-05594-9
    1. Pathology–Examinations, questions, etc.   I.   Title.
    [DNLM: 1.   Pathology–Examination Questions. QZ 18.2 D161pa 2009]
    RB119.P375 2009
    616.07076–dc22

                                                                    2008034795

Acquisitions Editor: Jim Merritt
Developmental Editor: Barbara Cicalese
Project Manager: Mary Stermel
Marketing Manager: Allan McKeown

Working together to grow
libraries in developing countries

www.elsevier.com | www.bookaid.org | www.sabre.org

ELSEVIER   BOOK AID International   Sabre Foundation

Printed in China

Last digit is the print number: 9   8   7   6   5   4   3   2   1

DEDICATION

To my grandchildren, Dania and Alden, two consummate practitioners of the Socratic method.

To remind them how they used to ask, "WHY, WHY, WHY," when they were small, and even after their exasperated grandma tried to stop them with the formulaic answer, "That's how it is in real life." (Just in case there is another more real or surreal life besides the "real one"!)

And to remind them of Grandpa's favorite quote from Kipling's *The Elephant's Child*:

> I keep six honest serving-men
> (They taught me all I knew);
> Their names are What and Why and When
> And How and Where and Who.

CONTENTS

CONTRIBUTORS

Ivan Damjanov, MD, PhD
Professor of Pathology, Department of Pathology and Laboratory Medicine, University of Kansas School of Medicine, Kansas City, Kansas

Snježana Dotlić, MD
Staff Pathologist, Clinical Hospital Center Zagreb, Zagreb, Croatia

Bruce A. Fenderson, PhD
Professor of Pathology, Department of Pathology, Anatomy, and Cell Biology, Jefferson Medical College, Thomas Jefferson University, Philadelphia, Pennsylvania

Zoran Gatalica, MD, DSc
Professor of Pathology, Department of Pathology, Creighton University School of Medicine, Omaha, Nebraska

Péter P. Molnár, MD, DSc
Professor of Pathology, Department of Pathology, University of Debrecen School of Medicine, Medical and Health Sciences Center, Debrecen, Hungary

Anamarija Morović, MD
Clinical Instructor, Department of Pathology and Laboratory Medicine, University of Cincinnati College of Medicine, Cincinnati, Ohio

Marin Nola, MD, PhD
Associate Professor of Pathology, Department of Pathology, University of Zagreb School of Medicine, Zagreb, Croatia

PREFACE

This book was prepared for medical students in the hope that they will use it as a study guide and a source of succinct information complementing other sources that have been made available to them by their professors. I also hope that the book will help them prepare for seminars and discussion groups, both in the standard medical school setting and in the new problem-based curriculum. Finally, I hope that some students will use it while reviewing the pathology material for the board examinations.

During the past 30 years, I have taught pathology in several medical schools and have thus had the privilege of interacting with many medical students. Many of them, assuming that I have gathered some experience in teaching, used to ask me how to study pathology. My usual answer was this: Try to develop your own style, find out what is the most efficient way of studying (i.e., discover whatever works best for you), and then apply this approach systematically by using all means that you have at hand.

Over the years, I learned that some medical students profit most from lectures, others from books, whereas still others need both the books and the lectures. Some students like to use atlases, whereas others like to study the pictures from the computers. Some students love to study microscopy slides and autopsy material, whereas others think that such exercises are a waste of time. In other words, there are no secret ways to learn pathology or, for that matter, anything else.

If there are no secrets to be offered on how to study pathology, what would then be a good reason to read a book titled *Pathology Secrets*? My answer to the astute student asking this question is simple: This book might help you see more clearly the "secret" pearls of wisdom contained in the "big books" (i.e., the prescribed textbooks of pathology), help you tackle the material presented during the course in various other formats, and help you concentrate on the "important" topics. It could also help you understand better the basic topics of pathology by presenting them from a different angle than you have seen than in the standard textbooks. In addition, because many questions in this book are answered in a concise, bulleted form, I thought that *Pathology Secrets* could help you acquire the essential concepts of pathology more easily and in a more systematic way than if you had to compile such an outline on your own. As an added bonus, I have also included a few mnemonics here and there and a few other tricks to help you memorize for the long term the important facts, information you could use later in the clinics.

This book contains close to 2000 questions dealing with the most important topics of pathology. Almost all these questions were classroom tested; that is, most of these questions were used in discussions with medical students. The answers provided to these questions are short and in a format that I would expect from my students attending seminars and discussion groups or in written essay–type examinations. I hope that my presentation of these answers conveys a clear message: Always cover the main topics; ignore the trivia and unnecessary details. Be systematic! Be concise! And remember: You do not have to know everything; nobody knows everything.

At the end of this Preface, I would like to acknowledge the input of all those medical students who have, in one form or another, helped me develop the Socratic course of pathology outlined here, formulate the questions, and summarize the answers. I must also acknowledge the contributions of my colleagues, or former students and collaborators from other universities in the United States and Europe, who helped me put this book together.

—Ivan Damjanov, MD, PhD

TOP 100 SECRETS

These secrets are 100 of the top board alerts. They summarize the concepts, principles, and most salient details of pathology.

1. The cell volume depends on the proper function of the cell membrane, which remains semipermeable only if properly energized with adenosine triphosphate (ATP).

2. Cell injury is accompanied by an increased concentration of free calcium ions in the hyaloplasm.

3. Cell death causes distinctive nuclear changes, including pyknosis, karyolysis, and karyorrhexis.

4. Necrosis is death of cells or tissues caused most often by ischemia or the action of toxic substances and infectious pathogens.

5. Although apoptosis is also called programmed cell death, it can be also induced by exogenous factors, such as viruses or drugs.

6. Hyperplasia is an increase in the size of a tissue or organ resulting from an increased number of constituent cells, whereas hypertrophy entails enlargement of individual cells.

7. Inflammation involves a vascular, a cellular, and a humoral response.

8. Mediators of inflammation are produced by many cells, including endothelial cells and inflammatory cells, and the liver, which is the main source of plasma proteins.

9. Hageman factor (clotting factor XII) plays a pivotal role in activating the kinin, complement, clotting, and fibrinolytic systems.

10. Cytokines are multifunctional polypeptides that modulate the function of other cells.

11. Polymorphonuclear leukocytes are the principal cells of acute inflammation, whereas lymphocytes, macrophages, and plasma cells participate in chronic inflammation.

12. Edema is accumulation of fluid in the interstitial spaces and the body cavities.

13. Thrombosis is a pathologic form of coagulation of circulating blood inside intact vascular spaces.

14. The Virchow triad includes three factors that promote thrombosis: changes in the vessel wall, changes in blood flow, and changes in the composition of blood.

15. Thromboembolism is the most common form of embolism.

16. Disseminated intravascular coagulation is a form of thrombosis in small blood vessels associated with uncontrollable bleeding because of consumption of coagulation factors in blood.

17. Infarct is an area of ischemic necrosis that is usually caused by occlusion of vessels or hypoperfusion of tissues with blood.

18. Shock, a condition caused by hypoperfusion of tissues with blood, can be classified as cardiogenic, hypovolemic, and distributive (related to vasodilatation).

19. Hypersensitivity reactions involve cell and tissue injury caused by antibodies or products of activated T lymphocytes

20. Autoimmune diseases are based on the immune reaction against self-antigens.

21. Acquired immunodeficiency syndrome (AIDS), an infectious disease caused by the human immunodeficiency virus (HIV), is characterized by profound suppression of the immune system and susceptibility to infections, neurologic disorders, and malignancies.

22. *Cancer* is a synonym for *malignant tumors*.

23. The main groups of malignant tumors are carcinomas, sarcomas, lymphomas, and gliomas.

24. Carcinogens are cancer-inducing factors that include physical forces, chemicals, viruses, and endogenous oncogenes.

25. Reactions of the host to the tumor can be classified as local or systemic and include various inflammatory, immune, hormonal, circulatory, and neural processes.

26. Teratogens are chemical, physical, or biological agents capable of inducing developmental abnormalities in a fetus.

27. Down syndrome, the most common autosomal chromosomal abnormality, is characterized by mental deficiency and characteristic facial and somatic features.

28. According to the laws of Mendelian genetics, single gene defects are inherited as autosomal dominant, autosomal recessive, or sex-linked dominant or recessive traits.

29. Atherosclerosis is a multifactorial disease that predominantly affects older people, but it can be accelerated by hypertension, hyperlipidemia, and smoking.

30. Arterial hypertension is a multifactorial disease of unknown etiology, but it can also be secondary to renal, endocrine, vascular, and neurologic diseases.

31. Vasculitis, an inflammation of vessels, is most often immunologically mediated.

32. Aneurysms are localized dilatations of the arteries most often caused by atherosclerosis and hypertension.

33. Cardiac failure may be caused by inherent heart disease or extracardiac causes, such as pressure overload in hypertension or volume overload in renal water retention.

34. Coronary heart disease is the most common cause of cardiac failure and the most common cause of death in the United States.

35. Myocardial infarction represents an area of myocardial cell necrosis caused by ischemia.

36. Arrhythmia is the most common complication of myocardial infarction.

37. Endocarditis is most often caused by bacteria.

38. Cardiomyopathy occurs in three forms known as dilatated, hypertrophic, and restrictive cardiomyopathy.

39. Ventricular septal defect, the most common noncyanotic congenital heart disease, is characterized by a left-to-right shunt.

40. Tetralogy of Fallot, the most common cyanotic congenital heart disease, includes four pathologic findings: ventricular septal defect, overriding dextraposed aorta, pulmonary artery stenosis, and right ventricular hypertrophy.

41. Hypochromic microcytic anemia is most often caused by iron deficiency and chronic blood loss.

42. Sickle cell anemia is a hereditary hemoglobinopathy caused by a mutation of the α-globin gene.

43. Lymphomas—malignant tumors of lymphoid cells—are most often of B-cell origin.

44. Leukemia is a malignancy of hematopoietic and lymphoid cells characterized by the appearance of malignant cells in the circulation.

45. Multiple myeloma, a malignancy of plasma cells, is associated with lytic bone lesions and monoclonal gammopathy.

46. Hodgkin disease, a form of lymph node malignancy characterized by the presence of Reed–Sternberg cells, occurs in several histologic forms.

47. Atelectasis is incomplete expansion of the lungs or the collapse of previously inflated lung parenchyma.

48. Adult respiratory distress syndrome (ARDS) is caused by diffuse alveolar damage resulting from injury of endothelial cells or pneumocytes forming the alveolar–capillary units.

49. Chronic obstructive pulmonary disease includes several diseases, the most important of which are emphysema and chronic bronchitis.

50. Bronchial asthma is a chronic relapsing inflammatory obstructive lung disease presenting with hyperreactivity of airways and periodic bronchospasm.

51. Acute pneumonia is an inflammation of lungs usually caused by viruses or bacteria.

52. Pneumoconioses are interstitial lung diseases caused by inhaled particles such as coal, silica, or asbestos.

53. Most lung cancers originate from the epithelium of the bronchi and are related to smoking.

54. Esophagitis is most often caused by gastroesophageal reflux disease (GERD).

55. Atrophic gastritis, the most common form of gastritis, is most often caused by *Helicobacter pylori*.

56. Peptic ulcers are prone to bleeding.

57. Carcinomas of the esophagus and stomach have poor prognosis.

58. Diarrhea can be classified as osmotic, secretory, exudative, malabsorptive, and mixed.

59. Malabsorption syndrome is characterized by steatorrhea and deficiency of fat-soluble vitamins.

60. Inflammatory bowel disease includes Crohn disease and ulcerative colitis, which share some features but also differ in many aspects.

61. Carcinoma of the large intestine is the third most common form of cancer and the third most common cancer-related cause of death in the United States. It occurs most often in the rectosigmoid area.

62. Jaundice can be classified as prehepatic (hemolytic), hepatic, and posthepatic (obstructive).

63. Cirrhosis is equivalent to end-stage liver disease characterized by loss of normal hepatic architecture, fibrosis, and the formation of regenerating nodules.

64. Hepatitis is most often caused by viruses, drugs, or immune mechanisms.

65. Chronic alcoholism may cause three pathologic changes in the liver: fatty liver, alcoholic hepatitis, and cirrhosis.

66. Alcohol and biliary disease account for 80% of all causes of acute pancreatitis.

67. Diabetes mellitus, a disease characterized by hyperglycemia, is caused by insulin deficiency or tissue resistance to insulin, and it occurs in two main forms called type 1 and type 2.

68. Uremia is a set of clinical and laboratory findings found in patients with end-stage kidney disease.

69. Glomerulonephritis is immunologically mediated in most instances.

70. Pyelonephritis is a bacterial kidney infection.

71. The most important tumors of the kidneys and the urinary tract are renal cell carcinoma, transitional cell carcinoma, and Wilms tumor.

72. Testicular tumors are derived from germ cells in 90% of cases and belong to two groups: seminomas and nonseminomatous germ cell tumors (NSGCTs).

73. Prostate carcinoma is the most common malignant tumor in males.

74. Carcinomas of the vulva, vagina, and cervix are linked to human papilloma virus (HPV) infection.

75. Endometrial adenocarcinoma is linked to hyperestrinism.

76. Leiomyomas are the most common benign tumors of the uterus.

77. Breast carcinoma is the most common malignant tumor in females.

78. Hyperthyroidism may be caused by autoimmune mechanisms (e.g., in Graves disease), tumors (e.g., follicular adenomas), or hyperfunctioning goiters.

79. Hyperparathyroidism, most often caused by parathyroid adenoma, is characterized by hypercalcemia.

80. Hypofunction of adrenal glands is the cause of Addison disease, whereas hyperfunction causes Cushing syndrome.

81. The three most important skin diseases caused by bacteria are impetigo, folliculitis, and acne.

82. Warts are caused by HPV infection.

83. Psoriasis is a common chronic skin disease of unknown etiology affecting 1% to 2% of the population.

84. Skin cancer is related to sun exposure.

85. Basal cell carcinoma of the skin, the most common malignant tumor, is only locally invasive and rarely metastasizes.

86. Pigmented skin lesions may be benign (such as freckles, lentigo, and nevus) or malignant (such as malignant melanoma).

87. Osteoporosis is a form of osteopenia characterized by a loss of both calcium salts and organic matrix of the bones (osteoid).

88. The two most important diseases of the joints are rheumatoid arthritis and osteoarthritis.

89. Osteosarcoma occurs most often in children and young people, whereas chondrosarcoma has its peak incidence in adults.

90. Duchenne muscular dystrophy is the most common genetic muscle disease.

91. The most important immunologic diseases of the muscle are polymyositis and myasthenia gravis.

92. Rhabdomyosarcoma is a malignant tumor of striated muscle.

93. The most important forms of intracranial bleeding are intracerebral hemorrhage in hypertension, subdural hematoma, subarachnoid hematoma, and epidural hematoma.

94. Infection of the brain and the meninges can occur through four main routes: vascular spread, direct extension, ascending neural route, and penetrating wounds.

95. Tabes dorsalis is a spinal cord lesion caused by syphilis.

96. Multiple sclerosis is a demyelinating autoimmune disease characterized by a chronic relapsing and remitting course.

97. Alzheimer's disease, an old-age neurodegenerative disease of unknown etiology, is the most common cause of dementia.

98. Most brain tumors are malignant.

99. Gliomas are malignant tumors of the central nervous system originating from astrocytes, oligodendroglia cells, and ependymal cells.

100. Diabetic neuropathy is the most common peripheral nerve disease encountered in general practice.

CELL PATHOLOGY

Ivan Damjanov, MD, PhD

CHAPTER 1

CELL INJURY

1. **Define cell injury.**
    Normal cells are in a state of homeostasis (i.e., an equilibrium with their environment). Injury is defined as a set of biochemical and/or morphologic changes that occur when the state of homeostasis is perturbed by adverse influences. Cell injury may be reversible or irreversible.

2. **What is the difference between reversible and irreversible cell injury?**
    The differences are mostly quantitative. Reversible injury is usually mild, and, following the removal of the adverse influences, the cell reverts to its normal steady state. If the cell cannot recover, the injury is considered to be irreversible.

3. **What could cause cell injury?**
    The causes of cell injury are classified as exogenous or endogenous. In principle, cell injury can occur due to the following factors:
    - Excessive or overly prolonged normal stimuli
    - Action of toxins and other adverse influences that could inhibit the vital cell functions (e.g., oxidative phosphorylation or protein synthesis)
    - Deficiency of oxygen and/or essential nutrients and metabolites

KEY POINTS: CELL INJURY ✔

1. Cell injury can be reversible or irreversible.

2. Hypoxia is the most important cause of cell injury.

3. Irreversible cell injury can be recognized by changes in the appearance of the nucleus and rupture of the cell membrane.

4. **Name some exogenous causes of cell injury.**
    Exogenous causes include physical, chemical, and biological factors, such as heat and cold, toxins and drugs, and viruses and bacteria.

5. **Name some endogenous causes of cell injury.**
    Endogenous causes include genetic defects, metabolites, hormones, cytokines, and other "bioactive" substances.

6. **What is hypoxia?**
    Hypoxia is a relative deficiency of oxygen recognizable as a disproportion between the need for oxygen and its availability. It may result from a reduced supply or increased demand that cannot be satisfied. Complete block in the oxygen supply is called anoxia.

7. **What could cause hypoxia or anoxia?**
Hypoxia and anoxia can result from the following:
- Inadequate supply of oxygen (e.g., low concentration of oxygen in air at high altitude)
- Obstruction of airways (e.g., strangulation and drowning)
- Inadequate oxygenation of blood in the lungs (e.g., lung diseases)
- Inadequate oxygen transport in blood (e.g., anemia)
- Inadequate perfusion of blood in the tissues (ischemia resulting from heart failure)
- Inhibition of cellular respiration—that is, blocked utilization of oxygen (e.g., cyanide poisoning of respiratory enzymes)

8. **How does hypoxia cause cell injury?**
Oxygen is essential for aerobic respiration. Hypoxia prevents normal oxidative phosphorylation, thus reducing the capacity of mitochondria to generate adenosine triphosphate (ATP). Without ATP, the cell cannot maintain its vital functions. Hypoxic cells swell. This change is called hydropic or vacuolar change and is typically reversible.

9. **How does ATP deficiency cause cell swelling?**
The cell volume depends on the proper functioning of the plasma membrane, which remains semipermeable only if properly energized with ATP. ATP provides fuel for the Na/K ATPase, which acts as a pump, keeping the high concentration of sodium in the intercellular fluid and the high concentration of potassium inside the cell. If this ATPase malfunctions because of an energy deficiency, an uncontrolled influx of sodium and water from the extracellular space occurs. A consequent net increase of the total fluid content in the cytoplasm results in cell swelling. The intracellular concentration of potassium declines because potassium leaks out of the cell.

10. **Where does water accumulate during hydropic change?**
Water accumulates in the hyaloplasm but also in the invaginations of the plasma membrane *(hypoxic vacuoles),* mitochondria, and the cisterns of rough endoplasmic reticulum (RER), causing their malfunction. Swollen mitochondria produce less energy, and the detachment of ribosomes from membranes of dilated RER results in reduced protein synthesis (Fig. 1-1).

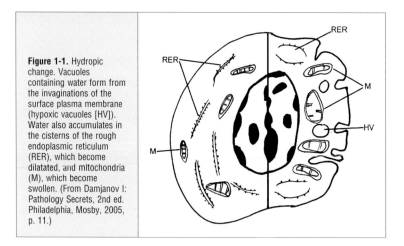

Figure 1-1. Hydropic change. Vacuoles containing water form from the invaginations of the surface plasma membrane (hypoxic vacuoles [HV]). Water also accumulates in the cisterns of the rough endoplasmic reticulum (RER), which become dilatated, and mitochondria (M), which become swollen. (From Damjanov I: Pathology Secrets, 2nd ed. Philadelphia, Mosby, 2005, p. 11.)

11. **What is the role of calcium in acute cell injury?**
Cell injury is accompanied by an increased concentration of free calcium ions in the hyaloplasm (cytosol). These calcium ions are derived from the extracellular fluid, from the mitochondrial

compartment, and from the cisterns of RER. Ionized calcium amplifies the adverse effects of hypoxia by activating several enzymes:

- **Lytic ATPase:** Degrades ATP and further reduces the energy stores.
- **Phospholipases:** These enzymes remove phospholipids from the plasma or mitochondrial membranes, further impairing their function.
- **Proteases:** These enzymes degrade cell membrane or cytoskeletal proteins.
- **Endonucleases:** These enzymes act on the RNA and DNA.

All of these changes are initially reversible, but if prolonged or intensified they may lead to irreversible cell injury (Fig. 1-2).

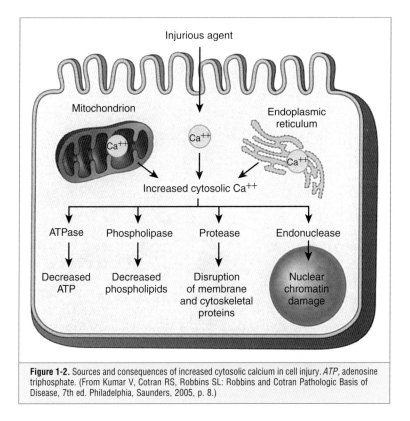

Figure 1-2. Sources and consequences of increased cytosolic calcium in cell injury. *ATP,* adenosine triphosphate. (From Kumar V, Cotran RS, Robbins SL: Robbins and Cotran Pathologic Basis of Disease, 7th ed. Philadelphia, Saunders, 2005, p. 8.)

12. **How does the cell compensate for the loss of aerobic respiration?**
    Breakdown of ATP is accompanied by an increase in adenosine monophosphate (AMP), which activates enzymes involved in anaerobic glycolysis. This leads to depletion of glycogen stored in the cytoplasm.

13. **Is the cytoplasm of injured cells acidic or alkaline?**
    Cell injury is accompanied by the lowering of intracellular pH from the normal neutral to the acidic range. For example, the inhibition of oxidative phosphorylation promotes anaerobic glycolysis, which is accompanied by accumulation of lactic acid in the cytoplasm. Phosphates released from phospholipids and ATP contribute further to the acidification of the cytoplasm. Acidic milieu inhibits the activity of most enzymes except those in the lysosomes, which function most efficiently in the acid pH. The release of acid hydrolases from the lysosomes may further contribute to cell injury.

14. **How does the reversible cell injury become irreversible?**
    The transition from reversible to irreversible cell injury is gradual and occurs when the adaptive mechanisms have been exhausted. A theoretical "point of no return" separating the reversible from irreversible injury cannot be precisely defined even under tightly controlled experimental conditions.

15. **What are the signs of irreversible cell injury?**
    Initially, the differences between the reversible and irreversible cell injury are only quantitative. For example, the hypoxic vacuoles become more numerous and larger. The mitochondria are swollen, and many are even ruptured. However, many of these changes are still reversible, and it is only when the plasma membrane ruptures and the nuclear changes ensue that one can be certain that an injury is irreversible and the cell is dead.

16. **Which mitochondrial changes are irreversible?**
    Swelling of mitochondria represents a reversible change. Irreversible changes include the following:
    - Rupture of double membrane
    - Fragmentation
    - Myelin figures (concentric curling up of damaged membranes)
    - Calcification

    Damaged mitochondria are taken up into autophagosomes and digested (Fig. 1-3).

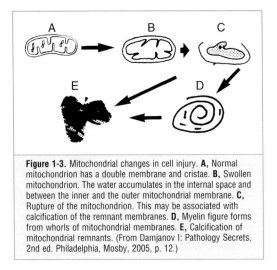

Figure 1-3. Mitochondrial changes in cell injury. **A,** Normal mitochondrion has a double membrane and cristae. **B,** Swollen mitochondrion. The water accumulates in the internal space and between the inner and the outer mitochondrial membrane. **C,** Rupture of the mitochondrion. This may be associated with calcification of the remnant membranes. **D,** Myelin figure forms from whorls of mitochondrial membranes. **E,** Calcification of mitochondrial remnants. (From Damjanov I: Pathology Secrets, 2nd ed. Philadelphia, Mosby, 2005, p. 12.)

17. **What are myelin figures?**
    Myelin figures are cytoplasmic bodies seen in damaged cells by electron microscopy. They are composed of concentric whorls of membranes derived from damaged cytoplasmic organelles, such as mitochondria, or RER. Myelin figures are prominent in neurons in Tay-Sachs disease and other inborn errors of metabolism damaging the cytoplasmic membranes. Like other remnants of damaged organelles, myelin figures are taken up into autophagosomes.

18. **Which nuclear changes are signs of cell death?**
    Dead cells show typical nuclear changes (Fig. 1-4):
    - **Pyknosis:** This term is derived from the Greek word *pyknos* meaning "dense," and it denotes condensation of chromatin.
    - **Karyolysis:** This change results from the lysis of chromatin due to the action of endonucleases.

- **Karyorrhexis:** This term is derived from the Greek word *rhexis* meaning "tearing apart" and denotes fragmentation of nuclear material. Colloquially, it is described as formation of "nuclear dust."

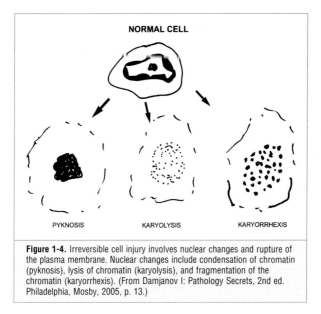

Figure 1-4. Irreversible cell injury involves nuclear changes and rupture of the plasma membrane. Nuclear changes include condensation of chromatin (pyknosis), lysis of chromatin (karyolysis), and fragmentation of the chromatin (karyorrhexis). (From Damjanov I: Pathology Secrets, 2nd ed. Philadelphia, Mosby, 2005, p. 13.)

19. **What are the clinical signs of irreversible cell injury?**
    Irreversible cell injury results in a loss of cell functions. For example:
    - **Myocardial cell injury:** loss of heart contraction
    - **Motor neuron:** muscle paralysis
    - **Islets of Langerhans:** diabetes

20. **Are there any clinically useful diagnostic laboratory signs of cell injury?**
    Severe cell injury is typically associated with a release of cytoplasmic enzymes into the blood. For example:
    - Creatine kinase may indicate cardiac or skeletal muscle cell injury.
    - Aspartate aminotransferase (AST) and alanine aminotransferase (ALT) are released from damaged liver cells.
    - Lactate dehydrogenase (LDH) is released from ruptured red blood cells and many other cells.

21. **Can cell injury caused by hypoxia or anoxia be reversed or repaired by providing the cells with adequate oxygen?**
    Irreversibly damaged cells cannot be revived by oxygen. On the other hand, the function of reversibly injured cells that are still living can be improved by oxygen. The reoxygenation must be performed carefully because if overly zealous, it may cause so-called *reperfusion injury*. This type of injury is caused by oxygen-derived free radicals that may form under such conditions. For example, reestablished blood flow to a myocardium made hypoxic by coronary obstruction may cause reperfusion injury of still-living myocardial cells at the marginal zone of a myocardial infarction.

22. **What are free radicals?**
    Free radicals are unstable, highly reactive atoms or molecules that have an unpaired electron in their outer orbit. After they are formed, they tend to self-propagate, forming new radicals in an

autocatalytic sequence of reactions. The best-known free radicals are derived from oxygen and include the following:

- Superoxide (O_2^-)
- Hydrogen peroxide (H_2O_2)
- Hydroxyl radical (OH^1)

23. How are oxygen radicals formed?
Oxygen radicals are formed in small quantities during normal cellular respiration. These oxygen radicals are neutralized by natural antioxidants and degraded by protective enzymes. If these normal defense mechanisms do not work, the free radicals may accumulate in toxic quantities. Oxygen radicals are also formed by leukocytes, which use these reactive molecules to kill bacteria.

24. How are free oxygen radicals neutralized?
Superoxide is inactivated by superoxide dismutase and hydrogen peroxide by catalase and glutathione peroxidase. Vitamin E and vitamin C also have antioxidant activity.

25. How do free radicals damage cells?
Free radicals damage cells through a variety of mechanisms, most notably by the following:

- **Lipid peroxidation:** This process leads to membrane damage.
- **Cross-linking of proteins:** This leads to inactivation of enzymes.
- **DNA breaks**: This injury may block DNA transcription and cause mutations.

IRREVERSIBLE CELL INJURY

26. What is necrosis?
Necrosis (from the Greek term *necros,* "dead") is localized death of cells, tissues, organs, or parts of the body in a living organism.

27. What are the histologic signs of necrosis?
The signs of necrosis are the same as those of irreversible cell injury—that is, cell membrane rupture and nuclear changes, such as pyknosis, karyolysis, and karyorrhexis.

28. What are the main forms of necrosis?
The main forms of necrosis are:

- Coagulative necrosis
- Liquefactive necrosis
- Caseous necrosis
- Fat necrosis
- Fibrinoid necrosis

29. What is the most common form of necrosis?
The most common form of necrosis is coagulative necrosis. It is typically found in myocardial infarction, as well as in infarcts of the kidney, the spleen, and many other organs. Even the infarcted tumors may undergo coagulative necrosis.

KEY POINTS: IRREVERSIBLE CELL INJURY ✓

1. Irreversible cell injury causes cell death, which is also known as necrosis.

2. Necrosis can occur in several forms recognizable by gross or microscopic examination of tissue.

30. **What are the features of coagulative necrosis?**
Coagulative necrosis is characterized by sudden cessation of basic cell function caused by a blockage of the action of most enzymes. Because the action of hydrolytic cytoplasmic enzymes is also blocked, there is no dissolution of tissue (i.e., there is little autolysis). Hence, the overall outline of the dead tissue remains preserved. The necrotic tissue appears paler than normal and resembles boiled meat.

31. **What is liquefactive necrosis?**
Liquefactive necrosis is characterized by softening of the necrotic tissue to the point at which it transforms into a pastelike mush or watery debris. Liquefaction of tissues occurs because of the action of hydrolytic enzymes released from dead cells, as in brain infarct, or from the lysosomes of inflammatory cells invading the tissue, as in an abscess.

32. **Provide a few examples of liquefactive necrosis.**
    - **Brain infarct:** The necrotic area softens *(encephalomalacia),* and the necrotic tissue debris is phagocytized by macrophages. The remaining cavity is filled by diffusion of fluid from surrounding interstitial spaces of the brain ("the body abhors a vacuum"). Such a fluid-filled pseudocyst may persist unchanged indefinitely.
    - **Abscess:** This is formed of localized purulent infection. Typically it presents as a cavity filled with pus—that is, liquefied tissue of the affected organ permeated with dead and dying neutrophils.
    - **Wet gangrene of extremities:** Typically seen in patients with diabetes, it is a form of coagulative necrosis with superimposed bacterial infection. The tissue becomes liquefied through the action of bacterial lytic enzymes.

33. **What is caseous necrosis?**
Caseous necrosis is typically found in tuberculous and fungal granulomas. On gross examination, it is soft and greasy, resembling cottage cheese. Histologically, the necrotic tissue has lost its normal structure and appears amorphous and finely granular.

34. **What is fat necrosis?**
This typically involves fat cells in and around the pancreas, the omentum, or the wall of the abdominal cavity. It is characterized by lipolysis that occurs when the fat cells are permeated by lipase and other lytic enzymes released from damaged pancreatic cells. This occurs typically in the course of acute pancreatitis. The fat tissue initially appears soft and gelatinous, but thereafter it transforms into chalky white patches composed of calcium soaps. Histologically, the fat cells lose their outlines and become indistinct. Deposition of calcium gives the necrotic fat cells a bluish tinge.

35. **What is fibrinoid necrosis?**
Fibrinoid necrosis is limited to small blood vessels. Typically, it involves small arteries, arterioles, and glomeruli affected by autoimmune diseases (e.g., systemic lupus erythematosus) or malignant hypertension. The walls of necrotic vessels or glomeruli are impregnated with fibrin and appear homogeneously red in routine hematoxylin-eosin (H&E)–stained slides. Detailed analysis would show that these deposits contain other plasma proteins as well; however, fibrin overshadows other proteins in histologic slides and gives the name to this lesion. Fibrinoid necrosis can be recognized only in histologic preparations and has no distinct macroscopic features.

36. **What is the outcome of necrosis?**
    - **Complete restitution:** This process is called *regeneration,* and the dead cells are replaced by almost parenchymal cell. Regeneration occurs in organs composed of facultative mitotic cells, such as the kidneys or liver.

- **Repair:** The dead cells are replaced by fibrous tissue forming microscopic or macroscopic scars. For example, in the heart dead myocardial cells are removed by phagocytes and replaced by a fibrous scar.
- **Calcification:** In some instances, the necrotic tissue is impregnated with calcium salts (dystrophic calcification).
- **Resorption of necrotic tissue:** In the brain, the necrotic tissue is removed by macrophages, and the infarct is transformed into a fluid-filled pseudocyst.

APOPTOSIS

37. **What is apoptosis?**
Apoptosis is a form of cell death based on sequential activation of "death genes" and "suicide pathway enzymes." It is also called *programmed cell death*.

38. **How is apoptosis initiated?**
Apoptosis may be initiated through several pathways. The two most important pathways are:
- **Extrinsic pathway:** This pathway is activated by the activation of the so-called death receptors on the surface of the cell membrane. Ligands for these receptors are proteins such as tumor necrosis factor or Fas ligand.
- **Intrinsic mitochondrial pathway:** This pathway is initiated by an increased permeability of mitochondria, which release proapoptotic molecules, such as cytochrome, that act on the initiator caspases, such as the extrinsic pathway.
Many other mechanisms can initiate apoptosis, such as radiation, drugs, hormones, immune mechanisms (e.g., cytotoxic T lymphocytes). Withdrawal of hormones and growth factors essential for the survival of the cell can also cause apoptosis. For example, castration is accompanied by a decrease of testosterone concentration in the blood, which leads to apoptosis of prostatic cells.

39. **How do apoptosis signals trigger cell death?**
The initial signal on the cell membrane or from the mitochondria activates the initiator caspases, which act on execution caspases. These then act on enzymes, nucleic acids, and the cytoskeletal proteins, thus leading to the fragmentation of the nucleus and cytoplasm into membrane-bound apoptotic bodies. Apoptotic bodies are phagocytized by neighboring cells or macrophages.

KEY POINTS: APOPTOSIS ✔

1. Apoptosis is programmed cell death that can result from endogenous or exogenous activation of cell suicide genetic pathways.

2. Apoptosis is important for fetal development and many normal processes during adult life, but it is also involved in many pathologic processes.

40. **How does apoptosis differ from necrosis?**
Apoptosis usually affects single cells, whereas necrosis involves larger groups of cells or tissues. During necrosis, there is no gene activity, and most of the cytoplasmic maintenance enzymes are inactivated; during apoptosis, there is sequential, genetically controlled enzyme activation and inhibition. During necrosis, cells swell (oncosis); during apoptosis, the cell cytoplasm and the nucleus fragment into apoptotic bodies. Necrotic cells elicit an inflammatory response and are phagocytized by neutrophils. Apoptotic bodies are phagocytized by nonprofessional phagocytes, such as neighboring cells, or macrophages.

41. **What will happen if genetically programmed apoptosis does not occur during fetal development?**
Apoptosis is essential for normal development of many organs, and if it does not occur, malformations may develop. For example, apoptosis mediates the disappearance of interdigital folds on fetal limbs. If apoptosis does not occur, the fingers will not develop normally (syndactyly).

42. **Can apoptosis be induced by viruses?**
Yes. The best example is the apoptosis of hepatocytes in viral hepatitis. Apoptotic hepatocytes appear as anuclear, round eosinophilic bodies. Similar apoptotic bodies seen in the liver of patients who have yellow fever are called Councilman bodies in honor of the scientist who described them first. Human immunodeficiency virus (HIV) kills CD4+ helper T lymphocytes by apoptosis.

43. **What is the role of antiapoptotic protein Bcl-2 in the pathogenesis of B-cell lymphoma?**
Bcl-2 is a protein normally suppressing apoptosis. It name stems from the fact that it was first identified in cells of B-cell lymphoma. It is encoded by a gene that is overexpressed in B-cell lymphoma cells. Bcl-2 prevents the death of lymphoma cells, thus making them "immortal." Such cells accumulate in lymph nodes and basically outlive the host, who will usually die overwhelmed by immortal tumor cells.

ADAPTATIONS

44. **What is the significance of cellular adaptations?**
The term *adaptation* is used to describe changes that occur in cells and tissues in response to prolonged stimulation, lack of oxygen and nutrients, or chronic injury. Adaptations are usually reversible, but in some cases they may become irreversible. The most important adaptations are shown in Fig. 1-5. They encompass several reversible processes, such as:

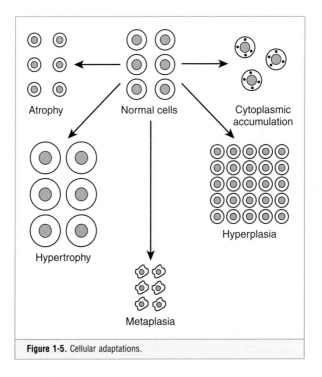

Figure 1-5. Cellular adaptations.

- Atrophy
- Hypertrophy
- Hyperplasia
- Metaplasia
- Intracellular accumulation of various substances

KEY POINTS: ADAPTATIONS ✓

1. Adaptations are usually reversible changes that result in increased, decreased, or altered functions of cells, tissues, and organs.

2. Adaptations can be physiologic or pathologic.

3. Adaptations may have many causes.

45. **What is atrophy?**
Atrophy is reduction in size of cells, tissue, or organs. Atrophic cells are smaller than normal because their nucleus and cytoplasm have shrunken in size. Tissues and organs composed of atrophic cells are obviously smaller. However, they can also decrease in size because of loss of cells. Such atrophy is also called *involution* and is usually an age-related, irreversible phenomenon.

46. **Is atrophy always pathologic?**
Atrophy can be physiologic or pathologic. Atrophy of the uterus after pregnancy is an example of physiologic atrophy. Atrophy (involution) of the thymus in adolescence or in early adult life is physiologic. Atrophy of the uterus occurs after the removal of the ovaries but may be reversed with hormonal therapy. Thymic involution is irreversible.

47. **What are the causes of pathologic atrophy?**
Pathologic atrophy can have several causes, such as:
- **Disuse:** Muscle atrophy occurs in people who do not use their muscles.
- **Denervation:** Transection or a loss of motor neurons results in atrophy of skeletal muscles.
- **Lack of trophic hormones:** Endocrine glands (e.g., thyroid, adrenal, and gonads) atrophy after resection of the pituitary.
- **Ischemia:** Reduced blood supply leads to atrophy of the brain or kidneys.
- **Malnutrition:** Protein-energy deficiency may cause atrophy of skeletal muscles and parenchymal organs.

48. **What is hypertrophy?**
Hypertrophy is increased organ size resulting from an increase in the size of constituent cells, without an increase in the cell number.

49. **Which organs can undergo pure hypertrophy?**
Pure hypertrophy without any hyperplasia occurs only in the heart and the skeletal muscle. Because the heart muscle is composed of terminally differentiated myocytes that cannot divide, an increased demand for action can be met only by enlarging the size of the muscle cells. Hyperplasia cannot occur in the heart. Skeletal muscles contain reserve cells that could theoretically divide and contribute to the muscle mass, but this never occurs in normal circumstances. Thus, a demand for additional work is met by muscle cell hypertrophy.

50. **What happens in heart cells undergoing hypertrophy?**
Hypertrophic cardiac myocytes enlarge. During this process, they acquire more cytoplasm and their nuclei enlarge as well. The cytoplasm contains more contractile proteins.

The amount of DNA and RNA in the nucleus is increased proportionately to the total cell mass. Hypertrophic cells express some genes that are not expressed in normal cells. The exact function of these genes—such as oncogenes (e.g., c-fos and c-jun) and genes for some proteins that were expressed only in fetal life (e.g., myosin heavy chain and atrial natriuretic factor)—is not known.

51. What triggers the hypertrophy of heart cells?
Hypertrophy results from a combined action of mechanical stimuli (increased workload) and vasoactive substances (e.g., angiotensin II). Calcium plays an important role as a secondary messenger.

52. Is cardiac hypertrophy a beneficial adaptive response?
Hypertrophy of the cardiac myocytes improves cardiac output but only as long as the increased heart mass can be adequately perfused with blood. A disproportion between the increased myocardial mass and coronary blood supply will cause cardiac ischemia and reduce the efficacy of the heart. Extreme hypertrophy of cardiac myocytes will reduce the efficacy of cardiac cells even if the blood supply is adequate. Hypertrophic hearts have a reduced capacity for adaptation and are prone to sudden block. The reasons for sudden death in people with hypertrophic hearts are not known.

53. What is hyperplasia?
Hyperplasia is an increase in the size of a tissue or organ caused by an increased number of constituent cells.

54. Is hyperplasia always pathologic?
No. Hyperplasia can also be physiologic. For example, the enlargement of the uterus in pregnancy is a physiologic event. Erythroid bone marrow hyperplasia in high altitudes is yet another example of a physiologic hyperplasia.

55. Can hyperplasia be combined with hypertrophy?
More often than not, hyperplasia is combined with hypertrophy. For example, thickening of an obstructed urinary bladder almost always entails both hypertrophy and hyperplasia of smooth muscle cells. In an enlarged uterus of pregnancy, myometrial smooth muscle cells are increased not only in number (hyperplasia) but also in size (hypertrophy).

56. Does the abbreviation BPH stand for benign prostatic hyperplasia or hypertrophy?
Prostatic enlargement, known as BPH, is predominantly caused by hyperplasia of prostatic glands and stromal smooth muscle cells. However, these cells are also enlarged, which justifies (to some extent) the common clinical practice of calling this disease benign prostatic hypertrophy. This is a rare example in which both pathologists and surgeons are right!

57. What is metaplasia?
Metaplasia is replacement of one mature cell type by another one. For example, replacement of bronchial stratified columnar epithelium by squamous epithelium is an example of squamous metaplasia that occurs in smokers. Intestinal metaplasia of the esophagus, called Barrett esophagus, is most often caused by chronic irritation by gastric juices in gastroesophageal reflux.

58. Is metaplasia reversible?
In most cases, metaplasia is reversible and the tissue reverts to its normal state after the stimulus or irritant has been removed. If the adverse circumstances persist, metaplasia may progress to dysplasia and then to frank neoplasia, which is irreversible.

59. **What substances can accumulate in cells?**

Substances accumulating inside the cells can be classified as exogenous or endogenous. Exogenous substances include, for example, carbon particles inhaled from polluted air accumulating in macrophages in anthracosis or pigment used for tattooing of skin. Endogenous substances accumulating in cells are as follows:

- **Lipids:** Accumulation of triglycerides in hepatocytes leads to formation of fatty liver (hepatic steatosis).
- **Proteins:** Accumulation of α_1-antitrypsinin hepatocytes results in the formation of cytoplasmic globules.
- **Glycogen:** Accumulates in the liver and many other organs in congenital glycogenoses.
- **Lipofuscin:** This lipid-rich brown pigment of aging accumulates in many organs during aging and in chronic diseases.
- **Hemosiderin:** This iron-rich brown pigment accumulates in the liver and many other organs in congenital hemochromatosis or in patients who have received multiple transfusions.

WEBSITES

1. http://www.ncbi.nlm.nih.gov/entrez/query.fcgi?db=PubMed
2. http://www-medlib.med.utah.edu/WebPath/webpath.html#MENU
3. http://www.pathguy.com
4. http://vlib.org/Science/Cell_Biology/apoptosis.shtml

BIBLIOGRAPHY

1. Adams JM, Cory S: Bcl-2-regulated apoptosis: mechanism and therapeutic potential. Curr Opin Immunol 19:488–961, 2007.
2. Bertazza L, Mocellin S: Tumor necrosis factor (TNF) biology and cell death. Front Biosci 13:2736–2743, 2008.
3. Burton JL, Underwood J: Clinical, educational, and epidemiological value of autopsy. Lancet 369:1471–1480, 2007.
4. Catalucci D, Latronico MV, Ellingsen O, Condorelli G: Physiological myocardial hypertrophy: how and why? Front Biosci 13:312–324, 2008.
5. Kinchen JM, Hengartner MO: Tales of cannibalism, suicide, and murder: programmed cell death in C. elegans. Curr Top Dev Biol 65:1–45, 2005.
6. Ritter O, Neyses L: The molecular basis of myocardial hypertrophy and heart failure. Trends Mol Med 9:313–321, 2003.
7. Wajant H: Death receptors. Essays Biochem 39:53–71, 2003.
8. Zong WX, Thompson CB: Necrotic death as a cell fate. Genes Dev 20:1–15, 2006.

CHAPTER 2

INFLAMMATION AND REPAIR

Ivan Damjanov, MD, PhD

1. What is the difference between cell injury and inflammation?
Cell injury can be induced in isolated single cells, monocellular organisms (e.g., amoeba), or cells grown in tissue culture. In contrast, inflammation cannot be induced in monocellular organisms or in cells cultured in vitro. An inflammatory response is a reaction to cell injury that can occur only in vascularized tissues of multicellular organisms. The same noxious stimuli that cause cell injury, however, can cause inflammation as well.

2. What is the aim of inflammation?
In general, the aim of inflammation is to eliminate or neutralize the cause of injury and repair its consequences. For example, the ultimate goal of an inflammatory response to bacteria is to destroy them and/or neutralize their adverse effects by limiting their spread inside the body. The inflammatory response is also important for repairing the tissues damaged or destroyed by bacteria. Not all inflammations have such an obvious aim, and in some instances the initial salutary effect of inflammation is overshadowed by unforeseen adverse outcomes.

3. What are the main components of inflammation?
Every inflammatory response is based on a coordinated activation and interaction of numerous components, which can be grouped under three major headings:
- Vascular response
- Cellular response
- Humoral response (chemical mediators of inflammation)

4. What is the difference between acute and chronic inflammation?
Acute inflammation is an immediate reaction to injury. Typically, as its name implies (Latin *acutus*, "sharp"), it has a sudden onset and is of short duration. It lasts a few hours or days. In contrast, chronic inflammation (Greek *chronos*, "time") lasts longer. Acute inflammation can become chronic, but the exact point of transition from one to another form of inflammation cannot be precisely defined. The onset of a chronic inflammation cannot be established in most cases.

Pathologic changes caused by acute inflammation differ from those caused by chronic inflammation. Acute inflammation is typically mediated by neutrophils. Chronic inflammation is mediated by macrophages, lymphocytes, and plasma cells, and it often involves fibroblasts, angioblasts, and other tissue components seen in repair reactions.

ACUTE INFLAMMATION

5. What are the three main sets of events taking place in tissues during acute inflammation?
Three main events in acute inflammation are:
- Hemodynamic changes
- Increased permeability of vessel walls
- Emigration of leukocytes from blood vessels into the tissues

6. **What is the difference between an exudate and a transudate?**
   See Table 2-1.

TABLE 2-1. DIFFERENCES BETWEEN TRANSUDATE AND EXUDATE		
	Transudate	Exudate
Appearance	Clear	Turbid
Specific gravity	<1.015	>1.020
Protein content	<3 g/dL	>3 g/dL
Cells	Scant	Numerous neutrophils

KEY POINTS: ACUTE INFLAMMATION ✓

1. Acute inflammation is a rapid response to injury involving a sequential change in blood flow, the interaction of intravascular leukocytes and endothelial cells, and migration of leukocytes toward the pathogens.

2. Inflammation is moderated by mediators of inflammation found in the plasma or secreted by cells. The most important of these are biogenic amines, coagulation factors, complement proteins, arachidonic acid derivatives, and cytokines.

7. **What is edema?**
   Edema (Greek *oidema*, "swelling") is an excess of fluid in tissues or serous body cavities. It may develop as a result of transudation or exudation.

8. **Why does edema develop in acute inflammation?**
   Inflammatory edema has three main causes:
   - **Increased hydrostatic pressure in microcirculation:** Arteriolar dilatation associated with an increased influx of blood promotes transudation of fluid in capillaries and venules.
   - **Increased permeability of blood vessels:** The vessel walls of capillaries and venules become leaky under the influence of mediators of inflammation, allowing the passage of plasma proteins and fluid. The loss of fluid leads to hemoconcentration, which promotes stasis of blood cells. Stasis is associated with increased blood pressure in venules, which in turn prevents the return of the fluids from the interstitial spaces into the bloodstream.
   - **Reduced oncotic pressure of the plasma:** The loss of proteins as a result of increased transudation or exudation will gradually reduce the oncotic pressure of the plasma. Decreased oncotic pressure of the plasma facilitates the passage of fluid into the interstitial space. At the same time, the return of water from the interstitial space into the circulating blood at the venular end of microcirculation is reduced.

9. **How does the permeability of small vessels increase during inflammation?**
   There are several mechanisms, the most important of which are the following:
   - **Formation of gaps between endothelial cells:** This is the most common form of increased permeability. In early stages of inflammation, it occurs predominantly in venules under the influence of histamine or bradykinin. In later stages of inflammation, it is mediated by cytokines. These mediators of inflammation cause widening of intercellular gaps as a result of retraction of endothelial cells.

- **Direct injury of endothelial cells:** Usually a sign of severe injury caused by a variety of agents, it occurs in arterioles, as well as capillaries or venules. The defect in the vessel wall cannot be repaired easily, thus allowing indiscriminate leakage of cells and plasma components into the interstitial spaces.
- **Leukocyte-mediated injury:** Adherence of neutrophils to endothelial cells, especially in pulmonary venules or glomerular capillaries, increases their permeability.
- **Increased transcytosis:** Vesicular transport of fluids across the cytoplasm of venules may occur under the influence of vascular endothelial growth factor (VEGF). VEGF is also a cause of increased leakiness of newly formed blood vessels in the granulation tissue and chronic inflammation.
  See Fig. 2-1.

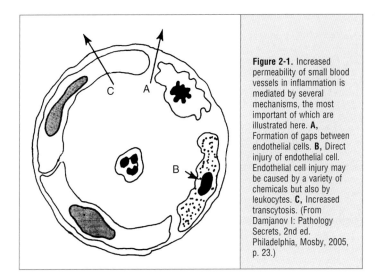

Figure 2-1. Increased permeability of small blood vessels in inflammation is mediated by several mechanisms, the most important of which are illustrated here. **A,** Formation of gaps between endothelial cells. **B,** Direct injury of endothelial cell. Endothelial cell injury may be caused by a variety of chemicals but also by leukocytes. **C,** Increased transcytosis. (From Damjanov I: Pathology Secrets, 2nd ed. Philadelphia, Mosby, 2005, p. 23.)

10. **What are the main events leading to transmigration of leukocytes across the vessel wall?**
    - **Margination:** The slowing of the blood flow allows the neutrophils to exit from the center of the bloodstream into the peripheral part and thus establish contact with endothelial cells.
    - **Rolling:** The leukocytes, which are normally found in the bloodstream, continue rolling over the endothelial cells. During this process, leukocytes and endothelial cells become activated and establish loose contacts with one another. These contacts are mediated by surface adhesion molecules called *selectins*.
    - **Adhesion:** Progressive activation of leukocytes and endothelial cells leads to expression of polypeptide adhesion molecules called *integrins*. Integrins on the surface of neutrophils attach to complementary integrins or endothelial cells, thus firmly binding these cells to each other.
    - **Transmigration:** Neutrophils attached to endothelial cells by integrins assume an amoeboid shape and begin actively crawling over the inside surface of venules until they reach the intercellular gaps. Finally, leukocytes squeeze through the intercellular gaps and enter the intercellular spaces outside the vessels.
      See Fig. 2-2.

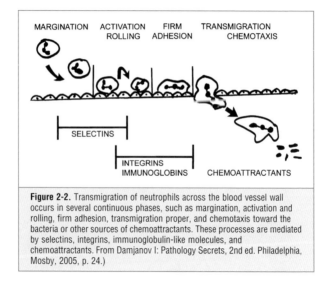

Figure 2-2. Transmigration of neutrophils across the blood vessel wall occurs in several continuous phases, such as margination, activation and rolling, firm adhesion, transmigration proper, and chemotaxis toward the bacteria or other sources of chemoattractants. These processes are mediated by selectins, integrins, immunoglobulin-like molecules, and chemoattractants. From Damjanov I: Pathology Secrets, 2nd ed. Philadelphia, Mosby, 2005, p. 24.)

11. **What is the difference between selectins and integrins?**
Selectins, found on the surface of leukocytes, platelets, and endothelial cells, are proteins that bind specifically to carbohydrates. Integrins, on the other hand, are found only on leukocytes. They bind to intercellular adhesion molecules of the immunoglobulin family (e.g., ICAM-1 and VCAM-1) and extracellular matrix (ECM) molecules, such as fibronectin or laminin.

12. **How are leukocytes activated?**
Activation of leukocytes is triggered by cell surface phenomena, which stimulate the receptors in the plasma membrane. Typically, this occurs following binding of leukocytes to endothelial cells or binding of interleukins to receptors on the plasma membrane of leukocytes. Signals transmitted from the cell surface receptors may activate phospholipase C, which in turn generates lipid-derived messengers, such as diacylglycerol (DAG) and inositol triphosphate (IP3). The ensuing metabolic changes lead to an increased concentration of cytosolic calcium ions. Calcium has a pivotal role in activating several intracellular processes, which are important for the action of leukocytes.

13. **What are the signs of leukocyte activation?**
Activated leukocytes differ from inactive leukocytes in several respects:
- **Expression of adhesion molecules:** Selectins and integrins appear on the cell surface or are expressed in higher numbers and show higher affinity for liquids.
- **Changes in the cytoskeleton:** Owing to the polymerization and redistribution of microtubules and microfilaments, the cell shape changes from round to flattened or amoeboid. Leukocytes form pseudopods and start moving actively toward the stimuli. Cytoskeletal changes also contribute to the formation of phagocytic vacuoles.
- **Degranulation:** The contents of cytoplasmic granules are released into phagocytic vacuoles or the extracellular spaces. Inside the phagocytic vacuoles, these enzymes participate in the digestion of bacteria. Enzymes released from the granules into the outer spaces act on ECM molecules and basement membranes, allowing the leukocytes to penetrate the tissues.
- **Oxidative burst:** Activated leukocytes generate free oxygen radicals, which are important for killing bacteria.
- **Protein synthesis:** Proteins are synthesized to replenish those excreted during degranulation, as well as those used up as a result of increased cellular activity.

14. **What is chemotaxis?**
Chemotaxis is active movement of cells along a chemical gradient generated by a chemoattractant.

15. **What are the most important chemotactic substances?**
Chemoattractants can be exogenous or endogenous. Exogenous chemoattractants are derived from bacterial polypeptides, which carry a terminal formulated-methionine sequence. Similarly, endogenous chemoattractants are generated from mitochondrial polypeptides released from damaged cells. Other important endogenous chemotactic substances include the following:
- Products of complement system activation (e.g., C5a)
- Arachidonic acid derivatives formed through the lipoxygenase pathway (e.g., leukotriene B4)
- Cytokines (e.g., IL-8)

16. **How do chemoattractants act on leukocytes?**
Like many other stimuli, chemoattractants activate leukocytes. Sequentially, this activation involves the following:
- Binding the chemoattractant to the cell membrane and the release of G proteins
- G protein–mediated activation of phospholipases, which leads to the production of secondary messengers, such as DAG and IP3
- Increased concentration of calcium ions in the hyaloplasm
- Calcium-mediated assembly of microfilaments

17. **What are pseudopods?**
Literally translated from Greek, the term *pseudopods* means "false feet." It refers to the extensions of the cell cytoplasm formed along the leading edge of activated leukocytes. Pseudopods contain aggregates of microfilaments composed of actin and myosin. Contraction of myosin leads to shortening of microfilaments, which act as ropes pulling the remainder of the cytoplasm toward the furthermost tip of the pseudopods.

18. **How do leukocytes kill bacteria?**
The killing of bacteria occurs in three stages and involves:
- Attachment of bacteria to the surface of the leukocyte
- Uptake of bacteria into phagocytic vacuoles
- Killing and degradation
  See Fig. 2-3.

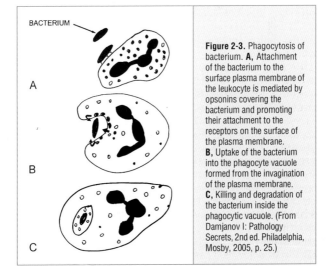

BACTERIUM

A

B

C

Figure 2-3. Phagocytosis of bacterium. **A,** Attachment of the bacterium to the surface plasma membrane of the leukocyte is mediated by opsonins covering the bacterium and promoting their attachment to the receptors on the surface of the plasma membrane. **B,** Uptake of the bacterium into the phagocyte vacuole formed from the invagination of the plasma membrane. **C,** Killing and degradation of the bacterium inside the phagocytic vacuole. (From Damjanov I: Pathology Secrets, 2nd ed. Philadelphia, Mosby, 2005, p. 25.)

19. **How do leukocytes attach to bacteria?**
Like any other particular material, bacteria attach nonspecifically to the surface of migrating leukocytes. To improve the attachment of leukocytes to potentially harmful bacteria, body fluids coat the bacteria with *opsonins* (Greek, "condiment" or "delicacy"). Leukocytes have receptors for opsonins, allowing them to attach with greater efficiency to opsonized bacteria than to other particles.

20. **What are the main opsonins?**
Opsonins are proteins normally found in the plasma and interstitial fluids, but they also may be formed nonspecifically in response to injury. The main opsonins are:
- Immunoglobulin G (IgG)
- C3b fragment formed during the activation of the complement cascade
- Collectins, such as mannose binding protein, which act as natural lectins (carbohydrate-binding proteins)

21. **How do leukocytes form phagocytic vacuoles?**
The formation of phagocytic vacuoles involves focal invagination of the cell surface membrane accompanied by the elongation of the cytoplasmic process laterally to that invagination. These cytoplasmic changes depend on restructuring of cytoskeleton and resemble those leading to the formation of pseudopods. Cytoskeletal changes rely on the activation of metabolic events that are identical to those that occur in activated leukocytes responding to chemotactic stimuli.

22. **What are the main bactericidal substances used by neutrophils?**
Bacteria can be killed through two mechanisms:
- **Oxygen-dependent killing:** This mechanism depends on the oxygen burst resulting from the activation of nicotinamide adenine dinucleotide phosphate (NADPH) oxidase. Oxidation of NADPH generates superoxide, which spontaneously transforms into hydrogen peroxide (H_2O_2). H_2O_2 is the substrate for myeloperoxidase, which links it to a chloride ion, generating hypochloric acid. Hypochloric acid, similar to household Clorox, is the most potent bactericidal chemical generated in the phagosomes.
- **Oxygen-independent killing:** Although less efficient than oxygen-dependent killing, this mechanism plays an important role in the fight against bacteria. It depends on the action of lysozyme, lactoferrin, and cationic proteins (e.g., defensin). The overall acidic environment inside the phagocytic vacuoles is toxic to some bacteria. Oxygen-independent killing of bacteria is especially important in people suffering from congenital deficiency of NADPH oxidase (chronic granulomatous disease) or myeloperoxidase deficiency.

23. **What are the clinical consequences of congenital defects of abnormal leukocyte functions?**
Congenital defects of phagocytosis, or bacterial killing, present as increased susceptibility to infections. Infants born with one of these defects are especially prone to opportunistic infections—that is, infections caused by ubiquitous, often saprophytic bacteria and fungi of low virulence that do not cause infections in people without these defects.

24. **What are the most important congenital defects of leukocyte function?**
Congenital defects of leukocyte function are rare, occurring in less than 1 in 10,000 infants. Nevertheless, these "experiments of nature" are significant because they provide insight into the pathophysiology of leukocyte functions and how these cells combat infections. The most important examples of abnormal leukocyte function are as follows:
- **Defects in leukocyte adhesion:** This category encompasses deficiencies of various leukocyte adhesion molecules, integrins, and enzymes that synthesize the carbohydrate ligands for the selectins.
- **Defects of phagocytosis:** Deficiency of C3 complement impairs opsonization. Chediak–Higashi syndrome, a defect in microtubule polymerization, is characterized by

defective leukocyte migration and phagocytosis. Neutrophils typically have giant granules and are unable to degranulate upon stimulation.

- **Defective bactericidal activity:** Deficiency of NADPH oxidase is the basic defect in children suffering from chronic granulomatous disease. In this disease, the leukocytes cannot generate superoxide, which impairs the oxygen-dependent killing of bacteria. These children are especially sensitive to infection with catalase-positive microbes such as *Staphylococcus aureus*. Catalase-negative streptococci are less dangerous. These bacteria produce peroxide that is used by the leukocytes to generate hypochloric acid and to kill the pathogens. Deficiency of myeloperoxidase is characterized by an inability of leukocytes to produce H_2O_2 and hypochloric acid. Affected children are prone to fungal infections.

25. **What are the most important plasma-derived mediators of inflammation?**
The most important mediators of inflammation are proteases that belong to one of several interrelated systems activated by Hageman factor (clotting factor XII):

- **Kinin system:** This results in the formation of kallikrein and bradykinin. Kallikrein itself is capable of activating Hageman factor and could play a role in autocatalytic propagation of the entire enzymatic cascade.
- **Clotting system:** This results in the formation of fibrin through the intrinsic clotting pathway.
- **Fibrinolysis system:** Activation of plasminogen into plasmin results in lysis of fibrin and also activation of the complement cascade.
- **Complement system:** This involves sequential activation of complement proteins C1 to C9 and their activators and inhibitors.
See Fig. 2-4.

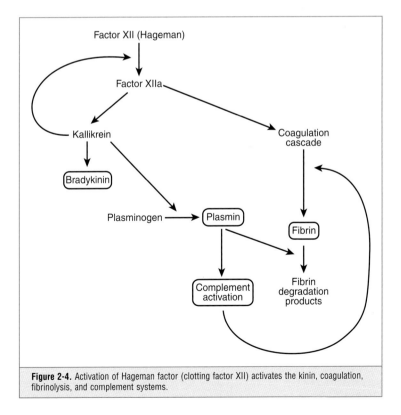

Figure 2-4. Activation of Hageman factor (clotting factor XII) activates the kinin, coagulation, fibrinolysis, and complement systems.

26. **What is bradykinin?**
Bradykinin is a low-molecular-weight peptide formed from a high-molecular-weight kininogen through the action of the enzyme kallikrein. Like histamine, bradykinin increases vascular permeability. The action of bradykinin is short lived because it is inactivated by kininases.

27. **What is histamine?**
Histamine is a low-molecular-weight biogenic amine stored in the granules of mast cells, basophils, and platelets. Upon release, it binds to the H1 receptor on endothelial cells, increasing the permeability of venules, which leads to edema.

28. **How is histamine released from mast cells?**
Mast cells release histamine in response to a number of stimuli, including mechanical stimulation, anaphylatoxins formed from complement, and certain neuropeptides.
In type I hypersensitivity reactions (e.g., hay fever), histamine is released as a result of the interaction of antigen and immunoglobulin E (IgE) bound to the plasma membrane of mast cells.

29. **What is complement?**
Complement proteins form a system that includes approximately 20 plasma enzymes. Activation of the complement system leads to the formation of biologically active fragments (e.g., C3a and C5b) and complexes (e.g., C567 and membrane attack complex [MAC]) that have an important role in inflammation.

30. **How is the complement system activated?**
The complement system can be activated by three convergent pathways known as the classical, alternative, and lectin-binding pathways.
- **Classical pathway:** This was named because it was first discovered many years ago during formation of antigen–antibody immune complexes.
- **Alternative pathway:** This pathway is activated by fragments of bacteria and fungi and other particulate foreign substances, toxins, and enzymes.
- **Lectin-binding pathway:** This pathway is initiated by the mannose-binding protein (MBP), a liver-derived plasma protein. MBP binds to mannose residues on the bacterial plasma membrane and is an important initiator of the inflammatory response to bacteria.

31. **What are the consequences of complement activation?**
Complement activation has four major biologic functions:
- **Opsonization of bacteria:** This is primarily accomplished by fragments such as C3b. Neutrophils and macrophages have receptors for C3, which allows them to bind firmly to opsonized bacteria and phagocytize them.
- **Chemotaxis:** Complement fragments such as C5a and intermediate complexes such as C567 attract neutrophils to the site of inflammation.
- **Anaphylatoxic action:** Complement fragments such as C5a are called *anaphylatoxins* because they bind to mast cells and stimulate them to release histamine, which then leads to increased permeability of blood vessels. This is typically seen in anaphylactic shock but also occurs in most other forms of localized inflammatory edema.
- **Cytolysis:** MAC formed from the aggregated complement proteins C5 to C9 inserts itself into the plasma membrane of target cells, causing their lysis. This is typically seen in immune hemolytic anemia.

32. **What are the main arachidonic acid–derived mediators of inflammation?**
Arachidonic acid, a lipid-derived eicosanoid, is formed from cell membrane phospholipids. After it is formed inside the cell, arachidonic acid is metabolized through two major pathways:

- **Cyclooxygenase pathway:** This pathway leads to the formation of prostaglandins (PG) of the PGD, PGE, and PGF series; prostacyclin (also known as PGI2); and thromboxane. Endothelial cells preferentially produce prostacyclin, which prevents the aggregation of platelets and acts as a potent vasodilator. Platelets, on the other hand, preferentially produce thromboxane, which favors aggregation of platelets and vasoconstriction. PGE2 stimulates smooth muscle cell contraction.
- **Lipoxygenase pathway:** Leukotrienes (LTC4, LTD4, and LTE4) formed by this pathway act on smooth muscle cells of bronchi and blood vessels. In asthma, they cause bronchoconstriction, vasoconstriction, and increased vascular permeability; thus, they are known as slow-reacting substances of anaphylaxis (SRS-A). LTB4 is a potent chemotactic factor. Lipoxins cause vasodilatation.

33. **What are the effects of inhibitors of arachidonic acid metabolism?**
Inhibitors of arachidonic acid metabolism have antiinflammatory effects. The most important inhibitors are:
- **Cyclooxygenase inhibitors:** Among these widely used drugs, one should mention aspirin, nonsteroidal antiinflammatory drugs (NSAIDs) such as indomethacin (Tylenol), and new COX-2 inhibitors.
- **Lipoxygenase inhibitors:** These drugs are mostly used in the treatment of asthma.
- **Corticosteroids:** These adrenal hormones inhibit phospholipase involved in the production of arachidonic acid but also act on several other enzymes involved in the metabolism of eicosanoids.

34. **What is the platelet-activating factor (PAF)?**
PAF, described first as a phospholipid-derived mediator of platelet aggregation and degranulation, is a multifunctional, biologically active molecule. It acts on many cells. It is synthesized by leukocytes, endothelial cells, and many other cells. Receptors for PAF are present on numerous cells, all of which can act when exposed to this mediator. For example, it can cause bronchospasm and vasospasm but also vasodilatation and increased vascular permeability.

35. **What are cytokines?**
Cytokines, originally isolated from lymphocytes and therefore called lymphokines, are multifunctional polypeptides that modulate the function of other cells. Cytokines comprise interleukins, numbered in sequence of their discovery (IL-1, IL-2, etc.); interferons (alpha, beta, and gamma); tumor necrosis factor (TNF) (alpha and beta); and a number of chemotactic polypeptides known as chemokines.

36. **What are the functions of cytokines?**
Cytokines have numerous functions and mediate the following:
- Synthesis and release of other mediators of inflammation, such as prostaglandins or nitric oxide
- Activation of leukocytes, stimulating chemotaxis, phagocytosis, adhesion of leukocytes to endothelial cells, and recruitment of leukocytes to the site of inflammation
- Endothelial cell reactions such as their anticoagulant or procoagulant activity
- Proliferation of fibroblasts and angioblasts and formation of the granulation tissue
- Fever
- Acute-phase reactant synthesis in the liver; this effect accounts for the increased erythrocyte sedimentation rate (ESR) in infectious diseases

37. **What are the oxygen-derived bactericidal and vasoactive mediators of inflammation?**
- **Oxygen-derived free radicals:** These are formed by neutrophils during the initial respiratory burst that occurs upon the internalization of the bacteria. The first oxygen derivative is

superoxide (O-2), which is then transformed into H_2O_2 through the action of superoxide dismutase on the cell surface and the phagolysosomes. H_2O_2 is reduced to hydroxyl radical in the presence of $Fe2+$ (Fenton reaction).

- **Hypochlorous acid (HOCl):** Myeloperoxidase from primary leukocytic granules transforms H_2O_2 in the presence of chloride into hypochlorous acid, the most potent of all bactericidal substances produced by leukocytes.
- **Nitric oxide (NO):** Nitric oxide synthetase (NOS) produces NO from l-arginine and molecular oxygen. Endothelial cells, which contain NOS, produce NO constitutively. NO is a potent vasodilatator. It also inhibits platelet adhesion in influx of leukocytes in the blood vessels of the inflamed area. NOS of macrophages is not constitutively expressed but can be induced by cytokines.

38. **Which mediators of inflammation act on blood vessels to cause their constriction, dilatation, or increased permeability?**
    - **Vasoconstriction:** This results from the action of thromboxane A2 and leukotrienes.
    - **Vasodilatation:** This results from the action of prostaglandins, lipoxins, and NO.
    - **Increased vascular permeability:** This results from the action of leukotrienes. Histamine leads to rapid but transient increased permeability of venules in early stages of inflammation. Bradykinin is a "slower" analog of histamine (remember that *brady* means "slow" in Greek). Leukotrienes and PAF also increase vascular permeability.

    Some mediators of inflammation have different effects on different vessels. Histamine causes dilatation of venules but constricts the arterioles. PAF can cause both vasodilatation and vasoconstriction.

39. **Which mediators of inflammation are chemotactic to leukocytes?**
    Chemotaxis of leukocytes is stimulated by complement fragments (C5a), leukotriene B4, lipoxins, and many interleukins.

40. **Which mediators of inflammation cause pain?**
    Prostaglandins and bradykinin.

41. **Which mediators of inflammation act as pyrogens?**
    Exogenous pyrogens (i.e., substances that cause fever) stimulate macrophages to produce endogenous pyrogens, such as IL-1, TNF-α, and IL-6. IL-1 stimulates the synthesis of PGE2, which acts on the hypothalamic thermoregulatory centers, raising the thermostat for body temperature. TNF-α and IL-6 act directly on the hypothalamus but also stimulate the production of IL-1.

42. **What is the outcome of acute inflammation?**
    - **Resolution:** In most instances, all signs of acute inflammation disappear without any consequences.
    - **Suppuration:** Excessive exudation of neutrophils accompanied by destruction of tissue-localized suppuration results from the cystic action of enzymes released from leukocytes and is called an abscess.
    - **Transition to chronic inflammation:** This usually occurs gradually, and the moment of transition usually cannot be established.
    - **Repair by fibrosis:** Following destruction of tissue by the inflammation, the damaged cells are removed by phagocytes and granulation tissue grows into the damaged area. The integrity of the tissue can be completely restored, as in an ulcerated mucosal lesion, or the entire area can become fibrosed and scarred.

CHRONIC INFLAMMATION

43. **What are the typical features of chronic inflammation?**
Any inflammation that does not heal on its own after a few days can be called chronic. Pathologically, such inflammation is mediated by macrophages, lymphocytes, and plasma cells. Typically, there is much more tissue destruction than in acute inflammation, and the damaged cells are replaced by fibrous scars. The entire area is often permeated by newly formed blood vessels.

KEY POINTS: CHRONIC INFLAMMATION ✔

1. Chronic inflammation can be a continuation of unresolved acute inflammation, or it may begin as such in response to certain stimuli, as in granulomas.

2. The principal cells of chronic inflammation are lymphocytes, plasma cells, and macrophages.

44. **How does chronic inflammation begin?**
Chronic inflammation occurs under the following conditions:
- Nonhealing or persistent acute inflammation, as in nonhealing bacterial pneumonia
- Persistent infections caused by pathogens that cannot be readily eliminated (e.g., viral hepatitis C or tuberculosis)
- Continuous exposure to noxious exogenous influences (e.g., tobacco smoke)
- Foreign material (e.g., surgical material left over in the wound)
- Autoimmune diseases: most diseases caused by endogenous antigens tend to run a prolonged course
- Transplant rejection: foreign antigens typically induce chronic immune reactions involving both the B and T lymphocytes
- Diseases of unknown origin: the cause of many chronic inflammatory diseases, such as chronic inflammatory bowel disease or usual interstitial pneumonitis, is unknown

45. **What are the mononuclear cells found in chronic inflammatory reactions?**
In contrast to acute inflammation, which is mediated by polymorphonuclear leukocytes that have a segmented nucleus, chronic inflammation is mediated by cells that have a nonsegmented single nucleus. The term *mononuclear cells* comprises macrophages, lymphocytes, and plasma cells.

46. **What attracts mononuclear inflammatory cells to the site of inflammation?**
Macrophages are descendants of blood-borne monocytes, which exit from blood vessels in response to the same chemotactic stimuli that attract the neutrophils. However, because the monocytes are less mobile than neutrophils, they arrive at the site of inflammation 24 to 48 hours later.

47. **What is the function of macrophages in chronic inflammation?**
Macrophages produce and secrete a number of biologically active substances, including:
- Cytokines, such as IL-1 and IL-2, which modulate the action of other cells
- Chemokines, which attract other macrophages and lymphocytes to the area
- Free oxygen radicals, which kill bacteria and other cells
- Growth factors, such as fibroblast growth factor (FGF) and platelet-derived growth factor (PDGF), which stimulate the growth of other cells, most notably fibroblasts and angioblasts in granulation tissue during wound healing

- Proteases, which remove the damaged tissue elements
- Arachidonic acid metabolites, which amplify the inflammation

48. What are granulomas?

Granulomas, the hallmarks of granulomatous inflammation, are aggregates of epithelioid macrophages and lymphocytes and occasional multinucleated giant cells. Epithelioid macrophages differ from the usual macrophages in that they have more abundant cytoplasm filled with vacuoles and lysosomes. Their cell borders are closely opposed to one another so that the entire structure appears "epithelioid" (i.e., it resembles the epithelial layer of the skin).

49. How are granulomas formed?

Granulomas form in response to bacteria and fungi that cannot be readily eliminated (e.g., *Mycobacterium tuberculosis* or *Histoplasma capsulatum*) or substances that initiate a cell-mediated, rather than humoral, type of hypersensitivity. Macrophages that arrive at the site of injury ingest the noxious material and become activated. Activated macrophages secrete chemokines to recruit new macrophages and lymphocytes. At the same time, under the influence of cytokines secreted by themselves and those produced by lymphocytes, macrophages transform into epithelioid cells, which become immobile and prefer to stay in the granulomas rather than wander. Under the influence of interferon-γ, some epithelioid cells fuse into multinucleated giant cells.

50. How are granulomas classified?

Granulomas can be pathogenetically subdivided into three groups:

- **Infectious granulomas:** This group comprises typical caseating granulomas found in tuberculosis and some deep fungal infections, such as histoplasmosis or blastomycosis; gummas of syphilis, which also contain plasma cells; and suppurative granulomas found in cat scratch disease or bartonellosis, which contain central areas of liquefactive necrosis caused by neutrophils.
- **Noninfectious granulomas:** These granulomas are found in delayed cell-mediated immune reactions (e.g., hypersensitivity pneumonitis) and diseases of unknown etiology (e.g., sarcoidosis). Granulomas are occasionally seen in lymph nodes draining an area involved by tumors. These granulomas are composed predominantly of epithelioid macrophages and a few scattered lymphocytes and do not show central caseating necrosis.
- **Foreign body granulomas:** These are granulomas that form around exogenous indigestible material such as surgical suture material, splinters of wood, ova of parasites, and so on. They contain numerous giant cells. Within these giant cells, it is often possible to identify the causative material; such cells are therefore called foreign body giant cells.

51. What is the outcome of granulomatous inflammation?

Granulomas persist for a long time. They may slowly resolve and disappear, leaving no signs of tissue injury, or they may fibrose and heal by scarring. Infectious necrotizing granulomas may coalesce and, by destroying tissue, form cavities filled with caseous material.

52. What are the main functions of macrophages?

Macrophages have numerous functions and participate in chronic inflammation, healing, and immune reactions. The most important functions of macrophages are as follows:

- **Phagocytosis:** Macrophages have surface receptors for IgG and C3 and thus phagocytize opsonized bacteria with ease.

- **Secretion of proteins and lipid-derived mediators:** Macrophages can produce complement proteins (e.g., C1–C5), coagulation factors (e.g., factor VIII), bactericidal substances (e.g., properdin and lysozyme), proteases, cytokines and chemokines, arachidonic acid derivatives, and oxygen radicals and NO.
- **Antigen processing:** Macrophages take up foreign antigens by phagocytosis or pinocytosis (if fluid) and present the processed material to T and B lymphocytes.

53. **What are Langhans giant cells (GCs)?**
Multinucleated giant cells found in granulomas of tuberculosis have traditionally been called Langhans GCs. However, similar GCs can be seen in other granulomas as well. Note that these cells are different from epidermal mononuclear macrophages known as Langerhans cells, named after the scientist who discovered the islets of Langerhans. Historically, they have been separated from other multinucleated GCs, such as Touton GC (found in xanthogranulomas) and Warthin–Finkeldey GC (found in measles). All these cells are formed through the fusion of epithelioid macrophages, and there is not much use in separating them from each other.

54. **What is the function of eosinophils?**
Eosinophils can participate in acute processes but are more prominent in chronic processes. The main functions of eosinophils are:
- **Bactericidal action:** Eosinophils arrive to the site of infection later than neutrophils but stay there longer. They kill bacteria less efficiently than either neutrophils or macrophages. Hence, they are considered slower and less efficient "cousins" of these phagocytes.
- **Antiparasitic action:** Eosinophils contain crystalloid granules filled with major basic protein (MBP), eosinophilic cationic protein (ECP), and other proteins that kill parasites. Infiltrates elicited by parasites typically are rich in eosinophils.
- **Participation in allergic reactions:** Eosinophils participate in allergic reactions to foreign antigens. Most prominently, they are found in atopic (type I hypersensitivity) reactions, such as hay fever and asthma. It is thought that they counterbalance the action of mast cells, which are the primary reactants to foreign antigens in these diseases.

55. **What are the systemic signs and symptoms of inflammation?**
Typical systemic signs of inflammation are the following:
- Fever with sweating and chills
- Tachycardia (heart rate >90/min)
- Tachypnea (respiratory rate >20/min)
- Constitutional symptoms (loss of appetite, tiredness, weakness, and drowsiness)
- Laboratory findings (leukocytosis, elevated ESR, etc.)

56. **What are the causes of leukocytosis in inflammation?**
Leukocytosis, defined as a two- or threefold increase in the number of leukocytes in the peripheral blood (usually >12,000 leukocytes per microliter), is caused by an accelerated release of leukocytes from the bone marrow. This bone marrow response is mediated by IL-1 and TNF-α derived from inflammatory cells at the site of inflammation. If the inflammation persists, macrophages and T lymphocytes will produce colony-stimulating factors (CSFs), which promote the formation of new leukocytes in the bone marrow.

57. **What accounts for the increased ESR in inflammation?**
ESR is easily determined by measuring the rate at which the red blood cells separate from plasma 1 and 2 hours after the blood was drawn. Because the sedimentation rate of erythrocytes depends on the concentration and the relative electric charge of plasma proteins, it is a rough measure of altered plasma protein composition, most notably of the

concentration of albumin and the so-called acute-phase reactants. Acute-phase reactants that increase in plasma are C-reactive protein, α1-antitrypsin, ceruloplasmin, fibrinogen, serum amyloid associated (SAA)–protein, and some others. There are sensitive biochemical tests that measure the concentration of C-reactive protein in blood. These tests can be used instead of the standard ESR.

MORPHOLOGY OF INFLAMMATION

58. **What determines the morphology of inflammatory reactions?**
    - **Etiology:** The morphology of lesions depends on the nature of the pathogen that has caused them. Pus-forming bacteria, such as *Staphylococcus aureus,* often cause abscesses. Caseous necrosis, a feature of tuberculosis, often leads to the formation of cavitary lung lesions.
    - **Location:** The anatomic features of the organ involved are among the most important determinants of the type of inflammation. For example, certain forms of inflammation, such as ulcer, occur only on the mucosal surface or the skin and do not appear in solid organs, such as the liver or kidneys. Catarrhal inflammation occurs only on mucosal surfaces containing mucus-secreting cells, such as nasal or bronchial mucosa.
    - **Duration of the inflammation:** Acute inflammation tends to be more exudative, whereas chronic inflammation is often associated with fibrosis and scarring.

59. **What is serous inflammation?**
    Serous inflammation is characterized by exudation of acellular, protein-poor, serumlike fluid. Typical examples are blisters on skin caused by herpes simplex virus or burns and pleural effusion related to viral infection of the lungs and pleura.

60. **What is fibrinous inflammation?**
    Fibrinous inflammation results from exudates rich in fibrin. Fibrinogen, a high-molecular-weight plasma protein, can exit only through large defects in the blood vessel wall, and thus fibrinous inflammation entails vessel wall injury or increased vascular porosity. Fibrinous exudates consist of a meshwork of fibrin (i.e., polymerized fibrinogen). The surface of the pericardial cavity has a "bread and butter" appearance because the fibrin in the exudate forms strands bridging the space between the epicardium and the pericardium. Fibrinous pericarditis can be caused by mycobacteria (e.g., *M. tuberculosis*) but also may be sterile and result from rheumatic fever, uremia, and even a transmural myocardial infarct.

61. **What is suppurative inflammation?**
    Suppurative or purulent inflammation is characterized by exudation of pus. Pus is defined as the semifluid, viscous material composed of dead and dying neutrophils, plasma proteins, and liquefied tissue detritus. Localized destruction of the tissue results in a pus-filled cavity, which is called an abscess. Empyema is a collection of pus in a preexisting body cavity (e.g., pleural cavity) or a hollow organ (e.g., empyema of the gallbladder). Such lesions also may carry anatomic designations such as pyosalpinx (pus in the fallopian tube), pyometra (pus in the uterine cavity), and pyonephrosis (pus in the renal pelvis and calices).

62. **What is ulceration?**
    An ulcer, a defect in the surface lining of the skin or mucosae, results from inflammation-induced necrosis of the superficial layers of the involved organ. In gastric or duodenal ulcers,

mucosal necrosis results from the action of the hydrochloric acid and pepsin in the digestive juices. In amebic colitis, ulcers result from the lytic action of amoebas in the lumen. The cause of confluent ulcerations of the large intestine typical of ulcerative colitis is not known.

63. What is pseudomembranous inflammation?

Pseudomembranous inflammation is a variant of ulcerative inflammation.

The mucosal injury, usually caused by bacterial toxins, begins as necrosis of the superficial cell layers. Necrotic mucosal cells slough off and become intermixed with mucus, bowel contents, and exudated fibrin to form a layer *(pseudomembrane)* that covers the remaining lower parts of the mucosa. This layer is called pseudomembrane to distinguish it from "true" anatomic membranes—that is, structures that normally cover the external surfaces of organs or form borders between the layers of multilayered organs. Such pseudomembranes can be scraped off during endoscopic examination, exposing a bleeding ulcerated surface underneath.

64. What is gangrenous inflammation?

Gangrene results when bacteria invade necrotic tissue. Typically, such inflammation occurs on the legs of diabetics who have diabetic microangiopathy and accelerated atherosclerosis and therefore suffer from hypoperfusion of the extremities. Gangrene may also occur in an infarcted intestine. In both instances, the infection is caused by saprophytic bacteria, which is normally present at the site of ischemia tissue necrosis.

REGENERATION AND REPAIR

65. Which injuries can be repaired by regeneration?

Extensive tissue injury can be repaired by regeneration only in organs that are composed of cells that are normally proliferating or can be induced to proliferate. Regeneration cannot take place in organs such as heart and brain, which are composed of terminally differentiated cells.

66. How are cells classified on the basis of their replicative potential?

During embryonic development, all organs are composed of dividing cells. In the adult organism, some cells retain the propensity to divide, whereas others become quiescent and exit from the mitotic cell cycle. Accordingly, there are three cell types:

- **Mitotic, continuously dividing cells:** These cells, also called labile cells, represent the stem cells of constantly renewing tissues such as the epidermis, the mucosal layer of internal organs, bone marrow, or seminiferous tubules of the testis. At a given time, tissues composed of mitotic cells contain more than 1.5% cells in mitosis throughout the entire adult life.
- **Facultative mitotic cells:** Also called stable cells, these cells are arrested in the G0 phase. They can enter the mitotic cycle in certain circumstances and divide into two daughter cells. Organs composed of stable cells have the capacity to regenerate and compensate the loss of parenchymal cells by equivalent newly formed cells. Stable cells form most parenchymal organs, such as the liver, kidneys, and endocrine organs. Endothelial cells, fibroblasts, and other connective tissue cells are also classified as stable cells.
- **Postmitotic, nondividing cells:** These cells, also called permanent cells, cannot reenter the mitotic cycle. These cells cannot be replaced, and an injury is usually repaired by replacing these terminally differentiated cells with cells that cannot perform their specific function. Brain and heart are the prototypes of organs composed of permanent cells. For practical purposes, skeletal muscle is also classified under this heading because the reserve cells inside the muscle cannot fully compensate for the loss of mature striated muscle fibers.

KEY POINTS: REGENERATION AND REPAIR ✓

1. Regeneration can occur in organs and tissues composed of mitotic and facultative mitotic cells, but the organs composed of postmitotic cells cannot regenerate.

2. Wound healing is the best prototype of repair in which the granulation tissue plays a crucial role.

3. Crucial components of wound healing are the cells, such as fibroblasts, macrophages, and angioblasts, and their products, including ECM proteins.

67. **How are quiescent cells induced to divide?**
Induction of cell division involves a sequence of events that includes several steps:
- Binding of growth factor to the plasma membrane receptor
- Activation of the receptor, which has tyrosinase kinase activity
- Transmission of signals through metabolic pathways and secondary messengers such as calcium ions
- Activation of nuclear transcription factors
- Entry of the cell into the cell cycle

68. **How many phases does a typical cell cycle have?**
The cell cycle has four phases:
- G1 (presynthetic gap)
- S (synthetic phase)
- G2 (postsynthetic gap)
- M (mitotic phase)

The mitotic cells are most often nondividing and thus in phase G0. The entry into the mitotic cycle and the progression of the cell cycle from one phase to another is regulated by cyclins labeled A through E and cyclin-dependent kinases. Each of these kinases has specific inhibitors that can block the mitotic cycle.

69. **Can the cell division be inhibited?**
Normal cells grown in tissue culture stop dividing as a result of contact inhibition, a control mechanism that is activated after the cells attain a certain density or reach the edges of the tissue culture flask. Transforming growth factor–beta (TGF-β) can stop the cell division by acting on cell cycle control proteins.

70. **What are growth factors?**
Growth factors (GFs) are polypeptides produced by a variety of cells. The terminology for various factors, reminiscent of alphabet soup, evolved over the years and is rather confusing. Epidermal growth factor (EGF), for example, was initially thought to act only on epidermal cells, but today it is known that it stimulates both epidermal and mucosal epithelial cells, as well as fibroblasts. PDGF was initially isolated from platelets, but today it is known that it is produced by other cells as well. Some growth factors do not carry the letters GF in their name (e.g., TNF). Many interleukins also have GF activity.

71. **What are the common features of growth factors involved in repair and regeneration?**
Growth factors are a heterogeneous group of polypeptides that nevertheless share some common features:
- **Receptors:** To act on cells, GFs must act on cellular receptors. Some receptors are ubiquitous, whereas others are only found on some cells. For example, PDGF acts on numerous mesenchymal cells, whereas the VEGF acts only on endothelial cells. Some GFs act on the same receptor, such as EGF and TGF-α.

- **Pleiotropism:** Although they are called growth factors, most GFs not only stimulate cell division but also mediate other cellular processes, such as synthesis and secretion of collagen, fibronectin, and other proteins and migration of cells.
- **Redundancy:** Because many GFs have the same function as some other GFs, a deficiency of one GF can be easily compensated by another one. However, deficiency of a specific receptor is more serious. For example, the congenital deficiency of the fibroblast growth factor receptor 3 results in achondroplastic dwarfism. It is worth noting that the contact of cell membrane with ECM can trigger similar growth stimuli and mimic the action of growth factors.

72. **What are the most important ECM components that are laid down during the repair of inflammatory lesions?**
Extracellular components laid down during repair can be grouped under three headings: (1) collagens, (2) adhesive proteins, and (3) proteoglycans.
- **Collagens:** This group includes 19 described fibrillar or nonfibrillar proteins. The most important among these are:
  ○ **Collagen type I:** This is the most abundant structural protein. It is the main component of connective tissues, tendons, and bones but is found also in most organs. It has a triple helical structure imparting strength and structure to tissues.
  ○ **Collagen type III:** This protein, abundantly found in pliable organs and blood vessels, is also copious in fetal tissues. In a healing wound or in repair, it is the first type of collagen to be laid down by fibroblasts.
  ○ **Collagen type IV:** This nonfibrillar collagen is found in basement membranes separating tissue compartments one from another in blood vessels and in the pericellular basement membranes that surround some cells, such as smooth muscle cells.
- **Adhesive proteins**
  ○ **Fibronectin:** This glycoprotein binds to other ECM molecules and cells, serving as a part of the scaffold, as well as glue, that holds the tissue together.
  ○ **Laminin:** This glycoprotein is an integral component of basement membranes but also serves as an adhesive substance in smooth and striated muscle cells.
- **Proteoglycans:** These negatively charged molecules are highly hydrophilic and can bind water on its side chains, which extend through the intercellular spaces. At the same time, proteoglycans serve as interstitial glue that holds together other elements.

WOUND HEALING

73. **What is granulation tissue?**
The term *granulation tissue* was used by ancient surgeons for the red, granular tissue filling the nonhealing wounds. With the advent of microscopy, it was discovered that granulation tissue occurs in all wounds during healing but that it may occur in chronic inflammation as well. It consists of fibroblasts surrounded by abundant ECM, newly formed blood vessels, scattered macrophages, and some other inflammatory cells.

74. **What are angioblasts?**
Angioblasts are connective tissue cells that form new blood vessels. Angiogenesis is promoted by growth factors acting on angioblasts. Several growth factors promote angiogenesis, but the most potent ones are VEGF and basic fibroblast growth factor (BFGF).

75. **What are myofibroblasts?**
Myofibroblasts have hybrid properties of fibroblasts and smooth muscle cells. In other words, these cells can produce collagens and other matrix proteins, but they can also contract. Myofibroblasts are found in the granulation tissue and are important for the contraction of wounds and the prevention of dehiscence.

76. **What is the role of macrophages in wound healing?**
    - **Cleanup of debris:** In the first stages of wound healing, macrophages phagocytize the cell debris and help the neutrophils in cleaning up the field.
    - **Recruitment of other cells:** Macrophages recruit other cells and are essential for the entry of fibroblasts and angioblasts into the wound.
    - **Stimulation of matrix production:** Macrophages are a potent source of growth factors and interleukins that stimulate fibroblasts and angioblasts to produce the ECM.
    - **Remodeling of the scar:** Macrophages secrete collagenases, stromelysin, and other lytic enzymes that degrade collagen and other matrix components, thus restructuring the entire field. At the same time, macrophages, as well as fibroblasts, secrete tissue inhibitors of metalloproteinases (TIMPs), which counteract the action of lytic enzymes so that the remodeling of the scar proceeds in a regulated manner.

77. **How do wounds heal by primary intention?**
    Clean surgical wounds heal by primary intention. Sequentially, the wound passes through several stages:
    - **Hematoma (day 1):** Initially, the wound is filled with coagulated blood and cell detritus. Influx of neutrophils, followed during the second day by an influx of macrophages, ensures that the extraneous material is removed.
    - **Inflammation and early granulation tissue (days 2–3):** Macrophages stimulate the ingrowth of fibroblasts and angioblasts, which start forming collagen type III. Epidermal cells form a bridge that seals off the defect.
    - **Fully developed granulation tissue (days 4–6):** Neovascularization reaches its peak, and the entire area seems swollen and red. In addition to numerous newly formed capillaries, the granulation tissue contains numerous fibroblasts that rapidly synthesize ECM molecules.
    - **Blanching (week 2):** Deposits of collagen compress and slowly replace the blood vessels and reduce the blood flow through the healing wound.
    - **Scar formation:** Macrophages become less prominent. During the next few weeks, the granulation tissue is gradually replaced by fibrous scar. During this period, collagen type III is slowly replaced by collagen type I and the wound acquires tensile strength. By the end of the third month, the tissue has approximately 80% of its original strength.
    - **Remodeling of the scar:** This process can take several months, during which the tissue acquires even more tensile strength.

78. **Which wounds heal by secondary intention?**
    Large, gaping wounds, as well those that are infected or contain foreign material, heal by secondary intention.

79. **Does the process of healing differ in wounds that heal by primary and those that heal by secondary intention?**
    The basic process of healing is the same in all wounds. In contrast to clean surgical wounds healing by primary intention, wounds healing by secondary intention:
    - Require more time to close because the edges are far apart
    - Show a more prominent inflammatory reaction in and around the wound
    - Contain more copious granulation tissue inside the tissue defect

80. **What is wound contraction?**
    Reduction in size of the wounds healing by secondary intention is called *wound contraction*. It occurs as a result of the action of myofibroblasts in the granulation tissue.

81. What is the most common cause of delayed wound healing?
The most common cause of delayed wound healing is infection. Other causes, such as foreign bodies in the wound, mechanical factors, nutritional deficiencies (e.g., protein or vitamin C deficiency), or excess corticosteroids, may also play a role.

82. What is wound dehiscence?
Dehiscence (Latin, "oplit apart") is opening of a healing or partially healed wound with separation of its edges. Often this occurs as a result of mechanical factors but it may also be related to infection or ischemic necrosis of the sutured edges.

83. What is a keloid?
Keloids are hyperplastic scars composed of irregularly deposited bundles of collagen in the dermis. They may appear as bulging masses extending beyond the confines of the original injury.

84. What is proud flesh?
Exuberant granulation tissue preventing the closure of the wound or proper epithelialization has historically been called proud flesh. Usually it must be removed by cautery to allow the wound to heal.

85. What are contractures?
Contractures are deformities of extremities caused by irregular scars formed over the joints. Such scars, most often related to extensive burns, limit the mobility of joints, and the affected part of the extremity usually cannot fully extend.

WEBSITES

1. http://www.ncbi.nlm.nih.gov/entrez/query.fcgi?db=PubMed
2. http://www-medlib.med.utah.edu/WebPath/webpath.html#MENU
3. http://vlib.org/Science/Cell_Biology/cell_adhesion_ecm.shtml
4. http://www.pathguy.com/lectures/inflamma.htm

BIBLIOGRAPHY

1. Akdis CA, Blaser K: Histamine in the immune regulation of allergic inflammation. J Allergy Clin Immunol 112:15–22, 2003.
2. Alisjahbana B, Netea MG, van der Meer JW: Pro-inflammatory cytokine response in acute infection. Adv Exp Med Biol 531:229–240, 2003.
3. Hantash BM, Zhao L, Knowles JA, Lorenz HP: Adult and fetal wound healing. Front Biosci 13:51–56, 2008.
4. Hinz B, Phan SH, Thannickal VJ, et al: The myofibroblast: one function, multiple origins. Am J Pathol 170:1807–1816, 2007.
5. James DG: A clinicopathologic classification of granulomatous disorders. Postgrad Med 76:457–465, 2000.
6. Kobayashi Y: The role of chemokines in neutrophil biology. Front Biosci 3:2400–2407, 2008.
7. Peters-Golden M, Henderson WR Jr: Leukotrienes: N Engl J Med 357:1841–1854, 2007.
8. Pober JS, Sessa WC: Evolving functions of endothelial cells in inflammation. Nat Rev Immunol 7:803–815, 2007.

CHAPTER 3

HEMODYNAMIC DISORDERS

Ivan Damjanov, MD, PhD

EDEMA

1. **How is body water distributed?**
   Body water is divided into two main compartments:
   - Intracellular, comprising two thirds of total body fluid.
   - Extracellular, comprising one third of total body fluid. The extracellular compartment is further divided into an interstitial compartment containing 75% of the extracellular fluid and an intravascular compartment, which contains 25% of the extracellular fluid.

2. **What is edema?**
   Edema is accumulation of fluid in the interstitial spaces and the body cavities.

3. **How is edema classified according to the distribution of the fluid?**
   Edema can be localized or generalized.
   - **Localized edema:** Typically, this involves one organ or part of the body. Clinically important examples of localized edema are brain edema, lung edema, or accumulation of fluid in the thoracic cavity (hydrothorax) or abdominal cavity (ascites).
   - **Generalized edema:** When edema involves the entire body, it is called anasarca.

KEY POINTS: EDEMA ✔

1. Edema is accumulation of fluid in tissue or body cavities caused by mechanisms that involve the blood flow, composition of plasma, the vessel wall, and the adjacent tissue.

2. Transudates differ from exudates in several respects, including their pathogenesis and physical and chemical properties.

3. The understanding of the pathogenesis of edema in various organs is important for the understanding of the symptoms and the treatment of such diseases.

4. **How are various forms of edema classified according to their pathogenesis?**
   Main causes of edema are:
   - Increased intravascular (hydrostatic) pressure
   - Increased permeability of vessel wall
   - Decreased oncotic pressure of the plasma
   - Sodium retention in the kidneys
   - Obstruction of lymph flow

5. **What is hydrostatic edema?**
   Hydrostatic edema results from increased intravascular pressure owing to:
   - **Impaired venous return:** Increased central venous pressure caused by heart failure leads to generalized edema, which is, however, more pronounced in the lower extremities. Obstruction of veins by thrombi may lead to localized edema (e.g., edema of the calf as a result of thrombosis of popliteal veins).
   - **Increased influx of arterial blood:** Arterial dilatation owing to heat or in the course of inflammation may cause or contribute to the formation of edema.

6. **What are the common causes of increased vascular permeability that lead to edema?**
   The most common cause of increased vascular permeability is inflammation. Inflammatory edema results from the action of mediators such as histamine, complement fragments (C3a and C5a), bradykinin, platelet-activating factor (PAF), and leukotrienes.

7. **What is oncotic edema?**
   Oncotic pressure of the plasma is primarily maintained by albumin. Reduced concentration of albumin in plasma (hypoalbuminemia) may result from:
   - **Decreased protein synthesis:** Most plasma proteins are synthesized in the liver. Hypoalbuminemia, as seen in end-stage liver disease, is the most important cause of generalized edema caused by reduced protein synthesis in chronic liver disease.
   - **Increased protein loss:** Loss of proteins may occur through the kidneys in nephrotic syndrome or in the stool in protein-losing enteropathy.
   - **Inadequate protein intake:** Low-protein diet, as in kwashiorkor, a malnutrition disease that occurs in African children on a protein-deficient diet, may result in generalized edema.

8. **How does sodium retention cause edema?**
   Retention of sodium plays a major role in the pathogenesis of cardiac edema. Heart failure is accompanied by reduced perfusion of the kidneys, which stimulates the juxtaglomerular apparatus to secrete renin. Renin activates the angiotensin system, resulting in an increased secretion of aldosterone from the adrenal cortex. Aldosterone acts on the distal convoluted tubules of the kidney, stimulating them to retain sodium. Retention of sodium is accompanied by water retention, which expands the intravascular volume, leading to increased hydrostatic pressure and hydrostatic edema.

9. **What is lymphedema?**
   Lymphedema results from obstruction of lymphatics and an impaired clearance of lymph from the interstitial spaces. Typically, this is a localized form of edema involving parts of the body, as in:
   - *Elephantiasis,* a term used to denote massive leg edema caused by obstruction of inguinal lymph nodes by filarial worms in filariasis
   - Edema of the arm that develops following surgical dissection of axillary lymph nodes involved by breast cancer; this surgical procedure may disrupt the normal lymph flow

10. **What is the difference between transudate and exudate?**
    Transudate is an ultrafiltrate of plasma that contains few, if any, cells and does not contain large plasma proteins, such as fibrinogen. Transudate results from increased hydrostatic or reduced oncotic pressure. Exudate, on the other hand, is a sign of inflammation and is typically a consequence of increased vascular permeability. Vascular changes permit diapedesis of white blood cells and the passage of large-molecular-weight proteins of the plasma. Accordingly, transudate resembles serum, whereas exudate resembles cell-rich plasma. Transudates do not coagulate, whereas exudates do. The main differences between transudate and exudates are listed in Table 2-1.

11. **What is pitting edema?**
Pitting edema is a clinical term used for subcutaneous leg edema typically found in patients suffering from heart failure. The name refers to the "pit" that can be induced by pressing the skin over the shin.

12. **What is the pathogenesis of pulmonary edema?**
Pulmonary edema is most often caused by increased pulmonary venous pressure secondary to left-heart failure. In adult respiratory distress syndrome, shock, or infections (pneumonia), pulmonary edema is caused by increased permeability of pulmonary capillaries. Pulmonary edema may also occur in generalized edema caused by hypoalbuminemia of end-stage liver disease or nephrotic syndrome.

13. **What is the pathogenesis of ascites of cirrhosis?**
Ascites, a common feature of cirrhosis (end-stage liver disease), represents a transudate that develops owing to:
   - **Hypoalbuminemia:** This results from reduced synthesis of albumin in the damaged liver.
   - **Portal hypertension:** This results from impeded blood flow through the fibrotic liver.
   - **Impaired lymph drainage:** Normally a liter or more lymph flows through the liver, and in cirrhosis this lymph flow is diverted so that the lymph is not drained into the major lymphatics but enters the abdominal cavity.
   - **Increased retention of sodium and water:** Kidneys retain water and salt because of compensatory hyperaldosteronism. After the fluid begins accumulating in the abdominal cavity, the water in the intravascular compartment is reduced, providing a signal for the activation of the renin–angiotensin system. Ultimately, this will cause secondary hyperaldosteronism and retention of sodium and water in the kidney.

14. **What are the causes of brain edema?**
Most acute and many chronic brain injuries can cause brain edema. Brain edema typically accompanies:
   - Infection (encephalitis or meningitis)
   - Brain infarcts and hemorrhage
   - Cranial or cerebral trauma
   - Cerebral tumors

HYPEREMIA AND CONGESTION

15. **What is the difference between active hyperemia and congestion?**
In hyperemia, which is an active process, the increased blood influx into the tissues results from dilatation of arterioles. Typically this occurs in inflammation. Adrenergic stimuli cause dilatation of arterioles of the face during blushing. Increased blood flow through the muscles during exercise is another example of active hyperemia.
   Congestion, also known as passive hyperemia, results from stagnation of blood in the capillaries caused by impeded outflow of blood on the venous end. Obstruction of veins with thrombi or backward pressure caused by heart failure is typically accompanied by congestion.

16. **What is the color of hyperemic and congested tissues?**
Hyperemic tissues contain increased amounts of oxygenated blood, and therefore such tissues appear bright red. In contrast, congested tissues contain increased amounts of deoxygenated venous blood and therefore appear dusky red or bluish. Hyperemic tissues are warm, whereas the congested tissues are clammy and cold.

KEY POINTS: HYPEREMIA AND CONGESTION ✔

1. Hyperemia is an active process involving dilatation of arterioles, whereas congestion refers to passive stagnation of blood in the veins.

2. Hyperemia and congestion occur under different conditions and have different clinical implications.

17. **How does acute congestion differ from chronic passive congestion?**
In acute congestion, the blood is inside the dilated veins and capillaries. Such an accumulation of blood may pass without serious consequences, but if it occurs rapidly, the ensuing hypoxia and mechanical compression of tissue around the dilated blood vessels may cause necrosis. In chronic passive congestion, there is invariably ischemia accompanied by loss of parenchymal cells, which are usually replaced by fibrosis.

18. **How does congestion affect the liver?**
Acute congestion leads to centrilobular stasis of blood that fills the central vein and the sinusoids around it. If the congestion develops suddenly and a large amount of blood is retained in the liver, the centrilobular hepatocytes will undergo necrosis. In chronic passive congestion, the hepatocytes die off and are replaced by fibrous tissue. The cut surface of the liver in such cases has the appearance of a nutmeg. The fibrosis may progress, and the nutmeg liver may transform into cardiac cirrhosis.

19. **How does chronic passive congestion affect the lungs?**
Chronic passive congestion of the lungs is typically a consequence of left heart failure. It is accompanied by extravasation of red blood cells (RBCs) into the alveolar spaces. These RBCs fall apart and are taken up by macrophages, which can be expectorated as "heart failure cells." Macrophages also enter the interstitial spaces, where they may die or stimulate fibroblasts to produce collagen. On gross examination at autopsy, such lungs appear brownish red, due to hemosiderin, and fibrotic, due to the deposition of collagen. The technical term for these changes is brown induration of the lungs.

20. **How does chronic passive congestion affect the legs?**
Prolonged stagnation of blood leads to dilatation of veins (varicose veins) and capillaries. RBCs leak out of the capillaries and die in the interstitial tissues of the subcutis. Hemosiderin formed from hemoglobin accounts for the brownish discoloration of the skin. Chronic ischemia of the skin impedes healing of minor traumatic injuries, and ulcers form. Such stasis ulcers tend to heal slowly or not at all.

HEMORRHAGE

21. **What is hemorrhage?**
Hemorrhage (bleeding) is escape of blood from blood vessels or the heart. Hemorrhages can be classified according to the site of origin:
- **Cardiac:** These are usually caused by penetrating wounds or rupture of ventricle as a result of myocardial infarction.
- **Arterial:** These are usually caused by trauma or rupture of an aneurysm.

- **Capillary:** These are usually caused by trauma or surgery, but they may also occur in a variety of diseases characterized by weakness of vessel walls (e.g., Ehlers–Danlos syndrome and vitamin C deficiency) or platelet disorders (e.g., idiopathic thrombocytopenic purpura).
- **Venous:** These are commonly caused by trauma or surgery.

22. **What are the differences between petechiae, purpura, and ecchymoses?**
   All three terms refer to hemorrhages into the skin and mucosae. Pinpoint hemorrhages smaller than 1 mm are called petechiae; those measuring 1 mm to 1 cm in diameter are called purpura; and those larger than 1 cm are called ecchymoses. This classification is arbitrary and has survived only by tradition. Note that petechiae often become confluent and become purpura or ecchymoses. To complicate matters, the term *purpura* is also used for several diseases characterized by widespread cutaneous hemorrhages (e.g., thrombotic thrombocytopenic purpura and Henoch–Schönlein purpura).

KEY POINTS: HEMORRHAGE ✔

1. The clinical symptoms depend on the source of hemorrhage.

2. Specific clinical–pathologic terms are used for various forms of hemorrhage.

23. **What is the color of a hematoma?**
   Hematoma is a grossly visible accumulation of extravasated blood in the tissue. First it is red, and then as the blood is deoxygenated, it becomes dusky and bluish red. As the RBCs fall apart, biliverdin forms, and the hematoma will appear greenish. Bilirubin formed from biliverdin will give it a yellow hue. After that, the remnants of the RBC may be resorbed and the tissue resumes its normal color, or the iron portion of heme pigment is taken up by macrophages and degraded into hemosiderin, which gives the tissues a brownish color.

24. **How are hemorrhages into body cavities named?**
   Hemorrhage can occur into any of the preexisting body cavities. Such hemorrhages are named by combining the prefixes *hem* or *hemato* (from Greek *haima*, "blood") and the anatomic site involved. Accordingly, most of these terms are self-explanatory. For example, terms such as *hematopericardium*, *hematothorax*, and *hemarthrosis* can be easily understood as denoting bleeding into the pericardial, pleural, or intraarticular space, respectively. Other terms are not so intuitively obvious. For example, *hematocephalus* denotes accumulation of blood in the ventricles of the brain. *Hematocolpos* signifies accumulation of blood in a vagina occluded by an imperforate hymen.

25. **What is hematuria?**
   Hematuria is appearance of blood in urine. It may be classified as microscopic (i.e., detectable by microscopic examination of urine) or macroscopic if visible to the naked eye. Hematuria may be a sign of kidney or urinary tract disease.

26. **What is hematemesis?**
   Hematemesis is vomiting of blood. Typically, it is a sign of esophageal and gastric hemorrhage. Common causes of hematemesis are ruptured esophageal varices and peptic ulcer of the stomach and duodenum.

27. **What is hematochezia?**
    Hematochezia is bleeding through the rectum. It is typically caused by diseases of the large intestine.

28. **What is melena?**
    Melena or black blood presenting as "coffee-ground" material in the stool is a sign of upper gastrointestinal bleeding. Such blood is partially digested by hydrochloric acid of the gastric juice and transformed into a black pigment called hematein. This pigment is not digested in the intestines and is passed in the feces.

29. **What is the difference between epistaxis and hemoptysis?**
    Epistaxis is bleeding from the nose. Hemoptysis is bleeding from the lungs; literally it means "spitting of blood."

30. **What is the difference between menorrhagia and metrorrhagia?**
    Menorrhagia is heavy menstrual bleeding. Metrorrhagia occurs at any time and is not related to menstrual bleeding. The term menometrorrhagia is used for a heavy menstrual bleeding that does not stop after a few days.

HEMOSTASIS AND THROMBOSIS

31. **How is hemostasis related to thrombosis?**
    Both processes are based on the coagulation of blood. Hemostasis ("stopping of hemorrhage") is the physiologic process designed to stop the bleeding from ruptured blood vessels. Thrombosis is a pathologic form of coagulation of circulating blood inside intact vascular spaces.

32. **What are the main components of the hemostatic process?**
    Both hemostasis and thrombosis depend on the interaction of numerous components, which can be grouped as related to the:
    - Vessel wall
    - Platelets
    - Coagulation proteins of the plasma

KEY POINTS: HEMOSTASIS AND THROMBOSIS

1. Thrombosis, like its normal counterpart hemostasis, depends on the interaction of the vessel wall, platelets, and the coagulation factors in the plasma.

2. The coagulation cascade includes three parts: an intrinsic, an extrinsic, and a common pathway.

3. Factors that predispose to thrombosis are found in the vessel wall, in the blood, or can be related to altered blood flow (so-called Virchow's triad).

4. Thrombi may resolve or change and cause a variety of secondary pathologic changes.

33. **How does endothelium of blood vessels act on the coagulation of blood?**
    Endothelial cells have both procoagulant and anticoagulant properties, and according to the needs of the body, they may either promote blood clotting or inhibit it.

34. **How does endothelium prevent blood clotting?**
   Anticoagulant functions of endothelial cells include:
   - **Inhibition of platelet aggregation:** Endothelial cells secrete prostacyclin (PGI2) and nitric oxide (NO), which dilatate blood vessels, thus increasing the blood flow and reducing the chance of adhesion of platelets to the vessel wall. Prostacyclin also directly inhibits the aggregation of platelets.
   - **Inhibition of platelet antithrombin activity:** This is mostly accomplished by thrombomodulin, which captures thrombin and submits it for degradation by the anticoagulant protein C.
   - **Fibrinolysis:** Endothelium secretes plasminogen activator, which generates plasmin from plasminogen. Plasmin lyses fibrin and prevents the growth of the clot.

35. **How does endothelium promote blood clotting?**
   Endothelial cells promote blood clotting through several mechanisms that are counterbalanced by the anticlotting forces. Procoagulant mechanisms include release of:
   - **von Willebrand factor from Weibel–Palade granules in the cytoplasm of endothelial cells:** This factor mediates the binding of platelets to surfaces and also serves as a carrier for the coagulation factor VIII.
   - **Thromboplastin (tissue factor, F III):** This promotes the extrinsic pathway of the coagulation cascade.
   - **Inhibitors of plasminogen activator (PAI)**.

36. **What are the essential components of platelets?**
   Platelets are derived from the fragmentation of the cytoplasm of megakaryocytes. Platelets have the following components that are essential for their participation in hemostasis and thrombosis:
   - **Granules (alpha granules and delta granules or dense bodies):** These granules contain a number of ready-made biologically active substances, including coagulation factors such as fibrinogen, mediators of inflammation such as histamine, and growth factors such as platelet-derived growth factor (PDGF).
   - **Cytoskeleton:** This is composed of tubulin, actin, and myosin filaments that allow the rapid extrusion of granules from the cytoplasm. Microfilaments and microtubules also mediate the change of the shape of platelets and account for the "clot retraction."
   - **Adhesion molecules and receptors:** These glycoproteins are expressed on the cell membrane of activated platelets, allowing them to adhere to fibrinogen and von Willebrand factor and also each other.
   - **Phospholipids:** These cell components (e.g., platelet factor 3) act with and calcium stored in dense granules as cofactors in the coagulation cascade.

37. **What happens after activation of platelets?**
   Activation of platelets is followed by four phases of clot formation. These phases, which partially overlap one another, include:
   - Adhesion of platelets to the surface of the vessel wall
   - Release of chemical mediators stored in granules
   - Aggregation with other platelets to form the primary hemostatic plug
   - Contraction and formation of the secondary hemostatic plug composed of firmly aggregated platelets and fibrin

38. **What is the role of coagulation proteins in hemostasis and thrombosis?**
   Coagulation factors are a group of plasma proteins that are activated by acting upon each other in a sequence known as the extrinsic and intrinsic pathway. These proteins lead to activation of thrombin, which plays a crucial role in the polymerization of fibrinogen into fibrin. Fibrin formed at the end of the coagulation cascade represents the meshwork skeleton of the clot and also serves as the glue that holds together platelets and other components of the clot. Deficiency of coagulation factors results in bleeding disorders.

39. **What is the difference between the intrinsic and the extrinsic coagulation pathway?**
    The intrinsic pathway is so called because it can be activated by pouring the blood into a test tube without adding any extrinsic material. The coagulation cascade is activated by the binding of Hageman factor (F XII) to negatively charged glass. The extrinsic pathway is activated by adding tissue factor, which activates factor VII.
    The mnemonic TEEN helps in remembering that the activation of factor X through the intrinsic pathway involves factors twelve, eleven, eight, and nine

40. **How is the coagulation activated in vivo?**
    The intrinsic pathway is activated by exposure to collagen or basement membranes denuded of endothelial cells or disrupted vessel walls. It can be activated by plasma proteins such as prekallikrein and platelets. The extrinsic pathway is activated by tissue factor (i.e., a number of thromboplastins released from damaged tissue).

41. **Which events occur in the common pathway of the coagulation cascade?**
    - The intrinsic and the extrinsic pathway converge, activating factor X.
    - Activated factor X forms interact with factor V, platelet factor 3, and calcium to form the prothrombin complex.
    - The prothrombin complex cleaves a portion of the prothrombin molecule leading to the formation of enzymatically active thrombin.
    - Thrombin is an enzyme that cleaves fibrinogen into fibrin monomers and fibrinopeptides A and B.
    - Under the influence of factor XIII, fibrin monomers polymerize into insoluble fibrin strands.

42. **Which plasma coagulation factors are vitamin K dependent?**
    Factors II (prothrombin), VII, IX, and X—proteins synthesized in the liver—cannot participate in the coagulation cascade and cannot interact with calcium and platelet factor 3 unless carboxylated in the presence of vitamin K. Anticoagulant proteins C and S are also vitamin K dependent.

43. **What are the main natural anticoagulants?**
    - **Antithrombins:** These serine protease inhibitors block the action of thrombin and other serine proteases (activated factors IX, X, XI, and XII).
    - **Proteins C and S:** These proteins inhibit factors VIII and V, thus blocking the intrinsic and extrinsic pathway.
    - **Plasmin:** This is formed from plasminogen; it acts on fibrin, cleaving it into fibrin degradation products D, E, X, and Y.

44. **Is heparin an important anticoagulant?**
    Heparin is a potent anticoagulant drug widely used in the treatment of coagulation disorders. Heparin combines with antithrombin III to form a complex that inhibits the action of thrombin. Heparin is stored in the granules of mast cells and basophils and may be released during the degranulation of these cells. It is, however, not normally present in the circulating plasma. Endothelial cells express on their surface heparin-like molecules that bind antithrombin III and have the same anticoagulant activity as heparin.

THROMBOSIS

45. **What is thrombosis?**

Thrombosis is a pathologic process characterized by intravascular clotting in a living person. Clots formed in circulating blood inside the blood vessels or cardiac chambers are called thrombi. Postmortem clots or coagula formed in a test tube are not called thrombi.

46. **What is Virchow's triad?**

In 1845 Rudolf Virchow, the famous German pathologist, suggested that three factors promote thrombosis:
- Changes in the vessel wall
- Changes of blood flow
- Changes in the composition of blood

47. **Why does the vessel wall predispose to thrombosis?**

There are two main reasons:
- Damaged endothelial cells produce or release procoagulant substances (e.g., thromboplastin, von Willebrand factor, PAF, and inhibitor of plasminogen activator), whereas the production of anticoagulant substances (e.g., thrombomodulin, antithrombin III, NO, and plasminogen activator) is reduced.
- Loss of endothelial cells exposes the underlying basement membrane or collagen in the wall of the blood vessels, allowing the binding of platelets to these structures. Binding of platelets to these surfaces, mediated by von Willebrand factor, leads to formation of platelet aggregates and initiates the formation of thrombi.

48. **What are the common and important causes of endothelial cell injury or loss that initiate thrombosis?**
- Hemodynamic injury (e.g., as a result of high blood pressure)
- Atherosclerosis
- Infection (e.g., thrombophlebitis)
- Autoimmune diseases (e.g., polyarteritis nodosa)
- Metabolic disorders (e.g., hyperlipidemia and homocystinemia)
- Trauma or surgery

49. **Which changes in the blood flow predispose to thrombosis?**

There are two principal changes in the blood flow that predispose to thrombosis:
- Stasis, typically found in dilated veins
- Turbulent flow, typically encountered in abnormally dilated heart chambers that are not contracting regularly (e.g., atrial fibrillation) or arterial aneurysms

50. **How do hemodynamic changes promote thrombosis?**

Altered blood flow may cause endothelial cell injury or increase the coagulability of the blood. Several mechanisms may play a role, such as the following:
- Turbulent flow may mechanically damage the endothelial cells.
- Turbulent flow or stasis may activate endothelial cells and stimulate them to secrete procoagulants at the expense of anticoagulant substances.
- Stasis or turbulent flow may bring platelets and leukocytes in contact with the endothelial cells and facilitate their attachment.
- Stasis may reduce the inflow of fresh blood that contains natural anticoagulants.
- Stasis may retard the removal of small platelet aggregates that would have floated away in normal circulation, thus allowing the buildup of the thrombus.

51. **What are the common causes of hemodynamic changes that promote thrombosis?**
    - Venous thrombi are most often a complication of varicose veins.
    - Arterial thrombi develop in aortic aneurysms and overulcerated atherosclerotic plaques.
    - Cardiac thrombi develop in irregularly contracting hearts (e.g., atrial fibrillation), over the damaged endocardium (e.g., mural thrombi over a myocardial infarct), and in an infected cardiac valve (e.g., bacterial endocarditis).

52. **How does changed composition of blood contribute to thrombosis?**
    Increased concentration of coagulation proteins or reduced concentration of natural anticoagulants lead to hypercoagulability of the blood. These hypercoagulable states fall into two large groups:
    - **Hereditary hypercoagulable states:** These genetic diseases (also known as thrombophilias) include congenital deficiency of antithrombin III, protein C, or protein S and mutation of the gene-encoding factor V (called factor V Leiden). Approximately 5% to 10% of all people have some genetic defect predisposing them to thrombosis.
    - **Acquired hypercoagulable states:** Increased coagulability of the blood may be encountered in many conditions. For example, tissue damage results in an increased release of thromboplastin and other procoagulants. Tumor cells may enter the circulation and initiate thrombosis. Bacteria and other pathogens may have the same effect. In chronic infections, the liver may increase the production of fibrinogen (one of the so-called acute-phase reactants) and reduce production of anticoagulants. Disseminated intravascular coagulation (DIC) is commonly encountered in many forms of shock. An increased tendency for thrombosis is encountered in obese people and those who smoke, although the exact pathogenesis of these hypercoagulable states is not known.

53. **How do immune mechanisms cause thrombosis?**
    Thrombi form in many immune diseases and can also develop in response to exogenous antigens:
    - **Polyarteritis nodosa:** This type III hypersensitivity reaction is characterized by fibrinoid necrosis of the wall of small- and medium-sized arteries. Thrombi readily form over such inflammatory lesions because of local accumulation of thromboplastin from damaged tissue and other procoagulant substances released from the inflammatory cells.
    - **Systemic lupus erythematosus (SLE):** This type III hypersensitivity reaction leads to the deposition of immune complexes in many sites. Among others, it damages glomeruli, which often contain microthrombi. Libman–Sacks endocarditis, a common feature of SLE, presents with thrombi on the mitral valve. These thrombi accumulate at the site of endocardial injury caused by immune mechanisms.
    - **Antiphospholipid antibodies:** A common finding in a variety of clinical conditions (e.g., strokes and infarcts), these antibodies are detectable by their reactivity with cardiolipin, a phospholipid antigen used in the Wasserman reaction for syphilis. These antibodies bind to the phospholipids of platelets (PF3), promoting formation of thrombi.
    - **Heparin-induced thrombocytopenia:** This form of low platelet count is found in approximately 5% of patients treated for prolonged periods of time for increased coagulability of blood with heparin. The exogenous heparin apparently induces formation of antibodies that bind to heparin platelet factor 4 complex and destroy platelets. These antibodies also cross-react with heparin-like substances on endothelial cells, causing endothelial cell injury and thus promoting thrombosis.

54. **What are the most important clinical conditions complicated by thrombosis?**
    - **Deep vein thrombosis (DVT):** Also known as phlebothrombosis, it most often involves the deep leg veins. It is the most common form of clinically diagnosed thrombosis. DVT may be related to varicose dilatation of calf veins, but often its causes are not apparent.
    - **Prolonged immobility and rest:** Lying in bed or sitting a long time in an airplane predispose to thrombosis.

- **Tissue damage:** Conditions that cause massive tissue destruction, such as crush trauma, burns, or surgery, are commonly complicated by thrombosis. Prolonged bed rest after such incidents may cause stasis of the blood and increase the risk for thrombosis.
- **Pregnancy and obstetrical complications:** Generally speaking, pregnancy predisposes to thrombosis. Oral contraceptives and steroid hormones increase the risk for thrombosis as well.
- **Circulatory disturbances:** Major circulatory disturbances such as myocardial infarction and stroke, are important risk factors.
- **Tumors:** Thrombosis is related to the release of thromboplastin, which promotes coagulation.

A mnemonic to remember common causes of thrombosis is THROMBI:

Tissue damage (trauma, fractures, burns, and surgery)
Hereditary conditions (factor V Leyden, deficiency of antithrombin, and protein C or S)
Rest (prolonged bed rest after surgery or in old age)
Obstetrics (normal pregnancy, eclampsia, and abruptio placentae)
Malignancy
Blood flow disturbances (varicose veins, myocardial infarct, aneurysms, and apoplexy)
Immune mechanisms (SLE, anti-phospholipid antibody, and polyarteritis nodosa)

MORPHOLOGY OF THROMBI

55. **What are the macroscopic features of thrombi?**
Large thrombi formed in the veins, arteries, and heart of a living person have typical features that distinguish them from postmortem clots:
- **Lines of Zahn:** Thrombi form by the deposition of platelets and fibrin, which forms a white layer. RBCs deposit on this layer, forming a red layer on which a new layer of fibrin and platelets is deposited. These alternating white and red lines are called *lines of Zahn*.
- **Friability:** Thrombi are held together with fibrin that does not permeate all layers uniformly but leaves cleavage lines between the white and red layers. Most thrombi will crumble along cleavage lines when bent or compressed with the finger. The friability of thrombi accounts for the fact that they may detach and embolize.
- **Attachment:** Thrombi are attached to the surface of the vessel or heart chamber in which they were formed.
- **Molding:** Thrombi formed inside veins typically retain the shape of the vessel in which they were formed and appear like casts of these veins and their tributaries. Veins filled with thrombi appear expanded and may be palpated during physical examination. At autopsy, such veins appear completely filled and widened.

56. **What is the appearance of postmortem clots?**
Postmortem clots form from the blood that does not circulate. Owing to the forces of gravity, the RBCs sediment and separate from plasma. Accordingly, the postmortem clots consist of a lower red part (colloquially described as resembling "currant jelly") and a yellow part (known as "chicken fat"). Postmortem thrombi are pliable and do not appear friable like the premortem thrombi. Such clots do not fill or expand the blood vessels in which they are found. Postmortem thrombi can be easily removed from the blood vessels at autopsy.

57. **What is the appearance of clots formed in a test tube?**
Clots formed in test tubes are red and resemble the currant jelly part of the postmortem clots. The lower red part is covered with a very thin "buffy coat" composed of white blood cells and platelets.

58. **What are mural thrombi?**
Mural (literally, "formed on the wall") are thrombi attached to the endothelial surface of aorta, large veins, or the endocardium of the heart chambers. Similar thrombi found on cardiac valves are called valvular thrombi. Valvular thrombi are also called vegetations.

59. What are occlusive thrombi?
Occlusive thrombi are found in smaller arteries, veins, and capillaries. They fill and thus completely occlude the lumen of these vessels.

OUTCOMES OF THROMBOSIS

60. What are the possible outcomes of thrombosis?
- **Resolution:** Fibrinolysis mediated by plasmin accounts for the dissolution of most thrombi. Because the endothelial cells lining the veins produce more plasminogen activator, venous thrombi are lyzed more readily than cardiac and arterial thrombi.
- **Propagation:** Thrombi that do not resolve by fibrinolysis tend to "grow" because of the deposition of additional platelets, fibrin, and red blood cells. Such growth is typically accompanied by the formation of a downstream "tail."
- **Embolization:** Thrombi may detach from the vessel wall and give rise to emboli carried downstream by the blood. Large thrombi may form fragments, which also may embolize.
- **Organization:** Ingrowth of granulation tissue from the vessel wall forms a firm link between the thrombus and the vessel wall. As in a healing wound, granulation tissue will slowly transform into a fibrous scar. A small "bump" inside the vessel may be the only residue of such an organized thrombus.
- **Recanalization:** The blood vessels in the granulation tissue organizing the thrombus may fuse into larger channels that bridge the thrombus, allowing the resumption of blood flow. *See* Fig. 3.1.

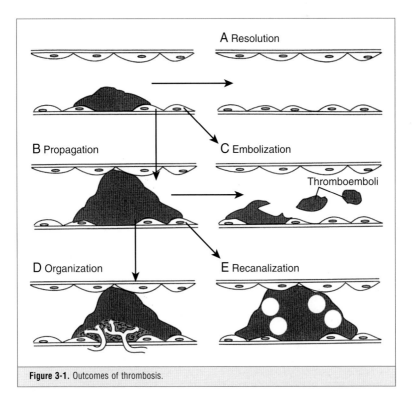

Figure 3-1. Outcomes of thrombosis.

KEY POINTS: EMBOLISM AND INFARCT ✓

1. Thrombi are clinically the most important source of emboli, but there are many other potential sources of embolism.

2. Infarcts develop as a result of obstruction of arterial and venous blood flow or hypoperfusion of tissues.

3. Infarcts of various organs have unique pathologic and clinical features.

61. **What are the possible complications of thrombosis?**
    - **Infarction:** Occlusive thrombi may completely interrupt the blood flow through an artery, causing ischemic necrosis of the tissue supplied by that vessel. This is a typical complication of arterial thrombosis (e.g., coronary artery thrombosis).
    - **Edema and obstruction of venous outflow:** This is typically seen in venous thrombosis.
    - **Emboli:** Thromboemboli are a common complication of thrombosis, regardless of whether the thrombi are venous, arterial, or cardiac.
    - **Infection:** Thrombi are a fertile soil for bacteria and are easily infected.
    - **Inflammation of the vessel wall:** Organization of infected venous thrombi elicits an inflammation in the vessel wall. This thrombophlebitis is associated with redness, swelling, and pain of tissues around a cordlike thrombosed vein.

62. **What is migratory thrombophlebitis?**
    Migratory thrombophlebitis is a feature of Trousseau syndrome associated with pancreatic and gastric carcinoma. It presents with the appearance of thrombi in superficial veins. These thrombi disappear spontaneously and reappear at some other site. Thrombi form because of the entry of thromboplastin released from the cancer cells into the circulation.

EMBOLISM

63. **What are emboli?**
    Emboli are particulate, fluid, or gaseous material carried by the bloodstream from the site of their origin or entry into the circulation to other parts of the body. Emboli are classified according to the material from which they are formed:
    - Thromboemboli
    - Air (gas) emboli
    - Fat emboli
    - Bone marrow emboli
    - Tumor emboli
    - Cholesterol emboli
    - Foreign body emboli
    - Amniotic fluid emboli

64. **What are the most common and clinically most important emboli?**
    Thromboemboli represent the most common and most important emboli. Thromboemboli are classified according to how they are carried by blood:
    - **Venous:** These originate in the veins and are carried by venous blood into the lungs.
    - **Arterial:** These emboli originate in the heart or aorta and large arteries and are carried by arterial blood into various organs, such as the brain, kidney, and spleen.

- **Paradoxical:** These emboli originate as venous emboli, but instead of reaching the lungs, they cross through a foramen ovale or some right-to-left shunt in the heart and thus reach the arterial circulation.

65. **What are pulmonary emboli?**
Pulmonary embolism (PE) is most often caused by venous thromboemboli originating in the veins of the lower extremities. Depending on the size of the thromboemboli and the extent of embolization, PE may present in several forms:
- Occlusion of the main pulmonary artery or its main branches may cause sudden death. Such a saddle embolus typically prevents influx of blood into the lungs.
- Occlusion of the branches of the pulmonary artery will cause infarcts. The lungs have dual circulation, and in normal circumstances the occlusion of pulmonary artery branches may be compensated by an influx of blood from the bronchial arteries. However, if PE is associated with heart failure and atherosclerosis of the aorta (a condition that prevents the compensatory blood supply through the bronchial arteries), ischemic necrosis of lung parenchyma will develop. When the blood from the bronchial arteries finally reaches the ischemic area, it will perfuse blood vessels that are necrotic and will leak into the alveolar spaces. Accordingly, pulmonary infarcts appear as red, airless, triangular areas.
- Nonocclusive emboli in branches of the pulmonary artery do not produce ischemia and may be clinically unrecognized. Over time, these thrombi become organized. This process narrows the lumen of pulmonary artery branches and over time may lead to pulmonary hypertension.

66. **Where do arterial emboli lodge most often?**
Arterial emboli may occlude any artery. Which artery will be occluded depends on the size of the thrombus. Large thrombi occlude large arteries, such as those of the legs and arms and those of celiac, mesenteric, renal, splenic, or cerebral arteries. Smaller emboli reach the branches of these arteries in various organs.

67. **What are septic thromboemboli?**
Septic emboli result from infected thrombi, such as valvular vegetations in bacterial endocarditis. Infarct caused by such emboli becomes infected by bacteria and transforms into an abscess.

68. **What is air embolism?**
Air embolism is caused by entry of atmospheric air into the circulation or by the appearance of intravascular nitrogen bubbles as a result of decompression. Air bubbles may occlude blood vessels or cause DIC. DIC is triggered by platelets that tend to adhere to nitrogen bubbles and become activated to initiate the coagulation cascade.

69. **Can air embolism kill?**
Small amounts of air are innocuous, but if more than 150 mL is injected, death can occur. The injected air fills the right ventricle, not allowing the influx of venous blood. Blood entering the right ventricle is transformed into a foamy air–fluid mixture that also obstructs the blood flow, rapidly causing death.

70. **How does air enter into the circulation?**
Air typically enters the venous blood during various procedures:
- Trauma or surgery on the neck accompanied by a tear in the wall of the jugular vein or the superior vena cava may lead to negative pressure in the thorax, which plays an important role in sucking the air into the venous blood.
- Childbirth or abortion may allow the entry of air into uterine veins.
- The cubital vein may serve as the entry point during blood transfusions given under positive pressure.

71. **What is decompression sickness?**

    Decompression sickness *(caisson disease)* is a form of gas embolism resulting from the appearance of nitrogen bubbles in the blood. Nitrogen is physically dissolved in the blood and is kept in the solution by normal atmospheric pressure. Decompression, as typically seen in divers who come to the surface from deep waters too fast or in pressurized caisson chambers, will allow nitrogen to come out of the solution in the form of gaseous bubbles. These gas bubbles occlude small blood vessels or initiate DIC. Occlusion of the small blood vessels in the joints, bones, and soft tissues causes painful muscle contractures ("the bends"). Occlusion of pulmonary vessels causes shortness of breath ("the chokes"). Severe ischemic necrosis may cause widespread infarcts and even death.

72. **What is fat embolism?**

    Fat embolism results from the entry of fat globules into the circulation. In most instances, the cause of fat embolism is fracture of long bones. Fat cells in the bone marrow rupture as a result of trauma, releasing their contents into the venous blood. Trauma of subcutaneous or breast fat cells usually does not cause fat embolism.

73. **How does fat embolism present clinically?**

    Symptoms of fat embolism appear 1 to 3 days after fracture of long bones of the extremities. These symptoms are related to ischemia caused by the occlusion of capillaries by fat globules. During the first 2 days, the patient typically has shortness of breath, which is caused by the occlusion of pulmonary capillaries. Small globules that are filtered through the lungs cause microscopic foci of necrosis accompanied by minute pericapillary hemorrhages that occur in both hemispheres. These microscopic infarcts present as mental, sensory, or motor disturbances. Fat globules also induce DIC, which may aggravate the already precarious condition of most patients. Approximately 10% of patients with fat embolism die.

74. **What are the autopsy findings in lethal fat embolism?**

    Fat globules filling the capillaries can be demonstrated in frozen sections of the lung, brain, and other organs. In the brain, the capillaries occluded with fat globules are surrounded by a ring of hemorrhage infiltrating the microscopic perivascular infarcts.

75. **What is bone marrow embolism?**

    Entry of bone marrow particles into the circulation may occur upon fracture of bones that contain hematopoietic bone marrow. Typically, it occurs during cardiopulmonary resuscitation of people who have had a cardiac arrest. Compression of the chest during this procedure may fracture the ribs, which allows the entry of bone marrow in the circulation. Bone marrow particles are carried by venous blood to the lungs, where they occlude small branches of the pulmonary artery. These emboli are of no clinical significance and are a sign of a vigorous resuscitation.

76. **What is tumor embolism?**

    Tumor cells may enter the circulation by migrating through capillary walls but also through the walls of larger vessels during surgery. Circulating tumor cells may be found in many tumor patients, but in only a minority of these patients will cells ultimately form emboli. Tumor cell emboli usually do not cause infarcts. Arrested tumor cells grow out of the vessel and form secondary tumor nodules. Tumor emboli are essential for the hematogenous dissemination of tumors and the formation of distant metastases.

77. **What are cholesterol emboli?**

    Cholesterol emboli result from the entry of cholesterol crystals from atherosclerotic lesions into the arterial bloodstream. Typically this occurs during catheterization of the aorta or a surgical procedure, but it may also be caused by spontaneous rupture of an atheroma. These crystals occlude capillaries causing microscopic infarcts. Cholesterol crystals occluding retinal arteries can cause loss of vision. Brain infarcts are usually microscopic and associated with so-called transient ischemic attacks characterized by mental, sensory, or motor deficiencies. Massive occlusion of renal arterioles and glomerular capillaries may result in acute renal failure.

78. **What is foreign body embolism?**
Foreign bodies entering the circulation may be carried to distant parts of the body by the circulation. Examples of such emboli are cotton, wool, or cloth fibers entering the blood flow during surgery, crystals of talc or starch injected by intravenous drug abusers, and bullets.

79. **What is amniotic fluid embolism?**
Amniotic fluid may enter into the uterine veins during childbirth. Fortunately, it is very rare (1:80,000 deliveries), but if it occurs, it is lethal in 80% of cases.
   Amniotic fluid contains lanugo hairs, vernix, and even meconium, which may occlude the pulmonary artery branches and cause sudden death. At autopsy of deceased women, all these particulate substances may be found in pulmonary capillaries. Amniotic fluid contains tissue debris that is highly thrombogenic. These substances may induce DIC, and in these cases, women die in shock. At autopsy, all major organs contain microscopic thrombi in small blood vessels.

80. **What is DIC?**
DIC is a form of microangiopathic thrombosis characterized by consumptive coagulopathy. Translated into colloquial English, this means that DIC represents a clotting disorder characterized by formation of thrombi in small blood vessels (arterioles, capillaries, and venules). Formation of these microthrombi consumes the platelets (resulting in thrombocytopenia) and leads to a depletion of fibrin (hypofibrinogenemia) and other coagulation proteins. Loss of coagulation proteins leads to bleeding, which cannot be stopped. This vicious cycle of thrombosis and bleeding, typical of DIC, cannot be interrupted easily.

81. **What are common causes of DIC?**
DIC can be triggered by many mechanisms, including:
- **Infections:** This is most often caused by gram-negative sepsis, but it may be caused by fungal infections, meningococcemia, and many other infections.
- **Neoplasms:** Most often the underlying causes are carcinomas of the gastrointestinal tract and promyelocytic leukemia.
- **Massive tissue injury:** The best-known examples are traffic trauma, burns, and extensive surgery.
- **Shock:** Any form of shock can result in DIC.
- **Obstetric complications:** DIC is typically a complication of amniotic fluid embolism, eclampsia, and abruptio placentae, it but may occur in many other pregnancy-related conditions.

82. **What is the pathogenesis of DIC?**
Intravascular coagulation can be initiated by three often interrelated pathways:
- Activation of Hageman factor initiating the intrinsic coagulation cascade
- Thromboplastins activating the extrinsic coagulation pathway
- Endothelial cell injury
   For example, massive tissue injury will release or activate enzymes that act on the Hageman factor and may injure or activate the endothelial cells. At the same time, tissue injury will release thromboplastins, which activate the extrinsic coagulation pathway. Lipopolysaccharides of gram-negative bacteria can also activate Hageman factor, act as thromboplastins, and injure endothelial cells.

83. **What are the pathologic findings in DIC?**
The most prominent findings are numerous fibrin thrombi in small vessels. These microthrombi are easily found in the heart, brain, glomeruli of the kidneys, and other sites. Microthrombi cause microscopic infarcts. Most patients die before such foci of ischemic necrosis become histologically apparent.

84. **What is Waterhouse–Friderichsen syndrome?**
This syndrome represents a DIC caused by *Neisseria meningitidis*. Typically it presents with purpura of the skin and hemorrhagic infarction of the adrenals.

85. **What are the laboratory findings in DIC?**
- All bleeding tests (prothrombin [PT] and activated partial thromboplastin time [aPTT]) are prolonged.
- Thrombocytopenia occurs.
- Fibrin degradation products appear in urine.

INFARCT

86. **What is the difference between an infarct and infarction?**
An infarct is an area of ischemic necrosis. Infarction is the process that leads to this ischemic necrosis.

87. **What are the causes of infarction?**
Infarction results from sudden reduction of blood supply to an area. Infarcts can be classified pathogenetically:
- **Arterial:** This is caused by obstruction of an artery.
- **Venous:** This is caused by obstruction of venous blood outflow.
- **Hypotensive:** This is caused by hypoperfusion of tissues by arterial blood that typically occurs in shock and is related to hypotension.

88. **What is the difference between red and white infarcts?**
According to their gross appearance at autopsy, infarcts can be classified as pale or red.
　　Pale infarcts (meaning paler than the normal tissue) reflect ischemia that has evolved owing to the obstruction of a nutrient artery or hypoperfusion of tissue in hypotension. Such infarcts develop in solid organs supplied by anatomically or functionally terminal arteries, as typically found in the heart, kidneys, and spleen. Terminal arteries in these organs do not have functioning anastomoses, and the occlusion of an arterial branch will deprive the tissue of blood and cause a pale infarct.
　　Red infarcts are suffused with blood and appear dark or bluish red. They occur in the following:
- Venous infarcts result from obstruction of vein. The blood cannot exit from the infarcted area, and therefore the area appears congested.
- Organs with double blood supply, such as the lungs, receive venous blood through the pulmonary artery and arterial blood through the bronchial arteries originating from the thoracic aorta. Obstruction of the branches of the pulmonary artery will cause an infarct, and the ischemic area will subsequently be flooded by blood from nutrient (bronchial) arteries. Similar events account for the red color of infarcts in the liver, which receives blood from the portal vein and the hepatic artery.
- Organs with well-developed anastomoses, such as the brain, receive blood from the branches of carotid and basilar arteries. Likewise small intestines receive the arterial blood from the arcuate internastomozing branches of the mesenteric arteries.

89. **What is a septic infarct?**
Septic infarcts result from arterial obstruction with infected (septic) thromboemboli. Bacteria enter the ischemic area from the infected thrombus and transform the infarct into an abscess.

90. **Is gangrene related to infarction?**
Gangrene is a term used to denote two forms of infarcts:
- **Dry gangrene:** This is characterized by mummification of the infarcted tissues and typically occurs on lower extremities. The leg, foot, or toes appear black and dry, like Egyptian mummies.
- **Wet gangrene:** This represents moist infected infarcts developing in parts of the body that normally contain saprophytic bacteria. Typically this occurs on the infarcted feet or toes of diabetics. Arterial or venous infarcts of the large intestines, which normally contain saprophytic bacteria, also appear gangrenous.

91. **What is the fate of patients with infarcts?**
The outcome of infarcts depends on the tissue and organ affected:
- **Fibrosis:** In the heart infarct, cardiac myocytes are replaced by fibrous tissue (scar).
- **Resorption:** In the cerebral infarct, the necrotic tissue becomes liquefied and is resorbed. The resulting empty space (pseudocyst) is filled with fluid.
- **Regeneration:** Infarcted liver cells are replaced by regenerating hepatocytes.

SHOCK

92. **What is shock?**
Shock is a condition caused by hypoperfusion of tissue with blood. It may be classified as:
- **Cardiogenic:** This typically occurs in heart failure and could be caused by "pump failure" as in infarction or an occlusion of ostia caused by valvular disease in endocarditis.
- **Hypovolemic:** This type of shock typically follows massive bleeding or any other form of fluid loss.
- **Distributive:** Also known as hypotensive shock, this results from peripheral vasodilatation as in massive sepsis or anaphylactic shock.
  Common to all these conditions is a circulatory collapse resulting from a disproportion between the volume of the circulating blood and the vascular space that it is supposed to fill. Ensuing tissue hypoxia or anoxia leads to multiple organ failure.

93. **What are the causes of cardiogenic shock?**
- Pump failure (ejection fraction <20%) caused by myocardial infarction or conduction disturbances (e.g., heart block and fibrillation) account for most cases.
- Obstructive heart failure caused by massive pulmonary emboli or valvular disease.

KEY POINTS: SHOCK ✔

1. Shock is an important clinical condition caused by circulatory collapse that occurs under many conditions, always resulting from a hypoperfusion of tissues.

2. Shock causes recognizable pathologic and clinical findings, which vary depending on the severity of shock.

94. **What are the causes of hypovolemic shock?**
- Loss of blood owing to an arterial wound, rupture of aneurysm, and so on.
- Loss of fluids as a result of burns, vomiting, diarrhea, and so on.

95. What causes peripheral hypotension?
Loss of peripheral vascular tonus and pooling of blood in peripheral circulation may result from:
- Vasodilatation caused by bacterial toxins
- Anaphylactic shock, mediated by histamine, and so on
- Neurogenic stimuli (e.g., severe pain and spinal cord or brain injury)

96. What are the typical pathologic findings in shock?
Pathologic findings are similar to those seen in DIC.
- Widespread microthrombi
- Multiple foci of ischemic necrosis
- Hemorrhage

97. Which organs are most often affected in shock?
- Lungs typically show signs of diffuse alveolar damage also known as acute respiratory distress syndrome (ARDS).
- Gastrointestinal tract shows widespread mucosal ischemia resulting in multiple hemorrhagic erosions or ulcerations.
- Kidneys show tubular necrosis.
- Liver shows acute centrilobular congestion and necrosis.
- Brain ischemia results in microscopic focal hemorrhages and edema.
- Adrenals show congestion of the inner cortex, hemorrhage, and focal cortical necrosis.

98. How is shock classified clinically?
Three stages of progressively worsening shock are recognized:
- Early or compensated shock
- Decompensated but still reversible shock
- Irreversible shock

99. What are the features of compensated shock?
The body is trying to compensate for loss of fluid or expansion of the peripheral vascular space by increasing the heart rate, constricting the arterioles, and reducing the loss of fluids in the urine. Typical clinical findings are:
- Tachycardia (a heart rate >100 beats/min)
- Skin pallor as a result of constriction of arterioles
- Reduced urine production

100. What are the features of decompensated but still reversible shock?
This stage evolves after the compensatory mechanisms of early shock have failed. It is characterized by:
- **Hypotension:** Both the systolic and diastolic pressure and the cardiac output drop.
- **Tachypnea and dyspnea (shortness of breath):** The lungs are trying to compensate for hypoxia. Pulmonary edema slowly develops, further impairing oxygenation.
- **Oliguria (urine volume <500 mL/day):** This develops because of massive constriction of renal arterioles and reduced glomerular filtration rate.
- **Acidosis:** Low pH of the blood is the consequence of decreased renal and pulmonary functions and anaerobic glycolysis in tissue favored by anoxia. Acidosis is partially metabolic and partially respiratory and is marked by an increased accumulation of lactic acid (product of anaerobic glycolysis).

101. What are the features of irreversible shock?
Complete circulatory collapse and marked hypoperfusion of vital organs lead to DIC, a loss of vital functions, and multiple organ failure. Clinical signs are:
- Marked hypotension and extreme tachycardia (filiform pulse)

- Respiratory distress not responding to oxygen therapy and assisted ventilation with a respirator
- Loss of consciousness progressing to coma
- Gastrointestinal bleeding
- Anuria, with elevated blood urea nitrogen (BUN) and creatinine in blood
- Severe acidosis
- Laboratory signs of DIC (prolonged PT, aPPT, thrombocytopenia, and microangiopathic hemolytic anemia)

WEBSITES

1. http://www.ncbi.nlm.nih.gov/entrez/query.fcgi?db=PubMed

2. http://www-medlib.med.utah.edu/WebPath/webpath.html#MENU

3. http://www.pathguy.com

BIBLIOGRAPHY

1. Bick RL: Disseminated intravascular coagulation: current concepts of etiology, pathophysiology, diagnosis, and treatment. Hematol Oncol Clin North Am 17:149–176, 2003.
2. Blickstein D, Blickstein I: Oral contraception and thrombophilia. Curr Opin Obstet Gynecol 19:370–376, 2007.
3. Brohi K, Cohen MJ, Davenport RA: Acute coagulopathy of trauma: mechanism, identification and effect. Curr Opin Crit Care 13:680–685, 2007.
4. Butenas S, Orfeo T, Brummel-Ziedins KE, Mann KG: Tissue factor in thrombosis and hemorrhage. Surgery 142 (4 suppl):S2–S14, 2007.
5. Furie B, Furie BC: In vivo thrombus formation. J Thromb Haemost 5(suppl 1):12–17, 2007.
6. Lensing AWA, Prandoni P, Prins MH, Buller HR: Deep-vein thrombosis. Lancet 353:479–485, 1999.
7. Levi M, Ten Cate H: Disseminated intravascular coagulation. N Engl J Med 341:586–593, 1999.
8. Slofstra SH, Spek CA, Ten Cate H: Disseminated intravascular coagulation. Hematol J 4:295–302, 2003.
9. Toh CH, Dennis M: Disseminated intravascular coagulation: old disease, new hope. Br Med J 327:974–977, 2003.

CHAPTER 4

IMMUNOPATHOLOGY

Zoran Gatalica, MD, DSc

1. **What are the main cells of the immune system?**
   - Lymphocytes
   - T lymphocytes
   - B lymphocytes
   - Natural killer cells
   - Macrophages
   - Dendritic cells

   Neutrophils, eosinophils, basophils, and platelets found in the blood are an important part of the body defense system but are not directly involved in recognition of foreign (nonself) stimuli and antigens, which is the primary function and characteristic of the cells of the immune system.

2. **List key facts about T lymphocytes.**
   - T lymphocytes are typically found in the following locations:
     - Paracortical areas of lymph nodes
     - Periarteriolar sheaths of the spleen
     - Thymus
     - Bone marrow and peripheral blood
   - T lymphocytes account for 60% to 70% of circulating lymphocytes in the blood.
   - The specific surface antigen is antigen-specific T-cell receptor (TCR), which can be composed of $\alpha\beta$ (95% of T cells) or $\gamma\sigma$ heterodimers. Each T cell has a unique TCR, reflecting a unique rearrangement of the genes (marker of clonality).
   - The common surface marker present on all T lymphocytes is nonvariable CD3 protein (pan T-cell marker).
   - There is functional diversity of T-cell populations; CD4+ helper/inducer cells constitute approximately 60% of mature T lymphocytes, and CD8+ suppressor/cytotoxic cells constitute approximately 30% of mature T lymphocytes. Furthermore, CD4+ cells differ in their ability to secrete cytokines: The TH1 subset secretes IL-2 and IFN-γ, whereas TH2 secretes IL-4 and IL-5.

3. **List key features of B lymphocytes.**
   - B lymphocytes are typically found in the following locations:
     - Superficial cortex of lymph nodes
     - Germinal centers and mantle zone of stimulated lymph nodes
     - Follicles of the white pulp of the spleen
     - Mucosa-associated lymphoid system (MALT) in intestines and the respiratory tract
     - Bone marrow and peripheral blood
   - B lymphocytes constitute 10% to 20% of circulating lymphocytes in the blood.
   - Antigen-specific surface immunoglobulin M (IgM) is the consequence of the unique gene rearrangements and a marker of B-cell clonality.

- Two more nonvariable transmembrane proteins (Igα and Igβ) form a heterodimer that is a part of the B-cell receptor complex.
- On antigenic stimulation, B cells form plasma cells that secrete antigen-specific immunoglobulins.

4. **List key features of natural killer (NK) cells.**
   - NK cells constitute approximately 10% to 15% of circulating lymphocytes.
   - They are CD3 negative and do not rearrange the CD3 gene but do express some surface T-cell markers. They express receptors for Fc of IgG (also known as CD16), which enables them to lyse IgG-coated target cells.
   - They can kill a variety of virus-infected cells and some tumor cells without prior sensitization (i.e., "natural" killer). NK cells express inhibiting receptors for class I major histocompatability complex (MHC) molecules present on all nucleated cells. If a virus or a neoplastic transformation altered the expression of MHC class I molecules, the inhibition is interrupted and the NK cell attacks the altered cell (causing cell lysis).

5. **What is the main function of macrophages in the immune response?**
   Macrophages belong to the class of antigen presenting cells (APCs), crucial for the activation of T lymphocytes. Macrophages take up the antigen, process it, and present it to T cells.

6. **What are dendritic cells?**
   Dendritic cells are APCs found in the germinal follicles (follicular dendritic cells), interstitium of many organs (interdigitating dendritic cells), and the skin (Langerhans cells).

7. **List key features of cytokines.**
   - Cytokines are soluble signaling molecules secreted by a variety of cells, both of the immune and the nonimmune system.
   - They can act on the same cell that secreted them (autocrine effect), on the cells in close proximity (paracrine effect), or on remote cells after being transported through the bloodstream (endocrine effect).
   - The best-known cytokines are interferons, interleukins (ILs), tumor necrosis factor, chemokines (chemoattractors), and colony-stimulating factors (hematopoietic growth factors).

8. **What are the characteristics of histocompatibility antigens?**
   They bind processed foreign proteins (e.g., viral particles during cell infection and phagocytized material) and are involved in presenting them on the cell surface to T cells.
   Class I antigens are expressed on all nucleated cells and are encoded by three closely linked gene loci (HLA-A, HLA-B, and HLA-C). Foreign protein (e.g., viral particles synthesized within the cell) is associated with MHC class I protein and transported to the cell surface, where it is recognized by CD8+ cytotoxic T cells bearing TCR specific for the antigen peptide.
   Class II antigen (HLA-DP, HLA-DQ, and HLA-DR) expression is restricted to APCs (macrophages and dendritic cells); they bind phagocytized antigens and present them on their surface, where they are recognized by CD4+ helper T lymphocytes.
   An association of certain diseases and specific HLA types (higher relative risk of developing certain disease) has been noticed. This may be because of the close proximity of HLA genes and the disease-causing gene on chromosome 6 or because of the type of HLA (so-called haplotype).

9. **How are the antigens classified?**
   - Exogenous (e.g., dust, pollens, chemicals)
   - Endogenous, formed within the body of the same individual (autologous) or genetically different individual of the same species (homologous)

10. **What is the pathogenesis of hypersensitivity reactions?**
    In certain individuals, repeated exposure to a specific antigen leads to adverse reactions (hypersensitivity) rather than an induction of a protective immune response (immunity). Several pathogenetic mechanisms underlie tissue destruction in hypersensitivity:
    - Release of vasoactive and spasmogenic mediators of inflammation (type I)
    - Binding of antibodies to the antigens on the cell surface, predisposing them to lysis of phagocytosis (type II)
    - Formation of antigen–antibody complexes capable of activation of the complement system (type III)
    - Sensitization of T lymphocytes after reaction with antigen leading to granulomatous inflammation initiated by CD4+ lymphocyte sensitization or leading to CD8+ killing of antigen-bearing cells (both examples of type IV hypersensitivity reaction)

11. **What are the characteristics of type I hypersensitivity (anaphylactic) reactions?**
    - Develop rapidly (within minutes) following exposure to the antigen in a previously sensitized individual
    - Based on a mast cell participation
    - Mediated by IgE in most instances

12. **Are the type I hypersensitivity reactions localized or systemic?**
    Type I hypersensitivity reaction may cause a localized or a systemic reaction.
    - **Localized reaction:** If the allergen is confined to the site of contact, localized edema and inflammation typically develop (e.g., hives and rhinitis). This reaction causes only minor discomfort, but it may also be life threatening if it involves the larynx or the bronchial tree (e.g., bronchial asthma).
    - **Systemic reaction:** A life-threatening anaphylactic shock may develop, especially if the antigen was introduced intravenously (e.g., antibiotic).

13. **What is the pathogenesis of localized type I hypersensitivity reactions?**
    These reactions involve the interaction of three cell types:
    - **B cells:** Virgin B cells stimulated by antigen (allergen) transform into IgE-secreting plasma cells.
    - **TH2 lymphocytes:** Helper T lymphocytes produce IL-4, which is necessary for stimulation of IgE-secreting B cells.
    - **Mast cells:** These cells bind IgE to their surface and act as effector cells.
      First exposure leads to a sensitization and priming of the T and B cells, which interact and produce IgE that binds to the surface of mast cells in tissues. Upon second exposure to the same antigen, cross-linking of IgE on the mast cells occurs. Cell surface changes stimulate two sets of reactions (Fig. 4-1).
    - **Immediate reaction:** This involves a rapid release of mediators stored in mast cell granules.
    - **Delayed reaction:** This reaction is mediated by substances that need to be synthesized, and their release occurs several hours after the initiation of the immune reaction.

14. **What occurs during the immediate degranulation of mast cells?**
    Antigen-triggered degranulation of mast cells leads to a release of preformed (primary) mediators of inflammation:
    - **Biogenic amines:** Histamine, the primary mediator of this group, will increase vascular permeability ($\rightarrow$ edema) and stimulate smooth muscle contraction (bronchospasm) and secretion of mucus or gastric juices.
    - **Enzymes:** Hydrolytic enzymes (e.g., chymase and tryptase) contribute to inflammation by activating kinins and the complement system. Fragments of complement proteins have a chemotactic action and recruit other cells to the site of inflammation.
    - **Proteoglycans:** The most important is heparin, which has an anticoagulant action.

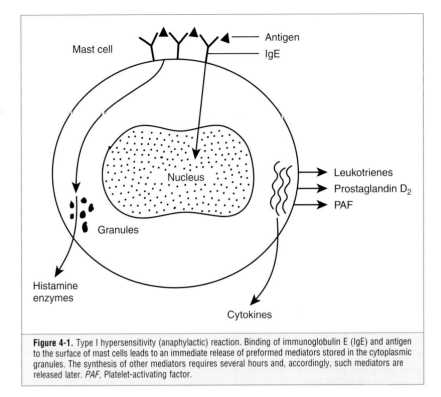

Figure 4-1. Type I hypersensitivity (anaphylactic) reaction. Binding of immunoglobulin E (IgE) and antigen to the surface of mast cells leads to an immediate release of preformed mediators stored in the cytoplasmic granules. The synthesis of other mediators requires several hours and, accordingly, such mediators are released later. *PAF*, Platelet-activating factor.

15. **Which mediators are released from mast cells in a delayed manner?**
    These mediators, known as secondary mediators and released 6 to 12 hours later, include:
    - **Lipid-derived mediators:** Antigen binding to mast cells triggers an activation of phospholipase A2 that generates arachidonic acid from intracellular lipids. Arachidonic acid is further metabolized into leukotrienes and prostaglandins. Platelet-activating factor (PAF) is also formed.
    - **Cytokines:** This response is characterized by the recruitment of inflammatory cells (neutrophils and eosinophils) that sustain the inflammation, causing further damage in the affected tissue.

16. **What are the symptoms associated with type I hypersensitivity reactions?**
    The symptoms depend on the route of exposure, dose of antigen, and the target organ sensitivity (Fig. 4-2).
    - **Systemic allergen presentation:** Typically this reaction occurs upon injection of drugs, hormones, or antisera into a previously sensitized person. Clinically, an anaphylactic shock develops, which is characterized by hypotension due to widespread vascular dilatation, widespread edema, difficulty breathing due to laryngospasm, laryngeal and pulmonary edema, and cardiac dysrhythmia.
    - **Localized reactions:** Antigen entering the body through the skin, by inhalation, or through ingestion evokes a reaction usually limited to one organ system.
        - **Upper respiratory tract reactions:** Seasonal upper respiratory allergies caused by pollens (>10 μm) evoke hay fever. Similar but prolonged allergic rhinitis may result from sensitization to dust mites. In both instances, there is nasal congestion, watery discharge, itching, sneezing, and cough.
        - **Gastrointestinal reactions:** Ingestion of allergens may lead to diarrhea, malabsorption syndrome, and protein-losing enteropathy. Massive hypoproteinemia may even cause shock.

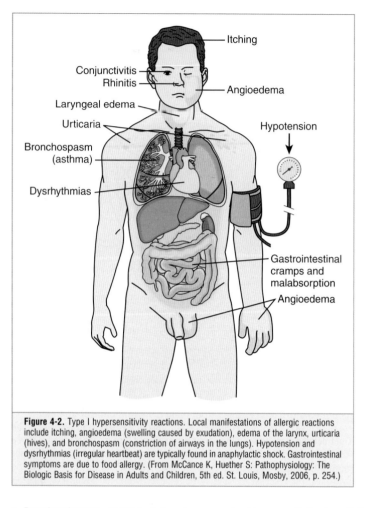

Figure 4-2. Type I hypersensitivity reactions. Local manifestations of allergic reactions include itching, angioedema (swelling caused by exudation), edema of the larynx, urticaria (hives), and bronchospasm (constriction of airways in the lungs). Hypotension and dysrhythmias (irregular heartbeat) are typically found in anaphylactic shock. Gastrointestinal symptoms are due to food allergy. (From McCance K, Huether S: Pathophysiology: The Biologic Basis for Disease in Adults and Children, 5th ed. St. Louis, Mosby, 2006, p. 254.)

○ **Bronchopulmonary reactions:** Asthma is an example of hypersensitivity of small airways to inhaled allergens. It presents with bronchospasm causing wheezing, hypersecretion of mucus, and coughing. Death due to asphyxia may result from extreme bronchoconstriction and plugging of bronchi with mucus (status asthmaticus).
○ **Skin reactions:** Atopic dermatitis, a common disease of childhood, is caused by prolonged exposure to and sensitization by foreign antigens.

17. **What are the characteristics of type II hypersensitivity (cytolytic) reactions?**
Antigen is present on the surface of the target cell. It may be intrinsic antigen (e.g., Rh D blood antigen) or antigen adsorbed on the cell surface from the environment (e.g., drugs acting as haptens). The antibody interaction with the antigen elicits three reactions (Fig. 4-3):
■ **Complement-activated cell lysis:** Binding of antibody (primarily IgM) to the antigen on the cell surface leads to an activation of complement-activated cell lysis and the formation of the cytolytic membrane attack complex (MAC), which destroys cells (e.g., acute hemolytic transfusion reaction).

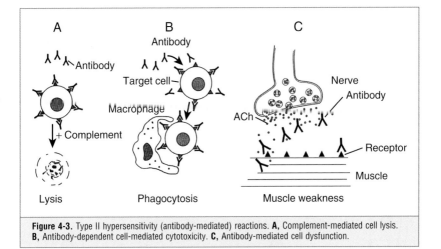

Figure 4-3. Type II hypersensitivity (antibody-mediated) reactions. **A,** Complement-mediated cell lysis. **B,** Antibody-dependent cell-mediated cytotoxicity. **C,** Antibody-mediated cell dysfunction.

- ○ **Antibody-dependent cell-mediated cytotoxicity (ADCC):** Binding of low-density (primarily IgG) antibodies that act as opsonins is followed by phagocytosis of damaged cells. ADCC typically mediates autoimmune hemolytic anemia and thrombocytopenia.
- ○ **Antibody-mediated cell dysfunction:** Binding of stimulatory antibodies to receptors for thyroid-stimulating hormone (TSH) on thyroid cells may stimulate hypersecretion of thyroid hormones in Graves disease. Binding of antiacetylcholine receptor antibodies at the neuromuscular junction may block nerve transmission and the cause of muscle weakness in myasthenia gravis.

18. **List important diseases caused by type II hypersensitivity cytotoxic reactions.**
    - ■ **Transfusion reaction:** This is caused by a mismatched blood transfusion. An infusion of blood of an A blood group donor into a B blood group recipient will result in a massive hemolytic reaction mediated by the natural anti-A blood group antigen in the recipient.
    - ■ **Hemolytic disease of the newborn (erythroblastosis fetalis):** This reaction occurs transplacentally and is mediated by maternal IgG antibodies to the fetal Rh+ positive red blood cells (RBCs). It occurs only in Rh− mothers who have been immunized to Rh blood group antigen during the first pregnancy by an Rh+ fetus.
    - ■ **Autoimmune hemolytic anemia:** This disease results from the production of anti-RBC antibodies that bind to RBC and cause hemolysis. The causes of such an immune reaction are not known.
    - ■ **Pemphigus vulgaris:** This blistering skin disease is caused by antibodies to the proteins forming the intercellular junctions (desmosomes) of the epidermis.
    - ■ **Goodpasture syndrome:** This pulmonary–renal disease is caused by antibodies that react with type IV collagen in the glomerular and pulmonary vascular basement membranes. One could call these antibodies cytotoxic, but the term *membranotoxic* seems more appropriate.

19. **What are the characteristics of immune complex–mediated hypersensitivity (type III) reactions?**
    - ■ Binding of antibody to the antigen forms complexes that are not cleared by the reticuloendothelial system but instead are deposited in tissues where they elicit an inflammatory reaction through activation of complement (Fig. 4-4).
    - ■ Complexes may be formed locally in the tissue or in the circulation and then deposited in various tissues. Either way, aggregated Fc regions of IgG antibodies activate the complement pathway, leading to increased vascular permeability, activation of neutrophils, and tissue necrosis.

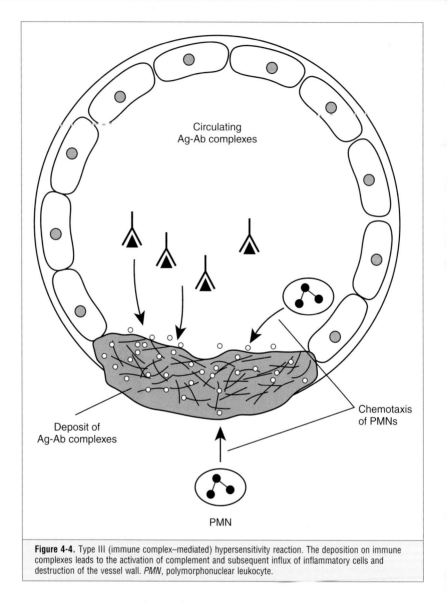

Figure 4-4. Type III (immune complex–mediated) hypersensitivity reaction. The deposition on immune complexes leads to the activation of complement and subsequent influx of inflammatory cells and destruction of the vessel wall. *PMN*, polymorphonuclear leukocyte.

- Antigens capable of inducing type III hypersensitivity reaction may be exogenous (e.g., streptococcal antigens, hepatitis B virus, and heroin) or endogenous (e.g., immunoglobulins and nuclear antigens).

20. **List the most important diseases caused by type III hypersensitivity reaction.**
   - **Systemic lupus erythematosus (SLE):** This disease is caused by circulating immune complexes that deposit in many organs, most often the skin, joints, and kidneys. Circulating blood cells are also often affected, resulting in anemia, leukopenia, and thrombocytopenia.

- **Polyarteritis nodosa:** This disease typically affects medium-sized arteries of internal organs, skin, eye, or peripheral nerves in an unpredictable manner.
- **Acute poststreptococcal glomerulonephritis:** This kidney disease typically follows a streptococcal throat infection and the formation of circulating antistreptococcal antibodies, which deposit in the glomerular basement membranes.
- **Membranous nephropathy:** In some forms of this immune-mediated glomerulopathy, there are circulating antigen-antibody complexes that deposit on the epithelial side of the glomerular basement membrane. The disease typically presents as nephrotic syndrome and massive proteinuria.
- **Serum sickness:** Injection of foreign serums may cause the formation of circulating immune complexes that are deposited in many organs. Most often it presents with a skin rash.

21. **What are the characteristics of cell-mediated (type IV) hypersensitivity?**
    - Primarily mediated through the interaction of TH1 helper CD4+ and cytotoxic CD8+ T lymphocytes.
    - A classic example is tuberculin reaction: In a previously sensitized individual (exposed to *Mycobacterium tuberculosis*), intracutaneous injection of purified protein derivate (PPD) of *M. tuberculosis* cultures will lead to delayed (8–12 hours) redness and induration at the site of injection. It reaches the peak in 24 to 72 hours, after which it slowly subsides.
    - Characterized by the accumulation of mononuclear cells (predominantly CD4+ T cells) around small vessels (cuffing).
    - If the antigen is nondegradable, perivascular lymphocytes are replaced by macrophages that resemble epithelium (epithelioid macrophages) and form a granuloma (Fig. 4-5).

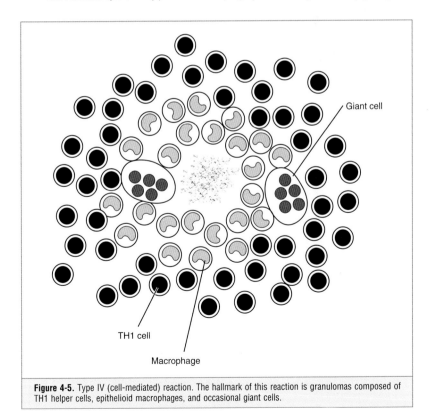

Figure 4-5. Type IV (cell-mediated) reaction. The hallmark of this reaction is granulomas composed of TH1 helper cells, epithelioid macrophages, and occasional giant cells.

22. **List the most important diseases caused by type IV hypersensitivity reaction.**
    - Contact dermatitis (poison ivy)
    - Tuberculosis
    - Sarcoidosis

23. **What kind of grafts (transplants) are there?**
    - Allograft: graft between genetically different individuals
    - Autograft: graft of one's own tissues
    - Isograft: graft from identical twin (also known as syngeneic graft)

24. **What are the features of a hyperacute transplant rejection?**
    - Occurs within minutes of transplantation
    - Mediated by preformed antidonor antibodies present in the recipient's circulation (e.g., ABO incompatibility)
    - Antigens in the endothelium of the transplanted organ are recognized by the preformed antibodies (IgM and IgG) capable of complement activation, resulting in thrombosis and fibrinoid necrosis and followed by ischemic necrosis of the transplanted organ.

25. **What are the characteristics of an acute transplant rejection?**
    - Occurs within days or months after the transplantation or at any time after the withdrawal of immunosuppressive therapy.
    - Mediated by both humoral (antibody-mediated) and cellular (T cell–mediated) mechanisms.
    - Vasculitis is a prominent feature. It is mediated by antidonor antibodies that attack the vessel wall, with subsequent thrombosis and thickening of the arterioles. Vascular changes cause an ischemia of the transplanted organ.
    - Interstitial accumulation of lymphocytes is a prominent feature. It is associated with parenchymal cell injury (e.g., tubular epithelium of kidneys or myocytes in the heart).

26. **What are the characteristics of chronic transplant rejection?**
    - Caused predominantly by vascular changes (intimal fibrosis) accompanied by ischemia and loss of parenchymal cells
    - Gradual and progressive decline in transplanted organ function over a period of months and years

27. **What is graft-versus-host disease (GVH)?**
    - Occurs when donor T lymphocytes recognize the recipient's HLA antigens as foreign and react against them.
    - Occurs with both bone marrow transplantation and solid organ transplantation, especially when these organs contain numerous lymphoid cells.
    - In acute GVH (occurring within the first 90 days), donor T lymphocytes attack the host's skin, biliary tract epithelium, and gut epithelium. This clinically manifests as maculopapular rash, secretory diarrhea, and signs of cholestasis.
    - The diagnosis is confirmed by a colon biopsy showing characteristic "exploding crypt lesions" (extensive death of epithelium of the crypts).
    - In chronic GVH (between 90 and 400 days), destruction of skin appendages, fibrosis of the dermis, and cholestatic jaundice are seen.

28. **How does immunologic tolerance develop?**
    - Tolerance is an inability to develop an immune response to a certain antigen.

- Self-tolerance is the normal state in which no immunologic response against self-antigens is present.
- Tolerance is the consequence of deletion of clones of self-reactive lymphocytes (T and B) early in life. It takes place centrally in the thymus and bone marrow (central tolerance) or in the peripheral tissues (peripheral tolerance).
- Activation of the Fas–Fas ligand (CD95/CD95L) apoptotic pathway plays an important role in the process of this clonal deletion, in both central and peripheral locations.
- Other mechanisms responsible for self-tolerance include clonal anergy, in which clones that escape deletion are rendered nonactive because they lack costimulatory factors necessary for activation (e.g., the CD28/B7 pathway). If this fails, there is a third mechanism of peripheral suppression by T cells in which these T cells suppress activation of certain autoreactive T cells.
- Some self-antigens are not presented to T cells during development (sequestered and cryptic self-antigens); hence, T cells specific for those antigens are not deleted.

29. **Define autoimmune disease.**
    Autoimmune diseases are caused by an immune reaction against self-antigens. They may involve a single organ or be multisystemic.

30. **How does autoimmunity develop?**
    Failure of peripheral tolerance: Activation of anergic clones later in life occurs because tissue damage has caused this antigen to present with costimulatory B-7 on APCs.
    Release of sequestered antigens: Antigens normally unavailable to the cells of the immune system become available and unmasking of cryptic antigens in the context of inflammation (to upregulate costimulatory pathways) occurs.
    Genetic predisposition may take several forms. Expression of certain HLA alleles confers higher susceptibility to the development of autoimmunity. Mutations (e.g., in Fas–Fas ligand) or polymorphisms in the genes responsible for the tolerance may lead to susceptibility to autoimmunity.
    Infections by viruses and other microbes may cause autoimmunity because of cross-reactivity, tissue necrosis (resulting in activation of anergic clones), or general stimulation (caused by the so-called superantigens) of the immune system.

31. **Why do some autoimmune diseases affect single organs, whereas others are systemic?**
    The outcome of an autoimmune reaction depends on the nature of the antigen. If the antigen is restricted in its expression to a single organ (e.g., TSH receptor on the thyroid gland), the autoimmune reaction will be limited to the cells of that organ. When more organs express the same antigen, more widespread disease ensues (multiorgan disease). Furthermore, several types of immune reactions against different self-antigens may be seen in systemic autoimmune disease.

32. **What are the criteria for the diagnosis of SLE?**
    SLE is an example of a systemic autoimmune disease capable of affecting virtually every organ in the body. It is characterized by a wide array of antibodies against self-antigens, neither organ- nor species-specific. SLE affects young women (in their 20s or 30s). A person is considered to suffer from SLE if at least 4 of 11 clinical and laboratory criteria are identified simultaneously or cumulatively at any interval of observation. These criteria are established by the American College of Rheumatology:
    1. Malar ("butterfly") rash over the face
    2. Discoid rash
    3. Photosensitivity (rash as a result of sun exposure)
    4. Oral ulcers

5. Arthritis (nondeforming polyarthritis)
6. Serositis (pleuritis and/or pericarditis)
7. Renal disorder (proteinuria of >0.5 g/day; cellular casts as signs of glomerulonephritis)
8. Neurologic disorder (seizures and/or psychosis)
9. Hematologic disorder (leukopenia, lymphopenia, thrombocytopenia, and hemolytic anemia)
10. Immunologic disorder (antibodies to native DNA or Smith antigen [anti-Sm]; antiphospholipid antibodies)
11. Antinuclear antibody (in the absence of drug-induced lupus)

During the flare-up of SLE, patients usually have fever, malaise, weight loss, and systemic signs of inflammation. Raynaud phenomenon, presenting as blanching of fingers and toes, is a common finding. Some patients have nonbacterial, sterile endocarditis (Libman–Sacks endocarditis), and occasionally some have neurologic and eye manifestations. Renal failure and infections are the most common cause of death.

33. **Are the antibodies against nuclear antigens (ANAs) diagnostic of SLE?**
Immunofluorescence test for ANAs is positive in almost all patients with SLE, but it may also be positive in many other autoimmune diseases, such as systemic sclerosis, Sjögren syndrome, and dermatomyositis. ANAs are also found in 5% to 15% of otherwise healthy people, and their incidence increases with age. This test has high sensitivity but low specificity for SLE.

34. **What is the best serologic test for diagnosing SLE?**
Antibodies to double-stranded DNA and to anti-Sm are virtually diagnostic of SLE but are seen in only 20% to 30% of patients. These tests have high specificity but low sensitivity for SLE.

35. **Why do patients with SLE frequently have positive VDRL and RPR tests for syphilis?**
Many SLE patients (40%–50%) have antiphospholipid antibodies, which often react with the cardiolipin antigen used as reagent in these serologic tests for syphilis. This cross-reactivity may account for the false-positive syphilis tests in SLE patients.

36. **What is lupus anticoagulant?**
SLE patients may have coagulation disorders that are often features of an antiphospholipid antibody syndrome. Antibodies found in this syndrome may lead to a prolongation of activated partial thromboplastin time (aPTT). Lupus anticoagulant can be demonstrated in the blood of these patients. Paradoxically, patients with antiphospholipid antibody syndrome suffer from recurrent venous and arterial thromboses.

37. **Does maternal SLE pose any danger to the offspring?**
SLE can be passed on to the offspring. Familial, twin, and ethnic studies suggest a genetic predisposition to SLE, which is inherited as a multifactorial disease. The incidence of the disease among infants born to mothers with SLE is in the range of 2% to 7%.

Neonatal lupus syndrome is a rare condition caused by the passive transplacental transfer of IgG autoantibodies from the mother with autoimmune disease. Skin rash, hematologic cytopenias, hepatosplenomegaly, myocarditis, and serositis are typically found. Symptoms mostly disappear within 6 to 8 months.

KEY POINTS: IMMUNOPATHOLOGY ✔

1. The immune system consists of B and T lymphocytes and accessory cells that react with foreign and endogenous antigens.

2. There are four hypersensitivity reactions that form the basis of most immunologic diseases.

3. Systemic lupus is the prototype of a systemic autoimmune disease, illustrating how tissue lesions develop and how autoantibodies can be used for diagnosis.

4. AIDS, an acquired immunodeficiency disease, is characterized by important secondary infections that typically develop in immunosuppressed people.

---

38. **What are the most characteristic microscopic findings in SLE?**
SLE is characterized by widespread deposition of immune complexes in tissues.
- **Skin:** Granular deposits of immune complexes along the epidermal–dermal basement membrane.
- **Kidneys:** Deposits of immune complexes are found in the glomeruli, in the blood vessels, and in the basement membranes of the tubules.
- **Heart:** Immune complex deposits are seen on the valves, most often on the mitral valve.

39. **What is the range of renal involvement in SLE?**
Nearly all patients with SLE have some signs of renal disease. The severity of the renal injury varies, and the kidney biopsy may be categorized into five classes:
- **Class I:** Normal biopsy (rare).
- **Class II:** Mesangial lupus glomerulonephritis. It is characterized by the expansion of the intercapillary matrix and a mild increase in the number of mesangial cells.
- **Class III:** Focal proliferative glomerulonephritis. It is characterized by segmental proliferation of endothelial and mesangial cells associated with neutrophilic infiltration in less than 50% of all glomeruli.
- **Class IV:** Diffuse proliferative glomerulonephritis. It is the most severe form of renal SLE. The majority of glomeruli show global hypercellularity, sometimes with crescents filling the urinary Bowman space.
- **Class V:** Membranous glomerulonephritis. It is principally characterized by the thickening of the capillary walls and a granular subepithelial deposition of immune complexes along the glomerular basement membranes.

40. **Describe the cardiac pathology of SLE.**
- Pericarditis (most common)
- Endocarditis (Libman–Sacks)
- Nonspecific myocarditis
- Accelerated coronary atherosclerosis

41. **What is discoid lupus erythematosus?**
Discoid lupus is a chronic skin disease characterized by well-demarcated, erythematous, discoid plaques, typically on the face and scalp but without systemic (extracutaneous) symptoms.
- Antibodies to double-stranded DNA are typically absent.
- There is a 5% to 10% risk of systemic disease (SLE).

42. **What is drug-induced lupus erythematosus?**
ANA test may become positive and typical symptoms of SLE may develop following administration of a variety of drugs (e.g., hydralazine for hypertension). Symptoms typically

disappear after discontinuation of the drug. Drug-induced lupus erythematosus differs from SLE in that:

- It is not associated with antibodies to double-stranded DNA.
- Antibodies to histones are present in 95% of affected people.
- Renal involvement is rare.
- Genetic susceptibility is indicated by a frequent association with HLA-DR4.

43. What is Sjögren syndrome?

Sjögren syndrome is caused by an autoimmune destruction of lacrimal glands, causing dry eyes (xerophthalmia), and salivary glands, causing dry mouth (xerostomia). It may occur as an isolated disorder (primary Sjögren syndrome) or as secondary Sjögren syndrome associated with other autoimmune diseases (RA, SLE, and scleroderma). The following are typical features:

- It affects mostly 35- to 45-year-old women (90% of patients are women).
- Antibodies against ribonucleoproteins (SS-A/Ro and SS-B/La) are found in approximately 80% of patients.
- Salivary and lacrimal glands are infiltrated with lymphocytes and enlarged.
- Patients with Sjögren syndrome are at high risk for developing lymphoma.

44. What is scleroderma?

Scleroderma, also known as systemic sclerosis, is a systemic disease characterized by microvascular injury and excessive fibrosis associated with signs of cellular and humoral autoimmunity affecting skin and many internal organs.

- An unknown triggering event leads to activation of lymphocytes. Cytokines produced by activated lymphocytes stimulate fibroblasts to produce collagen, resulting in fibrosis.
- An injury of the microvasculature leads to ischemic tissue injury.
- Autoantibodies are common and point to an immunologic nature of the disease.
  - ○ ANAs (50%) are of low specificity and found in other autoimmune diseases.
  - ○ Antibodies to DNA topoisomerase I (anti-Scl 70) found in 50% of patients are highly specific for systemic sclerosis.
  - ○ Antibodies to centromere (30%) are less specific but are found in 90% of patients who have the CREST subtype of systemic sclerosis (see question 46).

45. What are the pathologic findings in scleroderma?

- **Skin:** Atrophy and perivascular lymphocytic inflammation with edema followed by fibrosis, loss of skin appendages, and hyaline thickening of arterioles and capillaries.
- **Gastrointestinal system:** Esophagus and, to a lesser degree, small intestines are involved and show muscle atrophy and progressive fibrosis.
- **Musculoskeletal system:** Synovitis and myositis.
- **Kidneys:** The most striking changes involve interlobar arteries and arterioles. Intimal thickening with narrowing of the lumina with myxoid degeneration and fibrinoid necrosis.
- **Lungs:** Fibrosis and various degrees of vascular wall thickening.

46. What is CREST syndrome?

CREST syndrome is a form of limited scleroderma. Most patients (90%) have anticentromere antibodies. There is only minor involvement of internal organs. Typical features are:

- **C**alcinosis: calcification of the subcutis
- **R**aynaud phenomenon: spasm of digital arteries with acrocyanosis
- **E**sophageal dysfunction: loss of motility causing dysphagia
- **S**clerodactyly: clawlike flexion deformity of fingers
- **T**elangiectasia: dilatation of preexisting small skin vessels appearing as red macules

47. **Define inflammatory myopathies.**
This term comprises several autoimmune diseases characterized by inflammation of skeletal muscles (myositis) and muscle weakness. Autoantibodies, like ANAs, are found in 50% of patients but are of low specificity. Jo-1 antibody (antibody to histidyl-t-RNA synthetase) is more specific but is found only in 25% of patients. The most important entities are:
- Dermatomyositis
- Polymyositis
- Inclusion body myositis

48. **What is the difference between dermatomyositis and polymyositis?**
Polymyositis is an autoimmune disease involving the skeletal muscles. It may occur in an isolated form or in conjunction with skin lesions. In this case, the syndrome is called dermatomyositis. Common to both diseases are the following features:
- Preferential involvement of proximal parts of the extremities
- Pain and symmetrical proximal muscle weakness
- Histopathologic findings include infiltrates of lymphocytes and macrophages and muscle fiber injury
- Creatinine kinase (CK) is elevated in serum.
  Patients affected by dermatomyositis also show typical skin lesions. Dermatomyositis of childhood is associated with heliotrope rash (purple reddish discoloration, most prominently seen on the upper eyelids).

49. **List the main forms of polymyositis/dermatomyositis.**
- Primary polymyositis occurring in an isolated form
- Dermatomyositis
- Childhood dermatomyositis
  - Malignancy-associated dermatomyositis
  - Secondary polymyositis/dermatomyositis associated with other autoimmune diseases

50. **Define immunodeficiency.**
- Quantitative or qualitative defects of the immune system
- May involve the cells and components of:
  - Natural defense mechanisms (e.g., defects of the phagocytic and complement-mediated defense)
  - Acquired immunity involving the T and B lymphocytes
- Associated with an increased susceptibility to infection and lymphoproliferative diseases

51. **Classify immunodeficiencies.**
- **Primary:** This includes many congenital, mostly genetic deficiencies of one or more components of the immune system.
- **Secondary:** This includes numerous acquired deficiencies of one or more components of the immune system caused by infection, malnutrition, drugs, irradiation, cancer, or autoimmunity.

52. **What are the characteristic manifestations of primary immunodeficiencies?**
- Early onset, usually between 6 months and 2 years of age
- Recurrent infections

53. **How are primary immunodeficiencies classified?**
- B-cell deficiencies:
  - X-linked agammaglobulinemia (Bruton type)
  - Common variable immunodeficiency
  - Isolated IgA deficiency

- T-cell deficiencies:
  - Hyper-IgM syndrome
  - DiGeorge syndrome
- Severe combined immunodeficiency

54. **What are the characteristics of X-linked agammaglobulinemia of Bruton?**
    - Failure to assemble complete immunoglobulin molecules due to a mutation in the *btk* (Bruton tyrosinase kinase) gene located on the Xq21.2–22 chromosome
    - Absent or markedly decreased concentration of all classes of immunoglobulins (agammaglobulinemia)
    - Affects boys (X-linked disease)
    - Symptoms appear after 6 months of age. Typically, there is an increased incidence of otitis media, and skin and respiratory infections caused by *Haemophilus influenzae, Streptococcus pneumoniae,* or *Staphylococcus aureus*. During the first 6 months, the infant is protected by maternally acquired antibodies and the infections appear only after these antibodies have been cleared from the infant's body.

55. **What are the characteristics of common variable immunodeficiency?**
    - Late-childhood onset of hypogammaglobulinemia and recurrent infections
    - Boys and girls affected equally
    - High frequency of malignancies (gastric cancer and lymphoma) later in life

56. **What are the characteristics of isolated IgA immunodeficiency?**
    Isolated IgA deficiency is the most common congenital immunodeficiency, found in 1:850 people. Many of these men and women are asymptomatic. Because IgA is the major immunoglobulin found in mucosal secretions (respiratory, gastrointestinal, and urogenital tract), IgA deficiency is characterized by recurrent sinusitis, pulmonary and urinary infections, as well as recurrent diarrhea.

57. **What is the pathogenesis of X-linked hyper-IgM syndrome?**
    Affected people have high titers of IgM and IgD antibodies but low titers of IgG, IgA, and IgE antibodies, indicating that there is a defect in isotype switching.
    - The primary defect is in CD4+ T cells, which are responsible for production of cofactors necessary for stimulation of B-cell and isotype switching.
    - The cause is a mutation of X-chromosome gene encoding CD40L. This protein expressed on CD4+ lymphocytes acts as a ligand binding to a B-cell surface receptor (CD40). Binding of this ligand is important for the activation of B cells.
    - Patients suffer from pyogenic infections and are susceptible to infection with *Pneumocystis jiroveci.*

58. **What is DiGeorge syndrome?**
    - T-cell deficiency due to the abnormal development of thymus
    - Part of CATCH 22 syndrome: cardiac abnormality, T-cell deficit, cleft palate, hypocalcemia; syndrome is caused by a chromosome 22q11 deletion

59. **What are the characteristics of severe combined immunodeficiency (SCID)?**
    - Prominent susceptibility to severe, recurrent fungal *(Candida albicans),* viral, and bacterial infections
    - Both humoral (antibodies) and cellular (T cells) immune responses severely reduced
    - X-chromosome linked (boys are typically affected); mutation involves the gene encoding cytokine receptors

60. **What are the most common diseases resulting from deficiencies of the complement system?**
    - C2 deficiency results in increased susceptibility to infections and SLE-like syndrome.
    - C1-inhibitor deficiency gives rise to hereditary angioedema (episodes of edema of the mucosal surfaces).

61. **What is acquired immunodeficiency syndrome (AIDS)?**
    AIDS is an infectious disease caused by human immunodeficiency viruses (HIV). It is characterized by a profound suppression of the immune system and susceptibility to infections, neurologic disorders, and malignancies.

62. **What are the main characteristics of HIV?**
    Two genetically different but closely related forms of human pathogens are recognized: HIV-1 and HIV-2. Both are RNA viruses belonging to the retrovirus family. HIV expresses cell surface protein gp120, which binds to the CD4+ surface molecule of T helper lymphocytes. Proviral DNA synthesized by a reverse transcription in infected cells is integrated into the host's nuclear DNA.

63. **What are the modes of transmission of HIV?**
    - Sexual contact: homosexual (male) and heterosexual (male-to-female and female-to-male)
    - Parenteral inoculation: intravenous drug abusers and recipients of blood and blood products
    - Passage from infected mother to child: transplacental spread, transmission during the delivery, and breast-feeding

64. **What is the pathogenesis of AIDS?**
    - Primary targets for HIV are CD4+ T cells, but the viruses also invade macrophages and dendritic cells.
    - HIV binds to the CD4 molecule, which acts as a high-affinity receptor, but the infection requires coreceptors: CCR5 and CXCR4 (chemokine receptors).
    - After it is internalized, the viral genome undergoes reverse transcription, leading to formation of proviral DNA (cDNA).
    - In dividing cells, cDNA integrates into the host genome.
    - Upon antigenic stimulation, proviral DNA is transcribed and complete virus particles are produced, which may lead to cell death.
    - This results in a reduction in CD4+ T cells and persistent productive infection of macrophages, monocytes, and Langerhans cells.

65. **What is the natural history and what are the phases of HIV infection?**
    - **Early, acute phase:** Self-limited acute illness 3 to 6 weeks after the infection. High level of virus production and widespread infection of lymphoid organs.
    - **Middle, chronic phase:** No symptoms or persistent lymphadenopathy for several years. Minor infections.
    - **Final, crisis:** Long-lasting fever, severe opportunistic infections, secondary neoplasms, and neurologic disease. This usually develops after 7 to 10 years of the chronic phase.

66. **How is the clinically suspected diagnosis of AIDS confirmed?**
    - Laboratory tests are performed to detect antibodies against HIV proteins.
    - Seroconversion (the presence of antibodies against HIV in a previously nonreactive individual) usually occurs within 6 months of exposure to HIV.
    - Detection of infection during the serologic window before seroconversion requires detection of viral antigens or viral RNA.

67. **What are the common opportunistic infections in AIDS?**
    Opportunistic infections account for the vast majority of deaths in patients. These infections include:

- *P. jiroveci* pneumonia
- *C. albicans* infections of the mouth, esophagus, vagina, and lungs
- *Cytomegalovirus enteritis* and pneumonitis
- Atypical mycobacterial infection *(M. avium-intracellulare)* of the gastrointestinal tract
- *Cryptococcus neoformans* meningitis
- *Cryptosporidium enteritis*

68. **What are the most common neoplasms associated with HIV infections?**
    - Kaposi sarcoma
    - Non-Hodgkin lymphoma
    - Carcinoma of the uterine cervix
    - Squamous cell carcinoma of the skin

69. **What are the neurologic consequences of HIV infection?**
    Involvement of the central nervous system is common (clinically 40%–60%) and may present in several forms:
    - HIV-related diseases
      ○ Aseptic meningitis
      ○ AIDS dementia complex
    - Opportunistic infections: viral (cytomegalovirus and herpes simplex virus), fungal *(Coccidioides* and *Cryptococcus),* and protozoal *(Toxoplasma gondii)*
    - Neoplasms (lymphoma)

70. **What is amyloid?**
    Amyloid is a proteinaceous substance deposited between cells in various tissues and organs in a variety of clinical settings.
    - The name derives from its starchlike staining properties (PAS [periodic acid shift] positive).
    - Amorphous, eosinophilic, hyaline extracellular substance is seen under the microscope.
    - Amyloids are chemically diverse.
    - Amyloids have typical physical properties. All amyloids, irrespective of their biochemical composition, form nonbranching long fibrils (7.5–10 mm). By electron diffraction, they are arranged into b-pleated sheaths.
    - Congo red staining is typical. Under polarized light, Congo red-stained amyloid fibrils show an apple green birefringence.

71. **What are the three most common biochemical forms of amyloid?**
    - **AL:** This form of amyloid is formed from immunoglobulin light chains. It is found in multiple myeloma.
    - **AA:** This amyloid-associated protein is synthesized by the liver (in the form of the precursor serum amyloid A [SAA]). The form is seen in tissues of patients harboring chronic suppurative infections (e.g., bronchiectasis and osteomyelitis).
    - **Aβ:** This amyloid is found in Alzheimer disease (β-amyloid protein).

72. **What is amyloidosis?**
    Amyloidosis is a group of diseases characterized by a deposition of amyloid in various organs.
    - The deposition of amyloid may occur as a primary disease (e.g., in multiple myeloma) or in a secondary form during the course of chronic inflammatory or other diseases.
    - The disease may be limited (localized) to a single organ, or it may be systemic.
    - Some forms may be hereditary.

73. **What are the characteristics of primary amyloidosis?**
    - Systemic deposition of AL-type amyloid
    - Associated with plasma cell neoplasia and B-cell lymphoma
    - Monoclonal gammopathy (whole immunoglobulins or only light chains) found by electrophoresis of serum

74. **What are the features of secondary systemic amyloidosis?**
    - Underlying disease (e.g., tuberculosis, chronic ostoomyolitic, rheumatoid arthritis, and cancer) or condition (heroin abuse)
    - Widespread deposition of AA protein in many organs

75. **What are the characteristics of amyloidosis of aging?**
    - Systemic deposition of amyloid in elderly patients (seventh and eighth decades)
    - Frequent involvement of the heart (cardiac amyloidosis)

76. **What are the most severely affected organs in systemic amyloidosis?**
    - **Kidneys:** Both kidneys are enlarged, pale, and waxy. Glomerular mesangial, interstitial, and vascular wall depositions of amyloid are found.
    - **Spleen:** Splenomegaly presents with either nodular (follicular) depositions (sago spleen) or maplike (red pulp) depositions (lardaceous spleen).
    - **Liver:** Hepatomegaly, extracellular amyloid with pressure atrophy of hepatocytes.
    - **Small blood vessels:** Many organs show vascular deposits of amyloid, and, accordingly, the diagnosis may be made by biopsy of tissue from the fat pad, gingiva, or rectum.

WEBSITES

1. http://www.nlm.nih.gov/medlineplus/ency/article/000818.htm
2. http://www.merck.com/mmhe/sec16/ch184/ch184a.html
3. http://www.pathguy.com

BIBLIOGRAPHY

1. Akdis CA: Allergy and hypersensitivity: mechanisms of allergic disease. Curr Opin Immunol 18:718–726, 2006.
2. Cohn SE, Clark RA: Sexually transmitted diseases, HIV, and AIDS in women. Med Clin North Am 87:971–995, 2003.
3. Cooper MA, Pommering TL, Koranyi K: Primary immunodeficiencies. Am Family Physician 68:2001–2008, 2003.
4. D'Cruz DP, Khamashta MA, Hughes GR: Systemic lupus erythematosus. Lancet 369:587–596, 2007.
5. Kamradt T, Mitchison NA: Tolerance and autoimmunity. N Engl J Med 344:655–664, 2001.
6. Klein J, Sato A: The HLA system. First of two parts. N Engl J Med 343:702–705, 2000.
7. Lekstrom-Himes JA, Gallin JI: Advances in immunology: immunodeficiency diseases caused by defects in phagocytes. N Engl J Med 343:1703–1714, 2000.
8. Rosenwasser L: New insights into the pathophysiology of allergic rhinitis. Allergy Asthma Proc 28:10–15, 2007.
9. Stabinski L, Pelley K, Jacob ST, et al: Reframing HIV and AIDS. Br Med J 327:1101–1103, 2003.

CHAPTER 5

NEOPLASIA
Ivan Damjanov, MD, PhD

1. **Define neoplasia.**
   Neoplasia means "new growth." British pathologist Sir Rupert Willis defined it as follows:
   A neoplasm is an abnormal mass of tissue, the growth of which exceeds and is uncoordinated
   with that of normal tissues and persists in the same excessive manner after cessation of the
   stimuli that evoke the change.
   In contrast to normal cells, the growth of neoplastic cells is:
   - **Autonomous:** The growth of neoplastic cells is independent of growth factors and regulatory
     mechanisms operating inside the normal tissues.
   - **Excessive:** This excess may be evident in the size of the outgrowths and the duration of the
     proliferation.
   - **Disorganized:** The structures formed by tumor cells differ from normal tissues and do not fit
     into the general organization scheme of the normal body.

2. **Define other key words used in the study of neoplasia.**
   - **Tumor literally a swelling (tumefaction):** This term is used as a synonym for neoplasm.
     Clinically, tumors are classified as benign (good natured, innocuous) or malignant (bad,
     ominous, potentially lethal).
   - **Cancer:** This is a synonym for malignant tumors.
   - **Oncology:** This is the science dealing with the study of tumors (Greek term *oncos* is
     equivalent to the Latin term *tumor,* meaning "a swelling").

3. **What are hamartomas and choristomas?**
   - Hamartoma is a mass composed of cells and tissues native to the organ in which structures
     arose, usually during fetal development. Examples include the following:
     - **Mole (melanocytic nevus):** This skin hamartoma represents an aggregate of pigment cells
       that are normally dispersed in the skin.
     - **Pulmonary hamartoma:** This presents as a nodule composed of cartilage, bronchial
       epithelium, and smooth muscle cells.
   - Choristoma is a mass composed of normal cells or tissues found in a wrong location. It is
     also called ectopia. Examples include the following:
     - Pancreatic choristoma in the stomach or in the liver
     - Ectopic brain tissue in the nasal cavity

4. **Define dysplasia.**
   Dysplasia means abnormal growth and differentiation. The term may have a
   developmental pathology or oncologic meaning. In developmental pathology, it is used
   to describe morphogenetic abnormalities (e.g., dysplastic kidneys). In oncology, it is used
   to describe disorderly growth and maturation of cells that are not normal but that are not
   obviously malignant. This kind of dysplasia is a premalignant condition, a precursor of
   invasive neoplasia. Dysplasia can also be considered as a transitional stage linking neoplasia to
   hyperplasia or metaplasia. Examples include:

- **Squamous dysplasia of the cervix:** Dysplasia may be graded as mild, moderate, or severe (grade I, II, or III). Severe dysplasia cannot be reliably distinguished from carcinoma in situ. To avoid misunderstanding, dysplasia and carcinoma of the cervix are grouped together under the name *cervical intraepithelial neoplasia* (CIN), which is then graded as mild, moderate, or severe.
- **Liver cell dysplasia:** It is well known that liver cell carcinomas arise at an increased rate in cirrhosis caused by viral hepatitis B and C. Such pathologically altered liver may contain preneoplastic cells that can be recognized in histologic sections. Such cells have irregularly enlarged nuclei with prominent nucleoli.

5. **What is anaplasia?**
   Adult somatic cells are differentiated—that is, they express genes in a tissue-specific manner. Anaplasia of tumor cells is defined as lack of differentiation. Anaplastic tumor cells differ from normal cells and pathologists can recognize them as "atypical." Common features of anaplasia include:
   - **Pleomorphism:** variation in size and shape of nuclei
   - **Hyperchromatic nuclei:** the chromatin in the nuclei is increased in amount and irregularly distributed ("clumped")
   - **Atypical mitoses:** may be tripolar ("Mercedes logo like") or multipolar, in contrast to bipolar normal mitoses
   - **High nuclear cytoplasmic ratio:** thus resembling embryonic cells
   - **Bizarre cells:** including giant cells

KEY POINTS: NEOPLASIA ✔

1. Tumors are classified and named on the basis of their clinical and pathologic features, which must be correlated to determine the prognosis and the mode of therapy for each tumor.

2. Most tumors can be classified as either benign or malignant.

3. Metastasis, a unique feature of malignant tumors, is a complex process resulting in the transfer of tumor cells from the site of origin to distant organs.

6. **How are neoplasms classified clinically?**
   Neoplasms can be classified as benign or malignant on the basis of their clinical behavior. Benign tumors have a good prognosis, whereas malignant tumors have an unfavorable prognosis and are potentially lethal. A third category can be recognized for some tumor types, such as ovarian tumors. These tumors are called *borderline malignant* or *low-grade malignant tumors*. If recognized early and surgically resected, such borderline tumors have an excellent prognosis (>95% 5-year survival), but if untreated, they metastasize and will result in death.

7. **What is the basis of histologic or histogenetic classification of tumors?**
   Tumors often retain many of the histologic features of their tissue of origin. For example, a squamous cell carcinoma resembles normal squamous epithelium, whereas a transitional cell papilloma of the urinary bladder is lined by transitional epithelium resembling normal transitional epithelium. On the basis of such microscopic data, one can determine the composition of the tumors and in many instances theoretically reconstruct the histogenesis of most tumors (from Greco-Latin words *histo*, meaning "tissue," and *genesis*, meaning

"development"). The histologic–histogenetic classification of tumors is widely used to amplify the clinical classification. It serves as a basis for selecting treatment and for formulating the prognosis of the neoplastic disease in each particular case.

8. **What is the difference between carcinoma and sarcoma?**
Most human organs (except for the nervous system) are composed of epithelial cells, connective tissue cells, or both. Malignant tumors of epithelial origin are called carcinomas. Sarcomas are malignant tumors of connective tissue origin. Epithelial cells of carcinomas form nests surrounded by nonneoplastic connective tissue stroma. In sarcomas, the tumor cells are intermixed with the nonneoplastic stromal cells.
See Fig. 5-1.

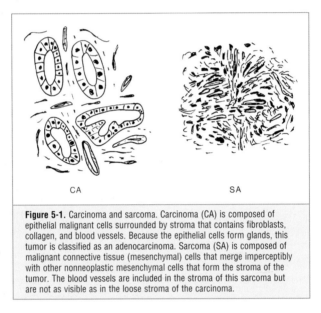

CA   SA

Figure 5-1. Carcinoma and sarcoma. Carcinoma (CA) is composed of epithelial malignant cells surrounded by stroma that contains fibroblasts, collagen, and blood vessels. Because the epithelial cells form glands, this tumor is classified as an adenocarcinoma. Sarcoma (SA) is composed of malignant connective tissue (mesenchymal) cells that merge imperceptibly with other nonneoplastic mesenchymal cells that form the stroma of the tumor. The blood vessels are included in the stroma of this sarcoma but are not as visible as in the loose stroma of the carcinoma.

9. **Are there any benign equivalents of carcinomas and sarcomas?**
Yes. The names for benign tumors are formed by adding the suffix *-oma* to the cell of their origin. Thus a benign tumor originating from fibroblasts is called fibroma, a tumor of fat cells is called lipoma, a tumor of smooth muscle cells is called leiomyoma, a tumor of striated muscles is called rhabdomyoma, a tumor of bone is called osteoma, and so on.
   Benign epithelial tumors could be called epitheliomas, but this term is not specific enough and is not used. Instead, benign epithelial tumors are known under a number of other names, such as:
- **Adenoma:** This tumor is composed of cells forming glands or tubules. Benign endocrine gland tumors are also called adenomas.
- **Papilloma:** This descriptive term is derived from the Latin word for the nipple. Papillomas appear as nipple-like protrusions on the surface of the skin or a hollow organ (e.g., urinary bladder). The surface of some papillomas may branch into smaller fronds, which give such tumors a cauliflower appearance.
- **Polyp:** This term is derived from the Greek term meaning "numerous feet" as seen in the octopus. These tumors may be attached to the surface of the skin or mucosa of hollow organs by a stalk. Other tumors form fingerlike epithelial protrusions broadly attached to the surface of their origin. Such tumors are called sessile polyps.
See Fig. 5-2.

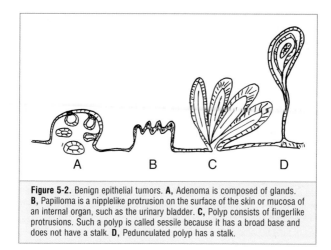

Figure 5-2. Benign epithelial tumors. **A,** Adenoma is composed of glands. **B,** Papilloma is a nipplelike protrusion on the surface of the skin or mucosa of an internal organ, such as the urinary bladder. **C,** Polyp consists of fingerlike protrusions. Such a polyp is called sessile because it has a broad base and does not have a stalk. **D,** Pedunculated polyp has a stalk.

10. **List the main histologic–histogenetic categories of human neoplasms.**
    On the basis of their histologic features and presumed cell or tissue of origin, neoplasms can be classified as:
    - **Epithelial tumors:** More than 80% of all human tumors are of epithelial origin. They can be benign or malignant. Depending on the type of epithelium, these tumors are classified as:
      - **Squamous cell tumors:** benign—squamous cell papilloma; malignant—squamous cell carcinoma
      - **Glandular tumors:** benign—adenoma; malignant—adenocarcinoma
      - **Transitional cell tumors:** benign—transitional cell papilloma; malignant—transitional cell carcinoma
    - **Connective tissue tumors:** Benign tumors include fibromas, lipomas, and osteomas, and so on; their malignant equivalents include fibrosarcomas, liposarcomas, osteosarcomas, and so on.
    - **Tumors of blood cells and lymphocytes:** All tumors in this category are malignant. They include entities such as lymphomas, leukemias, multiple myeloma, polycythemia rubra vera, Hodgkin disease, and others.
    - **Tumors of neural and glial cells and neural support structures:** This category includes tumors such as neuroblastoma, gliomas, and meningiomas.
    - **Germ cell tumors:** This category includes tumors such as seminoma, teratoma, teratocarcinoma, and choriocarcinoma.

11. **What are mixed tumors?**
    Mixed tumors are composed of both epithelial and connective tissue tumor cells. Benign mixed tumors composed of epithelial and myoepithelial cells and cells resembling cartilage cells are commonly found in the salivary glands. Malignant mixed tumors are called carcinosarcomas. Carcinosarcomas composed of adenocarcinoma and various sarcoma cells are most often found in the uterus. These uterine tumors are also called malignant mixed Müllerian tumors.

12. **What are teratomas?**
    Teratomas are tumors of germ cell origin. They are composed of tissues derived from three germinal layers: ectoderm, endoderm, and mesoderm. Thus in a teratoma one may find

ectodermal derivatives such as skin and neural tissue, endodermal derivatives such as intestine-like and bronchial-like structures, and mesodermal tissues such as bone or cartilage all intermixed in a haphazard manner. Malignant teratomas are called teratocarcinomas. These tumors consist of differentiated somatic tissues and malignant stem cells. These stem cells are developmentally equivalent to early embryonic cells and are called embryonal carcinoma cells.

13. **What is the difference between leiomyoma and rhabdomyoma?**
Leiomyomas are tumors composed of smooth muscle cells. Rhabdomyomas are tumors of striated muscle cells (i.e., cells forming the skeletal or heart muscle). Malignant tumors composed of the same cells are called leiomyosarcomas and rhabdomyosarcomas, respectively.

14. **What are blastomas?**
Blastomas are tumors composed of immature cells resembling those that form the fetal anlage or primordia of adult organs. Retinoblastoma is a tumor of the eye, neuroblastoma is a tumor composed of nerve precursors cells (neuroblasts), and a hepatoblastoma is a tumor composed of fetal hepatocytes.

15. **List the most well-known tumor eponyms.**
Eponyms (i.e., proper names used as designations) are applied to tumors that cannot be properly classified or whose histogenesis is controversial. The best-known tumor eponyms are:
- **Hodgkin disease:** a special form of malignant lymphoma
- **Ewing sarcoma:** a malignant bone tumor
- **Wilms tumor:** a malignant kidney tumor of childhood, also known as nephroblastoma
- **Kaposi sarcoma:** a blood vessel tumor of the skin and internal organs
- **Burkitt lymphoma:** a form of malignant lymphoma

16. **Is seminoma a benign tumor?**
The suffix -*oma* attached to the cell or tissue of origin of a specific tumor is commonly used to name benign tumors (e.g., osteoma and fibroma). There are, however, some important exceptions to this rule, and seminoma is one of them. Seminoma is a malignant tumor of the seminal epithelium in the testis. The equivalent tumor originating from the female germ cells in the ovary is called dysgerminoma.

17. **Give some other examples of malignant tumors ending in -oma.**
- **Glioma:** Almost all tumors derived from glia cells are malignant. This group includes tumors such as astrocytoma, oligodendroglioma, and ependymoma, all of which are actually malignant.
- **Lymphoma:** All lymphoid neoplasms are malignant. To emphasize this fact, it is customary to add an adjective and call these tumors malignant lymphomas.
- **Insulinoma, gastrinoma, somatostatinoma, and glucagonoma:** These endocrine pancreatic tumors originating from the islets of Langerhans may be either malignant or benign. Histologically, it is not possible to distinguish benign from malignant endocrine tumors.

18. **Is meningioma a benign tumor?**
Most meningiomas (96%) are biologically benign intracranial tumors of limited growth potential. Because of their intracranial location and the proximity to vital centers, meningiomas must be removed surgically because they can increase the intracranial pressure and compress the vital centers. Although biologically benign, such meningiomas may kill the host (i.e., act in a clinically "malignant" manner).

19. **What are the main differences between benign and malignant tumors?**
See Table 5-1.

TABLE 5-1. MAJOR DIFFERENCES BETWEEN BENIGN AND MALIGNANT TUMORS		
Feature	Benign	Malignant
Growth	Slow	Fast
	Expansive	Invasive
Gross appearance		
External surface	Smooth	Irregular
Capsule	Present	Not obvious
Cross section	Homogeneous	Variable
Color	Uniform	Variable
Microscopic		
Differentiation	Resembles tissue of origin	Anaplastic, does not resemble tissue of origin
Nuclei	Normal size and shape	Atypical, pleomorphic
		Hyperchromatic
Mitoses	Few	Numerous, often abnormal

20. **How are benign tumors distinguished from malignant tumors in practice?**
During the past 150 years, clinicians and pathologists have been correlating the clinical
behavior of various neoplasms with the histologic features of these tumors. Empirical
clinicopathologic criteria have been formulated on the basis of such studies and are used
to predict whether a tumor is benign or malignant. These criteria include:
- **Clinical findings:** Benign tumors tend to grow slowly and remain localized. Malignant tumors
tend to develop fast, disseminate through the body, and kill the patient.
- **Radiologic findings:** Benign tumors are circumscribed, whereas malignant tumors have
irregular outlines and invade the surrounding tissues. For example, mammographic
examination of the breast provides valuable data about breast tumors.
- **Gross features:** During surgery, one may assess tumors by direct inspection or palpation.
Surgeons can determine in many instances whether a tumor is most likely benign or
malignant.
- **Gross pathologic examination:** The previously mentioned criteria are often used by
pathologists to predict whether a tumor is benign or malignant.
- **Cytopathologic features:** Tumors can be examined by fine needle aspiration biopsy.
A needle is inserted, and a small sample of single cells is obtained by aspiration.
These cells can be examined microscopically and the diagnosis established in most cases.
- **Histologic examination:** Microscopic examination of tumors in most instances provides
the final proof that a tumor is malignant. In some instances, even the histologic
examination cannot indicate whether a tumor is benign or malignant. The best example
of such tumors is endocrine tumors, such as pituitary, thyroid follicular neoplasms, and
parathyroid tumors. In such cases, the diagnosis of malignancy can be made only if
the tumor is found to be clinically malignant (i.e., has metastasized, extensively invaded,
and destroyed tissue or killed the patient).

21. **What is the difference between tumor invasion and metastasis?**
Malignant tumors invade locally and extend into the surrounding normal tissues.
In contrast, metastasis is a spread of tumors to sites that are anatomically separate
from their site of origin.

22. **How do tumors metastasize?**
Tumors can metastasize three ways:
- **Lymphatic spread:** Tumor cells invade the lymphatics and spread to local lymph nodes.
- **Hematogenous spread:** Tumor cells invade the blood vessels and are carried by blood to distant sites.
- **Seeding of body cavities:** Tumor cells enter the cavities and float in the serous fluid to attach on the surface of the peritoneal or pleural cavity.

23. **Which tumors metastasize through the lymphatics, and which ones metastasize hematogenously?**
Previously, it was thought that carcinomas metastasize through the lymphatics and sarcomas through blood vessels. This rule is only partially correct, and there are many exceptions. Tumors of organs that are rich in lymphatics, such as the breast and the large intestine, metastasize preferentially through the lymphatics. Such tumors may metastasize hematogenously as well, but blood-borne metastases usually occur in later stages of the disease. Tumors originating in organs that are well vascularized but contain few lymphatics, such as bones, tend to metastasize hematogenously. This fact accounts for the high rate of hematogenous metastases of bone sarcomas.

24. **Which carcinomas metastasize more often hematogenously than through the lymphatics?**
Carcinomas of the liver and the kidney, two organs that have more blood vessels than lymphatics, metastasize more often hematogenously than lymphogenously.

25. **Do all malignant tumors metastasize?**
No. Malignant tumors of the brain usually kill the patient before the tumor has the chance to metastasize. The fact that brain tumors do not have metastases does not automatically mean that the cells of these tumors cannot metastasize. Evidence that brain tumors can metastasize includes the following:
- **Drop metastases in the spinal cord:** These metastases develop occasionally from cerebellar medulloblastoma cells carried to distant sites by the cerebrospinal fluid.
- **Lymph node metastases in patients who have had brain surgery:** It is assumed that the surgery has breached the blood–brain barrier and thus allowed the tumors to metastasize.
- **Metastases through shunts:** Some brain cancer patients whose cerebrospinal fluid is drained into the abdominal cavity by a tube have developed distant metastases. Such metastases arise from tumor cells carried by the cerebrospinal fluid through the manmade shunt.

26. **Which tumors spread primarily by seeding of body cavities?**
Peritoneal seeding is common in patients with ovarian cancer. Malignant tumors originating from the surface epithelium of the ovary tend to detach and float away in the peritoneal fluid. Such floating cells may attach to the serosal surfaces covering the abdominal wall or abdominal organs.

27. **What is the difference between staging and grading of tumors?**
Staging is used to determine the extent of spread of a tumor. It is based on correlating all the available clinical data with the pathologic findings. For example, the size of the tumor is assessed radiologically and on gross examination during surgery and in the pathology laboratory. The lymph nodes are examined to establish whether the tumor has spread to local and distant lymph nodes. Radiologic and radioisotope studies can be used to establish whether there are distant metastases.

Grading of tumors is based on microscopic examination of tumor tissues obtained at the time of operation or by biopsy. Tumors are graded on a scale from I to III, or descriptively as well differentiated, moderately well differentiated, or poorly differentiated. Although grading is important, overall, staging is much more predictive of the tumor behavior and is thus more valuable for prognosis.

28. **What is the TNM system?**
The TNM system is used for staging of tumors. T stands for the size of the tumor, which is expressed according to defined criteria for each anatomic site on a scale from 1 to 4. N (from 0 to 3) stands for lymph node involvement, and M (0 negative, 1 positive) stands for distant metastases. Thus a small tumor that has not metastasized is designated as T1, N0, M0. A small tumor that has metastasized to lymph nodes and distant sites is designated as T1, N1, M1.

29. **Are there other staging systems besides the TNM system?**
Yes. TNM is not a perfect system, and many other systems have been developed by cancer societies and even major medical centers. Some tumor staging systems were devised even before the TNM system was proposed and are still used in clinical practice. Probably the best-known staging system is the Dukes system for staging colon cancer.

CANCER EPIDEMIOLOGY

30. **Define cancer epidemiology.**
Cancer epidemiology deals with the occurrence of tumors in human populations. By studying cancer incidence, prevalence, and specific mortality, epidemiologists try to identify environmental and genetic causes of cancer and thus contribute to better diagnosis, treatment, and prevention.

31. **Define epidemiologic terms: incidence, prevalence, and mortality.**
   - Incidence of cancer is the number of new cases of a specific cancer registered over a specified period in a defined population. For example, the yearly incidence of cancer of the thyroid has increased in Japan since the atomic bomb explosions in 1945.
   - Prevalence of cancer is the number of all cases of cancer—both new and old—registered within a defined population at a given point in time. For example, the prevalence of cancer may have increased because of an environmental carcinogen but also because of improved treatment and longer survival of cancer patients.
   - Mortality of cancer is the number of deaths from a given form of cancer during a specified period of time in a defined population.

32. **How are epidemiologic data used to detect environmental carcinogens?**
Epidemiologic data may point to a cause-and-effect relationship between a cancer and a potential carcinogen. For example, a high incidence of lung cancer among smokers provided the first indication that lung cancer may be related to tobacco smoking. These initial data were corroborated by showing that there is a dose–response relationship and that the risk of cancer is directly proportional to the number of years and the number of cigarettes smoked ("pack years"). Finally, it was shown that tobacco tar contains carcinogenic polycyclic hydrocarbons. These carcinogens can produce malignant tumors in experimental animals and are the most likely cause of cancer in tobacco smokers.

KEY POINTS: CANCER EPIDEMIOLOGY ✔

1. Tumor incidence, prevalence, and mortality vary among populations and in different areas of the world.

2. The knowledge of epidemiologic data is important for medical practice and for the understanding of causes of tumors.

33. **What are the most common forms of cancer in men and women?**
    The most common tumors in men and women are skin neoplasms. The three most common malignant tumors of internal organs are as follows:

Men	Women
Prostate (31%)	Breast (31%)
Lung (14%)	Lung (13%)
Large intestine (10%)	Large intestine (11%)

34. **What are the most common causes of cancer-related death?**

Men	Women
Lung cancer (31%)	Lung cancer (25%)
Prostate cancer (11%)	Breast cancer (15%)
Large intestine cancer (10%)	Large intestine cancer (11%)

35. **List the most common cancers that show a geographic variation and the country where these cancers have the highest prevalence.**
    See Table 5-2.

TABLE 5-2. GEOGRAPHIC VARIATIONS OF COMMON CANCERS		
Organ System	**Type of Cancer**	**Country with Highest Prevalence**
Alimentary system	Esophagus	Iran, China, Africa
	Stomach	Japan, Chile, Iceland
	Liver	Sub-Saharan Africa, Southeast Asia
	Colon	United States, Western Europe
Skin	Melanoma	Australia, United States (south)
	Squamous	Australia, United States (south)
Breast	Ductal/lobular	United States, Western Europe
Genital system	Penis	South America
	Prostate	United States, Western Europe
Lymphoid	Burkitt lymphoma	Sub-Saharan Africa

36. **Has the incidence of some cancers increased during the past 50 years?**
    Yes. The best example is the increased incidence of lung cancer, especially in women. It is related to smoking. The incidence of prostate cancer has also increased, probably because of the widespread use of serologic tests for prostate-specific antigen in screening of elderly men, as well as improved diagnosis. The incidence of Kaposi sarcoma among male homosexuals increased with the acquired immunodeficiency syndrome (AIDS) epidemic.

37. **Has the incidence of some cancers decreased during the past 100 years?**
    The incidence of gastric cancer has decreased in the United States, probably because of widespread use of refrigeration, preventing the contamination of food. A decreased

incidence of invasive carcinoma of the cervix is related to the use of Pap smears for diagnosing preinvasive stages of the tumor. A decreased incidence of liver cancer in Japan has been noticed recently. It is attributed to the widespread use of vaccination against hepatitis virus B.

38. **List the important diseases that are associated with an increased incidence of cancer.**

Disease	Type of Cancer
Solar keratosis of the skin	Squamous carcinoma
Cirrhosis	Hepatocellular carcinoma
Ulcerative colitis	Colic adenocarcinoma
Reflux esophagitis/Barrett esophagus	Esophageal adenocarcinoma
Atrophic gastritis	Gastric adenocarcinoma
Paget disease of bone	Osteosarcoma
Immunodeficiency disorders	Lymphoma
Gonadal dysgenesis	Germ cell tumors

39. **List important infectious diseases associated with an increased incidence of some cancers.**

Disease/Pathogen	Type of Cancer
Epstein-Barr infection	Burkitt lymphoma, nasopharyngeal cancer (especially in China)
Viral hepatitis B and C	Hepatocellular carcinoma
Human papilloma virus infection	Carcinoma of cervix
Human T-cell lymphoma/leukemia	T-cell lymphoma/leukemia leukemia virus
AIDS	Lymphoma, Kaposi sarcoma

40. **List the most important hereditary tumor syndromes associated with increased incidence of cancer.**
    - **Familial adenomatous polyposis coli:** multiple adenomatous polyps of the large intestine that undergo malignant transformation into adenocarcinomas
    - **Neurofibromatosis type 1:** multiple neurofibromas that give rise to neurofibrosarcomas
    - **von Hippel–Lindau syndrome:** angiomas of the retina and hemangioblastoma of cerebellum, with a high risk for developing renal carcinoma

41. **List some hereditary syndromes with an increased incidence of cancer.**
    - **Li–Fraumeni syndrome:** This familial syndrome is characterized by an increased incidence of carcinomas of the breast, colon, and ovary, leukemia, sarcomas, and brain tumors.
    - **Ataxia telangiectasia:** This childhood disease presents with cerebellar ataxia (related to a loss of Purkinje cells), immunodeficiency, and vascular lesions (telangiectatic dilatation of small blood vessels). The disease is associated with an increased incidence of lymphoma.
    - **Wiskott–Aldrich syndrome:** This X-linked immunodeficiency disease affects only boys who have long-standing eczema and thrombocytopenic purpura. The disease is associated with an increased incidence of lymphoma.

42. **List three autosomal recessive disorders of DNA repair mechanism or increased chromosomal fragility associated with an increased incidence of cancer.**
    - **Xeroderma pigmentosum:** This defect in the repair of DNA breaks is related to a genetic defect of nucleotide excision enzymes. This enzyme deficiency is associated with an increased susceptibility to ultraviolet (UV) irradiation. Affected people develop skin cancer at an early age.
    - **Bloom's syndrome:** This chromosomal fragility syndrome is also associated with telangiectasia and immunodeficiency. The karyotype shows a large number of nonrandom chromosomal translocations. Patients develop gastrointestinal tumors and lymphoma at an increased rate.
    - **Fanconi anemia:** This chromosomal fragility syndrome is accompanied by development of lymphomas, hepatocellular carcinomas, and squamous cell carcinomas.

43. **List examples of cancers showing racial differences in their incidence.**
    - **Prostate cancer:** high incidence in white Americans but even higher in African Americans; low incidence among Japanese
    - **Skin cancer:** increased incidence in fair-skinned people of northern European origin; low incidence in highly pigmented persons
    - **Breast cancer:** high incidence in European and North American women; low incidence in Japan and many other Asian and African countries
    - **Multiple myeloma:** 3 or 4 times higher incidence in African Americans than in Americans of other races

44. **List some cancers that are more common in men than in women.**
    - Alimentary tract cancers: carcinoma of the oropharynx, esophagus, and stomach
    - Liver cancer
    - Bladder cancer
    - Lung cancer

45. **List some cancers that are more common in women than in men.**
    - Thyroid cancer
    - Carcinoma of the gallbladder
    - Meningioma

46. **Which tumors show peak incidence in older people?**
    Most malignant tumors occur more often in older people. Among the common cancers, it is only the incidence of carcinoma of the prostate and colon that increases progressively with advancing age. The incidence of other cancers levels off and may even decrease after the age of 75.

47. **Which tumors show peak incidence in infancy and early childhood?**
    Tumors that occur most often in children aged younger than 5 years are:
    - Acute lymphoblastic leukemia/lymphoma
    - Wilms tumor
    - Retinoblastoma
    - Neuroblastoma
    - Yolk sac tumor of the testis
    - Rhabdomyosarcoma

48. **Which tumors show peak incidence in late childhood and adolescence?**
    Tumors that have a peak incidence in the 6- to 15-year age group are:
    - Osteosarcoma
    - Ewing sarcoma
    - Primitive neuroectodermal tumor (PNET)
    - Medulloblastoma

49. **Which tumors have peak incidence in the 25- to 40-year age group?**
    Testicular germ cell tumors have a peak incidence in the 25- to 40-year age group and are an important cause of morbidity among middle-aged men.

50. **Which tumor has a biphasic peak age incidence?**
    Hodgkin disease has two peaks: one in the early 20s and the other at approximately 60 years.

MOLECULAR BASIS OF CANCER

51. **Are malignant tumors monoclonal or polyclonal?**
    Most malignant tumors are monoclonal (i.e., result from the malignant transformation of a single cell). Monoclonality of tumors can be best shown in malignant hematopoietic neoplasms. The cells of these neoplasms all express the same surface markers. Cells of multiple myeloma all secrete the same immunoglobulin (monoclonal gammopathy).

52. **How can one reconcile the theory of monoclonality with the fact that many tumors are composed of heterogeneous cell populations?**
    The experimental data suggest that most tumors are of monoclonal origin. Nevertheless, as the tumors grow, new clones may emerge due to new mutations. Diversity and heterogeneity of tumor cell populations overshadow the initial monoclonality. Similar events probably occur in human tumors. Despite their heterogeneity, most cell populations of these tumors retain some ancestral genetic markers that point to a common precursor (i.e., the original cell that has undergone malignant transformation). Some tumors are polyclonal from the onset. It is assumed that a "field effect" leads to malignant transformation of more than one normal cell, each of which gives rise to a specific tumor cell population. The field effect also accounts for the occurrence of multiple tumors in the same organ system (e.g., in the ureter and the urinary bladder) or closely juxtaposed organs, such as the mouth, larynx, and pharynx.

53. **How many cell divisions occur from the time of malignant transformation until the tumor becomes clinically detectable?**
    A precise answer cannot be given, but it is known that approximately 30 cell duplications must occur before 1 gram of tumor is formed and the earliest tumor mass becomes detectable.

KEY POINTS: MOLECULAR BASIS OF CANCER ✔

1. Most tumors develop because of the action and interaction of exogenous carcinogens, endogenous oncogenes, and tumor suppressor genes.

2. Carcinogens are mostly chemical factors, physical factors, or biologic agents.

3. Oncogenes and tumor suppressor genes are important causes of neoplasia.

54. **What are carcinogens?**
    Carcinogens are cancer-inducing factors that can be classified as:
    - Physical forces—UV light, x-rays, and gamma radiation
    - Chemicals
    - Viruses
    - Endogenous oncogens

55. **Define the main concepts of chemical carcinogenesis: initiation, promotion, and progression of tumors.**
   - **Initiation:** This is the first step that will induce the irreversible but not lethal change in the genetic material of the affected cell.
   - **Promotion:** This is the second step required for the formation of tumor. It promotes the replication of the initiated cells. Promoters cannot induce cancer on their own. Some carcinogens may act as initiators and promoters.
   - **Progression:** This is the third phase of tumor formation in which the growth of tumor becomes autonomous.

56. **What is the difference between direct-acting and indirect carcinogens?**
   - **Direct-acting carcinogens (e.g., nitrogen mustard and some metals such as nickel):** capable of binding to the DNA and directly causing genetic damage.
   - **Indirect carcinogens:** must be metabolized into an active form (proximal carcinogen) that can bind to the DNA. Typical examples are:
     - Polycyclic hydrocarbons from cigarette smoke are metabolized by cytochrome P450 into DNA-binding epoxides in the bronchial epithelium.
     - Aromatic amines ingested in food are metabolized in the liver, and the proximal carcinogens are excreted in urine. These carcinogens act on the transitional epithelium of the urinary bladder.

57. **List some important environmental carcinogens and neoplasms they may cause.**
   - **Polycyclic aromatic hydrocarbons:** found in tobacco smoke and tar; may cause lung cancer and skin cancer
   - **Aromatic azo dyes:** urinary bladder cancer in workers in aniline dye industry
   - **Benzene:** leukemia in chemical-industry workers
   - **Aflatoxin B-1:** toxin produced by *Aspergillus flavus* that grows on moldy grains and peanuts; suspected as cause of liver cancer in underdeveloped countries
   - **Nickel:** cancer of nasal cavity and lungs in mine workers
   - **Arsenic:** skin cancer in vineyard workers
   - **Asbestos:** mesothelioma in shipyard and insulation workers

58. **How are human carcinogens identified?**
   - Epidemiologic studies (Increased incidence of cancer in certain populations is often the first indication. Such studies have helped identify asbestos as the cause of mesothelioma and tobacco smoking as the cause of lung cancer.)
   - Isolation of chemicals
   - Study of potential carcinogens in experimental animals
   - Testing of potential carcinogens on cells in tissue culture
   - Mutagenesis testing in bacteria (Ames test)

59. **Why is scrotal cancer important for the understanding of human carcinogenesis?**
   Scrotal cancer is rare. Nevertheless, the story about it is instructive because it shows how a clinical epidemiologic observation may lead to a discovery of a carcinogen. The story spans more than 200 years:
   - Sir Percival Pott, a British physician, noticed in the 1770s a high incidence of scrotal cancer in chimney sweeps and suggested that soot may be the cause.
   - One hundred years later, German physicians noted an increased incidence of skin cancer in chemical-industry workers and suspected that soot contains carcinogens.
   - Japanese scientists Yamagiwa and Ishikawa reported in 1915 that tar applied in soluble form to rabbits' ears produced skin tumors.
   - Dibenzanthracene was isolated from tar in 1929 as the proximal chemical carcinogen.

- The discovery of dibenzanthracene led to the identification of other polycyclic hydrocarbon carcinogens. Polycyclic hydrocarbons were found to cause cancer in experimental animals and produce malignant transformation of normal cells in tissue culture.
- Molecular biologists working in the last quarter of the 20th century discovered that polycyclic hydrocarbons interact with DNA, causing specific mutations associated with malignant transformation of normal cells.

60. **What is the evidence that viruses cause human cancer?**
Most evidence is indirect, and the only definitely proved human oncogenic virus is the RNA retrovirus (HTLV-1) causing human T-cell leukemia/lymphoma. The following are other viruses associated with a high incidence of cancer:
- Human papilloma virus (HPV) subtypes 16 and 18 are implicated in the pathogenesis of carcinoma of the cervix and the lower female genital tract.
- Epstein-Barr virus has been associated with Burkitt lymphoma and nasopharyngeal carcinoma.
- Hepatitis virus B and C chronic liver disease has been associated with an increased incidence of hepatocellular carcinoma.
- Herpes virus 8 has been isolated from cells of Kaposi sarcoma.

61. **What is the evidence that UV radiation causes cancer?**
We are all constantly exposed to UV light, which is part of sunlight. The following facts support the view that UV light is a major skin carcinogen:
- Exposure to UV light promotes skin cancer in a dose-related manner. The more time one spends in the sun, the more one is at risk for developing skin cancer.
- The incidence of all major skin cancers—basal cell carcinoma, squamous cell carcinoma, and melanomas—is increased on sun-exposed surfaces of the human body.
- In the United States, the incidence of skin cancer is higher in southern than northern states.
- Skin cancer develops more often in fair-skinned than highly pigmented people.
- Skin cancer can be experimentally induced by exposing nude mice to UV light over prolonged periods of time.

62. **Which tumors have been linked to exposure to x-rays and ionizing radiation?**
X-rays and ionizing radiation can also cause skin cancer. Other cancers linked to ionizing radiation are:
- Leukemia/lymphoma
- Thyroid cancer (e.g., following atomic bomb blasts and Chernobyl atomic plant disaster)
- Osteogenic sarcoma (e.g., radioactive phosphorus dial painters in watch factories in the early 20th century)
- Lung cancer (e.g., uranium miners)
- Liver angiosarcoma (e.g., following radioactive Thorotrast use as a radiologic imaging contrast material)

63. **How does cancer begin?**
Cancer begins with malignant transformation of a normal cell involving an irreversible alteration of its DNA. Cancer-inducing genetic alterations involve normal genes involved in cell replication and death. Four types of genes are typically affected:
- Genes encoding growth factors, growth factor receptors, and signaling proteins involved in various steps of cell division
- Genes regulating apoptosis
- Genes belonging to the family of tumor suppressor genes
- Genes encoding DNA repair enzymes

64. **What are oncogenes?**
Oncogenes are cancer-inducing genes derived from normal cellular genes called protooncogenes. Human oncogenes, named cellular oncogenes (c-oncogenes), are homologous to viral oncogenes (v-oncogenes), known for some time to cause cancer in animals. All these genes are involved in cell proliferation and differentiation and are classified on the basis of their function into four groups. These functional groups and the representative protooncogenes and c-oncogenes are listed in Table 5-3.

TABLE 5-3. FUNCTIONAL GROUPS AND THEIR REPRESENTATIVE PROTOONCOGENE AND C-ONCOGENE

Function	Protooncogene	c-Oncogene
Growth factor	Platelet-derived growth factor	*sis*
Growth factor receptor	EGF-receptor	*erb-B2*
Signal transduction protein	Tyrosine kinase	*abl*
DNA-binding proteins	Transcription activator	*myc*

EGF, epidermal growth factor.

65. **How are protooncogenes activated to become oncogenes?**
Protooncogenes can be transformed into oncogenes through four basic mechanisms:
- **Point mutation:** A single base substitution in the DNA chain results in a miscoded protein. Point mutation of the ras oncogene is found in approximately 30% of common human cancers, such as carcinoma of the lung, large intestine, and pancreas.
- **Gene amplification:** This lesion is associated with an increased number of copies of a protooncogene. The best example is amplification of c-myc in neuroblastomas. The more c-myc is amplified, the more malignant are these childhood tumors.
- **Chromosomal rearrangements:** Translocations and deletions of parts of chromosomes lead to a juxtaposition of genes that are normally not in close proximity to one another. These rearrangements form new gene complexes, in which one gene acts as the promoter for the other. For example, translocation of the c-myc gene (normally located on chromosome 8) onto chromosome 14 positions this protooncogene next to the immunoglobulin heavy chain gene. The immunoglobulin gene is activated in B lymphocytes and acts as a promoter for the c-myc gene. This chromosomal rearrangement is the basis of malignant transformation of lymphocytes in Burkitt lymphoma.
- **Insertional mutagenesis:** This form of oncogene activation occurs because of an insertion of a viral gene into the mammalian DNA, resulting in genetic dysregulation. The best example of such an event may be found in hepatitis virus B–infected human liver cells.

66. **What is Philadelphia chromosome?**
Philadelphia chromosome is the first tumor-specific chromosomal change discovered by Nowell and Hungerford in 1960. It was named after the city in which it was discovered. It is a shortened chromosome 22 resulting from a reciprocal translocation of parts of chromosomes 22 and 9. This translocation leads to a juxtaposition of protooncogene *c-abl* (tyrosine kinase encoding gene on chromosome 9) and *bcr* on chromosome 22. The fusion protein p210 bcr–abl is thought to play a role in the malignant transformation of white blood cell precursors in the bone marrow. Philadelphia chromosome is found in 90% of all cases of chronic myelogenous leukemia.

67. **What are double minutes in tumor cells?**

    Double minutes are abnormal paired fragments of chromosomes found in some tumor cells. They contain amplified genes, some of which may be oncogenes. Other cytogenetic signs of gene amplification are homogeneous staining regions (HSRs) and abnormal banding regions of chromosomes stained with special stains.

68. **What are tumor suppressor genes?**

    Tumor suppressor genes are regulatory genes that act as autosomal dominant genes, preventing the abnormal division of cells. Loss of heterozygosity due to deletion or mutation of a tumor suppressor gene allows the cell to proliferate and is important for the initiation of malignant tumors.

69. **What is the role of the retinoblastoma suppressor gene *(Rb)*?**

    Rb is a tumor suppressor gene found on chromosome 13. It encodes a protein that binds to DNA, regulating gene expression. Dephosphorylated *Rb* gene inhibits cell division. When the *Rb* gene is phosphorylated, cell division takes place. Loss of *Rb* results in uncontrolled cell proliferation and formation of eye tumors known as retinoblastomas.

70. **What is the difference between sporadic and familial retinoblastoma?**

    Normal people have two alleles of the *Rb* gene. Sporadic retinoblastoma develops only if both of these genes are lost or inactivated. This loss of *Rb* typically occurs in two steps, as originally proposed by Alfred Knudsen in his famous "two hit" theory of carcinogenesis. Sporadic retinoblastomas are rare tumors and occur at a rate of 1:30,000.

    Familial retinoblastomas develop in genetically predisposed people who have only one active allele of the *Rb* gene. The second *Rb* allele has either been lost because of a deletion of a portion of the long arm of chromosome 13 or inactivated by a mutation. Accordingly, such people need only "one hit" to develop retinoblastomas. Predisposition to retinoblastoma is inherited in an autosomal dominant manner. Familial retinoblastomas develop at an earlier age than sporadic retinoblastomas and are often bilateral.

71. **Are retinoblastoma patients at risk for other tumors?**

    Retinoblastoma patients surviving treatment of an early-childhood ocular tumor are at risk of developing osteosarcomas in adolescence.

72. **List other important tumor suppressor genes.**

    - *p53:* Inactivation of this tumor suppressor gene on chromosome 17 is found in many common malignant tumors, such as carcinoma of the large intestine, lung, and breast.
    - *APC:* This gene, identified in familial adenomatous polyposis coli, is inactivated in tumors that develop in large bowel cancer and that occur in this syndrome and in Gardner syndrome (polyposis coli with osteomas, epidermal cysts, and fibromatosis).
    - *NF1:* It is inactivated in neurofibromatosis type 1.
    - *NF2:* It is inactivated in people who have bilateral acoustic schwannomas.
    - *WT-1:* It is inactivated in Wilms tumors of the kidney.
    - *VHL:* It is inactivated in renal cell tumors that develop in the von Hippel–Lindau syndrome but also in renal cancers unrelated to this syndrome.

73. **Which tumor suppressor gene plays a role in the pathogenesis of breast carcinoma?**

    Two breast carcinoma susceptibility genes have been identified in familial forms of this neoplasm: *BRCA1* and *BRCA2*. These tumor suppressor genes have a role in the pathogenesis of familial forms of ovarian cancer as well.

74. **Which tumor suppressor gene is most often mutated in human malignant tumors?**

    p53 mutations are the most common genetic abnormalities found in human cancers. It is mutated in approximately 80% of all colon cancers and 30% to 50% of cancers of the lungs, breast, and others sites. This gene is also the main defect in the Li–Fraumeni multicancer family syndrome.

75. **What are mutator genes?**

    Mutator genes belong to a group of recently identified cancer genes. These genes, also known as caretaker genes, ensure the integrity of the cellular genome. Cells with dysfunctional mutator genes accumulate genetic mutations, which make them more susceptible to malignant transformation. This usually occurs when the mutation of mutator genes is combined with the action of oncogenes or defective tumor suppressor activity.

76. **What are the best-known tumor mutator genes?**

    Mutator gene defects have been best documented in:
    - **Hereditary nonpolyposis colon cancer (HNCC or Lynch syndrome):** This familial condition is characterized by an increased incidence of colon, small intestine, stomach, and, in women, carcinoma of the endometrium and ovary. Because of the defective function of the mutator gene (one of four DNA mismatch repair genes), these patients accumulate numerous mismatched errors in DNA replications. These mutations, which would be excised in normal circumstances, accumulate over time and by adulthood are found 1000 times more often than in other people. Microsatellite instability is seen in 90% of the tumors that develop in these patients.
    - **Ataxia telangiectasia:** This hereditary syndrome presents with cerebellar ataxia, immunodeficiency, and dilatations of small blood vessels. Lymphoma and carcinoma of the stomach and breast develop at an increased rate. These patients carry a mutated *AT* gene called *ATM* (ataxia telangiectasia mutated). Normal *AT* is a mutator gene encoding a nuclear phosphoprotein that is involved in the control of DNA replication. Patients carrying *ATM* have a reduced capacity to repair DNA breaks and are prone to accumulating numerous genetic mutations over time. The *ATM* is found at a rate of 1% in the population at large and may play a major role in the pathogenesis of breast and stomach cancer.

77. **What is the role of telomerase in cancer?**

    Each chromosome has a terminal part that consists of nucleotide repeats forming so-called telomere complexes. The telomere complex serves as an internal clock and also prevents the end-to-end fusion of chromosomes during mitosis. With each cell division, the telomeres shorten, and by the time the entire complex has been eliminated, the cell stops dividing. This is one of the causes of the limited replication of adult cells explanted in culture. Cancer cells have an upregulated telomerase activity, and this enzyme prevents the naturally programmed shortening of the telomere complexes. Activated telomerase probably contributes to the "immortalization" of cancer cells.

78. **How does dysregulation of apoptosis contribute to neoplasia?**

    Normal cells are programmed to die after a limited life span. This is achieved through a complex genetic mechanism, the so-called suicide pathway, responsible for the programmed cell death or apoptosis. Mutation of apoptosis genes may contribute to immortalization of cells as has been noticed in many human neoplasms.

79. **Give an example of how defective apoptosis can contribute to the formation of neoplasia.**

    The best example is a defect of the apoptosis gene *bcl-2*. This gene is mutated in chronic lymphocytic leukemia/lymphoma. Lymphoma cells do not die but accumulate in the lymph nodes, bone marrow, and the blood circulation.

80. **What are the most common chromosomal abnormalities in human tumor cells?**
Chromosomal abnormalities occur very often in tumor cells. They may be classified as random—that is, specific for a particular tumor type (e.g., the Philadelphia chromosome is specific for chronic myelogenous leukemia [CML])—or nonrandom. Karyotypic abnormalities include:
- Deletions (e.g., deletion of a segment of the long arm of chromosome 13 in retinoblastoma)
- Translocations (e.g., translocations in Burkitt lymphoma and CML)
- Amplifications of chromosomal regions (e.g., in neuroblastoma) evidenced as:
  - Homogenous staining regions (HSRs)
  - Double minutes

HOST RESPONSE TO TUMORS

81. **How does the host react to neoplasia?**
Host reaction can be considered under two headings:
- Local tissue reaction, such as formation of tumor stroma
- Systemic reaction, such as immune response

82. **What is meant by desmoplasia?**
Desmoplasia (derived from Greek words *desmos*, meaning "connective," and *plasia*, meaning "formation") is a term for the formation of connective tissue in response to tumors. This connective tissue accounts for the rock-hard texture of tumors such as scirrhous breast carcinoma or carcinoma of the prostate.

83. **Is desmoplasia promoting or limiting the growth of tumor cells?**
We do not know the correct answer. On one hand, desmoplasia may be a defense mechanism used by the body to wall off the tumor and limit the invasive growth of tumor cells. On the other hand, the connective tissue stroma provides a framework for the growth of tumors and protects them mechanically from outside damage. Stroma also contains blood vessels that are essential for the nourishment of tumor cells. It is not known why some tumors are desmoplastic and others do not elicit a desmoplastic reaction.

KEY POINTS: HOST RESPONSE TO TUMORS ✓

1. Tumors cause local changes in the organs of their origin and systemic changes mediated by a variety of mechanisms.
2. The understanding of the host's response to tumors is important for diagnosis of tumors and their treatment.

84. **What role does angiogenesis play in the formation of tumors?**
Angiogenesis (i.e., the formation of new blood vessels) is a common host reaction to malignant tumors. Formation of blood vessels and lymphatics is essential for the inflow of nutrients into the tumor and the survival of tumor cells.

85. **How do malignant tumors stimulate angiogenesis?**
Tumor cells secrete cytokines that stimulate the ingrowth of angioblasts in a manner similar to the formation of granulation tissue in healing wounds. Angiogenic factors include a variety of growth factors, such as platelet-derived growth factor (PDGF) and basic fibroblast growth

factor (bFGF). These factors may be derived from tumor cells but also from the host's inflammatory cells (e.g., macrophages) infiltrating the tumor.

86. **How do tumor cells invade the host tissues?**
Tumor cells secrete lytic enzymes that digest the basement membranes and various components of the extracellular matrix. The most important enzymes are matrix metalloproteinases:
- **Interstitial collagenases:** degrade collagen types I to III
- **Gelatinases:** degrade collagen type IV in basement membranes
- **Stromelysins:** degrade collagen type IV and proteoglycans
Lytic enzymes secreted by tumors are neutralized by tissue inhibitors of metalloproteinases (TIMPs), which limit invasiveness of tumor cells.

87. **How do tumor cells metastasize?**
Metastasis is a multistep process that allows tumor cells to move from one site to another. These steps include:
- Detachment of invasive cells from the main tumor mass
- Invasion of the basement membrane and the connective tissue
- Intravasation (i.e., entry of tumor cells into the vessel)
- Dissemination of tumor cells in the intravascular fluid (blood or lymph)
- Anchorage (i.e., attachment of tumor cells to endothelial cells at a distant site)
- Extravasation (i.e., emigration of tumor cells through the vessel wall)
- Proliferation at the distant site

88. **Do all tumor cells that have entered the blood circulation form metastatic foci?**
No. It has been shown that many tumor cells enter circulation at the time of surgery. Most of these cells will die and will not form metastases. It is not known why some tumor cells die and others survive and are capable of forming metastases.

89. **How does immunosurveillance against tumors work?**
Immunosurveillance against tumors is based on both natural and acquired immunity. The body has numerous mechanisms for eliminating unwanted and potentially dangerous neoplastic cells. Most neoplastic cells formed because of spontaneous or induced mutations are thus eliminated, and such cells are not allowed to develop into clinically detectable tumors.

90. **Which cells act against tumor cells?**
Essentially all inflammatory cells can be mobilized in the body's defense against tumors. The most important among these cells are:
- **Natural killer cells:** These cells have innate antitumoral activity and can kill tumor cells without previous sensitization. Lymphokine activated killer cells (LAKs) are even more potent than native natural killer cells.
- **Macrophages:** These cells are also part of the nonspecific natural immune response to tumor cells.
- **Cytotoxic cells (CD+8):** T lymphocytes react to tumor antigens and are the most important tumoricidal cells of the acquired immune response.
Antibodies to tumor cells are important for antibody-dependent cell-mediated or complement-mediated cytotoxicity.

91. **What are tumor markers?**
Tumor markers are substances that are secreted by tumor cells or released from the surface of tumor cells into the circulation. These substances can be classified as:
- Oncofetal glycoproteins found on tumor cells and fetal cells (e.g., carcinoembryonic antigen [CEA])
- Serum proteins (e.g., alpha-fetoprotein)
- Enzymes (e.g., lactate dehydrogenase and prostate-specific antigen)

- Hormones (e.g., human chorionic antigen, insulin, and calcitonin)
- Biogenic amines (e.g., norepinephrine and vanillylmandelic acid)

92. **List some clinically useful tumor markers.**
    Tumor secretory products or antigens released into the blood may be detected serologically (i.e., with antibodies as in a radioimmunoassay). The most important tumor markers currently used are listed in Table 5-4.

TABLE 5-4. MAJOR TUMOR MARKERS

Tumor Marker	Function	Tumor
Alpha-fetoprotein	Fetal serum protein	Hepatocellular carcinoma, g germ cell tumor
Chorionic gonadotropin	Placental hormone	Germ cell tumor, choriocarcinoma
Carcinoembryonic antigen	Oncofetal glycoprotein	Adenocarcinoma (colon, etc.)
Calcitonin	Hormone	Medullary carcinoma of the thyroid
Prostate-specific antigen	Enzyme of seminal	Prostate carcinoma fluid

93. **List some local adverse effects of tumors.**
    - Mass effect (e.g., palpable breast mass deforming the breast)
    - Compression of normal tissue with loss of function (e.g., pituitary atrophy and hypopituitarism due to pituitary adenoma)
    - Pain due to compression of nerves
    - Destruction of normal tissue (e.g., punched-out bone lesions in multiple myeloma) or perforation of a hollow organ (e.g., gastric cancer)
    - Obstruction of hollow organ (e.g., obstruction of large intestine by carcinoma)
    - Irritation and inflammation (e.g., bronchial cancer causing coughing)
    - Bleeding due to erosion of blood vessels (e.g., vaginal bleeding)
    - Necrosis (e.g., ischemic necrosis due to obstruction of a nutrient vessel)

94. **List some systemic adverse effects of tumors.**
    - Nonspecific symptoms, such as loss of appetite, fatigue, and weakness
    - Cachexia and weight loss
    - Fever and night sweats
    - Paraneoplastic syndromes

95. **What is cachexia?**
    Cachexia is loss of body weight accompanied by weakness and exhaustion. It may be caused by large tumors that act as parasites draining energy and nutrients. In other cases, tumors inhibit nutrition (e.g., carcinoma of the esophagus prevents swallowing). Other tumors secrete cytokines, such as tumor necrosis factor, which promote catabolism and loss of fat tissue and muscles.

96. **What are paraneoplastic syndromes?**
    Paraneoplastic syndromes include signs and symptoms caused by remote tumor effects. Essential features of paraneoplastic syndromes are as follows:
    - Unrelated to the mechanical effects of the tumor mass or distant metastases
    - May result from substances released from tumor cells but not found in the normal cells from which the tumor has originated

- May result from a series of immunologic and other host reactions to tumor
- May have a complex and not fully understood pathogenesis

97. **How are paraneoplastic syndromes classified?**
    - Endocrine
    - Neuromuscular
    - Hematologic
    - Dermatologic
    - Renal

98. **List three endocrine paraneoplastic syndromes.**
    - Cushing syndrome caused by adrenocorticotropic hormone (ACTH)–secreting small-cell carcinoma of the lung
    - Hypercalcemia due to the secretion of parathyroid-like polypeptide by squamous cell carcinoma of the lung
    - Hypoglycemia due to the secretion of insulin-like growth hormone by leiomyosarcoma of the uterus

99. **List three hematologic paraneoplastic syndromes.**
    - Polycythemia due to erythropoietin-secreting renal cell carcinoma
    - Migratory thrombophlebitis (Trousseau syndrome) due to the release of thromboplastins from carcinoma of the pancreas
    - Anemia due to cold autoantibodies in patients with lymphoma

100. **List two neuromuscular paraneoplastic syndromes.**
    - Myasthenia gravis associated with thymoma
    - Lambert–Eaton syndrome (muscular weakness) due to antibodies to neuromuscular junction proteins in patients with small cell carcinoma of the lung

101. **List two dermatologic paraneoplastic syndromes.**
    - Acanthosis nigricans—hyperpigmentation on the neck and intertriginous areas in patients with gastric carcinoma
    - Dermatomyositis associated with a number of cancers

102. **Name a renal paraneoplastic syndrome.**
    Nephrotic syndrome caused by the deposition of tumor antigen–antibody immune complexes in the glomerular basement membranes.

WEBSITES

1. http://www.ncbi.nlm.nih.gov/entrez/query.fcgi?db=PubMed

2. http://library.med.utah.edu/WebPath/webpath.html

3. http://www.cancer.gov

4. http://www.mic.ki.se/Diseases/C04.html

BIBLIOGRAPHY

1. Albertson DG: Gene amplification in cancer. Trends Genet 22:447–55, 2006.

2. Albertson DG, Collins C, McCormick F, Gray JW: Chromosome aberrations in solid tumors. Nature Genet 34:369–376, 2003.

3. Cheung AL, Deng W: Telomere dysfunction, genome instability and cancer. Front Biosci 13:2075–2090, 2008.

4. Eccles CA, Woloh DR: Metastasis: recent discoveries and novel treatment strategies. Lancet 369:1742–1757, 2007.

5. Jemal A, Siegel R, Ward E, et al: Cancer statistics, 2007. CA Cancer J Clin 57:43–66, 2007.

6. Piris A, Mihm MC Jr: Mechanisms of metastasis: seed and soil. Cancer Treat Res 135:119–127, 2007.

7. Rutherford GC, Dineen RA, O'Connor A: Imaging in the investigation of paraneoplastic syndromes. Clin Radiol 62:1021–1035, 2007.

8. Schinzel AC, Hahn WC: Oncogenic transformation and experimental models of human cancer. Front Biosci 13:71–84, 2008.

9. Smith RA, von Eschenbach AC, Wender R, et al: American Cancer Society guidelines for the early detection of cancer: update of early detection guidelines for prostate, colorectal, and endometrial cancers. CA Cancer J Clin 51:38–75, 2001.

10. Tlsty TD, Coussens LM: Tumor stroma and regulation of cancer development. Annu Rev Pathol 1:119–150, 2006.

CHAPTER 6

DEVELOPMENTAL AND GENETIC DISEASES

Bruce A. Fenderson, PhD

1. **How common are birth defects?**
   Developmental and genetic diseases account for half of all infant mortality in the United States. It is estimated that 1 in 50 children worldwide is born with a major birth defect. Approximately 1 in 100 has a single gene defect, and 1 in 200 has a major chromosomal defect. If one also considers diseases with polygenic patterns of inheritance (e.g., atherosclerosis and hypertension), the lifetime risk of genetic disease may be as high as 65 in 100.

2. **What are the major causes of birth defects?**
   The causes of most birth defects are unknown (70%). Approximately 25% are due to cytogenetic or hereditary diseases. The remaining birth defects (5%) are associated with maternal exposure to chemicals, radiation, or infections or are related to maternal metabolic factors or birth trauma. The major causes of birth defects can be classified as follows:
   - Errors of morphogenesis
   - Chromosomal abnormalities
   - Single gene defects
   - Polygenic defects
   - Transplacental and birth injury

3. **Define hereditary, familial, and congenital disease.**
   - Hereditary diseases are passed from parents to their offspring. The risk of inheritance depends on whether the trait is carried on a sex chromosome or autosome and on whether the trait is dominant or recessive.
   - Familial diseases run in families and represent examples of multifactorial (polygenic) inheritance. There is no reliable pattern of inheritance because of the low probability of inheriting all of the mutations necessary for clinical disease. If an individual is a member of a family with a history of a familial disease, he or she has a greater probability than the general population of inheriting this disease. For first-degree relatives of affected individuals, the risk is 5% to 10%.
   - Congenital diseases are present at birth. They may be due to structural changes in DNA (mutations) or by direct injury to the fetus in utero.

4. **List congenital malformations that occur at least once in 1000 newborn children.**
   - Anencephaly (0.3/1000 in the United States and 5–6/1000 in Wales and Ireland)
   - Fetal alcohol syndrome (1–3/1000 in the United States and Europe)
   - Down syndrome (1/1000 for women up to their mid-30s; 1/30 for women age 45)
   - Klinefelter syndrome (1/1000 males)
   - TORCH complex (1–5/1000 of all live-born infants in the United States)
   - Cleft lip with or without cleft palate (1/1000)

ERRORS OF MORPHOGENESIS

5. **What are teratogens?**

   Teratogens are chemical, physical, or biologic agents that are able to induce developmental abnormalities. Some teratogens are toxic and cause necrosis, whereas others trigger programmed cell death (apoptosis). Teratogens may also induce developmental abnormalities by altering patterns of gene expression, inhibiting cell interactions, or blocking morphogenetic cell movements.

6. **List proved human teratogens.**
   - Radiation (atomic weapons and radioiodine)
   - Infections (cytomegalovirus, herpes virus, syphilis, *Toxoplasma*, and rubella virus)
   - Maternal metabolic factors (alcoholism, diabetes, folic acid deficiency, and endemic cretinism)
   - Drugs (aminopterin, busulfan, cocaine, coumarin anticoagulants, cyclophosphamide, lithium, mercury, thalidomide, and retinoic acid)

7. **List basic principles of teratology.**

   Approximately 5% of birth defects are linked to maternal exposure to chemicals, drugs, or radiation or linked to maternal metabolic disturbances or infections. The biochemical mechanisms of teratogenesis in these cases are varied. Indeed, exposure to a proved teratogen does not always cause a congenital malformation. General principles of teratology include the following:
   - Teratogens produce growth retardation or malformation. The outcome depends on complex interactions between the mother, placenta, and fetus.
   - Genes of the mother and fetus determine susceptibility to a teratogen (e.g., there is variable susceptibility to the effects of alcohol).
   - Most teratogens are harmful only during a critical window of development (e.g., thalidomide is teratogenic only between days 28 and 50 of pregnancy).
   - Teratogenic agents inhibit specific receptors or enzymes or disrupt specific developmental pathways (e.g., some agents show neurotropism or cardiotropism).
   - Effects of teratogens are dose-dependent. A "safe" dosage may exist; however, in the absence of certain knowledge, teratogens should be avoided by pregnant women.

8. **Define agenesis, aplasia, hypoplasia, dysraphic anomaly, involution failure, division failure, atresia, dysplasia, ectopia, and dystopia.**
   - Agenesis is the complete absence of an organ or lack of specific cells within an organ (e.g., lack of germ cells in "Sertoli cell only syndrome").
   - Aplasia is the absence of an organ with retention of the organ rudiment (e.g., aplasia of the lung).
   - Hypoplasia is incomplete development of an organ (e.g., microphthalmia and microcephaly).
   - Dysraphic anomaly is caused by failure of opposed structures to undergo adhesion and fusion (e.g., spina bifida and anencephaly are dysraphic anomalies of the neural tube).
   - Involution failure is persistence of an embryonic structure that normally disappears during development (e.g., persistent thyroglossal duct).
   - Division failure is incomplete cleavage of embryonic tissues owing to lack of programmed cell death (e.g., incomplete separation of digits in syndactyly).
   - Atresia is failure of an organ rudiment to form a lumen (e.g., esophageal atresia).
   - Dysplasia is abnormal organization of cells in a tissue (e.g., congenital cystic renal dysplasia).
   - Ectopia is an error of morphogenesis in which an organ is located outside its correct anatomic site (e.g., ectopic parathyroid glands can be located within the thymus).
   - Dystopia is an error of morphogenesis in which an organ is retained at a site where it resided during a stage of development (e.g., cryptorchidism occurs when dystopic testes are retained in the inguinal canal).

9. **What is Potter complex?**

   Potter complex is an example of a "developmental sequence anomaly" in which multiple disorders lead to the same birth defect through a common pathway. Signs of Potter complex include pulmonary hypoplasia and abnormal position of hands and legs (signs of fetal compression). These abnormalities are caused by reduced amniotic fluid level (oligohydramnios). Because fetal urine serves to maintain the normal volume of amniotic fluid, the causes of oligohydramnios include renal agenesis and urinary tract obstruction. Oligohydramnios may also be caused by chronic leakage of amniotic fluid through the cervical plug.

10. **List dysraphic anomalies of the neural tube.**

    Dysraphic anomalies are caused by a failure of apposed edges of the presumptive neural plate to fuse properly during early development (days 25–35). Neural tube defects follow multifactorial (polygenic) inheritance. Maternal serum alpha-fetoprotein levels and ultrasonography are used to diagnose dysraphic anomalies in utero. Examples of dysraphic anomalies include the following:
    - Spina bifida is incomplete closure of the spinal cord and vertebral column. It occurs most frequently in the lumbar region and represents a defect in neural tube closure on days 25–30.
    - Meningocele is a herniation of the meninges through a defect in the vertebral column in patients with spina bifida.
    - Myelomeningocele is a herniation of both the meninges and the spinal cord through a defect in the vertebral column in patients with spina bifida.
    - Acrania is complete or partial absence of the cranium.
    - Anencephaly is the absence of the cranial vault with reduced or missing cerebral hemispheres.
    - Craniorachischisis is a more extensive dysraphic anomaly that may extend from the cranium to the vertebral column.

11. **Explain the role of folic acid in the pathogenesis of neural tube defects.**

    Pharmacologic doses of folic acid have been shown to reduce the incidence of neural tube defects by lowering plasma levels of homocysteine. Homocysteine is a teratogen for the central nervous system and heart. Women with reduced activity of 5,10-methylenetetrahydrofolate reductase exhibit elevated plasma levels of homocysteine and are at risk for bearing children with neural tube and other birth defects.

12. **What are the typical clinical features of thalidomide-induced malformations?**

    Thalidomide is a sedative (derivative of glutamic acid) that has been found to cause birth defects when used by women between days 28 and 50 of pregnancy. Approximately 3000 children were born with birth defects during the 1960s to women who used thalidomide during early pregnancy. Clinical features of thalidomide-induced birth defects include:
    - Phocomelia (foreshortening of the arms)
    - Amelia (lack of arms)
    - Microtia (small ears)
    - Anotia (lack of ears)
    - Congenital heart disease

13. **What are the typical clinical features of fetal alcohol syndrome?**

    Clinical features of fetal alcohol syndrome include facial dysmorphology, growth retardation, and mental deficiency/emotional instability. Specific anatomic findings include microcephaly, epicanthal folds, short palpebral fissure, maxillary hypoplasia, thin upper lip, micrognathia, poorly developed philtrum, and septal defects of the heart. Most children with fetal alcohol syndrome have IQs below 85. Additional psychological findings include short memory spans, impulsiveness, and emotional instability.

14. **Is fetal alcohol syndrome a common cause of mental retardation?**
    Yes. Fetal alcohol syndrome has an incidence of 1 to 3 in 1000 live births in the United
    States. It is a major cause of mental retardation and emotional instability. Studies in animal
    models indicate that ethanol triggers massive, programmed cell death (apoptosis) in the
    developing central nervous system.

15. **What is the TORCH complex?**
    TORCH is an acronym that refers to the signs and symptoms of congenital infection with
    Toxoplasma, others, rubella, cytomegalovirus, and herpes. Syphilis, tuberculosis, Epstein-Barr
    virus, varicella-zoster virus, and human immunodeficiency virus (HIV) are included in the
    "other" category. This acronym was coined to alert pediatricians to the fact that a search for
    one etiologic agent should include a search for all TORCH agents.

16. **How common is the TORCH complex?**
    The TORCH complex is seen in 1% to 5% of all live births in the United States, so it is a major
    cause of infant mortality and morbidity. Congenital syphilis is estimated to affect 1 in 2000
    live-born infants in the United States. Infants infected with TORCH agents may be asymptomatic
    at birth but develop typical signs and symptoms over the ensuing months.

17. **What are the typical clinical features of the TORCH complex?**
    Signs and symptoms of TORCH infections in the fetus or newborn include ocular defects
    (microphthalmia, glaucoma, cataracts, retinitis, and conjunctivitis), brain lesions (focal
    cerebral calcification and microcephaly), cardiac anomalies (patent ductus arteriosus and
    septal defects), and other systemic manifestations (pneumonitis, hepatomegaly, splenomegaly,
    petechiae, purpura, and jaundice). Late complications of congenital syphilis include rhinitis
    (snuffles), skin rash, pneumonia, vascularization of the cornea (interstitial keratitis), notched
    incisors, inflammation of the periosteum, meningitis, and deafness. The clinical finding of
    notched incisors, deafness, and interstitial keratitis is referred to as Hutchinson triad.

CHROMOSOMAL ABNORMALITIES

18. **What is the normal human karyotype?**
    Somatic cells of the human body possess 22 pairs of autosomes and two sex chromosomes
    (46,XX or 46,XY). The normal karyotype is diploid (two copies of each chromosome). Sperm
    and eggs carry 23 chromosomes and are haploid (one copy of each chromosome). Sperm
    determines genotypic sex by contributing either an X or a Y chromosome during fertilization.

19. **How is karyotype analysis used in medical genetics?**
    Cytogenetic studies are routinely performed on fetal cells collected from amniotic fluid
    (amniocentesis) or from chorioallantoic villus sampling. Cultured cells are treated with
    colchicine to obtain metaphase chromosome spreads. Chromosomes are stained with dyes
    (e.g., Giemsa) to reveal banding patterns under the microscope (G bands). These bands permit
    the identification of both numeric and structural chromosomal abnormalities. Fluorescence
    in situ hybridization (FISH) is also used for cytogenetic studies. In this assay, fluorescent
    dye-conjugated DNA probes are used to mark interphase chromosomes, map structural defects,
    and identify specific genes. Karyotype analysis can be used to determine:
    - Genotypic sex (i.e., identification of X and Y chromosomes)
    - Ploidy (i.e., euploid, aneuploid, or polyploid)
    - Chromosomal structural defects (e.g., translocation, isochromosome, and deletion)

20. **Define haploid, diploid, euploid, polyploid, aneuploid, monosomy, and trisomy.**
    - Haploid (n) refers to a single set of chromosomes (23 in humans). Postmeiotic germ cells (sperm and eggs) are haploid.
    - Diploid (2n) refers to a double set of chromosomes (46 in humans). Somatic cells are diploid.
    - Euploid refers to any multiple of the haploid set of chromosomes (from n to 8n).
    - Polyploid refers to any multiple of the haploid set of chromosomes greater than diploid (>2n).
    - Aneuploid refers to karyotypes that do not have multiples of the haploid set of chromosomes
    - Monosomy refers to an aneuploid karyotype with one missing chromosome (e.g., monosomy X in Turner syndrome).
    - Trisomy refers to an aneuploid karyotype with one extra chromosome (e.g., trisomy 21 in Down syndrome).

KEY POINTS: CHROMOSOMAL ABNORMALITIES ✓

1. Chromosomal abnormalities can be classified as structural or numeric.

2. Down syndrome is an autosomal trisomy characterized by mental retardation and characteristic facial features, as well as several abnormalities of internal organs.

3. Klinefelter syndrome and Turner syndrome are the two most important numeric abnormalities of sex chromosomes.

21. **How are chromosomal abnormalities classified?**
    Chromosomal abnormalities are classified as either structural or numeric. They affect both sex chromosomes and autosomes. Examples of structural abnormalities include deletion and translocation. The most common cause of numeric chromosomal abnormalities is nondisjunction, resulting in either monosomy or trisomy. Chromosomal abnormalities may arise during somatic cell division (mitosis) or gametogenesis (meiosis). Abnormalities that originate during gametogenesis are transmitted to all somatic cells of the offspring. Chromosomal abnormalities are common and usually result in spontaneous abortion during early pregnancy. Major chromosomal abnormalities are incompatible with life.

22. **List structural abnormalities of chromosomes.**
    - Deletion is loss of a portion of a chromosome. Examples include cri du chat syndrome (5p-), Wilms tumor aniridia syndrome (11p-), and retinoblastoma (13q-).
    - Reciprocal translocation is exchange of chromatin (crossing over) between nonhomologous chromosomes. Balanced translocations do not result in the loss of genetic material. Most carriers of balanced translocations have a normal phenotype.
    - Robertsonian translocation is centric fusion of two acrocentric chromosomes resulting in the formation of one large metacentric chromosome and one small fragment. This fragment is usually lost during subsequent cell divisions.
    - Isochromosomes are formed by faulty division of the centromere. If the centromere divides in a plane perpendicular to the long axis of the chromosome, pairs of isochromosomes are formed. One pair is composed of two short arms; the other pair is composed of two long arms. Approximately 15% of women with Turner syndrome have an isochromosome of the long arm of the X chromosome and are monosomic for genes on the missing short arm.
    - Inversion is the breaking of a chromosome at two points, followed by rejoining of the broken ends.
    - Ring chromosome involves breaking both telomeric ends of a chromosome, followed by end-to-end fusion of the centric portion. Ring chromosomes usually have no phenotypic consequence.

23. **Explain chromosomal breakage syndromes.**
Chromosomal breakage and translocation may be acquired or hereditary. Acquired chromosomal breakage and translocation is commonly associated with development of leukemias and lymphomas. Examples include chronic myelogenous leukemia t(9;22) and Burkitt lymphoma t(8;14). Hereditary syndromes associated with DNA damage and loss of cellular growth control include xeroderma pigmentosum, Bloom syndrome, Fanconi anemia, and ataxia telangiectasia. These hereditary syndromes exhibit autosomal recessive inheritance.

24. **What is nondisjunction, and how does it cause a numeric chromosomal abnormality?**
Nondisjunction is failure of paired chromosomes to move to opposite poles of the spindle during mitosis or meiosis. If nondisjunction occurs during meiosis, the resulting embryo inherits an extra chromosome (trisomy) or lacks a chromosome (monosomy). Nondisjunction occurs more commonly in people with structural chromosomal abnormalities, such as nonbalanced translocations. The incidence of nondisjunction increases dramatically with maternal age.

25. **List the most common birth defects caused by a numeric chromosomal abnormality.**
Most numeric chromosomal abnormalities are caused by nondisjunction. Examples include:
- **Down syndrome (trisomy 21):** The incidence is 1 in 1000 for women up to their mid-30s, but 1 in 30 for women at age 45 years. Most cases are accounted for by nondisjunction during the first meiotic division (meiosis I) of oogenesis.
- **Klinefelter syndrome (sex chromosome trisomy, XXY):** The incidence is 1 in 1000 in newborn males. Most cases are accounted for by maternal nondisjunction during the first meiotic division of oogenesis.
- **Turner syndrome (monosomy X):** Turner syndrome is one of the most common chromosomal abnormalities; however, most fetuses are aborted spontaneously. The incidence in newborn females is 1 in 5000. The missing X is usually of paternal origin.
- **Edward syndrome (trisomy 18):** The incidence is 1 in 8000. Most children die in infancy.

26. **What are the typical clinical features of Down syndrome?**
Down syndrome (trisomy 21) is the most common cause of mental retardation. The incidence strongly correlates with advancing maternal age, increasing to 1 in 30 by age 45. Two thirds of all conceptions with the trisomy 21 karyotype end in spontaneous abortion. Typical clinical features of Down syndrome are summarized as follows:
- The face and occiput tend to be flat, with a low-bridged nose, reduced interpupillary distance, oblique palpebral fissures, epicanthal folds, Brushfield spots of the iris, and a protruding tongue.
- Children suffer severe mental retardation and exhibit a progressive decline in IQ with age (from 70 to 30 by age 10).
- One third of children suffer from congenital heart disease. Anomalies include atrioventricular canal, ventricular and atrial septal defects, tetralogy of Fallot, and patent ductus arteriosus.
- Children are small, with shorter than normal bones of the ribs, pelvis, and extremities. Hands exhibit a simian crease, and the fifth finger usually curves inward (clinodactyly).
- Duodenal stenosis, imperforate anus, and congenital megacolon (Hirschsprung disease) occur in 2% to 3% of children.
- Men are sterile because of arrested spermatogenesis. Some women with Down syndrome have given birth, and 40% of these children exhibit trisomy 21.
- Children are at high risk of developing leukemia. For children younger than 15 years, the risk is approximately 15-fold greater than normal.
- Morphologic lesions characteristic of Alzheimer's disease (neurofibrillary tangles and senile plaques) appear in all patients with Down syndrome by age 35.

27. **What is the life expectancy for patients with Down syndrome?**
The most common causes of death in patients with Down syndrome are congenital heart disease and leukemia. With a normal heart, only 5% of children with Down syndrome die before age 10. After age 10, the estimated life expectancy is 55 years.

28. **Describe two forms of chromosomal change in Down syndrome.**
Chromosome 21 is the smallest human autosome and encodes approximately 225 genes. The region critical for the development of Down syndrome has been mapped to a small segment of the long arm (21q). The most common forms of chromosomal change in Down syndrome are:
   - Nondisjunction arising during the first meiotic division of gametogenesis (95% of cases); the incidence increases dramatically with maternal age, from 1 in 1000 during early reproductive years to 1 in 30 by age 45
   - Translocation of an extra long arm of chromosome 21 to another chromosome (5% of cases)

29. **How do the X and Y chromosomes regulate sex differentiation?**
The presence of a Y chromosome determines male phenotypic sex, regardless of the number of X chromosomes. Thus individuals with Klinefelter syndrome (47,XXY) are phenotypically male despite the presence of an extra X chromosome. The SRY gene on the Y chromosome is known to encode a transcription factor (SIP-1), which serves as a master switch to turn on male-determining genes that are present on the autosomes. Without an SRY gene, the phenotype is female.

30. **What are Barr bodies?**
Female embryos randomly inactivate either the paternal or the maternal X chromosome during embryogenesis to achieve dosage compensation for critical genes on the X chromosome. Thus females are mosaics for the maternal and paternal X chromosomes. X inactivation involves DNA methylation, gene repression, and chromatin condensation. Hyperchromatic X chromatin can be viewed under the light microscope and is referred to as a Barr body. In this connection, patients with Klinefelter syndrome (47,XXY) show a Barr body in all somatic cells, despite the fact that they are phenotypically male.

31. **What are the typical clinical features of Klinefelter syndrome?**
Klinefelter syndrome is an important cause of male hypogonadism and infertility. It affects approximately 1 in 1000 newborn males. It is defined as the presence of one or more extra X chromosomes in a phenotypic male (e.g., 47,XXY). The principal clinical features during childhood are behavioral. Klinefelter syndrome should be suspected in all boys with some degree of mental deficiency or behavioral abnormality. As they mature, boys with Klinefelter syndrome exhibit a eunuchoid body habitus (tall and thin) and develop certain feminine characteristics, including a high-pitched voice, gynecomastia, and female escutcheon. Testes and penis remain small. After puberty, the testes begin to atrophy, with loss of germ cells and Sertoli cells. Aspermia and peritubular fibrosis lead to infertility. Leydig cell function is impaired, leading to low serum levels of testosterone (increased estradiol-to-testosterone ratio). Follicle-stimulating hormone and luteinizing hormone levels are high, indicating that the pituitary gland is functioning normally. Testosterone can be used to virilize these patients, but it cannot restore fertility.

32. **What are the typical clinical features of Turner syndrome?**
Turner syndrome is defined as complete or partial monosomy of the X chromosome in a phenotypic female (e.g., 45,X). The principal clinical features of Turner syndrome are primary amenorrhea and sterility. Other features include short stature, webbed neck, low posterior hairline, wide carrying angle of the arms (cubitus valgus), broad chest with widely

spaced nipples, multiple pigmented nevi, and hyperconvex fingernails. Cardiovascular anomalies (e.g., coarctation of the aorta and bicuspid aortic valve) occur in 50% of patients. Ovaries lose oocytes and are converted to fibrous streaks during early childhood. Children with Turner syndrome have an excellent prognosis when treated with growth hormone and estrogens. Turner syndrome is a common cause of primary amenorrhea (one third of cases).

33. **What is a multi-X female?**
Approximately 1 in 1250 newborn females is born with one or more X chromosomes due to meiotic nondisjunction. Multi-X females may have amenorrhea or mild mental retardation, but most are normal.

34. **What is the difference between hermaphroditism and pseudohermaphroditism?**
Hermaphroditism is a disorder of genotypic sex in which patients have gonads with both ovarian and testicular tissue (ovotestes). Pseudohermaphroditism is a disorder of phenotypic sex in which patients have normal male or female gonads but ambiguous external genitalia. Male pseudohermaphroditism can result from androgen insensitivity of peripheral organs (testicular feminization) or defects in testosterone biosynthesis. Female pseudohermaphroditism is an autosomal recessive disorder associated with adrenal hypersecretion of androgens.

35. **Define genetic mosaicism.**
Chromosomal abnormalities and gene mutations may occur during any mitotic or meiotic cell division. If these changes occur in somatic cells during embryogenesis, clones of cells will be generated with different patterns of gene expression. Such cases are referred to as mosaics. In rare instances, germline mosaicism can result in the transmission of mutations, despite the fact that the parents show no manifestation of disease. Mosaicism due to mitotic nondisjunction is a common cause of Turner syndrome (20% of cases) and a rare cause of Down syndrome (2% of cases). In mosaics with Turner syndrome, 15% are 45,X/46,XX, and 5% are 45,X/46,XY.

36. **What is a gene?**
Genes are segments of DNA that contain information necessary to synthesize a polypeptide. The human genome is estimated to encode 30,000 genes (3 billion base pairs). Changes in gene expression mediate growth, development, and differentiation. Single genes may define phenotypic traits that follow the classical Mendelian laws of inheritance.

KEY POINTS: SINGLE GENE ABNORMALITIES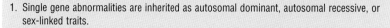

1. Single gene abnormalities are inherited as autosomal dominant, autosomal recessive, or sex-linked traits.

2. Autosomal dominant diseases usually affect structural proteins and receptors.

3. Autosomal recessive diseases usually affect enzymes.

4. Cystic fibrosis is the most common autosomal recessive disease.

5. Lysosomal storage diseases include sphingolipidoses, mucopolysaccharidoses, and glycogenosis type II.

6. The most important X-linked recessive diseases are fragile X syndrome, Duchenne–Becker muscular dystrophy, and hemophilia.

37. **Explain the transmission patterns of single gene defects (Mendelian traits).**
    Mendelian traits reflect the expression of two copies (alleles) of the same gene present on homologous chromosomes. Single gene defects (Mendelian traits) may be caused by the inheritance of one or both defective alleles, depending on the nature of the gene product. Autosomal genes are present on 1 of the 22 autosomes. Sex-linked genes are located on the X chromosome. The three most important forms of Mendelian inheritance are the following:
    - Autosomal dominant traits require the expression of only one allele of a homologous pair (i.e., the phenotype is present when alleles are heterozygous or homozygous).
    - Autosomal recessive traits require the expression of both alleles of a homologous pair (i.e., the phenotype is present when alleles are homozygous).
    - Sex-linked recessive traits require the expression of both alleles on the X chromosome (i.e., the phenotype is present when X-linked alleles are homozygous). Sex-linked recessive traits are most commonly seen in males (46,XY).

38. **Define single gene (Mendelian) traits.**
    Single gene (Mendelian) inheritance implies a specific risk of disease based on the transmission of defective alleles. The risk is 50% for inheritance of one defective allele and 25% for inheritance of two defective alleles. More than 5000 Mendelian disorders have been described.

39. **Define polygenic traits.**
    Polygenic traits are determined by multiple genes located on more than one chromosome. Multifactorial inheritance represents the additive effects of many abnormal genes and environmental factors (e.g., obesity, hypertension, atherosclerosis, and diabetes). Multifactorial disorders tend to run in families. The probability of occurrence is approximately 5% to 10% for first-degree relatives.

40. **How are chromosomal abnormalities inherited?**
    Most numeric abnormalities result in embryonic lethality. Individuals with monosomy or trisomy syndromes are almost always sterile. Examples include Down syndrome (trisomy 21), Klinefelter syndrome (trisomy XXY), and Turner syndrome (monosomy X). Structural chromosomal abnormalities that do not result in loss of chromatin (i.e., balanced translocations) typically show no phenotypic abnormality and may be transmitted to offspring.

41. **Discuss allelic polymorphism.**
    Most genes are carried in multiple sequences in a population. It is estimated that 1 in 250 base pairs in the human genome is variable (polymorphic). Polymorphisms typically reflect silent (nonlethal) mutations; however, polymorphic alleles may exhibit differences in protein function. For example, a single base substitution is known to convert the human blood group A enzyme (GalNac transferase) to the blood group B enzyme (Gal transferase).

42. **Explain codominance and pleiotropy.**
    Codominance refers to the expression of polymorphic alleles resulting in a new phenotype. For example, genes encoding the ABH blood group system show codominant inheritance. Two glycosyltransferase genes (A and B) determine four blood group types: A, B, AB, and O.
    Pleiotropy refers to the production by a single mutant gene of apparently unrelated, multiple effects. For example, mutant HbS protein predisposes red blood cells to lysis in patients with sickle cell anemia but also causes a wide variety of vascular complications, including thrombosis, infarction, and fibrosis.

43. **Explain the biochemical basis of a mutation.**
   Mutations are structural changes in DNA that may affect protein expression and function. Mutations occur spontaneously and provide the basis for the evolution of life on Earth. Mutations that occur in the germline are transmitted to future generations. Those that occur in somatic cells may contribute to the pathogenesis of neoplasia. Drugs, chemicals, and physical agents that increase the rate of mutation act as carcinogens and teratogens. Mutations occur within both coding and noncoding sequences. The following are major types of genetic mutations:
   - Point mutations are single base substitutions that can change a codon from one amino acid to another (missense mutation) or introduce a premature stop codon (nonsense mutation).
   - Frameshift mutations are base pair insertions or deletions that change the codon reading frame.
   - Large deletions can result in loss of a gene or juxtapose genes to create a hybrid encoding a new "fusion" protein.
   - Expansion of a trinucleotide repeat can arise in genes that have repeated sequences. The normal repeat size is 10 to 30, but affected patients can have hundreds or thousands of repeats.

44. **List examples of genetic diseases associated with expansion of a trinucleotide repeat.**
   - Huntington disease is a fatal neurodegenerative disease associated with expansion of a CAG trinucleotide repeat within the Huntington gene. It is an autosomal dominant disease with an incidence of 1 in 15,000.
   - Fragile X syndrome is the most common inherited cause of mental retardation, is associated with expansion of a CGG trinucleotide repeat that silences the promoter of the FMR1 gene, and is an X-linked recessive disease with an incidence of 1 in 1250 in males and 1 in 2500 in females.
   - Myotonic dystrophy is the most common cause of adult muscular dystrophy. It is associated with expansion of a CTG trinucleotide repeat within a protein kinase. It is an autosomal dominant disease with an incidence of 1 in 7000.
   - Friedreich ataxia is the most common inherited ataxia. It is associated with expansion of a GAA repeat in the frataxin gene. It is a rare, autosomal recessive disease with an incidence of 1 in 50,000.

45. **List mechanisms through which mutations cause genetic disease.**
   Mutations can affect both quantitative and qualitative aspects of gene expression.
   - Mutations in promoter sequences can suppress transcription.
   - Mutations near intron/exon boundaries can affect mRNA splicing and protein domain structure.
   - Nonsense mutations can block translation.
   - Point mutations, frameshift mutations, and deletions can lead to the production of abnormal proteins. Abnormal proteins may exhibit loss of function or gain of function. If the protein is part of a metabolic pathway, mutations can block synthesis of key components or lead to the buildup of intermediary metabolites. Gaucher disease is an example of a lysosomal storage disease in which macrophages accumulate glucosylceramide (an intermediary metabolite) because the appropriate glucosyl hydrolase is lacking.

46. **Explain the main features of autosomal dominant inheritance.**
   - Inheritance of one defective allele is sufficient to cause disease.
   - Males and females are affected equally because the defective allele resides on an autosome.
   - Children of a heterozygous parent have an approximately 50% chance of inheriting the disease.

- Unaffected children do not transmit disease to their offspring.
- If the disease interferes with reproductive capacity, most cases represent new mutations.
- Diseases may exhibit reduced penetrance and variable expressivity.
- Homozygous recessive individuals encountered (e.g., familial hypercholesterolemia). See Fig. 6-1.

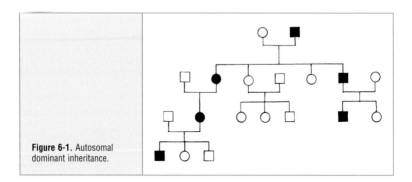

Figure 6-1. Autosomal dominant inheritance.

47. **Explain the concepts of reduced penetrance and variable expressivity.**
Penetrance refers to the percentage of individuals with a defective gene who actually show phenotypic manifestations of the disease. Some deleterious mutations remain silent (reduced penetrance) owing to the modifying effects of other genes and environmental conditions.
    Expressivity refers to variability in the clinical presentation or manifestation of disease.

48. **List the most common autosomal dominant diseases and their incidence.**
See Table 6-1.

TABLE 6-1. MAJOR AUTOSOMAL DOMINANT DISEASES AND THEIR INCIDENCE	
Disease	Frequency
Familial hypercholesterolemia	1:500
Adult polycystic kidney disease	1:1,000
Hereditary elliptocytosis	1:2,500
Neurofibromatosis type I	1:3,500
Hereditary spherocytosis	1:5,000
Ehlers–Danlos syndrome	1:5,000
von Willebrand disease	1:8,000
Familial adenomatous polyposis coli	1:10,000

49. **List the most common autosomal dominant disorders affecting the musculoskeletal system.**
See Table 6-2.

TABLE 6-2. MAJOR AUTOSOMAL DOMINANT DISORDERS AFFECTING THE MUSCULOSKELETAL SYSTEM

Disease	Frequency
Ehlers–Danlos syndrome type III	1:5,000
Myotonic dystrophy	1:7,000
Marfan syndrome	1:10,000
Osteogenesis imperfecta	1:10,000
Achondroplasia	1:15,000

50. **Explain why autosomal dominant diseases usually affect structural proteins and receptors rather than enzymes.**
Structural proteins and receptors are associated with dominant inheritance because they typically interact to form multimeric complexes. The presence of defective protein in patients with one mutant allele may be sufficient to render the entire complex nonfunctional. For example, patients with osteogenesis imperfecta synthesize an abnormal collagen chain that blocks the assembly of trimeric collagen fibrils. In contrast, enzymes are commonly associated with recessive inheritance because a 50% reduction in enzyme activity in patients with one mutant allele is typically corrected by increasing substrate concentration. Complete (100%) reduction in enzyme activity in patients with two mutant alleles cannot be corrected and is associated with clinical evidence of disease.

51. **What are the typical clinical features of Marfan syndrome?**
Marfan syndrome is an autosomal dominant disease associated with mutations in the gene coding for fibrillin-1. One third of cases are due to new mutations. Fibrillins are a family of collagen-like proteins that form microfibrils in the extracellular matrix. Microfibrils are thought to control the organization of elastin-rich fibers, which provide the resiliency of elastic tissues. Lack of fibrillin is associated with developmental abnormalities of the skeletal system, cardiovascular system, and eye.

- Patients with Marfan syndrome are typically tall and slender. Their fingers are thin and long (arachnodactyly), and they may exhibit a long skull (dolichocephaly). Additional skeletal manifestations include pectus excavatum, pectus carinatum, hyperextensible joints, and kyphoscoliosis. Patients are predisposed to dislocations and hernias.
- Cardiovascular disease is the most common cause of death in patients with Marfan syndrome. Without proper elasticity, the media of the ascending aorta weakens, leading to dilatation and dissecting aneurysm. Dilatation of the aortic ring may cause aortic regurgitation. Dissecting aneurysms may rupture into the peritoneal cavity or retroperitoneal space. Mitral valve prolapse and congestive heart failure are additional complications of Marfan syndrome.
- Dislocation of the lens is frequently seen because the ciliary zonules that suspend the lens are composed of fibrillin. Myopia and retinal detachment are additional complications.
- Without treatment, patients with Marfan syndrome die of cardiovascular disease by age 30 to 40. Proper treatment (blood pressure medication and aortic grafts) allows most patients to live a normal life span.

52. **What are the typical clinical features of Ehlers–Danlos syndrome?**
Ehlers–Danlos syndrome (EDS) comprises a group of autosomal dominant disorders associated with hyperelasticity and fragility of the skin. More than 10 types of EDS have been described. A common feature of all types is a defect in collagen, including defects in collagen synthesis,

secretion, and posttranslational modification. EDS types I through IV, VII, and X are associated with synthesis of an abnormal collagen protein. EDS types VI and IX are associated with defects in collagen processing enzymes (e.g., lysyl oxidase). EDS type IV (lack of collagen type III) is associated with the most life-threatening complications. Typical clinical features of EDS include:

- Skin hyperelasticity and fragility
- Joint hypermobility ("human pretzel")
- Bleeding diathesis
- Dehiscence of surgical incisions
- Spontaneous rupture of the large arteries, bowel, and gravid uterus (EDS type IV)
- Kyphoscoliosis and blindness (EDS type VI)
- Bladder rupture and skeletal abnormalities (EDS type IX)

53. **What are the typical clinical features of osteogenesis imperfecta?**
Osteogenesis imperfecta (brittle bone disease) is an autosomal dominant disease associated with mutations in the gene coding for collagen type I. Four subtypes are described:
- Type I infants appear normal at birth but develop multiple bone fractures during infancy. Children have blue sclera and develop hearing loss.
- Type II is usually fatal in utero or soon after birth.
- Type III is associated with short stature and skeletal deformities visible at birth.
- Type IV is similar to type I but shows a variable phenotype and normal sclera.

54. **What are the typical clinical features of neurofibromatosis?**
Neurofibromatosis (NF) type I is an autosomal dominant disease characterized clinically by the development of multiple, cutaneous neurofibromas. These benign tumors of Schwann cell origin are intimately associated with peripheral nerves. The NF1 gene encodes a GTPase activating protein, neurofibromin, which serves to suppress (switch off) the activity of the ras protein. Without neurofibromin, ras signaling leads to unrestrained cell proliferation and the development of benign polyclonal tumors. NF1 acts as a tumor suppressor gene in a manner similar to Rb, WT1, and p53. NF1 has a high mutation rate, and half of all cases are due to new (spontaneous) mutations. Clinicopathologic features of NF type 1 include:
- Multiple, cutaneous neurofibromas arising in late childhood
- Plexiform neurofibromas that infiltrate internally and cause disfigurement
- Neurofibrosarcomas arising in approximately 5% of patients
- Café-au-lait spots (light brown patches on the skin)
- Lisch nodules (pigmented nodules on the iris)
- Skeletal lesions, such as scoliosis and pseudarthrosis
- Mild mental impairment
- Risk of leukemia in children (>200 times normal)
    Neurofibromatosis type II (Central neurofibromatosis) This is a rare, autosomal dominant disease associated with mutations in the NF2 gene. The incidence of NF type II is 1 in 50,000, whereas the incidence of NF type I is 1/3500. Most patients with NF type 2 present with bilateral intracranial acoustic nerve schwannomas.

55. **What are the typical clinical features of achondroplasia?**
Achondroplastic dwarfism is a common autosomal dominant disease affecting epiphyseal chondroblast growth and differentiation. Patients have short limbs with a normal head and torso. The face is small with a bulging forehead, and the bridge of the nose is deeply indented. The pathogenesis of achondroplasia is related to gain-of-function mutations in the FGF-3 receptor. Constitutive activation of this growth factor receptor suppresses epiphyseal cartilage growth and prevents enchondral bone formation. Patients have normal intelligence and live a normal life span.

56. **What are the typical clinical features of familial hypercholesterolemia?**

Familial hypercholesterolemia is a common autosomal dominant disease associated with mutations in the gene for the low-density lipoprotein (LDL) receptor. Patients with familial hypercholesterolemia have high levels of LDL in the blood and exhibit increased rates of cholesterol deposition in arteries, tendons, and skin. The mean serum cholesterol level in heterozygotes is 350 mg/dL (normal, < 200 mg/dL), whereas the mean serum cholesterol level in rare homozygotes may be as high as 1000 mg/dL. Tissue macrophages internalize excess cholesterol and form nodules of lipid-rich "foam cells" in the skin (xanthomas) and arteries (atheromas).

Patients with familial hypercholesterolemia show evidence of accelerated atherosclerosis. Heterozygotes develop severe, atherosclerotic coronary artery disease by age 40. Most homozygotes die of myocardial infarction by age 30. Liver transplantation is an effective therapy for patients with familial hypercholesterolemia because LDL receptors are expressed primarily on the surface of hepatocytes.

Several classes of mutations are recognized on the basis of distinct biochemical mechanisms of disease:

- Class 1 mutations are the most common type and represent large deletions in the LDL receptor gene (i.e., null allele).
- Class 2 mutations prevent transport of the nascent LDL receptor polypeptide chain to the Golgi apparatus and cell surface.
- Class 3 mutations generate receptors on the cell surface that fail to bind LDL.
- Class 4 mutations allow LDL to bind to the receptor, but these receptors are unable to be clustered into coated pits and internalized by endocytosis.
- Class 5 mutations prevent recycling of the LDL receptor back to the membrane.

57. **Explain the main features of autosomal recessive inheritance.**

- Phenotype is present in homozygotes with two mutant alleles.
- Both parents are typically heterozygous carriers without symptoms.
- Twenty-five percent of the offspring of homozygous carriers are expected to be homozygotes with disease.
- Fifty percent of the offspring of heterozygous parents are expected to be heterozygotes and carriers of the mutant allele.
- Disease is transmitted by heterozygous carriers because most homozygotes die before reaching reproductive age.
- Disease phenotype is transmitted equally to males and females.
- Disease can occur in consanguineous matings because of increased carrier frequency.
- Recessive traits are commonly seen in children, whereas dominant traits are more commonly seen in adults.

See Fig. 6-2.

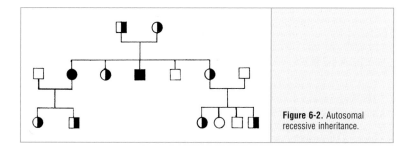

Figure 6-2. Autosomal recessive inheritance.

58. **Discuss the biochemical basis of autosomal recessive disorders.**

Autosomal recessive disorders are typically caused by mutations in enzymes that result in decreased production of a metabolic product and accumulation of an unmetabolized substrate.

Loss of one allele does not typically cause an abnormal phenotype because compensatory mechanisms can overcome an enzyme deficiency by increasing substrate concentration. However, compensatory mechanisms cannot overcome lack of enzyme activity in homozygotes with two mutant alleles. Thus diseases caused by an accumulation of unmetabolized substrate are typically associated with autosomal recessive inheritance.

59. List the most common autosomal recessive diseases and their incidence. See Table 6-3.

TABLE 6-3. MAJOR AUTOSOMAL RECESSIVE DISEASES AND THEIR INCIDENCE	
Disease	Frequency
Sickle cell anemia	High
Beta-thalassemia	High
Alpha-thalassemia	High
Hereditary hemochromatosis	1:400
Gaucher disease	1:1000
Myeloperoxidase deficiency	1:2000
Cystic fibrosis	1:2500

60. What are the typical clinical features of cystic fibrosis?
Cystic fibrosis (CF) is a common autosomal recessive disease associated with an abnormal chloride channel (cystic fibrosis transmembrane regulator) and impaired electrolyte transport in epithelial cells. Without chloride secretion, a viscid mucus forms in secretions in many organs in the body. As a result, patients with CF develop chronic pulmonary disease and CF of the exocrine pancreas. CF is diagnosed by measuring increased concentrations of electrolytes in the sweat (sweat chloride test). The skin of children with CF is said to "taste salty." CF is the most common autosomal recessive disease among the white population, with an estimated carrier frequency of 1 in 25. Clinical features of CF are most notable in the lungs, pancreas, gastrointestinal tract, and reproductive system.
- Chronic pulmonary disease is the most common cause of morbidity and mortality in patients with CF. Loss of the mucociliary ladder and airway obstruction are conducive to secondary infections, which cause chronic bronchitis, bronchopneumonia, lung abscesses, and bronchiectasis. The most common microorganisms found in the lungs of patients with CF are *Staphylococcus* and *Pseudomonas*. Patients develop respiratory failure and right-sided heart failure (cor pulmonale).
- Inspissated mucus causes most patients with CF to develop chronic pancreatitis and lose exocrine pancreatic function (i.e., loss of acinar cells and cystic fibrosis). Secondary biliary cirrhosis also occurs due to blockage of the biliary ducts.
- Small bowel obstruction (meconium ileus) is typically seen in infants with CF, due to lack of pancreatic enzymes and increased viscosity of the intestinal secretions. Malabsorption syndrome appears in early postnatal life. It presents with steatorrhea (foul-smelling, fatty stools), nutritional deficiencies, and growth retardation.
- Most males with CF are infertile due to fibrosis of the vas deferens, epididymis, and seminal vesicles. Most females are infertile due to amenorrhea and thickening of cervical mucous plugs.

61. List examples of inborn errors of amino acid metabolism.
- Phenylketonuria (PKU) is associated with mental retardation due to hyperphenylalaninemia.
- Tyrosinemia is associated with liver disease in patients with hypertyrosinemia.

- Alkaptonuria is associated with darkening of urine due to oxidation of homogentisic acid.
- Albinism is associated with hypopigmentation of skin due to insufficient synthesis of melanin.

62. **What are the typical clinical features of PKU?**
PKU is an autosomal recessive disease that can result (if untreated) in severe brain damage in infants and children. Brain damage is caused by increased blood levels of dietary phenylalanine (hyperphenylalaninemia) owing to a deficiency of phenylalanine hydroxylase in the liver. Phenylalanine is an essential amino acid that is normally obtained from the diet and oxidized in the liver to tyrosine by phenylalanine hydroxylase. In the absence of this liver enzyme, phenylalanine is converted to phenylketones. The name PKU derives from the fact that these phenylketones (e.g., phenylpyruvic acid) can be detected in the patient's urine.
Phenylalanine causes irreversible brain damage because it inhibits neurotransmitter synthesis and amino acid transport. This leads to a lack of neuronal development and defective myelin biosynthesis. Children with PKU are intellectually normal at birth. However, once phenylalanine is introduced into their diet, these infants exhibit irreversible mental retardation, with IQ levels dropping to 50 within 1 year. Children with PKU tend to exhibit blond hair and blue eyes because phenylalanine cannot be converted to tyrosine to form melanin. A "mousy" odor is also evident because of the formation of phenylacetic acid. Treatment of PKU involves elimination of phenylalanine from the diet.

63. **What are the typical clinical features of alkaptonuria?**
Alkaptonuria (ochronosis) is a rare autosomal recessive disease caused by mutations in the gene that encodes homogentisic acid oxidase. This enzyme deficiency blocks the metabolism of phenylalanine and leads to the accumulation of homogentisic acid in collagen-rich connective tissue throughout the body. Excretion of homogentisic acid causes the urine to darken upon standing (oxidation). Clinical features of alkaptonuria relate primarily to degenerative arthropathy caused by deposition of homogentisic acid in cartilage of the joints and vertebral column.

64. **What are the typical clinical features of albinism?**
Albinism comprises a group of hereditary disorders associated with hypopigmentation due to a defect in melanin biosynthesis. The most common form is oculocutaneous albinism (OCA), an autosomal recessive trait characterized by deficiency of melanin in the skin, hair follicles, and eyes. There are two major types:
- Tyrosinase-positive OCA is the most common type in both whites and blacks. The biochemical defect is unknown. Infants are born with complete albinism, but pigmentation increases with age.
- Tyrosinase-negative OCA is the second most common type of OCA. It is characterized by complete absence of tyrosinase. Tyrosinase converts tyrosine to form melanin. Therefore these patients lack melanin and exhibit snow-white hair, pink skin, blue eyes, and red pupils. These patients suffer from photophobia, strabismus, nystagmus, and decreased visual acuity. The incidence of squamous cell carcinoma is also increased.

65. **Explain the pathogenesis of lysosomal storage diseases.**
Lysosomal storage diseases comprise a large group of autosomal recessive traits (>40) characterized by the accumulation of unmetabolized substrates within lysosomes. These diseases are caused by mutations in genes that encode lysosomal acid hydrolases or their activating proteins. Without a catabolic enzyme, lysosomes swell with unmetabolized substrate, and cellular functions are eventually impaired. Macromolecular substrates are derived either from cellular components (autophagy) or extracellular sources (heterophagy). Lysosomal storage diseases are classified according to the type of material that is stored. Major categories include sphingolipidoses, mucopolysaccharidoses, and glycogenoses.

66. **List examples of lysosomal storage diseases.**
    Sphingolipidoses
    - Gaucher disease
    - Tay–Sachs disease
    - Niemann–Pick disease
    Mucopolysaccharidoses
    - Hurler disease (It is caused by deficiency of iduronidase and storage of unmetabolized dermatan or heparan sulfate. It presents with skeletal deformities, dwarfism, and mental retardation.)
    - Hunter disease (It is caused by deficiency of iduronate sulfatase and storage of unmetabolized dermatan or heparan sulfate.)
    Glycogenosis
    - Pompe disease (It is caused by deficiency of alpha-glucosidase and storage of glycogen.)

67. **What are the typical clinical features of Tay–Sachs disease?**
    Tay–Sachs disease is an autosomal recessive disease characterized by the inability to degrade ganglioside GM2 owing to a deficiency of N-acetyl-galactosaminidase (hexosaminidase). Ganglioside GM2 is abundant in cells of the central nervous system and accumulates within the lysosomes of neurons and macrophages. Clinical features of Tay–Sachs disease include a cherry-red spot on the retina, blindness, and mental retardation. This disease is common among Jews of East European ancestry (Ashkenazi), for whom the carrier frequency is approximately 1 in 30. Tay–Sachs disease presents in infancy (6–10 months) with mental and motor retardation. Seizures and blindness follow. Most children with Tay–Sachs disease die before age 4 years.

68. **What are the typical clinical features of Gaucher disease?**
    Gaucher disease is an autosomal recessive disease characterized by mutations in the gene for glucocerebrosidase. Glucosylceramide (cerebroside) is derived from the degradation of glycosphingolipids, which are abundant in the plasma membranes of neurons and blood cells. Cerebroside is cleaved to glucose and free ceramide by the action of glucocerebrosidase. Deficiency of this enzyme results in the accumulation of cerebroside in lysosomes of phagocytic cells throughout the body. There are two major forms of Gaucher disease: type I (adult onset) and type II (infantile). Type I is the most common form of Gaucher disease (99% of cases). It is a chronic disease that primarily affects the spleen and bone. Typical clinical features include hepatosplenomegaly, pancytopenia, thrombocytopenia, bone pain, and bone fractures. Macrophages engorged with stored lipid (Gaucher cells) can be seen in the spleen, liver, lymph nodes, and bone marrow. Infants with rare type II Gaucher disease show a complete absence of glucocerebrosidase enzyme activity. These infants suffer progressive central nervous system degeneration and early death.

69. **What are the typical clinical features of mucopolysaccharide storage diseases (mucopolysaccharidoses)?**
    Mucopolysaccharidoses comprise a group of autosomal recessive diseases of glycosaminoglycan metabolism. Glycosaminoglycans are high-molecular-weight polysaccharides associated with proteoglycans. They include dermatan sulfate, keratan sulfate, chondroitin sulfate, and heparan sulfate. These macromolecules are especially abundant in the ground substance of connective tissue. Mucopolysaccharidoses are chronic diseases affecting the liver, spleen, bone marrow, blood vessels, and heart. Clinical features include coarse facial features, joint stiffness, and mental retardation. Congestive heart failure and myocardial infarction are important causes of death.

70. **What are the typical clinical features of glycogen storage diseases (glycogenoses)?**
    Glycogenoses comprise a group of autosomal recessive diseases of glycogen metabolism. Glycogen is a highly branched polymer of glucose that is broken down enzymatically to yield free

sugars for energy production via glycolysis. Clinical features of glycogenoses vary greatly according to the specific enzyme deficiency, from organ-specific to systemic disease. Some enzyme defects cause hepatomegaly and hypoglycemia, whereas other enzyme defects are associated with muscle cramping after exercise.

71. Explain the main features of X-linked recessive inheritance.
    - The disease occurs only in males.
    - Heterozygous females are carriers without evidence of disease.
    - Sons of women who are carriers have a 50% chance of inheriting the disease.
    - Daughters of women who are carriers are asymptomatic, but 50% are expected to be carriers of the disease.
    - Daughters of affected fathers are all asymptomatic carriers.
    - Sons of affected fathers are free of the trait and cannot transmit the disease to their offspring.
    - Symptomatic homozygous females result only from the rare mating of an affected male with an asymptomatic carrier female.

    See Fig. 6-3.

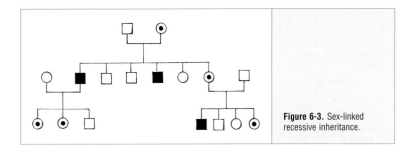

Figure 6-3. Sex-linked recessive inheritance.

72. List the most common X-linked recessive diseases and their incidence.
    See Table 6-4.

TABLE 6-4. MAJOR X-LINKED RECESSIVE DISEASES AND THEIR INCIDENCE	
Disease	Frequency in Males
Fragile X syndrome	1:1,000
Duchenne-Becker muscular dystrophy	1:3,500
Hemophilia A (factor VIII deficiency)	1:10,000
Lesch–Nyhan syndrome (HPRT deficiency)	1:10,000

73. What are the typical clinical features of muscular dystrophy?
    Muscular dystrophy is a common X-linked recessive disease caused by mutations in the gene encoding dystrophin. Dystrophin is a cytoskeletal protein that links muscle cells to laminin in the extracellular matrix. Defects in dystrophin lead to membrane damage and muscle cell necrosis. Small deletions in the N-terminal domain of dystrophin lead to mild disease symptoms (Becker type), whereas large deletions in the C-terminal domain lead to the more severe Duchenne type. Clinical features of Duchenne muscular dystrophy include muscle weakness (first evident in toddlers), pseudohypertrophy of calf muscles, cardiomyopathy, and progressive decline in IQ. Congestive heart failure is a common cause of death. Mean age at death is 17 years.

74. **What are the typical clinical features of hemophilia A?**
    Hemophilia A is an X-linked recessive disease caused by mutations in the gene encoding clotting factor VIII. Without this clotting factor, patients exhibit spontaneous bleeding into joints and internal organs. Disease symptoms vary from mild to severe depending on the amount of clotting factor activity in the blood. Complications of hemophilia include deforming arthritis, hematuria, intestinal obstruction, and respiratory decline. Treatment of hemophilia with clotting factor isolated from pooled human blood led to the transmission of HIV during the early years of the acquired immunodeficiency syndrome pandemic. Patients are now treated effectively and safely with recombinant clotting factors, which do not carry a risk of transmitting infectious disease.

75. **What are the typical clinical features of fragile X syndrome?**
    Fragile X syndrome is an X-linked recessive disease associated with expansion of a trinucleotide repeat (CGC) within the FM1 gene. This mutation results in the creation of an inducible fragile site that can be readily observed by karyotype analysis (light microscopy). Fragile X syndrome is the second most common cause of mental retardation after Down syndrome. It affects approximately 1 in 1250 males and 1 in 2500 females. Clinical signs and symptoms of fragile X syndrome in males include:
    - Increased head circumference and facial coarsening
    - Joint hyperextensibility
    - Enlarged testes (macro-orchidism)
    - Abnormalities of the heart valves
    - Mental retardation with IQ scores between 20 and 60

76. **How is fragile X syndrome inherited?**
    Although this syndrome represents a single gene defect, it exhibits nonclassical inheritance:
    - Approximately 20% of males with a fragile X site are phenotypically normal and serve as nonsymptomatic carriers.
    - Approximately 50% of heterozygous (carrier) females exhibit some degree of mental retardation. This feature may relate to patterns of X inactivation during embryogenesis.
    - Clinical symptoms often increase as the trait is passed from generation to generation. This feature, referred to as *anticipation,* is thought to be due to progressive expansion of the trinucleotide repeat during maternal meiosis. The severity of clinical symptoms is related to the number of trinucleotide repeats.

MITOCHONDRIAL INHERITANCE

77. **How do mutations in mitochondrial genes cause systemic disease?**
    Mitochondria are primordial symbionts in eukaryotic cells that generate adenosine triphosphate (ATP) through electron transport and oxidative phosphorylation. Mitochondria contain their own circular DNA, which accounts for approximately 1% of the human genome. Because sperm do not contribute mitochondria to the egg during fertilization, all mitochondrial genes (and diseases) are inherited from the mother. Mutations that interfere with ATP biosynthesis principally affect tissues with high energy requirements (e.g., the central nervous system, heart, and skeletal muscle).

78. **List diseases caused by mutations in mitochondrial genes.**
    - Leber hereditary optic neuropathy
    - Kearns–Sayre syndrome
    - Myoclonus epilepsy with ragged red fibers (MERRF) syndrome

GENETIC IMPRINTING

79. **What is genetic imprinting?**
Genetic imprinting refers to the fact that some diseases show phenotypic differences depending on whether they are inherited from the mother or the father. During meiosis, male and female genes are "imprinted" with instructions for expression during development. These instructions are complementary so that normal development only occurs when a male and female pronucleus combine. The biochemical basis for this phenomenon is believed to be methylation of cytosine-guanine base pairs within the GC-rich promoter regions of developmentally regulated genes. This epigenetic phenomenon results in the reversible silencing of transcription. Mutations in imprinted genes do not follow classical rules of Mendelian inheritance.

80. **List examples of diseases associated with defects in genetic imprinting.**
Phenotype associated with paternal inheritance:
   - Prader–Willi syndrome (hypotonia, obesity, hypogonadism, and mental retardation)
   - Familial glomus tumor (painful tumor of endothelial cell origin)
   Phenotype associated with maternal inheritance:
   - Angelman syndrome (hyperactivity, inappropriate laughter, and seizures)
   - Fragile X syndrome (mental retardation, facial coarsening)

MULTIFACTORIAL INHERITANCE

81. **Explain the main features of multifactorial inheritance.**
Most human traits (e.g., body height and intelligence) do not follow classical rules of Mendelian inheritance. These traits, and most chronic diseases, are determined by the interaction of multiple genes with a wide variety of environmental factors. Principal features of polygenic inheritance include the following:
   - The degree of clinical symptoms is directly proportional to the number of mutant genes.
   - Close relatives have a greater chance of showing symptoms because they share more mutant genes. The risk in first-degree relatives is estimated to be 5% to 10%.
   - Environmental factors influence the expression of clinical symptoms.
   - The risk is doubled if older siblings show symptoms of disease.
   - The more severe the symptoms, the greater the risk of transmitting this trait to offspring.
   - Some diseases show sex predilection (e.g., congenital pyloric stenosis occurs 5 times more frequently in males than females).

82. **List common polygenic diseases.**
   - Cleft lip and cleft palate
   - Neural tube defects (e.g., anencephaly, meningomyelocele, and spina bifida)
   - Diabetes mellitus type II
   - Hypertension
   - Psychiatric disorders (e.g., manic depression and schizophrenia)
   - Congenital heart disease
   - Atherosclerosis
   - Pyloric stenosis
   - Gout

DIAGNOSIS OF GENETIC DISORDERS

83. **List the principal methods used for prenatal diagnosis of genetic disorders.**
Methods for prenatal diagnosis of genetic disease require the isolation of fetal cells, followed by analysis of DNA. Methods for collecting embryonic or fetal cells include:

- Preimplantation embryo dissection to remove a single blastomere
- Amniocentesis to obtain fetal skin cells exfoliated in the amniotic fluid
- Chorionic villus biopsy to obtain extraembryonic fetal cells in the placenta
- Umbilical cord blood sampling to collect nucleated fetal blood cells

Preimplantation genetic diagnosis is an emerging technology that is currently offered at more than 50 fertility clinics worldwide. Removal of a blastomere from an eight-cell preimplantation embryo does not perturb embryogenesis and permits identification of genetic diseases before embryo transfer to the mother. Thus preimplantation genetic diagnosis can be used to select healthy embryos (i.e., embryos lacking lethal mutations) before implantation.

Principal methods used for the prenatal diagnosis of genetic diseases include the following:

- Karyotype analysis is used to identify chromosomal abnormalities. Cells are cultured in the presence of growth factors to induce mitosis and then treated with colchicine to obtain metaphase chromosome spreads. Metaphase chromosomes are stained with special dyes (e.g., Giemsa) to reveal unique banding patterns and then examined under high magnification for structural and numerical chromosomal abnormalities.
- FISH analysis is used to mark chromosomes and identify specific gene mutations, including deletions, translocations, and point mutations. DNA probes that are tagged with fluorescent dyes hybridize with specific DNA sequences, thereby "painting" chromosomes and marking specific gene mutations. Unlike karyotype analysis, FISH analysis can be applied to interphase nuclei.

84. **Discuss the role of molecular biology in the diagnosis and investigation of genetic disorders.**

Recombinant DNA techniques are used routinely to identify single gene mutations. The sensitivity of these methods has been dramatically improved by the use of the polymerase chain reaction (PCR), through which DNA and RNA samples can be amplified several million–fold. Molecular biology (molecular diagnostics) can be used to:

- Identify known point mutations, translocations, and deletions
- Infer mutations on the basis of restriction fragment length polymorphisms
- Investigate the pathogenesis of genetic diseases; for example, it can be used to:
  - Clone genes using direct and positional cloning methods (Direct methods rely on an understanding of the abnormal gene product [e.g., abnormal globin in patients with thalassemias]. Positional cloning relies on insights concerning the location of a gene on a particular chromosome.)
  - Produce pure proteins through recombinant DNA technology (e.g., human clotting factors for hemophiliacs)
  - Analyze patterns of gene expression using DNA chip technology (By analyzing the expression of thousands of genes, researchers can gain insights into the role of the entire genome in controlling cellular and organismal phenotype.)

WEBSITES

1. http://www.ncbi.nlm.nih.gov/entrez/query.fcgi?db=PubMed
2. http://www-medlib.med.utah.edu/WebPath/webpath.html#MENU
3. http://medgen.genetics.utah.edu/thumbnails.htm
4. http://www.ncbi.nlm.nih.gov/disease/index.html

BIBLIOGRAPHY

1. Bahado-Singh R, Cheng CC, Matta P, et al: Combined serum and ultrasound screening for detection of fetal aneuploidy. Semin Perinatol 27:145–151, 2003.

2. Berkowitz GS, Papiernik E: Epidemiology of preterm birth. Epidemiol Rev 15:414–443, 1993.

3. Clayton-Smith J: Genomic imprinting as a cause of disease. BMJ 327:1121–1122, 2003.

4. Leonard JV, Morris AAM: Inborn errors of metabolism around time of birth. Lancet 356:583–587, 2000.

5. Meikle PJ, Hoopwood JJ, Clague AE, Carey WF: Prevalence of lysosomal storage diseases. JAMA 281:249–254, 1999.

6. Mennuti MT, Driscoll DA: Screening for Down's syndrome—too many choices? N Engl J Med 349:1471–1473, 2003.

7. Wald NJ, Watt HC, Hackshaw AK: Integrated screening for Down's syndrome based on tests performed during the first and second trimesters. N Engl J Med 341:461–467, 1999.

THE BLOOD VESSELS

Ivan Damjanov, MD, PhD

CHAPTER 7

1. **What are the most important diseases of the blood vessels?**
    - Arteriosclerosis, which includes changes induced by aging and hypertension
    - Atherosclerosis, a multifactorial disease
    - Vasculitis, an inflammatory disease that occurs in several clinicopathologic forms
    - Varicose veins
    - Vascular tumors

2. **Do vascular diseases occur at any age?**
    Yes, but they occur most often in the elderly.

3. **What are the consequences of vascular diseases?**
    The most important consequences include disturbances of blood flow, such as hypoxia and infarction.

ARTERIOSCLEROSIS

4. **What is the difference between arteriosclerosis and atherosclerosis?**
    Arteriosclerosis is a generic term used for hardening of arteries and arterioles. Atherosclerosis is a multifactorial disease of arteries affected by atheromas.
    It should be noted that atherosclerosis affects only the aorta and its major branches. Arteriosclerosis may involve any artery in the body and also may affect arterioles.

5. **List some causes of arteriosclerosis.**
    - Atherosclerosis is the most common cause of hardening of the aorta and the major arteries providing blood to the heart, brain, and intestines.
    - Mönckeberg medial calcific sclerosis is characterized by idiopathic calcification of the media of muscular arteries. It is of limited clinical significance. For example, calcification of mammary arteries may be seen in mammograms and may be confused with calcification related to breast cancer.
    - Arteriolosclerosis is a multifactorial disease related to aging. It can be accelerated by hypertension and diabetes.

6. **What are the histologic features of arteriolosclerosis?**
    Arteriolosclerosis occurs in two histologic forms:
    - **Hyaline arteriolosclerosis:** It is characterized by thickening of the arteriolar wall due to the accumulation of homogeneous material that stains pink in hematoxylin and eosin-stained slides. The nature of this hyaline is unknown. Hyaline arteriolosclerosis is typically found in the kidneys of patients who have diabetes mellitus or benign arterial hypertension.
    - **Hyperplastic arteriolosclerosis:** It is characterized by thickening of the arteriolar wall due to the concentric proliferation of smooth muscle cells, giving the arterioles an "onion skin" appearance. These changes represent an adaptive response of arterioles to severe ("malignant") hypertension. Arteriolar damage caused by sudden onset of malignant hypertension may cause fibrinoid necrosis.

ATHEROSCLEROSIS

7. **What is the hallmark lesion of atherosclerosis?**
It is called atheroma, a term derived from the Greek word for porridge and a suffix, *-oma,* used to denote tumors (e.g., melanoma) and other tumefactions (e.g., hematoma).

8. **How does a typical atheroma appear?**
A typical atheroma appears as an induration of the vessel's wall. In an aorta opened at autopsy, it looks like a yellow bump or elevation of the intima. On cross-sectioning, it consists of a soft, lipid-rich center covered with a fibrotic capsule. Atheromas are often partially calcified.

KEY POINTS: ARTERIOSCLEROSIS AND ATHEROSCLEROSIS ✓

1. Arteriosclerosis, a generic term for hardening of the arteries and arterioles, is used for several chronic arterial diseases, the most important of which are atherosclerosis and hypertension.

2. Atherosclerosis is a multifactorial disease characterized by formation of atheromas.

3. Risk factors, classified as those that can and those that cannot be modified, accelerate the formation of atheromas.

4. The reaction to injury hypothesis provides the best explanation for the pathogenesis of atherosclerosis, but other theories may also elucidate some aspects of this disease.

9. **What are the earliest recognizable lesions of atherosclerosis?**
Experimental data and autopsy studies indicate that atherosclerosis may begin in two ways: as a fat streak or an intimal smooth muscle cell mass.
   - **Fatty streaks:** Fatty streaks develop from lipid that enters the blood vessel wall from the plasma. This insudation leads to the deposition of lipids in the stroma of the blood vessel, where it is oxidized by free oxygen radicals released from macrophages. Oxidized lipids are taken up by macrophages and smooth muscle cells, which transform into fat-laden foam cells. Accumulation of extracellular and intracellular lipids in the intima accounts for the appearance of fatty streaks that are visible to the naked eye as well as histologically in freshly frozen arteries sectioned with a cryostat.
   - **Intimal smooth muscle cell masses:** These masses are formed from medial smooth muscle cells that grow into the intima. This sequence of events can be induced in animals, and if animals are fed a lipid-rich diet, the smooth muscle cells become lipidized, contributing to the formation of fat streaks. Similar intimal smooth muscle cell masses are seen in humans at the site of arterial branching or bifurcation. It is assumed that these intimal cushions develop in response to injury caused by turbulent blood flow as it passes from one vessel into another of smaller caliber.

10. **What happens to fully developed atheromas in the human aorta?**
Atheromas may remain unchanged for extended periods of time, and there is evidence that in certain circumstances they can even regress. However, in most cases atheromas will evolve further and show a number of secondary complications, including:
   - **Expansion:** Enlarging atheromas become confluent, and ultimately the entire aorta is covered with atherosclerotic lesions.

- **Fibrosis and calcification:** Scarring transforms "soft" atheromas into "firm" atheromas, which calcify and become extremely hard and brittle.
- **Ulceration and thrombosis:** Rupture of the fibrous cap will typically release all the semiliquid material from the central portion of the atheroma. Because this material contains thromboplastin, it will trigger blood clotting, and a thrombus will develop at the site of intimal ulceration.
- **Aneurysmatic dilatation:** Atheromas may weaken the vessel wall by destroying the elastic tissue and the smooth muscles that maintain the integrity of the normal aorta. Under the influence of blood pressure, such weakened vessel walls will bulge outside and form an aneurysm.

11. **How do atheromas cause infarcts?**
    - **Thrombotic occlusion of arteries:** Thrombi that form over an ulcerated atheroma may occlude the blood vessel and thus interrupt the blood flow through it. This typically occurs in coronary or cerebral arteries.
    - **Thromboemboli:** Thrombi formed over ulcerated aortic atheromas are not large enough to interrupt the blood flow, and such thrombi do not cause infarcts. However, fragments of aortic thrombi may detach and form emboli, which can cause obstruction of smaller peripheral arteries.
    - **Cholesterol emboli:** Cholesterol crystals released into the arterial circulation during rupture of an aortic atheroma may cause a "shower" of small emboli and numerous microscopic infarcts in various tissue distal to the ruptured atheroma.
    - **Release of thromboplastin:** Thromboplastin released from atheromas may precipitate intravascular coagulation and formation of multiple microthrombi. Such a "localized" disseminated coagulation (DIC) may also cause infarcts by occluding arterioles and capillaries.

12. **What are the risk factors for atherosclerosis?**
    Risk factors can be classified as major or minor. Major factors can be further subdivided into those that are fixed (unavoidable) and those that can be modified.
    - Major fixed risk factors include age, male gender, family history of atherosclerosis, and genetic defects in the metabolism of lipids.
    - Major risk factors that can be modified include hypertension, hyperlipidemia, diabetes, and smoking.
    - Minor risk factors (i.e., factors that contribute to atherosclerosis but on their own have not been proved to cause the disease) are a diet rich in saturated fats and carbohydrates, obesity, physical inactivity, type A personality, and stress.
    The most important risk factors for atherosclerosis are included in the mnemonic *atheroma*:
    - **A**rterial hypertension
    - **T**obacco
    - **H**eredity (familial hypercholesterolemia)
    - **E**ndocrine (diabetes, postmenopausal estrogen deficiency, and hypothyroidism)
    - **R**educed physical activity (sedentary life)
    - **O**besity
    - **M**ale gender
    - **A**ge

13. **What is the evidence that hypertension is a major risk factor for atherosclerosis?**
    - **Epidemiologic evidence:** Hypertension is the most important risk factor for atherosclerosis in people older than 45 years. Such people have a 5 times higher incidence of ischemic heart disease than normotensive age-matched control subjects.
    - **Therapeutic trials:** Treatment of hypertension reduces the risk of atherosclerosis.

14. **What is the evidence that hyperlipidemia is a major risk factor for atherosclerosis?**
    - **Epidemiologic evidence:** Hyperlipidemia and especially hypercholesterolemia are the most important risk factors in people younger than age 45 years. Hypercholesterolemia is associated with accelerated development of atherosclerotic lesions, which appear earlier in life and are more pronounced than in people who have normal cholesterol blood levels.
    - **Genetic studies:** Genetic disorders involving various aspects of lipid metabolism are associated with severe atherosclerosis. For example, in familial hypercholesterolemia, an autosomal dominant disease, homozygotes are much more affected than heterozygotes. Homozygotes, who have blood cholesterol concentrations in the range of 600 to 1000 mg/dL, show first clinical signs of atherosclerosis by the time of puberty and if untreated will die by the time they reach 20 years. Heterozygotes, who have cholesterol levels ranging from 250 to 500 mg/dL, develop signs of atherosclerosis by age 40 years.
    - **Pathologic studies:** Atheromas contain large amounts of cholesterol, which presumably plays a role in the evolution of arterial lesions.
    - **Experimental data:** Animals given a high-cholesterol diet develop atherosclerosis more often than those fed a normal diet.
    - **Therapeutic data:** The treatment of hypercholesterolemia can slow the development of atherosclerotic lesions.

15. **How do various lipoproteins contribute to hypercholesterolemia?**
    Low-density lipoprotein (LDL) is the main determinant of the total cholesterol concentration.

16. **What are lipoproteins, and how are they classified?**
    Lipoproteins are spherical particles composed of apoproteins, phospholipids, cholesterol and cholesteryl esthers, and triglycerides. The concentration of cholesterol in various lipoproteins varies, but approximately 70% of total blood cholesterol is contained in low-density lipoproteins (LDL).
    Major classes of lipoproteins can be distinguished by ultracentrifugation of plasma:
    - High-density lipoproteins (HDLs), which contain less than 25% cholesterol, sediment the fastest.
    - LDLs, which contain 70% cholesterol, form a band just above the HDLs.
    - Very low-density lipoproteins (VLDLs), which contain 60% endogenous triglycerides and 25% cholesterol, form a band above the LDLs.
    - Chylomicrons, which contain 90% dietary triglycerides and 10% cholesterol, are the biggest particles that float on the top of the centrifuged plasma.

17. **List the key facts about lipoproteins.**
    - Chylomicrons are formed in the small intestine. Their main function is to transport lipids from the gastrointestinal tract. Lipoprotein lipase of endothelial cells acts on chylomicrons, releasing from them some triglycerides, which enter peripheral fat tissue and muscles. Chylomicron remnants containing cholesterol and the remaining triglycerides are taken up by the liver.
    - VLDLs secreted by the liver into the circulation carry triglycerides and cholesterol from the liver into the periphery. Lipoprotein lipase acts on VLDLs, releasing triglycerides that enter fat cells and other cells, leaving behind intermediate-density lipoproteins (IDLs), which are short-lived lipoproteins that transform into LDLs.
    - LDLs are the main vehicle for the transport of cholesterol from the liver to the peripheral cells. LDL is removed from blood by receptors on the surface of many cells, such as smooth muscle cells, fibroblasts, and adrenal cortical cells. LDL receptors are expressed on the surface of liver cells, which are instrumental in removing LDL from blood and reinserting it into the intermediary metabolism in the liver cell.

- HDLs are synthesized by the liver and the small intestine. They represent the main reservoir of apoproteins. In addition to donating apoproteins for the synthesis of other lipoproteins, HDLs are important carriers of cholesterol, transporting it from the peripheral tissues into the liver for excretion from the body in bile.

18. **What is the difference between "good" and "bad" lipoprotein?**
In common parlance, HDL is called good lipoprotein, and LDL is called bad lipoprotein. Approximately 70% of total blood cholesterol is contained in LDL. A high concentration of LDL has been associated with an increased risk of atherosclerosis, whereas high levels of HDL reduce this risk. HDLs mobilize the cholesterol from the periphery and are instrumental in its transport to the liver for excretion from the body.

19. **How could one raise HDL levels in blood?**
Exercise and alcohol in moderate amounts raise HDL, whereas smoking and obesity lower it. Exercise also reduces blood triglycerides, probably by increasing the activity of lipoprotein lipase.

20. **How are hyperlipoproteinemias classified?**
Hyperlipoproteinemias are classified into five groups on the basis of laboratory findings. Each group includes congenital and acquired hyperlipoproteinemias. The most common among these five groups are type II hyperlipoproteinemia, characterized by an increased concentration of LDL, and type IV hyperlipoproteinemia, characterized by an increased concentration of VLDL and low HDL.
  - **Type II hyperlipoproteinemia:** It is characterized by marked hypercholesterolemia. It includes several genetic diseases, such as familial hypercholesterolemia due to mutation of the gene for the LDL receptor and some diseases that may lead to the elevation of LDL and cholesterol. Secondary causes include cholesterol-rich diet, biliary tract obstruction, nephrotic syndrome, and hypothyroidism. Type II hyperlipoproteinemia is a major risk factor for coronary heart disease.
  - **Type IV hyperlipoproteinemia:** It is the most common form of hyperlipidemia, marked by hypertriglyceridemia and moderate hypercholesterolemia. It includes several genetic disorders of lipid metabolism, but more often it is secondary to another disorder. Secondary causes include alcohol abuse, diabetes, exogenous and endogenous steroids, oral contraceptives, pregnancy, and stress in general. It poses a moderate risk for coronary heart disease.

21. **How does hypertension promote atherosclerosis?**
Epidemiologic evidence indicates that hypertension promotes development of atherosclerosis, but the exact mechanism of this effect is not understood. In experimental animals, hypertension promotes the formation of smooth muscle cells and the insudation of lipid into the vessel wall. It may also cause endothelial cell injury. Injured endothelial cells may be more permeable to lipids. At the same time, they may also lose their capacity to control the proliferation of smooth muscle cells after vascular wall injury.
  It should be noted that hypertension affects smaller blood vessels and arterioles as well. Even pulmonary hypertension is accompanied by the appearance of fatty streaks in lung arteries. In normal circumstances, the pulmonary artery is not affected by atherosclerosis, in part because of low blood pressure inside this blood vessel.

22. **Besides lipoproteins, are there any other clinical laboratory findings that could predict development of atherosclerosis and some of its major complications?**
Clinical studies have identified a number of laboratory findings that are abnormal in people suffering from coronary heart disease and other complications of advanced atherosclerosis.

These tests may be used as predictors of coronary artery disease. The most promising tests under study are those measuring blood levels of:

- C-reactive protein
- Homocysteine
- Lipoprotein Lp(a)
- Plasminogen activator inhibitor-1
- Apolipoprotein E

23. **What are the most popular theories of atherosclerosis?**

Atherosclerosis is a multifactorial disease, and its pathogenesis is not fully understood. There is no theory that explains fully the pathogenesis of this disease. The following are the most important hypotheses:

- **Insudation hypothesis:** This hypothesis takes into account the fact that hypercholesterolemia plays a major role in atherogenesis. This hypothesis postulates that the insudation of lipid from the blood represents the primary event that ultimately leads to atherosclerosis.
- **Hemodynamic hypothesis:** This hypothesis is based on the fact that hypertension plays an important role in atherogenesis. Hemodynamic stress may cause endothelial injury and also promote the proliferation of smooth muscle cells in the injured intima. Hypertension also promotes the insudation of lipids.
- **Coagulopathy hypothesis:** This hypothesis postulates that the clotting abnormalities and adhesion of platelets to the endothelium initiate changes that will ultimately lead to the formation of atheromas. Indeed, platelets attached to the endothelium release a number of potentially damaging factors, including platelet-derived growth factor (PDGF), which stimulates the proliferation of smooth muscle cells. Preventive intake of aspirin, a drug that blocks the adhesion of platelets to the endothelium, may prevent the development of atherosclerosis.
- **Monoclonal proliferation hypothesis:** Cell biologists have discovered that the intimal cell masses consist of smooth muscle cells that are monoclonal (i.e., all derived from the same precursors). In this respect, these lesions resemble tumors. It is conceivable that atheromas and tumors have the same pathogenesis and are caused by the same growth-promoting factors. It is well known that growth factors, such as PDGF and basic fibroblast growth factor, have properties equivalent to viral and cellular oncogenes, but there is not enough evidence that atherosclerosis is a neoplastic disease.
- **Unifying reaction to injury hypothesis:** This hypothesis is the most popular explanation of atherogenesis.

24. **How does science explain the pathogenesis of atherosclerosis according to the reaction to injury hypothesis?**

According to this hypothesis, atherosclerotic lesions develop through several distinct phases (Fig. 7-1):

- Endothelial injury may be induced by mechanical, metabolic, and other adverse influences.
- Endothelial dysfunction or death results from the initial injury. Dysfunctional endothelial cells are presumably more permeable to lipids and other metabolites and have lost their capacity to control the growth of smooth muscle cells or interact with macrophages. Insudation of lipid and an invasion of the vessel wall by macrophages may ensue.
- Accumulation and attachment of platelets to the vessel wall: platelets degranulate, releasing growth factors and permeability factors, and also help recruit macrophages into the site of vascular injury.
- Proliferation of smooth muscle cells results in their ingrowth into the intima.
- Oxidation of lipids deposited in the stroma: macrophages releasing reactive free oxygen radicals play an important role in this process.
- Uptake of oxidized lipids into the cytoplasm of macrophages and smooth muscle cells results in the formation of foam cells.

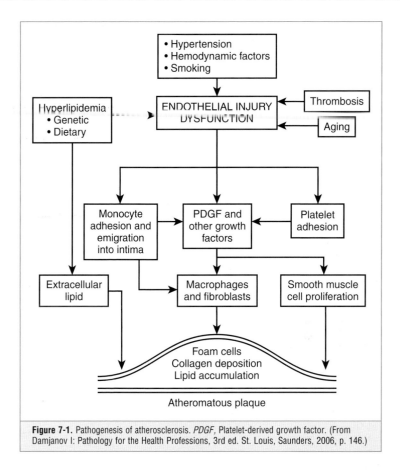

Figure 7-1. Pathogenesis of atherosclerosis. *PDGF,* Platelet-derived growth factor. (From Damjanov I: Pathology for the Health Professions, 3rd ed. St. Louis, Saunders, 2006, p. 146.)

- Foam cells die and release cell debris, enzymes, and lipids that form the semiliquid core of atheromas.
- Smooth muscle cells change their phenotype and become collagen-producing cells that form the capsule of atheroma.

25. **What are the main clinical manifestations of atherosclerosis?**
    - **Aorta—loss of elasticity contributes to hypertension:** Aneurysms develop most prominently in the abdominal aorta. Thrombi over ulcerated atheromas serve as a cause of thromboemboli. Cholesterol emboli result from ruptured atheromas.
    - **Coronary arteries—progressive narrowing causes ischemic heart disease:** Sudden occlusion by thrombi over an ulcerated atheroma causes infarct.
    - **Carotid arteries—narrowing causes cerebral ischemia:** Thrombi and ulcerated lesions give rise to cerebral and ocular infarcts.
    - **Cerebral arteries—stroke resulting from cerebral infarcts:** Transient ischemic attack and multiinfarct dementia result from slowly progressing atherosclerosis involving more than one blood vessel.
    - **Major intestinal arteries—ischemic bowel disease results from progressive narrowing:** Acute obstruction leads to massive intestinal infarcts.

- **Renal artery stenosis:** Renal ischemia is associated with reduced renal function and hypersecretion of renin and hypertension.
- **Iliac, femoral, and popliteal arteries:** Intermittent claudication or ischemic gangrene is seen.

HYPERTENSION

26. **How is hypertension defined?**
Hypertension is defined clinically as elevation of systolic pressure over 140 mmHg and diastolic pressure over 90 mmHg.

27. **What are the determinants of blood pressure?**
Blood pressure depends on the cardiac output and peripheral resistance. Blood pressure may result from increasing the cardiac output or peripheral vascular resistance:
- **Factors increasing cardiac output:** Increased heart rate (hyperthyroidism); water and sodium retention
- **Factors increasing peripheral resistance:** Neural alpha-adrenergic effect on arterioles; catecholamines, angiotensin II, aldosterone, and atrial natriuretic factor

28. **What is the difference between primary and secondary hypertension?**
The cause of primary hypertension (also known as idiopathic or essential hypertension) is not known. It accounts for 95% of all cases of hypertension. Secondary hypertension can be related to an underlying disease. In most instances, secondary hypertension is related to diseases of the kidneys, endocrine glands, neural disorders, and diseases of the aorta.
   To remember causes of secondary hypertension, use the mnemonic *renal*:
- **R**enal
- **E**ndocrine (adrenal cortical hyperfunction, pheochromocytoma, and hyperthyroidism)
- **N**eurologic (intracranial hypertension caused by brain tumor and encephalitis)
- **A**ortic (atherosclerotic rigidity of the aorta and coarctation)
- **L**abile (psychogenic, stress related, and postoperative)

KEY POINTS: HYPERTENSION ✔

1. Hypertension can be classified as primary (95%) and secondary.

2. Primary hypertension is a multifactorial disease of unknown etiology and pathogenesis.

3. Secondary hypertension is most often a complication of renal diseases.

29. **What is the pathogenesis of hypertension caused by renal ischemia?**
Renal hypoperfusion (e.g., narrowing of renal artery stenosis) stimulates release of renin from juxtaglomerular cells. Renin acts on angiotensinogen, which is converted to angiotensin I and thereafter to angiotensin II. This compound constricts arterioles, increasing peripheral resistance. At the same time, it stimulates the release of aldosterone from the adrenal cortex. Aldosterone stimulates sodium and water retention, increasing cardiac output. Hypertension is thus in part caused by increased peripheral resistance and in part by increased cardiac output.

30. **What are complications of hypertension?**
The most commonly affected organs are the heart, aorta, brain, eyes, and kidneys:
- Hypertrophy of the left ventricle and hypertensive heart disease
- Aortic dissection and aneurysms

- Hypertensive cerebral hemorrhage (stroke)
- Rupture of cerebral berry aneurysm with subarachnoid hemorrhage
- Hypertensive encephalopathy with headaches and mild cerebral dysfunction
- Hypertensive retinopathy
- Hypertensive renal disease

To remember the most important complications of hypertension, use the mnemonic *heart:*

- **H**eart hypertrophy
- **E**ye changes (retinopathy)
- **A**ortic dissection and aneurysm
- **R**enal disease
- **T**halamic hemorrhage (stroke)

VASCULITIS

31. **What is vasculitis?**
    Vasculitis (also known as angiitis) is inflammation of vessels (Fig. 7-2). It can be classified according to:
    - **Etiology and pathogenesis:** as infectious, immunologic, and radiation induced
    - **Anatomic site involved:** as aortitis, arteritis, capillaritis, venulitis, or phlebitis
    - **Distribution:** as localized or systemic
    - **Duration:** as acute or chronic

32. **Which infectious diseases cause vasculitis?**
    - **Bacterial sepsis:** Bacteria circulating in the blood may invade the endothelium, especially if the blood vessel is damaged or made ischemic by an infected thrombus. Such an infection may spread into the infarcted tissue, which leads to formation of an abscess. Bacterial infection eating through the wall of an artery may lead to the formation of a pseudoaneurysm, also known as mycotic aneurysm. In contrast to true aneurysms, which represent a dilatated portion of the vessel delimited by a thinned arterial wall, the cavity of a pseudoaneurysm represents a periarterial cavity (an abscess) formed by the lysis of tissue by bacterial enzymes.
    - **Bacterial thrombophlebitis:** Bacteria in an infected venous thrombus may invade the wall of the vein and cause inflammation. Because the veins have a thin wall, such infection may easily spread into adjacent soft tissues. Likewise, an infection in the soft tissues may spread into the wall of the vein and cause thrombosis.
    - **Rickettsial infections:** Rocky Mountain spotted fever, as its name indicates, is characterized by widespread purpura. *Rickettsia rickettsii,* the cause of this disease, tends to invade endothelial cells, causing vasculitis and disrupting small blood vessels. Pinpoint bleeding into the skin and many internal organs results from small blood vessel damage caused by the pathogen. Other rickettsial infections cause similar vasculitis and often present with purpura.
    - **Syphilis:** Treponema pallidum infection is typically accompanied by chronic inflammation of small blood vessels. In tertiary syphilis, infiltrates of lymphocytes and plasma cells surround the vasa vasorum of the aorta, causing aortic aneurysms. Perivascular infiltrates of plasma cells and lymphocytes in the meninges lead to tabes dorsalis and the syphilitic paresis of the insane.
    - **Fungal vasculitis:** Deep fungal infections, especially those caused by *Aspergillus* and *Rhizopus* species, are often complicated by an invasion of blood vessels by fungi. Invasion of blood vessels is accompanied by thrombosis and subsequent infarction of the tissue perfused by that blood vessel.

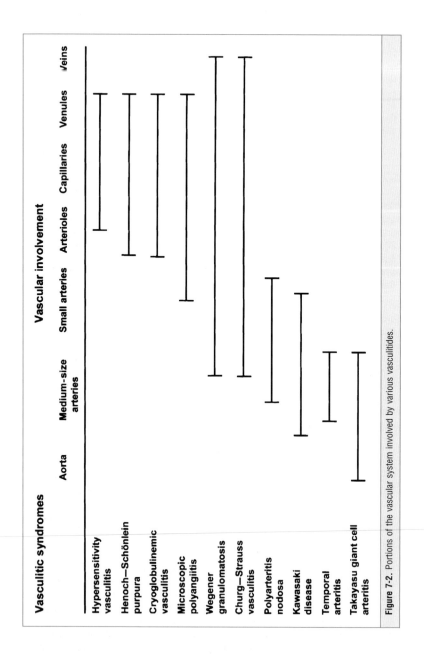

Figure 7-2. Portions of the vascular system involved by various vasculitides.

KEY POINTS: VASCULITIS ✓

1. Vasculitis may have many causes, but most often it is immunologically mediated.

2. The clinicopathologic classification of vasculitides is primarily based on the anatomic distribution of the lesions and the type and size of vessels involved.

33. **What is the pathogenesis of immunologically mediated vasculitis?**
    - **Local immune complex formation in the vessel wall:** Immune complexes are formed in the vessels in the course of polyarteritis nodosa. This disease is a clinical equivalent of the experimental Arthus phenomenon, which is induced by injecting the antigen into the perivascular space of an immunized animal. The antigen diffusing into the vessel wall encounters the antibody entering the vessel wall from the circulation. Antigen and antibody meeting in the vessel wall form immune complexes, which activate the complement system. Activated complement forms chemotactic fragments that attract neutrophils, thus causing an inflammation in the vessel wall.
    - **Deposition of circulating immune complexes in the vessel wall:** Immune complexes circulating in the blood of patients suffering from systemic lupus erythematosus (SLE) may be deposited in the wall of small blood vessels. These deposits activate complement, attract leukocytes, and incite vasculitis.
    - **Deposition of cryoglobulins:** Viral RNA found in the blood of patients infected with hepatitis C virus forms complexes with immunoglobulin G, which precipitates in cold and is thus called cryoglobulin. Deposits of cryoglobulin are accompanied by injuries of small blood vessels and purpura.

34. **What is the most common immunologically mediated acute vasculitis?**
    Hypersensitivity vasculitis, an allergic reaction to drugs and other unidentified exogenous antigens, is the most common form of immunologic acute vasculitis. It is assumed that some drugs may act as haptens and attach to an endogenous protein. Thus complexed, the hapten evokes an immune reaction. Specific antibodies react with the protein carrying the hapten and form immune complexes that are typically deposited in the wall of venules. Vasculitis is most prominent in the skin, in which the rupture of small vessels leads to purpura. Histologically, the vessels are infiltrated with neutrophils and surrounded by extravasated red blood cells leaking into the tissue across the damaged vessel wall (leukocytoclastic vasculitis).

35. **How do antineutrophil cytoplasmic autoantibodies (ANCA) cause vasculitis?**
    Antibodies reacting with cytoplasmic components of neutrophils are found in a number of autoimmune diseases, such as microscopic polyarteritis or Wegener granulomatosis. Although these antibodies are useful in the diagnosis of these diseases, it is not known how ANCA injures blood vessels. It is assumed that the antibodies bind to cytoplasmic components of neutrophils in vivo. Vascular injury presumably results from the release of enzymes from activated neutrophils.

36. **What is the difference between circulating ANCA and perinuclear ANCA?**
    Circulating ANCA (cANCA) are antibodies that in an indirect immunofluorescence microscopy test react diffusely with the cytoplasm of fixed neutrophils. The antigen causing the production of these antibodies has been identified as proteinase 3 (PR3), a component of cytoplasmic granules in neutrophils. cANCA is found in patients affected by Wegener granulomatosis.

    Perinuclear ANCA (pANCA) are antibodies that bind to the cytoplasm of neutrophils in a perinuclear pattern. These antibodies react with myeloperoxidase. These antibodies are typically seen in patients with microscopic polyangiitis and Churg–Strauss syndrome.

37. **What are the typical features of temporal (giant cell) arteritis?**
    - The most common form of chronic vasculitis
    - An old-age disease—rare before the age of 50 years
    - Granulomatous arteritis with giant cells involving short segments of head arteries, most often involving temporal arteries but also ophthalmic or vertebral arteries
    - Palpable nodularity of tortuous temporal arteries is typical
    - Symptoms include headaches, visual symptoms, and constitutional symptoms such as fever fatigue, and weight loss
    - Diagnosis requires biopsy of the affected blood vessel
    - Because of the segmental nature of inflammation, biopsy is negative in 30% cases

38. **What are the typical features of Takayasu arteritis?**
    - Also known as giant cell aortitis or "pulseless disease"
    - Most often affects young adult women (<40 years) of East Asian descent
    - Affects aortic arch (30%) and its branches but also other parts of the aorta and even the pulmonary artery; affected vessels have a thickened wall and narrowed lumen
    - Histologically presents as granulomatous giant cell arteritis, similar to temporal arteritis
    - Symptoms of ischemia—visual and neurologic symptoms and the absence of pulse
    - Pulmonary hypertension may be present because of the involvement of pulmonary artery
    - Clinically the course may be variable—rapid downhill course, 1 or 2 years, or slowly progressive course

39. **What are the typical features of polyarteritis nodosa?**
    - Systemic chronic vasculitis involving medium-sized and small arteries
    - Etiology unknown in most cases—30% have chronic viral hepatitis B
    - May involve any artery, but most often renal arteries
    - Important negatives: does not involve pulmonary arteries and does not produce glomerulonephritis
    - Segmental inflammation of arterial vessel wall with fibrinoid necrosis, similar to the experimental Arthus phenomenon
    - Perivascular inflammation results in nodularity (hence its name)
    - Microaneurysms, which are seen by angiography in 50% of cases
    - Intraluminal thrombosis may cause infarcts
    - Hypertension common if kidneys are involved
    - Classical feature: all stages of inflammation and healing are present at the same time in various blood vessels, reflecting the fluctuating nature of the disease
    - Good response to corticosteroids or cyclophosphamide

40. **What is Kawasaki disease?**
    - Also known as mucocutaneous lymph node syndrome
    - Affects predominantly children younger than 4 years
    - Arteritis involving large and medium-sized and smaller arteries associated with mucosal ulcerations, rash, and lymph node enlargement
    - May involve coronary arteries (20%) and cause aneurysms
    - Pathology varies from mild to severe transmural inflammation
    - Self-limited course in most instances; 20% have cardiovascular complications; 1% die

41. **What is the difference between classic polyarteritis nodosa and microscopic polyarteritis?**
    Both diseases involve medium-sized and smaller arteries. In microscopic polyarteritis, inflammation involves not only medium-sized and smaller arteries but also smaller vessels

and glomeruli. All lesions are in the same stage of inflammation. Furthermore, most patients have pANCA. However, the affected blood vessels do not contain deposits of immunoglobulins.

42. **What is Churg-Strauss syndrome?**
    - Also known as allergic granulomatosis and angiitis
    - Angiitis involving medium-sized and small arteries (as in polyarteritis nodosa) and small vessels and glomeruli (as in microscopic polyangiitis)
    - Associated with asthma, rhinitis, and eosinophilia
    - pANCA are found in 70% cases

43. **What is Wegener granulomatosis?**
    - Necrotizing arteritis involving respiratory tract and kidneys
    - Ulceration of respiratory mucosa, nasopharynx, and sinusitis
    - Necrotizing pulmonary lesions (irregularly shaped "geographic necrosis")
    - Necrotizing, crescentic glomerulonephritis
    - cANCA present in 70% cases
    - Renal failure develops quickly in untreated people
    - Responds well to cyclophosphamide

44. **What is Buerger disease?**
    - Also known as thromboangiitis obliterans
    - Affects predominantly young males (20–35 years) who smoke cigarettes
    - More common in men of Jewish, Japanese, and Indian origin
    - Involves medium-sized and small arteries of extremities
    - Acute and chronic inflammatory infiltrates in the vessel walls accompanied by formation of thrombi that contain microabscesses
    - Inflammation spreads through the vessel wall to adjacent veins and nerves
    - Smoking cessation may halt the progression of disease, but in other cases amputation of infarcted extremities must be performed

45. **What is the difference between Raynaud disease and Raynaud phenomenon?**
    Raynaud disease is a functional vasculopathy of unknown etiology. It is characterized by sudden vasoconstriction of peripheral arteries of the extremities and acral parts, such as the ears or nose. The cause of the unusual hyperreactivity of smooth muscle cells in small arteries and arterioles is unknown, but it is unrelated to any visible pathologic changes in the vessel wall. Raynaud phenomenon is used to describe the same symptoms in a person who has an underlying arterial disease, such as atherosclerosis, SLE, scleroderma, or Buerger disease.

ANEURYSMS

46. **What are aneurysms?**
    An aneurysm is a localized dilatation of an artery. Aneurysms may occur in the ventricles of the heart. Dilatations of the veins are called varicosities rather than aneurysms.

47. **What is the difference between a true aneurysm and a pseudoaneurysm?**
    Aneurysms have a wall typically formed of a pathologically altered segment of the affected vessel. Pseudoaneurysms are cavitated hematomas or abscesses formed because of a rupture in the wall of the artery. The lumen of the pseudoaneurysm communicates with the lumen of the artery through a vessel-wall defect. A fibrous capsule may form over time, delimiting the

lumen of the pseudoaneurysm from the adjacent soft tissue. This capsule represents either a portion of an organized hematoma or the capsule of an abscess.

48. **How are aneurysms classified morphologically?**
Aneurysms (Fig. 7-3) can be descriptively classified as:
- Fusiform aneurysm (symmetrical spindle-shaped dilatation)
- Cylindroid or tubular (lengthy dilatation in the form of a cylinder)
- Saccular aneurysm (sacklike bulging on one side of the artery)
- Berry aneurysm (small saccular aneurysm the size of a berry)

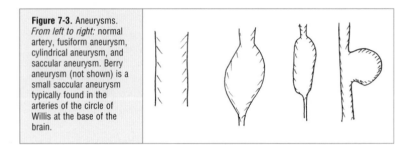

Figure 7-3. Aneurysms. *From left to right:* normal artery, fusiform aneurysm, cylindrical aneurysm, and saccular aneurysm. Berry aneurysm (not shown) is a small saccular aneurysm typically found in the arteries of the circle of Willis at the base of the brain.

KEY POINTS: ANEURYSMS ✓

1. The dilatations of arteries are called aneurysms and the dilatations of veins are called varices.

2. Aneurysms can be classified morphologically according to their shape or etiologically according to their causes.

49. **How are aneurysms classified etiologically?**
- Congenital aneurysms (e.g., cerebral "berry" aneurysms on the circle of Willis)
- Atherosclerotic aneurysms
- Syphilitic aneurysms
- Immunologically mediated aneurysms (e.g., in polyarteritis nodosa)

50. **Where are most atherosclerotic aneurysms located?**
Atherosclerotic aneurysms occur most often in the abdominal aorta.

51. **Where are most syphilitic aneurysms located?**
Most syphilitic aneurysms involve the ascending aorta and its arch.

52. **What is aortic dissection?**
Aortic dissection, previously called dissecting aortic aneurysm, results from forceful separation of the layers of the aortic wall due to the entry of blood between the layers. It results from a tear in the intima that allows the blood to penetrate into the vessel wall and produce an intramural hematoma dissecting between the intima and the media or the media and the adventitia or through the layers of the media.

53. **What are the common causes of aortic dissection?**
    - Aortic dissection most often occurs in older people who have atherosclerosis.
    - Hypertension is a major risk factor, and it probably plays a crucial role in propelling the blood through an intima defect between the layers of the vessel wall.
    - In people who do not have atherosclerosis, the aorta usually shows cystic medial necrosis. This disease is characterized by fragmentation of elastic fibers and an accumulation of acid mucopolysaccharides in the media. The nature of this degenerative disease is not fully understood. Similar degenerative changes are seen in the aorta of patients with Marfan disease and some other diseases based on the mutation of genes encoding intercellular matrix proteins, such as Ehlers–Danlos syndrome or osteogenesis imperfecta.

54. **What is the outcome of aortic dissection?**
    Aortic dissection is accompanied by high mortality. The defect in the vessel wall may lead to fatal exsanguination into the retroperitoneal spaces or the abdominal and thoracic cavity. Dissection of the initial intrapericardial portion of the aorta may cause cardiac tamponade.

55. **What is the difference between aneurysms and varices?**
    Aneurysms occur in arteries, whereas varices (Latin singular is *varix*) are dilatations of veins caused by prolonged stagnation of blood. Clinically important varices are:
    - Varicose leg veins, typically found in people who spend much time standing
    - Varices of the esophagus, typically found in portal hypertension accompanying cirrhosis of the liver
    - Hemorrhoids, representing the varices of the internal or external hemorrhoid plexus of the rectum
    - Varicocele, representing varicosities of the pampiniform plexus of the scrotum

TUMORS

56. **What is the most common benign vascular tumor?**
    Hemangioma, the most common vascular tumor, is one of the most common tumors in the human body. Hemangiomas are most often seen on the skin but may occur in any internal organ as well. Histologically, there are several subtypes (e.g., capillary hemangioma and cavernous hemangioma). Hemangiomas are of limited clinical significance, except for those that are located in a vital organ such as the brain. Such lesions may bleed and cause neurologic problems. Congenital hemangiomas may be of large size and may cause considerable disfigurement of the face or other parts of the body.

57. **What is the most important malignant vascular tumor?**
    Angiosarcoma, the most important malignant vascular tumor, occurs most often in soft tissues but may involve the bones, internal organs, and essentially any part of the body. These tumors are composed of malignant endothelial cells forming irregular anastomozing channels or solid nests. The prognosis depends on the size of the lesions and the extent of spread at the time of operation.

58. **What is Kaposi sarcoma?**
    Kaposi sarcoma is a vascular tumor presenting typically in the form of dark red and bluish skin plaques and nodules. It can also affect internal organs. It is caused by herpes virus type 8. Previously, it was considered to be a rare low-grade sarcoma affecting the extremities of elderly people of Eastern European and Mediterranean descent. However, with the spread of human immunodeficiency virus infection, Kaposi sarcoma has become epidemic, affecting most notably male homosexuals engaging in anogenital sexual intercourse.

KEY POINTS: TUMORS ✓

1. Benign tumors of blood vessels (hemangiomas) are common, whereas malignant tumors (angiosarcomas) are rare.

2. Kaposi sarcoma, a malignant tumor related to infection with herpes virus type 8, occurs at an increased rate in male homosexuals with AIDS.

59. **What are the four clinicopathologic forms of Kaposi sarcoma?**
   - **Classic sporadic form:** It presents as locally invasive, recurrent hemorrhagic lesions on the legs of elderly men. It may be associated with some other internal malignancy.
   - **Acquired immunodeficiency syndrome (AIDS)–associated epidemic form:** It affects male homosexuals suffering from AIDS. It involves the skin, lymph nodes, and internal organs, most notably the gastrointestinal tract.
   - **Posttransplantation Kaposi sarcoma:** These tumors present a few months to many years after solid organ transplantation. Tumors may be localized to the skin or involve the internal organs as well.
   - **Endemic African Kaposi sarcoma:** This tumor affects children in areas of sub-Saharan Africa. It presents with rapidly developing lymphadenopathy and a downhill course.

WEBSITES 🌐

1. http://www.ncbi.nlm.nih.gov/entrez/query.fcgi?db=PubMed

2. http://www-medlib.med.utah.edu/WebPath/webpath.html#MENU

3. http://www.americanheart.org

4. http://vasculitis.med.jhu.edu/typesof/polyarteritis.html

BIBLIOGRAPHY

1. Alberts WM: Pulmonary manifestations of the Churg–Strauss syndrome and related idiopathic small vessel vasculitis syndromes. Curr Opin Pulm Med 13:445–450, 2007.

2. Erickson VR, Hwang PH: Wegener's granulomatosis: current trends in diagnosis and management. Curr Opin Otolaryngol Head Neck Surg 15:170–176, 2007.

3. Ferrari AU, Radaelli A, Centola M: Invited review: aging and the cardiovascular system. J Appl Physiol 95:2591–2597, 2003.

4. Jennette JC, Falk RJ: Nosology of primary vasculitis. Curr Opin Rheumatol 19:10–16, 2007.

5. Jennette JC, Falk RJ: The role of pathology in the diagnosis of systemic vasculitis. Clin Exp Rheumatol 25(1 Suppl 44):S52–46, 2007.

6. Lucas AD, Greaves DR: Atherosclerosis: role of chemokines and macrophages. Expert Rev Mol Med 3:1–18, 2001.

7. Ross R: Rous–Whipple award lecture. Atherosclerosis. A defense mechanism gone awry. Am J Pathol 143:987–1002, 1993.

8. Sinclair D, Stevens JM: Role of antineutrophil cytoplasmic antibodies and glomerular basement membrane antibodies in the diagnosis and monitoring of systemic vasculitides. Ann Clin Biochem 44:432–442, 2007.

9. Widlansky ME, Gokce N, Keaney JF Jr, Vita JA: The clinical implications of endothelial dysfunction. J Am Coll Cardiol 42:1149–1160, 2003.

CHAPTER 8

THE HEART

Ivan Damjanov, MD, PhD

1. **What are the main heart diseases?**
   - Ischemic (coronary) heart disease
   - Valvular heart disease (e.g., endocarditis and rheumatic heart disease)
   - Myocardial diseases (myocarditis and cardiomyopathy)
   - Pericardial diseases
   - Congenital heart diseases
   - Neoplasms

2. **Define heart failure.**
   Heart failure is a condition in which the heart cannot meet the functional needs of the body. It may be of sudden onset (acute) or chronic. It elicits a number of hemodynamic, neural, hormonal, and renal responses, and it is clinically assessed as compensated or decompensated.

   In broad terms, the diseases causing heart failure can be classified into two main groups:
   - **Cardiac diseases:** This group includes all primary and secondary heart diseases, such as coronary heart disease, endocarditis, cardiomyopathies.
   - **Extracardiac causes of heart failure:** The main extracardiac causes of heart failure can be classified further as:
     - Pressure overload (e.g., hypertension)
     - Volume overload (e.g., hypervolemia due to water and sodium retention)
     - Increased demand (e.g., increased metabolism in hyperthyroidism)

3. **What are the most common cardiac causes of heart failure?**
   - **Pump failure:** This category includes numerous diseases that damage the myocardium and reduce its contractility:
     - Ischemic coronary heart disease
     - Electrical disorders (e.g., ventricular fibrillation)
     - Myocarditis
     - Cardiomyopathies (e.g., metabolic and hereditary)
   - **Valvular diseases:** The most important diseases in this group are:
     - Endocarditis (e.g., bacterial and immunologic diseases)
     - Degenerative diseases (e.g., calcific aortic stenosis of old age)
     - Metabolic disorders (e.g., Marfan syndrome and floppy mitral valve)
   - **Restrictive/constrictive diseases:** These diseases prevent dilatation of cardiac chambers in diastole:
     - Myocardial infiltration with amyloid, endomyocardial fibrosis, and so on
     - Pericarditis

KEY POINTS: THE HEART ✓

1. Coronary atherosclerosis accounts for the vast majority of heart disease in adults.

2. Heart failure can develop because of either cardiac or extracardiac disturbances, leading to right ventricular, left ventricular, or biventricular pump failure.

3. Symptoms and signs of heart failure are seen in the rest of the body and in most organ systems.

4. **What is the difference between forward and backward heart failure?**
   - Forward failure includes signs and symptoms of ischemia due to reduced systolic output.
   - Backward failure includes signs of congestion due to inadequate emptying of the heart chambers.

   In most clinical conditions, there are signs of both forward and backward failure.

5. **What is high-output heart failure?**
   This subset of heart failure is characterized by a high cardiac output (high systolic ejection fraction) caused by increased demand. It is typically encountered in conditions such as anemia, thyrotoxicosis, beriberi, and pregnancy. Prolonged ventricular overload leads ultimately to overexhaustion of the heart and heart failure.

6. **What are the features of right heart failure?**
   - Increased venous pressure
   - Congestion and edema of internal organs and soft tissues
     - Hepatomegaly ("nutmeg liver" at autopsy)
     - Congestive splenomegaly
     - Pitting edema of lower extremities (or the back in recumbent patients)
     - Hydrothorax, ascites, and anasarca

7. **What are the features of left heart failure?**
   - Increased pulmonary venous pressure
   - Congestion and edema of the lungs
   - Right heart failure (left ventricle failure is the most common cause of right ventricle failure)
   - Forward failure evidenced by hypoperfusion of major organs, followed by dysfunction of these organs and adaptive measures:
     - Renal hypoperfusion—oliguria: activation of the renin-angiotensin-aldosterone system and compensatory hypertension
     - Cerebral ischemia—somnolence, loss of mental functions, and syncope
     - Intestinal hypoperfusion—ischemic necrosis and hemorrhage into the lumen
     - Hepatic hypoperfusion—metabolic disturbances and jaundice

8. **What is cyanosis?**
   Cyanosis is bluish discoloration of the skin, mucosa or both due to reduced oxygenation of the blood. Clinically, it becomes evident when the oxygenation of hemoglobin falls below 85%. Two forms of cyanosis are recognized:
   - **Central cyanosis:** Both the skin and the mucosa are bluish. Typically, it occurs when the oxygenation of blood is impeded (e.g., adult respiratory distress syndrome), there is shunting of unoxygenated venous blood into the arterial circulation (e.g., cyanotic congenital heart diseases), or hemoglobin cannot take up oxygen (e.g., methemoglobinemia).
   - **Peripheral cyanosis:** Also known as acrocyanosis, it is characterized by bluish discoloration of the skin of the fingers and toes or the nose. It is best observed under cold weather conditions.

Peripheral cyanosis also occurs in chronic passive congestion. It is related to increased oxygen desaturation that occurs in stagnant blood. Hypovolemic shock is accompanied by cyanosis because of the shunting of blood from the skin into the internal organs.

9. **What is cardiac dyspnea?**
Dyspnea, or shortness of breath, results from pulmonary congestion and edema caused by left ventricle failure. Stagnant blood cannot be adequately oxygenated and does not reach the periphery to meet the oxygen demands. The edema fluid inside the alveoli forms a barrier that further impedes the gas exchange. To compensate for the resultant hypoxia followed by hypercapnia, the respiratory centers increase the rate of respiration (tachypnea). Orthopnea refers to dyspnea that occurs in the lying position and is relieved by sitting up or raising the head and chest with pillows. Dyspnea so severe that it would wake up the patient from sleep is called paroxysmal nocturnal dyspnea.

10. **What is cor pulmonale?**
Cor pulmonale is dilatation and hypertrophy of the right heart in response to pulmonary hypertension.
- **Acute cor pulmonale:** This sudden right heart failure may be caused by a saddle embolus obstructing the pulmonary artery or sudden overload of a chronic cor pulmonale by pneumonia.
- **Chronic cor pulmonale:** This form of chronic right heart failure is a consequence of chronic pulmonary hypertension. The right ventricle is dilatated, and its wall is thickened. The most common cause of chronic cor pulmonale is left heart failure. Other causes of chronic cor pulmonale are mostly related to various lung diseases. Alveolar hypoxemia is a potent stimulator of pulmonary vascular constriction, and this ultimately leads to irreversible changes in the vessel wall and narrowing of the pulmonary artery tree. Destruction of alveolar septa and the reduction of the capillary bed in the lungs are other important mechanisms.

11. **What are the most important diseases causing cor pulmonale?**
- Chronic obstructive pulmonary disease (COPD)
- Chronic lung disease (e.g., cystic fibrosis, bronchiectasis, and interstitial fibrosis)
- Recurrent thromboemboli
- Primary pulmonary hypertension (a disease of unknown etiology affecting mostly young women; female:male ratio, 5:1)
- Kyphoscoliosis and neuromuscular diseases affecting respiratory muscles

ISCHEMIC HEART DISEASE

12. **How common is ischemic heart disease?**
- Ischemic heart disease (IHD) is common.
- Cardiovascular diseases are the leading cause of death in the United States, accounting for approximately 1 million deaths per year.
- IHD accounts for approximately 50% of all cardiovascular diseases and is thus the most common cause of death in the United States.

13. **What are the main clinical forms of IHD?**
IHD is a consequence of atherosclerosis and develops when the coronary blood flow is inadequate to meet the needs of the myocardium. Ischemia that results from narrowing or obstruction of coronary arteries may be relative or absolute and will present itself in several clinical conditions:
- Angina pectoris
- Chronic heart failure
- Myocardial infarction
- Sudden death

14. **What are the risk factors for IHD?**
    Risk factors can be divided into two groups: those that cannot be modified (e.g., age, male sex, and familial predisposition [usually multifactorial]) and those that can be modified or avoided (e.g., hypertension, smoking, obesity, diabetes, and sedentary lifestyle).
    A mnemonic for the risk factors for IHD is *has lipids:*
    - **H**ereditary
    - **A**ge
    - **S**ex (male)
    - **L**ipidemia
    - **I**ncreased weight (obesity)
    - **P**ressure (arterial)
    - **I**nactivity (sedentary lifestyle)
    - **D**iabetes
    - **S**moking

15. **What is angina pectoris?**
    Angina is episodic pain or discomfort in the substernal area of the chest precipitated by exercise or excitement and relieved by rest. It represents a sign of relative myocardial ischemia caused by:
    - Atherosclerotic narrowing of the coronary arteries (90% of all cases)
    - Vasospasm of coronary arteries (5%)
    - Small blood vessel disease of the myocardium (e.g., diabetes)
    - Aortic valvular disease (aortic stenosis or insufficiency)

16. **What are the common clinical forms of angina?**
    Three forms of angina are recognized:
    - **Stable angina:** This most common form of angina, is precipitated by exercise or excitement. It is related to ischemia caused by atherosclerotic narrowing of coronary arteries.
    - **Unstable or crescendo angina:** This is also called preinfarction angina because it may progress to an infarct. It is characterized by pain that becomes increasingly more severe and is precipitated by increasingly less effort. It is caused by coronary atheromas prone to rupture. Rupture of atheromas results in intimal defects that are covered with thrombi, causing severe narrowing of the lumen. Peripheral emboli from ruptured atheromas also contribute to the ischemia.
    - **Prinzmetal variant angina:** It occurs at rest and is related to the spasm of coronary arteries. It responds well to vasodilator therapy (e.g., nitroglycerin). During the attack, the electrocardiogram (ECG) shows a transient elevation of the S-T segment.

17. **What are the pathologic findings in the myocardium caused by angina?**
    Stable angina and Prinzmetal angina do not cause any significant myocardial cell necrosis, and accordingly there are no microscopic changes in the heart. Unstable angina may be accompanied by focal myocyte necrosis, which is repaired by foci of fibrosis.

18. **Define myocardial infarction.**
    Myocardial infarction is anoxic necrosis of the myocardial cells caused by ischemia. Two types of infarcts are recognized:
    - **Transmural infarcts:** These localized areas of necrosis are found in specific anatomic areas corresponding to the portion of the myocardium supplied by the occluded coronary artery or its major branches. The necrosis involves the entire thickness of the ventricular wall from the endocardium to the subepicardial fat tissue. These infarcts are usually (90%) caused by occlusive thrombi forming in the artherosclerotic coronary arteries. In a small number of cases, they are related to thromboemboli or vasospasm, or their cause remains unknown.

- **Circumferential subendocardial infarcts:** These infarcts involve circumferentially the subendocardial area of the left and sometimes the right ventricle. These infarcts are caused by hypoperfusion of the myocardium and are not caused by coronary occlusion. Typically these infarcts occur in hypotensive shock. By ECG, these infarcts show changes typical of the so-called no-Q wave infarction (in contrast to Q wave infarcts, which are transmural).

19. **What is the anatomic distribution of myocardial infarcts?**
Most myocardial infarcts involve the left ventricle. The left coronary artery is more often occluded than the right coronary artery. The anatomic distribution of transmural infarcts depends on the site of occlusion.
    - **Left anterior descending coronary:** The infarct involves the anterior part of the left ventricle and anterior part of the interventricular septum.
    - **Left circumflex artery:** The infarct is in the lateral wall of the left ventricle.
    - **Right coronary artery:** The infarct is in the right ventricle, the posterior wall of the left ventricle, and the posterior part of the interventricular septum.

20. **List the common symptoms of a myocardial infarct.**
    - Substernal pain persisting for more than 30 minutes and not relieved by nitroglycerin
    - Pain may occur at rest but is often precipitated by work or exercise; occurs most often in the morning hours (catecholamine burst after awakening)
    - Severe distress marked by symptoms such as nausea, sweating, and vomiting
    - Dyspnea (shortness of breath)

21. **Which tests are helpful for the diagnosis of myocardial infarcts?**
ECG changes are found in most (85%) cases, but often they are nonspecific. Diagnostic ECG changes are found in 50% to 65% of cases during the first 2 days of onset of the infarction. Laboratory findings in serum that become positive after occlusion of coronaries are:
    - Troponin I or troponin T—4 hours (the most reliable test)
    - Myoglobin—2 to 4 hours (very nonspecific; any muscle injury may cause elevation)
    - Creatine kinase—6 hours (MB isoenzyme useful for distinguishing myocardial infarction from muscle diseases)
    - Aspartate aminotransferase—12 hours (nonspecific; found in liver diseases and many other diseases)
    - Lactate dehydrogenase—24 hours (nonspecific; any cell injury may cause it)
Echocardiography—useful for demonstrating abnormally contracting parts of the ventricular myocardium and visualizing thrombi or ruptures in the wall of the myocardium

22. **What are the pathologic findings in the myocardium in a typical myocardial infarct?**
    - **First day:** Myocardium is pale on gross examination. No histologic changes are seen, but there may be some eosinophilia of necrotic fibers.
    - **Second day:** Necrotic myocardial cells are surrounded by a few neutrophils.
    - **Third day:** Fragmentation of necrotic myocytes and numerous neutrophils are seen.
    - **Fourth day:** Macrophages appear, which slowly replace the neutrophils and remove the dead myocardial cells.
    - **End of first week:** Ingrowth of angioblasts marks the beginning of granulation tissue formation.
    - **Second week:** Granulation tissue has begun to replace the necrotic myocardium.
    - **Third week:** Granulation tissue slowly transforms into a fibrous scar.
    - **Six weeks:** A fibrous scar has formed.

23. **What is the outcome of myocardial infarction?**
Myocardial myocytes cannot regenerate, so the necrotic cells must be replaced by fibrous tissue. Fibrous scars are thus invariably found at the site of all healed infarcts.

However, the patient may die before the infarct heals. These patients most often die because of electrical disturbances, and the examination of the heart at autopsy will reveal the typical macroscopic and microscopic features of an infarct at various stages of evolution or healing.

KEY POINTS: ISCHEMIC HEART DISEASE ✔

1. Ischemic heart disease is related to complications of coronary atherosclerosis.

2. Coronary artery disease may cause only functional disturbances, as seen in angina pectoris and congestive heart failure, or it may present with pathologic changes in the heart and other organs, as in myocardial infarction.

3. Myocardial infarction is associated with characteristic pathologic, clinical, and biochemical changes, which change during the course of the disease.

24. **What are the typical complications of myocardial infarcts?**
   - **Arrhythmia:** This is the most common complication and the most common cause of death in the early as well as later postinfarction period.
   - **Sudden death:** Most often this occurs because of arrhythmia and other electrical disturbances.
   - **Cardiogenic shock:** Weakening of the myocardium leads to "pump failure" and acute backward and forward heart failure.
   - **Rupture of the myocardium:** This complication occurs during the first week postocclusion of coronary artery. During that time, the necrotic myocardium is very soft (because of the action of neutrophils infiltrating the area).
   - **Rupture of the free wall of the left ventricle:** The hole in the wall of the ventricle allows the blood to escape from the left ventricle into the pericardial cavity. The high pressure in the left ventricle will "blow out" the surrounding necrotic myocardium and enlarge the hole. Massive bleeding into the pericardial sac is called hemopericardium. The patient dies of cardiac tamponade.
   - **Rupture of the papillary muscles:** Because the damaged papillary muscle cannot contract, it will typically cause mitral insufficiency.
   - **Rupture of the interventricular septum:** The hole in the septum allows the blood from the left ventricle to enter the right ventricle. This shunt will overburden the right ventricle and cause acute right ventricular failure and pulmonary hypertension.
   - **Mural thrombosis:** It forms in the ventricle.
     - **Ventricular thrombi:** These thrombi are attached to the endocardium overlying the infarcted area of the ventricle.
     - **Atrial thrombi:** These thrombi develop usually because of irregular blood flow inside the dilatated and irregularly contracting left atrium (atrial fibrillation and atrial flutter).
   - **Extension or reinfarction:** They are found adjacent to the original infarct.
   - **Pericarditis:** Subepicardial necrosis of the myocardium leads to a sterile inflammation of the epicardium and exudation of fibrin. Rubbing of the epicardium and the pericardium further promotes the inflammation, which may lead to obliteration of the pericardial cavity and formation of fibrous adhesions in the healing stage of the disease.
   - **Ventricular aneurysm:** This complication develops several weeks and months after the infarction. Typically it develops at the site of large myocardial scars. The connective tissue of the scar does not contract and actually bulges out little by little during each systole until an aneurysm is formed. The lumen of these aneurysms often contains mural thrombi.

A convenient mnemonic to remember the most important complications of myocardial infarct is *appear:*

- **A**rrhythmia (e.g., atrial or ventricular fibrillation, cardiac block, asystole)
- **P**ump failure
- **P**ericarditis
- **E**mboli (from mural thrombi in ventricle or atria)
- **A**neurysm of the ventricle
- **R**upture (free wall of the ventricle, septum, or papillary muscle)

25. **What is Dressler syndrome?**

Dressler syndrome is a complication of transmural myocardial infarcts clinically presenting with pericardial pain associated with pericardial friction rub. Although the pathogenesis of this complication is not known, it is thought to be immunologically mediated. Pericarditis is presumably caused by the development of antibodies to proteins released from the necrotic myocardial cells. These patients have fever, pleural effusion, and joint pains (i.e., symptoms suggestive of serum sickness), all of which may also be caused by autoantibodies. Cortisone treatment is beneficial, also supporting an immunologic explanation.

26. **What is the pathogenesis of chronic IHD after an infarction?**

Myocardial infarctions typically develop in people who usually have generalized atherosclerosis. Accordingly, one can expect that the occluded coronary artery is not the only abnormal vessel and that other coronary arteries are also narrowed to some extent. Loss of myocardium in the infarcted area is accompanied by increased demand for work by the remaining uninfarcted myocardium. Because the blood to this normal myocardium flows through narrowed and calcified arteries, which cannot dilatate, the increased demand generates relative ischemia. Chronic pump failure develops over time.

27. **What are the pathologic findings in sudden cardiac death?**

The most common finding is thrombosis of coronary arteries. Typically, it develops over a ruptured "soft" atheroma—that is, an atheroma that has a soft central core (composed of semiliquid lipid-rich debris) covered with a fibrous cap. The rupture of the fibrous cap will release the atheromatous material into the coronary vessel. Because this material acts as thromboplastin, it will initiate local coagulation of the blood and result in the formation of thrombus. Other causes of sudden cardiac death are coronary diseases (e.g., vasculitis and coronary artery aneurysm), cardiac diseases not clinically recognized (e.g., cardiomyopathies and myocarditis), and valvular disease (e.g., mitral valve prolapse and aortic stenosis).

28. **Describe a hypertrophic heart.**

The hypertrophic heart appears enlarged. At autopsy, such hearts weigh 500 g or more. The walls of the left and the right ventricle is thickened. Extremely enlarged hearts weighing more than 600 g are colloquially called "cor bovinum" because they resemble bovine hearts.

Histologically, the cardiac myocytes are hypertrophic (i.e., in longitudinal sections they have a "boxcar" appearance). The nuclei are enlarged and are polypoid.

29. **What are the most common causes of cardiac hypertrophy?**

The most common causes are:

- Hypertension
- Aortic valvular disease (stenosis > insufficiency)
- Mitral insufficiency
- Cardiomyopathy

VALVULAR HEART DISEASE

30. **What are the main forms of endocarditis?**
    - Immunologically mediated endocarditis (e.g., rheumatic and systemic lupus erythematosus [SLE])
    - Bacterial endocarditis
    - Nonbacterial thrombotic endocarditis
    - Metabolically mediated endocarditis
    - Degenerative valvular disease of old age

31. **What is rheumatic endocarditis?**
    Rheumatic endocarditis is an aspect of rheumatic fever (RF). Because the incidence of RF has decreased dramatically in the United States and most industrialized countries, rheumatic endocarditis has become relatively rare. Currently the incidence of RF is only 1:100,000 in the United States. The decrease in the incidence of RF correlates with the widespread use of antibiotics in the treatment of various infections. The disease is still widely prevalent in underdeveloped countries, where it often occurs in an epidemic form. There is an epidemiologic correlation between the incidence of RF and poverty and overcrowding in some underdeveloped countries.

32. **What is RF?**
    RF is an immunologic complication of some infections caused by group A beta hemolytic streptococci. In most instances, the infection involves the oropharynx (strep throat), but it may also occur in skin wounds or other anatomic sites. Clinical signs and symptoms of acute RF appear 2 or 3 weeks following the infection. Chronic RF includes predominantly cardiac consequences of the acute RF.

33. **What is the evidence that RF is an immunologically mediated disease?**
    The exact pathogenesis of RF is not understood, and the disease cannot be reproduced experimentally. Nevertheless, all data indicate that it is based on a set of immunologic hypersensitivity reactions. The most important findings pointing to an immunologic nature of RF are:
    - Antibodies to streptococcal antigens, such as streptolysin O (ASO), DNAase, and hyaluronidase. These antibodies are not involved in the pathogenesis of tissue injury. ASO is a widely used test for proving that an infection was caused by streptococci.
    - Antibodies to streptococcal capsular M protein. Antibodies to M protein cross-react with some proteins in human connective tissue and are thought to play a pathogenetic role in RF.
    - Aschoff bodies are granulomas of a peculiar form found in the heart of most patients with RF. These histologic structures consist of a central area of fibrinoid necrosis surrounded by macrophages and lymphocytes. Macrophages have nuclei with centrally clumped chromatin that gives the nuclei a peculiar appearance—"owl-eyed" in cross-sections and "caterpillar-like" in longitudinal sections.

34. **What are the features of acute RF?**
    RF is diagnosed clinically using Jones criteria, which are divided into two groups: major and minor. The diagnosis is established when two major and one minor or one major and two minor criteria are present. These criteria (with the rate of occurrence included in parentheses) are listed in the mnemonic cardiac RF:
    - **C**arditis (35%)
    - **A**rthritis (75%)
    - **R**andom (involuntary) movements (chorea) (5%)
    - **D**ermatologic signs (erythema marginatum and nodosum) (10% each)
    - **I**nflammatory laboratory indices (increased erythrocyte sedimentation rate and C-reactive protein) (minor criterion)
    - **A**rthralgia (minor criterion)

- **C**ardiogram (ECG) (minor criterion)
- **R**ecurrent attack (previous RF) (minor criterion)
- **F**ever (minor criterion)

35. **What are the features of acute rheumatic carditis?**
RF involves the entire heart (i.e., it is a pancarditis). It includes
- **Endocarditis:** In the acute stages of the disease, the valves are swollen and focally covered with fibrin-rich exudate that forms nodular excrescences ("vegetations"). Because these vegetations are anchored to the valve by the underlying granulation tissue in the inflamed valves, they rarely detach to give rise to emboli.
- **Myocarditis:** RF may involve any part of the myocardium. Histologically, the myocardium contains Aschoff bodies, which heal over time and transform into fibrotic scars.
- **Pericarditis:** Inflammation of the epicardial and pericardial surfaces of the pericardial sac is accompanied by the formation of a fibrin-rich exudate. Fibrin covering the heart can be mechanically separated at autopsy from the fibrin on the inner surface of the pericardial sac, giving the heart the shaggy appearance of a butter-covered inside of a sandwich ("bread and butter" appearance).
- **Fibrinous pericarditis:** This may progress to fibrous pericarditis in which connective tissue adhesions develop between the two layers of the pericardial sac.
- **Constrictive pericarditis:** This is a rare late complication.

36. **What are the clinical features of acute rheumatic carditis?**
Vegetations and swelling of the inflamed heart valves alter the blood flow through the cardiac valves. These changes are accompanied by murmurs that can be heard on auscultation.
   Cardiac involvement may cause tachycardia, arrhythmias, and irregular ventricular contractions. Heart failure may occur, but rarely.
   Pericarditis presents with pericardial friction rub and chest pain.

37. **What is the usual outcome of acute RF?**
Acute RF heals without any sequelae in most instances. However, all those who once had RF are at increased risk of recurrence and exacerbation of cardiac lesions following another streptococcal infection. Chronic rheumatic carditis develops in only 1% of all cases.

38. **What are the most important features of chronic rheumatic carditis?**
The most important and the most common features of chronic RF are seen on the valves. The valves of the left ventricle (the aortic and mitral valves) are affected more often than those on the right side. Pathologically altered valves show:
- Deformities of the cusps
- Shortening and fusion of chordae tendineae
- Residual fibrinous vegetations, which often become infected with bacteria
- Superimposed infection, which may cause ulcerations of the cusps, perforation of valves, and rupture of chordae tendineae

39. **What are the functional consequences of valvular deformities in chronic rheumatic carditis?**
Valvular dysfunctions are classified as:
- **Valvular stenosis:** The orifice is narrowed because the valves cannot open completely.
- **Valvular insufficiency:** The valves do not close completely, thus permitting reflow of blood from one chamber to another (regurgitation).

40. **Explain the consequences of mitral stenosis.**
The mitral valve is supposed to be open during diastole and closed during systole. In mitral stenosis, the valve cannot open fully during diastole, and the normal inflow of the blood from the

left atrium into the left ventricle is impeded. The blood pressure in the left ventricle is increased, causing increased pulmonary and right ventricular pressure in a retrograde manner. Anatomic consequences include pulmonary congestion and brown induration and hypertrophy of the left atrium and the right ventricle (cor pulmonale). The left ventricle receives less blood than under normal conditions and is smaller than normal.

Clinically, the turbulent blood flow through the narrowed mitral valve presents with a diastolic murmur.

41. **Explain the consequences of mitral insufficiency.**
A mitral valve that cannot close during diastole is considered to be insufficient. The deformity allows a reflux of blood from the left ventricle into the left atrium and a backpressure into the lungs and the right ventricle. The left ventricle is overburdened and is typically hypertrophic and dilatated. The left atrium and the right ventricle undergo similar dilatation and hypertrophy. The lungs show signs of chronic congestion.

Clinically, regurgitation of the blood across the incompetent mitral valve presents with a systolic murmur.

42. **What are the consequences of aortic stenosis?**
Aortic stenosis does not allow the outflow of blood from the left ventricle into the aorta during systole. The left ventricle, straining to overcome the narrowing, undergoes hypertrophy. The blood pressure inside the left ventricle is increased, but it cannot be transmitted into the aorta. Hence, the aortic and peripheral arterial pressures are lower than normal, and the pulse range is reduced. Pulmonary backflow does not occur in the early stages of disease. However, when the left ventricle starts failing, backpressure occurs, and the lungs become congested. Ultimately, cor pulmonale develops as in any other form of left heart failure.

Clinically, aortic stenosis presents with a high-pitched systolic murmur.

KEY POINTS: VALVULAR HEART DISEASE ✓

1. Valvular diseases result from various inflammatory, immunologic, and degenerative diseases affecting the aortic, mitral, pulmonary, and tricuspid valves.

2. Valvular diseases cause functional disorders broadly classified as valvular stenosis or insufficiency.

3. Thrombi formed on the inflamed or damaged valves may give rise to arterial emboli that cause infarctions in many organs.

43. **What are the consequences of aortic insufficiency?**
Aortic valves are supposed to be closed during diastole. If the valves cannot close completely, blood regurgitation will occur during diastole. The left ventricle must work harder and will typically undergo hypertrophy and dilatation.

44. **What are the causes of infective endocarditis?**
Infective endocarditis can be caused by gram-negative or gram-positive bacteria and fungi, but most often it is caused by streptococci and staphylococci. Three groups of patients are recognized:
- **Patients with native valve endocarditis:** The valves of these patients are most often (70%) infected with alpha-hemolytic *Streptococcus viridans* species, which live in oropharynx as commensals. *Staphylococcus aureus* and *Staphylococcus epidermidis* infections account for 25% of cases, whereas all other bacteria and fungi account for the remaining 5% of cases.

- **Endocarditis in drug addicts:** Infection is most often caused by *S. aureus* (55%), group A *Streptococcus* (15%), and gram-negative bacteria (15%).
- **Endocarditis on prosthetic valves:** Staphylococci account for more than 50% of infections that occur within 2 months of surgery. Late-onset endocarditis is most often caused by *S. viridans* (40%) and staphylococci (30%).

45. **Which heart diseases predispose to infective endocarditis?**
Bacterial endocarditis develops without any obvious predisposing conditions in approximately 30% of cases. In the remaining 70% of cases, one of the following preexisting diseases plays a pathogenetic role:
- Chronic rheumatic endocarditis
- Congenital heart disease
- Calcific aortic stenosis
- Mitral valve prolapse

46. **What is the difference between acute and subacute endocarditis?**
In the preantibiotic era, it was relatively easy to distinguish the rapidly evolving acute bacterial endocarditis (ABE) from the subacute bacterial endocarditis (SBE) of insidious onset. Today such separation of these two forms of endocarditis is not always possible. Features favoring one over the other diagnosis are as follows:
- **Clinical features:** SBE is a slowly evolving disease that usually presents with nonspecific symptoms, such as fever, night sweats, and weight loss.
- **Cardiac symptoms:** Symptoms such as tachycardia, murmurs, and systemic symptoms related to emboli may or may not be present. In ABE, the symptoms are more pronounced and develop much faster. There are, however, no strict criteria for separating clinically SBE from ABE.
- **Bacteriology:** SBE is most often caused by bacteria of low virulence, such as beta-hemolytic streptococcus, whereas ABE is most often caused by highly virulent *S. aureus*. However, there are many exceptions, and it is not possible to predict which infection will cause which form of endocarditis.
- **Pathology:** ABE is characterized by large fragile vegetations associated with ulceration of the valves, perforation of valves, and rupture of chordae tendineae. The vegetations found in SBE are smaller, less friable, and associated with fewer destructive lesions.

47. **What is the pathogenesis of complications of bacterial endocarditis?**
Complications result from four sets of events:
- **Destruction of valves:** Endocarditis may impede the flow of blood and cause turbulence (reflected in murmurs). As the disease advances, bacteria may destroy parts of the valve, cause perforation, rupture of chordae tendineae, or abscesses at the base of the cusps. All these pathologic changes adversely affect the function of the valve and may cause insufficiency. Stenosis may also develop, even though more often it is found in the healing stages of the disease, characterized by fibrosis and calcification of cusps.
- **Dissemination of bacteria:** The entry of bacteria into the circulation results in bacteremia. The patient typically has symptoms of sepsis. Blood culture will reveal bacteria as the cause of these relatively nonspecific systemic symptoms.
- **Embolization:** Fragments of infected endocardial vegetations are carried by the blood, lodging in terminal arteries. Such emboli interrupt the blood supply to the affected area and cause localized ischemic necrosis (infarcts). Bacteria residing in the emboli enter the ischemic area and transform infarct into abscesses.
- **Immune complexes:** Antibodies form against antigens constantly released from bacteria in the infected endocardial vegetations. These immune complexes circulate in the blood and are deposited in the wall of glomeruli and small blood vessels. Symptoms of glomerulonephritis or vasculitis develop.
See Fig. 8-1.

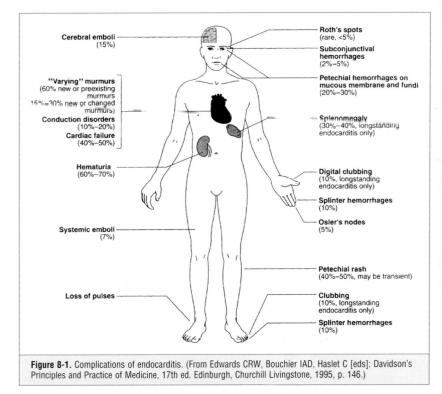

Figure 8-1. Complications of endocarditis. (From Edwards CRW, Bouchier IAD, Haslet C [eds]: Davidson's Principles and Practice of Medicine, 17th ed. Edinburgh, Churchill Livingstone, 1995, p. 146.)

48. **Which valves are most often affected by endocarditis?**
    Endocarditis more often affects the valves in the left than those in the right heart. The mitral valve is most often affected, followed by the aortic, tricuspid, and the pulmonic valve.

49. **Which conditions predispose to endocarditis of the right heart?**
    Right-sided endocarditis is most often found in association with:
    - Intravenous drug abuse (tricuspid valve affected in 50% of cases)
    - Indwelling venous catheters
    - Cardiac surgery
    - Ventricular septal defects
    - Carcinoid syndrome

50. **How does carcinoid syndrome affect the heart?**
    Intestinal carcinoids often secrete biogenic amines (e.g., serotonin) and polypeptide hormones (e.g., vasoactive intestinal polypeptide, somatostatin, and glucagon). These substances are carried by the portal venous blood to the liver, where they are inactivated and metabolized. However, if a carcinoid tumor metastasizes to the liver, its cells will secrete the bioactive substances into the hepatic venous blood, bypassing the liver. Serotonin and other vasoactive substances that have not been inactivated reach the heart and damage the endocardium. Chronic endocardial fibrosis develops in the form of plaques over the mural and valvular endocardium of the right atrium and ventricle, most often over the tricuspid valve. The valves of the left ventricle are less commonly affected because the potentially dangerous bioactive substances are inactivated while the blood is passing from the right ventricle through the lungs to the left ventricle.

51. **Can endocarditis develop on prosthetic heart valves?**

Prosthetic valves used to replace pathologically altered cusps are of two kinds: mechanical valves made of plastic and metal and bioprostheses of animal origin (e.g., pig valves). Infections typically occur at the base of these valves (i.e., in the interface between the valves and the traumatized cardiac tissue to which they are attached). Thrombi that develop on the artificial valves may also become infected.

52. **How common is endocarditis on prosthetic heart valves?**

Prosthetic valve endocarditis accounts for approximately 20% of all clinically diagnosed cases of endocarditis. It occurs in two forms:
- **Early-onset endocarditis:** This form is diagnosed within the first 2 months after surgery, occurs in 2% or 3% of patients who have had heart valve surgery, and is caused by intraoperative contamination with drug-resistant pathogens (e.g., *S. epidermidis, S. aureus,* and gram-negative bacteria or fungi).
- **Late-onset endocarditis:** It occurs at a rate of 0.5% per year after surgery. It is usually related to transient bacteremias.

53. **What are the other complications of heart valve replacement?**

Complications result from surgery as well as from the foreign nature of the material implanted. Neither the mechanical nor the bioprosthetic valves are exact replicas of the original valves, and both are associated with some potential complications. The most common complications are:
- Thrombosis
- Infection
- Paravalvular leaks
- Mechanical malfunction
- Mechanical deterioration (rupture of valves, calcification of bioprostheses, etc.)
- Mechanical hemolysis with hemoglobinuria and anemia

54. **What is nonbacterial thrombotic endocarditis?**

Nonbacterial thrombotic endocarditis (NBTE), also known as marantic endocarditis, is characterized by the formation of sterile vegetations on cardiac valves. These excrescences, composed of fibrin, platelets, and red blood cells, resemble thrombi. The exact pathogenesis of NBTE is not known, but the thrombi form on sites of minute mechanical injuries of the endothelium. Such injuries occur normally but are repaired by endothelial regeneration. In debilitated people (e.g., those who have terminal cancer or chronic infection), normal repair mechanisms are defective, and the endothelial defect is filled in with platelets and fibrin. Small thrombi that are not removed by plasminogen and other fibrinolytic substances grow and transform into larger excrescences. Hypercoagulability of the blood typically found in patients with gastrointestinal cancer is especially prone to NBTE.

55. **What is the significance of NBTE?**

Endocardial vegetations of NBTE may become infected and are potential precursors of bacterial endocarditis. Larger friable vegetations may fragment and give rise to emboli.

NBTE may produce embolic phenomena similar to those seen in bacterial endocarditis, but in NBTE blood cultures are typically sterile. Because NBTE requires treatment with anticoagulants, which are contraindicated in bacterial infective endocarditis, it is important to distinguish these two diseases.

56. **What is Libman–Sacks endocarditis?**

Libman–Sacks endocarditis is a feature of SLE. It presents in the form of multiple small wartlike excrescences on the mitral valve and less commonly tricuspid valve. These vegetations result from immune complex–mediated injury of the valvular endocardium, followed by thrombus formation. These vegetations can be identified in living patients by echocardiography, but usually these lesions are clinically of limited significance.

57. **Compare the endocardial vegetation in various forms of endocarditis.**
See Table 8-1.

TABLE 8-1. ENDOCARDIAL VEGETATION IN VARIOUS FORMS OF ENDOCARDITIS			
Feature	Rheumatic Fever	Infective Endocarditis	NBTE
Vegetation size and site	Small; surface of the leaflet	Large; free margins, base or chordae	Small or medium; surface of leaflet
Valvular inflammation	Chronic inflammation	Acute inflammation (PMNs), bacteria	No inflammation
Emboli	Rare	Common—septic	Rare—sterile
Valvular changes	Fibrosis, calcification	Ulceration, perforation, rupture	No significant changes
Blood tests	ASO (+)	Blood culture (+)	No diagnostic tests

ASO, antistreptolysin O antibodies; *NBTE*, Nonbacterial thrombotic endocarditis; *PMN*, polymorphonuclear.

58. **What is the cause of calcific aortic stenosis?**
Calcification of aortic valves is a common finding in the elderly. It is a form of dystrophic calcification involving the ring or the leaflets of the valve. The disease is often described as a "degeneration," in essence meaning that its causes are unknown. Calcific valves become progressively narrowed and malfunction, causing predominantly narrowing (stenosis) of the orifice but also some degree of regurgitation.

59. **What is the cause of valvular calcification in middle-aged people?**
Although idiopathic valvular degeneration with calcification can occasionally occur even in young people, one must exclude other causes of calcification, such as:
- **Rheumatic heart disease:** This usually affects both the mitral valve and the aortic valve.
- **Congenital bicuspid aortic valves:** This congenital defect is found in approximately 1% of all people. It remains asymptomatic until a person reaches the age of 60 to 70 years, when the valves become calcified and stenotic.

MYOCARDIAL DISEASES

60. **What is the difference between myocarditis and cardiomyopathy?**
Myocarditis is an inflammatory disease, whereas cardiomyopathy includes a variety of noninflammatory diseases also affecting the myocardium. In clinical practice, and even at autopsy, the distinction between these two entities is not clear. One should only consider viral myocarditis in acute stages of the disease; the myocardium is infiltrated with numerous mononuclear cells, but these cells disappear and are not found in late stages. Pathologically, chronic viral myocarditis is indistinguishable from other forms of dilatated noninfectious cardiomyopathy.

61. **List the most important causes of myocarditis.**
- Viruses (e.g., coxsackie B or influenza virus). Human immunodeficiency virus (HIV) may also cause myocarditis, but some patients with autoimmune deficiency syndrome (AIDS) have myocardial inflammation even though myocytes are not infected.
- Bacteria (e.g., staphylococci and *Borrelia burgdorferi* [Lyme disease])
- Parasites (e.g., *Trypanosoma cruzi*)

- Immunologic diseases (e.g., rheumatic fever and SLE)
- Sarcoidosis
- Idiopathic myocarditis

62. **What is the most common proved cause of myocarditis in the United States?**
The cause of myocarditis diagnosed at autopsy or by biopsy remains unknown in most cases.
It is thought that viruses account for the majority of cases. The most commonly identified
pathogens are coxsackie B virus, influenza, and echo and childhood exanthema viruses
(measles, varicella, and mumps).

63. **Which parasite causes myocarditis in South America?**
Trypanosoma cruzi, the cause of South American trypanosomiasis or Chagas disease, tends to
invade cardiac myocytes and provoke myocarditis.

64. **How does diphtheria cause myocarditis?**
Corynebacterium diphtheriae infection of the throat may be accompanied by myocarditis.
Myocardial injury is caused by toxins released from the bacteria into the circulation. The
myocardium does not contain bacteria. Macrophages infiltrating the damaged myocardium
represent scavengers sent in to remove the necrotic myocytes.

65. **What is Fiedler myocarditis?**
Fiedler myocarditis is an idiopathic form of myocardial inflammation characterized by infiltrates
composed of lymphocytes, macrophages, and giant cells.

66. **What are the pathologic features of myocarditis?**
Myocarditis caused by bacteria may present in the form of abscesses in the wall of the
heart chambers. Most other forms of myocarditis produce no distinct macroscopic changes.
At autopsy, the heart is usually enlarged and flabby. Microscopic examination will usually
reveal interstitial edema separating the myocardial cells one from another. Inflammatory
cells are seen in early stages of the disease, whereas fibrosis predominates in chronic
stages.

67. **How useful are microscopic findings for the diagnosis of myocarditis?**
The presumptive clinical diagnosis of myocarditis is made by excluding other myocardial
disease (e.g., myocardial infarct and rheumatic carditis). The definitive diagnosis can be made
only by combining microbiologic findings with histopathologic data. Myocardial biopsy must
be performed, but often the diagnosis is established only postmortem at autopsy.
   The following are microscopic findings found in various forms of myocarditis:
- **Abscess and infiltrates of neutrophils:** typically found in bacterial infections; bacterial
  myocarditis occurs in sepsis or in immunosuppressed people
- **Mononuclear infiltrates (Ly, Mf, and Pla):** typically found in viral myocarditis
- **Giant cells:** idiopathic Fiedler myocarditis
- **Trypanosomes in myocardial cells:** Chagas disease
- **Noncaseating granulomas:** sarcoidosis

68. **How are cardiomyopathies classified etiologically?**
Cardiomyopathies are classified etiologically into two major groups:
- **Primary—due to a primary heart disease, such as congenital cardiomyopathy:** The cause
  of primary cardiomyopathy may remain unknown. At autopsy, the diagnosis of primary
  cardiomyopathy is made after all other possible causes have been excluded.
- **Secondary—due to an identifiable cause of myocardial injury or a systemic disease:** The
  most important causes of secondary cardiomyopathy are hemochromatosis, amyloidosis,
  alcohol, and thiamine deficiency.

69. **What are the main clinicopathologic forms of cardiomyopathy?**
    Three forms are recognized (Fig. 8-2):
    - **Dilatated cardiomyopathy:** The heart is dilatated and enlarged, weighing more than 500 g. Histologically, there are numerous small fibrotic scars replacing focally myocardial cells (replacement fibrosis). Heart chambers are dilatated and may contain mural thrombi.
    - **Hypertrophic cardiomyopathy:** The ventricles show marked hypertrophy, which may reduce the volume of their lumen. In some cases, there is asymmetric hypertrophy of the ventricular septum leading to subaortic stenosis of the left ventricle.
    - **Restrictive cardiomyopathy:** The ventricles are infiltrated with extraneous material that prevents their dilatation.

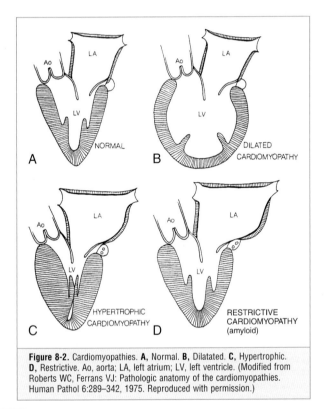

Figure 8-2. Cardiomyopathies. **A,** Normal. **B,** Dilatated. **C,** Hypertrophic. **D,** Restrictive. Ao, aorta; LA, left atrium; LV, left ventricle. (Modified from Roberts WC, Ferrans VJ: Pathologic anatomy of the cardiomyopathies. Human Pathol 6:289–342, 1975. Reproduced with permission.)

70. **List the most important facts about dilatated cardiomyopathy.**
    - It is the most common form of cardiomyopathy (nevertheless, it is still a rare disease).
    - Primary occurs more frequently than secondary cardiomyopathy (the cause is unknown in most cases). Secondary cardiomyopathy may be related to alcohol, thiamine deficiency (beriberi heart disease), and rare diseases such as Friedreich ataxia.
    - It is also called congestive cardiomyopathy.
    - It presents with systolic failure—increased end systolic pressure and diastolic volume.
    - Death occurs 2 years from onset of symptoms. Treatment is cardiac transplantation.

71. **List the most important facts about hypertrophic cardiomyopathy.**
    - Hypertrophy of the ventricles impedes diastolic filling.
    - More than 50% of all hypertrophic cardiomyopathies are familial.
    - Several gene mutations have been identified, but the most common is the mutation involving the b-cardiac myosin heavy chain.
    - Asymmetric septal hypertrophy is in most instances inherited as an autosomal dominant trait.

72. **List the most important facts about restrictive cardiomyopathy.**
    - Infiltration of the myocardium by extraneous substances impedes diastolic dilatation and systolic contraction.
    - In adults, it is most often caused by amyloidosis and hemochromatosis.
    - In infants, it may be found in mucopolysaccharidoses, glycogenosis type II (Pompe disease), and endomyocardial fibrosis.

73. **Is sarcoidosis a myocarditis or cardiomyopathy?**
    Sarcoidosis is a granulomatous myocarditis. Granulomas infiltrating and destroying the myocardium cause symptoms of restrictive cardiomyopathy, and accordingly in some books sarcoidosis is listed as a cardiomyopathy. This indicates that the separation of myocarditis and cardiomyopathy is often based on arbitrary criteria.

KEY POINTS: MYOCARDIAL DISEASES ✔

1. Inflammatory diseases of the heart muscle are called myocarditis, whereas all others are grouped under the term cardiomyopathy.

2. Myocarditis is most often caused by viruses.

3. Cardiomyopathy occurs in three forms: dilatated, hypertrophic, and restrictive.

PERICARDITIS

74. **What are the main forms of pericarditis?**
    Pericarditis is a common disease, which in most instances is mild and passes unrecognized. It may occur in an acute or a chronic form. Etiologically, pericarditis can be classified as:
    - Infectious—may be acute, as in viral infections, or chronic, as in tuberculosis.
    - Immunologic—occurs in RF and SLE.
    - Postinfarctional (i.e., related to a myocardial infarction)
    - Uremic
    - Radiation induced
    - Tumor related (metastases to the pericardium)

75. **What are the main pathologic forms of acute pericarditis?**
    Pericarditis is typically associated with an exudate in the pericardial cavity. Several pathologic forms of pericarditis are recognized:
    - **Serous pericarditis:** In most instances, it is caused by viral infection. The clear serous fluid must be distinguished from a transudate, which typically accumulates in the pericardial sac in heart failure or anasarca.
    - **Fibrinous pericarditis:** "Bread and butter" type of exudate is typically found in RF and SLE but also in uremic pericarditis and tuberculosis. Clinically it is recognized as a pericardial friction rub.

- **Purulent pericarditis:** Pus accumulates in the pericardial sac infected with pyrogenic bacteria. *Streptococcus pneumoniae, S. aureus,* and gram-negative bacilli may invade the pericardial cavity from adjacent infected thoracic organs (e.g., from pneumonia) or during sepsis.
- **Hemorrhagic pericarditis:** Bleeding into the pericardial cavity is usually of a noninfectious nature (e.g., following cardiac surgery), but it may also evolve during severe bacterial infection (fibrinohemorrhagic pericarditis). Previously, it was a common feature of tuberculous pericarditis.

76. **What are the pathologic forms of chronic pericarditis?**
    - **Chronic effusive pericarditis:** In this condition, the serous fluid persists inside the pericardial cavity. The amount of fluid varies from 50 mL to 1 L or more. It is most often idiopathic, but it also may be a residue of an acute infectious pericarditis.
    - **Adhesive pericarditis:** Healing of serous pericarditis usually results in no consequences, but it also may result in focal fibrous adhesions. Such adhesions usually cause no clinical symptoms.
    - **Fibrotic pericarditis:** Extensive scarring that develops from granulation tissue in the pericardial cavity is the end result of severe exudative pericarditis.
    - **Fibrocalcific pericarditis:** Extensive scarring with calcification of the fibrous tissue is an important complication of tuberculous pericarditis. Calcifications can be recognized by x-rays. This form is rare today.

77. **What is constrictive pericarditis?**
    Fibrotic or fibrocalcific pericarditis may prevent the dilatation of the heart chambers during diastole. Congestive heart failure, similar to heart failure of restrictive cardiomyopathy, develops. In contrast to cardiomyopathy, the heart is small.

78. **What is cardiac tamponade?**
    This term is used for the compression of the heart by fluid accumulating in the pericardial cavity. The fluid may accumulate insidiously, as in chronic effusive pericarditis, or suddenly, as in acute hematopericardium. Compression of the heart prevents diastolic dilatation of atria and ventricles. Heart failure results in increased back pressure in the lungs and the systemic venous circulation.

    Beck triad (hypotension, increased jugular venous pressure, and muffled heart sounds) is a typical clinical finding, but more often patients show only signs of cardiac shock, such as hypotension, tachycardia, dyspnea, and increased venous pressure. Pulsus paradoxus is recognized as decreased systolic pressure (>10 mmHg) during inspiration.

79. **What are the causes of hematopericardium?**
    Acute hematopericardium may cause cardiac tamponade and death, whereas chronic intrapericardial bleeding may be indistinguishable from effusive pericarditis. The causes of bleeding into the pericardial cavity include:
    - **Arterial dissection involving the root of the aorta:** One should remember that the first part of the aorta lies within the pericardial sac. Accordingly, a rupture of the aortic wall may cause intrapericardial bleeding.
    - **Trauma:** Vehicular accidents and other high-speed injuries may rupture the root of the aorta or the heart.
    - **Surgery:** Small amounts of blood are regularly found in the pericardial cavity after cardiac surgery (postcardiotomy states), but massive bleeding is uncommon.
    - **Bleeding disorders:** Thrombocytopenia that accompanies leukemia is probably the most common cause, but bleeding may also occur in aplastic anemia, following radiation and even severe vitamin C deficiency.

- **Neoplasms:** Malignant tumors invading the pericardial cavity (e.g., lung or esophageal cancer extending into the pericardium), metastases involving the epicardium, and rare epicardial primary tumors may be accompanied by serous or hemorrhagic effusions.

NEOPLASM

80. **How common are heart tumors?**
Primary heart tumors are so rare that they are not included in official statistics, and their real incidence is not known. Metastases are much more common, but even these secondary tumors are rare.

81. **What is the most common primary cardiac tumor?**
Myxomas account for more than 50% of all primary heart tumors. Most myxomas are sporadic, but some occur as part of Carney syndrome (skin and endocrine tumors and schwannomas).

82. **List the most important facts about myxomas.**
   - They are most often (80%) found in the left atrium.
   - They typically arise from the atrial septum around the fossa ovalis.
   - Most are pedunculated, but some are broad based and sessile. The size varies, but most are 5 mm to 5 cm.
   - On gross examination, myxomas appear gelatinous ("myxoid").
   - Histologically they are composed of spindle-shaped cells surrounded by loose myxoid matrix.

83. **What are the clinical features of cardiac myxomas?**
   - Symptoms may be nonspecific (e.g., fever, anemia, and elevated erythrocyte sedimentation rate) and are often described as protean (varied).
   - Tumor may fragment and give rise to arterial emboli.
   - Tumor may have a ball-valve effect and partially obstruct the mitral valve. Mitral obstruction results in symptoms that are indistinguishable from those caused by mitral stenosis.
   - Echocardiography is the most useful technique for visualizing the tumors.

84. **What are rhabdomyomas?**
Rhabdomyomas—benign striated muscle tumors of the myocardium—are the second most common primary heart tumor. These tumors are typically found in infants and children.

85. **What are the most common malignant tumors of the heart?**
Primary malignant tumors of the heart are extremely rare. Histologically, these tumors are sarcomas (angiosarcoma) or mesotheliomas. Metastases of malignant tumors originating in other organs are approximately 50 to 100 times more common than either primary benign or malignant cardiac tumors. Most often, these metastases originate in primary malignant tumors of the lung and breast. Malignant melanomas also tend to metastasize to the heart. Metastases may grow in any part of the heart, but most often they are found in the pericardium.

KEY POINTS: PERICARDITIS ✓

1. Pericarditis can be acute or chronic.

2. Pericarditis can be classified according to etiology (e.g., viral, bacterial, and immunologic) or according to the pathology (e.g., serous and purulent).

3. Acute hematoperitoneum causes tamponade of the heart and death.

CONGENITAL HEART DISEASE

86. **How common are congenital heart diseases?**

    Developmental anomalies of the heart and the major blood vessels are common and are found in 6 to 8 per 1000 newborns. Congenital heart diseases (CHDs) represent the most common form of heart disease in children.

87. **Do all CHDs become clinically apparent in childhood?**

    Some congenital defects become clinically apparent at birth or in infancy, others are recognized in early childhood, whereas others remain asymptomatic most of the life and are recognized only later in life. The best examples of CHDs that are diagnosed after infancy and childhood are:

    - **Bicuspid aortic valve stenosis:** It is found in 1% or 2% of the total population. Because of hemodynamic changes related to the valvular abnormality, bicuspid aortic valves tend to degenerate and calcify and are an important cause of calcific aortic stenosis in late adult life.
    - **Mitral valve prolapse ("floppy mitral valve"):** This occurs in approximately 2% to 3% of all adults and is usually diagnosed in adolescence or early adulthood.

88. **What are the most common CHDs of infancy and childhood?**

    Although there are hundreds of CHDs, 12 major diseases account for almost all those that are clinically recognized during infancy and childhood. Among these, the most common are:

    - Ventricular septal defect (30%)
    - Tetralogy of Fallot (10%)
    - Atrial septal defect (8%)
    - Patent ductus arteriosus (8%)
    - Coarctation of the aorta (6%)
    - Transposition of the great arteries (5%)

89. **List key facts about the causes of CHDs.**

    - The cause is unknown in more than 90% of cases.
    - Familial cases suggest polygenic inheritance in some instances.
    - Intrauterine exposure to *Rubella* virus (rare today in the United States) and alcohol.
    - Increased incidence in chromosomal syndromes (e.g., Down syndrome and Turner syndrome) suggests an association between chromosomal abnormalities and heart malformations.

90. **How are CHDs classified clinically?**

    Three groups of defects are recognized depending on whether there are defects in the septum between the two sides of the heart and whether shunting of blood occurs:

    - Malformations with a left-to-right shunt (acyanotic)
        - Atrial septal defect
        - Ventricular septal defect
    - Malformations with a right-to-left shunt (early cyanosis)
        - Tetralogy of Fallot
        - Malformations without shunts
    - Coarctation of the aorta

91. **List five CHDs that present with early cyanosis at the time of birth or soon thereafter.**

    Five diseases, all beginning with T, present with early cyanosis:

    - Tetralogy of Fallot (most common)

- Transposition of the great arteries (aorta arising from the right ventricle and pulmonary artery arising from the left ventricle)
- Truncus arteriosus communis (aorta and pulmonary artery are not separated from each other and form a single vessel overriding both ventricles)
- Tricuspid valve atresia (usually with atrial septal defect)
- Total anomalous return of the pulmonary veins (oxygenated blood returns to the right instead of the left atrium)

KEY POINTS: NEOPLASMS ✔️

1. Heart tumors are rare.

2. The most common primary benign tumor of the heart is myxoma of the left atrium, whereas pericardial metastases are the most common malignancy.

92. **What are the features of ventricular septal defect?**
    - This is the most common CHD (30%).
    - It most often involves the upper part (i.e., the membranous part) of the septum (80%). Muscular septal defects are less common but may be multiple.
    - Small defects (50% of all) are recognized by high-pitched holosystolic murmur (Roger disease). They tend to close spontaneously in the first 2 years of life.
    - The shunt is initially left to right, leading to pulmonary hypertension and right ventricular hypertrophy.
    - Reversal of the shunt occurs when the pulmonary hypertension exceeds the pressure in the aorta.
    - Reversal of the shunt from left to right to right to left (Eisenmenger syndrome) leads to cyanosis (cyanose tardive)

93. **What are the features of atrial septal defect (ASD)?**
    - ASD accounts for 10% of all CHDs.
    - It may present in several forms depending on which part of the septum is involved.
    - Ostium secundum defect occurs at the fossa ovalis and represents the most common form of ASD (90%).
    - Ostium primum defect involves the lower portion of the septum and may be associated with deformities of the mitral valve.
    - Sinus venosus–type defect is located at the entry level of the superior vena cava into the right atrium.
    - Shunt is left to right and causes fewer problems than ventricular septal defect (VSD).
    - Pulmonary hypertension and heart failure occur in 10% of cases.
    - ASD is usually diagnosed in early adult life (probably the most common CHD to be diagnosed in adult life).

94. **What are the anatomic components of tetralogy of Fallot?**
    As the name implies, this anomaly comprises four pathologic findings (Fig. 8-3):
    - VSD
    - Pulmonary artery stenosis
    - Overriding aorta sitting over the VSD
    - Right ventricular hypertrophy

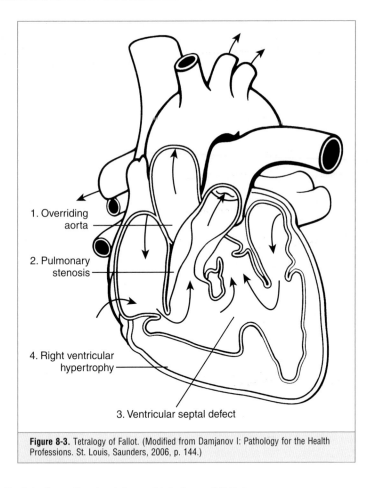

1. Overriding aorta
2. Pulmonary stenosis
4. Right ventricular hypertrophy
3. Ventricular septal defect

Figure 8-3. Tetralogy of Fallot. (Modified from Damjanov I: Pathology for the Health Professions. St. Louis, Saunders, 2006, p. 144.)

95. **Explain the pathophysiology of tetralogy of Fallot.**
    The narrowing of the pulmonary artery does not allow the entry of venous blood into the lungs. Instead, the unoxygenated venous blood passes through the VSD into the aorta that is overriding the VSD and thus receives the blood from both ventricles. The entry of the venous blood into the aorta leads to cyanosis and generalized hypoxia. In addition to the complex cardiologic findings, other clinical features include:
    - Cyanosis (Bluish discoloration of the skin and mucosa may be evident at birth. In some infants, cyanosis develops at variable rates after birth, but in most children it is evident by age 4 months.)
    - Hypoxemic spells (These spells are marked by deepening cyanosis or dyspnea. The children may faint or lose consciousness.)
    - Retarded growth
    - Squatting position frequently assumed by older children
    - Clubbing of fingers

96. **What is the prognosis of tetralogy of Fallot?**
    Some children may die in the first year of life. Those who survive show signs of initial improvement, but the condition usually deteriorates during the second and third decades of life.

Death occurs because of protracted anoxia, infections that occur at an increased rate, and cerebrovascular accidents related to thromboemboli. Patients with mild cases of the disease, called the acyanotic variety, may have a relatively normal life. Surgery is recommended as the treatment of choice for most cases, but it is associated with a 3% to 15% mortality rate.

97. **What is coarctation of the aorta?**
Coarctation of the aorta is characterized by narrowing of the aorta. It occurs in two forms:
- **Infantile form:** In this condition, the aortic arch and the ascending aorta are markedly narrowed. Ductus arteriosus does not undergo atresia, and it serves as the conduit for the blood to the aorta below the narrowing. Most infants do not survive without surgical correction of the defect. The head and the upper extremities are hypoxic, whereas the lower parts of the body (receiving the venous blood through the open ductus arteriosus) are cyanotic.
- **Adult type:** The narrowing of the aortic arch occurs opposite the insertion of the ductus arteriosus, which undergoes normal atresia. Because of aortic narrowing, there is hypertension in the head and upper extremities (i.e., parts of the body supplied by the arteries originating from the arch of the aorta). The parts of the body below the obstruction are hypoxic, and the blood pressure measured on the legs is lower than the pressure measured on the arms. Collateral circulation develops through internal mammary arteries so that the arterial blood from the branches of the subclavian arteries may provide oxygen to the aorta beyond the obstruction. Collaterals that involve the intercostal arteries cause notching of the ribs.

98. **What is patent ductus arteriosus?**
Ductus arteriosus is a normal fetal blood vessel allowing the blood from the venous system to bypass the lungs. After birth, ductus undergoes atresia and transforms into a narrow strand of connective tissue. Delayed occlusion of the ductus is a common finding in prematurely born infants. Ductus is kept open by prostaglandin (PGE2), and closure can be accelerated by injecting inhibitors of PGE2, such as indomethacin.
If the ductus arteriosus does not close, it will provide a venue for the reflow of arterial blood from the aorta into the pulmonary artery. This left-to-right shunt is associated with a loud "machinery murmur." Pulmonary hypertension develops.

KEY POINTS: CONGENITAL HEART DISEASE ✓

1. Congenital heart diseases are an important form of heart disease in infants and children.

2. Congenital heart diseases are classified into three major groups: those with left-to-right shunt, called acyanotic; those with right-to-left shunt, called cyanotic; and those that do not have any shunts between the right and left part of the heart.

3. The most common acyanotic heart disease is ventricular septal defect, whereas the most common cyanotic heart disease is tetralogy of Fallot.

99. **What are the common clinical findings in children with CHD?**
- Heart failure—defective hearts cannot function as efficiently as normal hearts. Furthermore, these hearts are often overburdened and must work harder.
- Chronic ischemia—inadequate perfusion of tissues and hypoxia due to inadequate oxygenation of blood cause growth retardation, easy fatigability, and somnolence.
- There is increased incidence of endocarditis.
- There is increased incidence of thrombosis.

WESTITES

BIBLIOGRAPHY

1. Burke A, Jendy J Jr, Virmani R: Cardiac tumours: an update: Cardiac tumours. Heart 94:117–123, 2008.

2. Burke AP, Virmani R: Pathophysiology of acute myocardial infarction. Med Clin North Am 91:553–572, 2007.

3. Goyle KK, Walling AD: Diagnosing pericarditis. Am Fam Physician 66:1695–1702, 2003.

4. Hurst RT, Lee RW: Increased incidence of coronary atherosclerosis in type 2 diabetes mellitus: mechanisms and management. Ann Intern Med 139:824–834, 2003.

5. Klatt EC: Cardiovascular pathology in AIDS. Adv Cardiol 40:23–48, 2003.

6. Kolodgie FD, Burke AP, Nakazawa G, Cheng Q, Xu X, Virmani R: Free cholesterol in atherosclerotic plaques: where does it come from? Curr Opin Lipidol 18:500–507, 2007.

7. Kolodgie FD, Nakazawa G, Sangiorgi G, Ladich E, Burke AP, Virmani R: Pathology of atherosclerosis and stenting. Neuroimaging Clin N Am 17:285–301, 2007.

8. Lusis AJ: Genetic factors in cardiovascular disease. 10 questions. Trends Cardiovasc Med 3:309–316, 2003.

9. Oakley CM: Myocarditis, pericarditis and other pericardial diseases. Heart 84:449–454, 2000.

10. Sexton DJ, Spelman D: Current best practices and guidelines. Assessment and management of complications in infective endocarditis. Infect Dis Clin North Am 16:507–521, 2002.

11. Stollerman GH: Rheumatic fever. Lancet 349:935–942, 1997.

CHAPTER 9

THE HEMATOPOIETIC AND LYMPHOID SYSTEMS

Marin Nola, MD, PhD, and Snježana Dotlić, MD

1. **What are the most important diseases of the hematopoietic and lymphoid systems?**
   - Anemia
   - Polycythemia
   - Leukemia
   - Leukopenia
   - Non-Hodgkin lymphoma
   - Hodgkin lymphoma
   - Multiple myeloma
   - Lymphopenia and immunodeficiency diseases
   - Bleeding disorders

RED BLOOD CELL DISORDERS

2. **Define anemia.**
   Anemia can be defined as a decrease in the red blood cell (RBC) mass and the hemoglobin content in the blood. It may be diagnosed by the demonstration of decreased values of certain parameters:
   - Hemoglobin concentration
   - Hematocrit
   - Erythrocyte count
   One should note that overhydration due to fluid retention may expand plasma volume, and fluid loss may contract plasma volume. These conditions are called hemodilution and hemoconcentration, respectively. Hemodilution should not be confused with anemia.

3. **What are the best hematologic tests for diagnosing anemia?**
   - RBC count
     - Hemoglobin
     - Hematocrit
   - RBC indices
     - Mean cell volume (MCV)
     - Mean corpuscular hemoglobin (MCH)
     - Mean corpuscular hemoglobin concentration (MCHC)
   - RBC distribution width
   - White blood cell (WBC) count
   - Platelet count
   - Cell morphology

- Reticulocyte count
- Iron supply studies
  - Serum iron
  - Total iron-binding capacity
  - Serum ferritin, marrow iron content
- Bone marrow examination
  - Aspirate
  - Biopsy

4. **List three major groups of anemia according to their etiology and pathogenesis.**
- Anemia due to blood loss
  - Acute blood loss: massive bleeding from ruptured vessels, wounds, and trauma
  - Chronic blood loss: bleeding lesions of gastrointestinal tract and gynecologic disturbances
- Anemia due to increased rate of RBC destruction (hemolytic anemia)
  - Intrinsic (intracorpuscular) abnormalities of red cells:
    - Hereditary
      - Red cell membrane disorder: hereditary spherocytosis
      - Red cell enzyme deficiencies: glucose-6-phosphate dehydrogenase deficiency
      - Disorders of hemoglobin synthesis: sickle cell disease and thalassemia syndromes
    - Acquired
      - Paroxysmal nocturnal hemoglobinuria
  - Extrinsic (extracorpuscular)
    - Antibody mediated: transfusion reaction, erythroblastosis fetalis, and immunohemolytic anemia
    - Mechanical injury of RBCs: microangiopathic hemolytic anemia
- Anemia due to impaired RBC production
  - Disturbance of proliferation and differentiation of stem cells; aplastic anemia and pure RBC aplasia
  - Disturbance of proliferation and maturation of erythroblasts
    - Defective DNA synthesis: megaloblastic anemia
    - Defective hemoglobin synthesis: iron deficiency and thalassemia
    - Unknown or multiple mechanisms: anemia of chronic infections and myelophthisic anemia

5. **How are anemias classified according to the red cell size and shape and their hemoglobin content?**
- According to red cell size
  - Microcytic (small)
  - Normocytic (normal)
  - Macrocytic (large)
- According to degree of hemoglobinization, reflected in the color of red cells
  - Hypochromic (decreased)
  - Normochromic (normal)
- According to the red cell shape
  See Table 9-1 and Fig. 9-1.

TABLE 9-1. ABNORMAL RED BLOOD CELL (RBC) MORPHOLOGY

Abnormality	Features	Significance
Anisocytosis	Variation in RBC size	Nonspecific
Poikilocytosis	Variation in RBC shape	Nonspecific
Target cells	Targetlike appearance	Thalassemia, hemoglobinopathics
Sickle cells	Bipolar (sickle) or hollyleaf	Sickle cell anemia RBCs
Schistocytes	RBC fragments	Microangiopathic hemolytic anemia
Teardrops	Tennis racket RBCs	Myelofibrosis, severe anemias
Spherocytes	Spherical RBCs with dense hemoglobin content	Hereditary spherocytosis, alcoholism
Bite cells	Smooth semicircle taken from one edge	G6PD deficiency

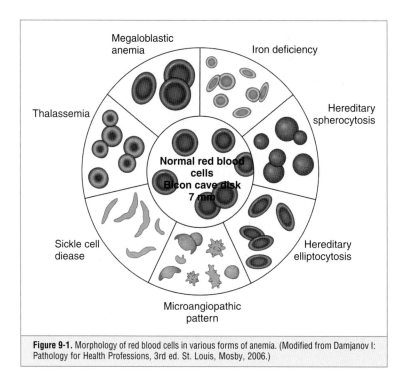

Figure 9-1. Morphology of red blood cells in various forms of anemia. (Modified from Damjanov I: Pathology for Health Professions, 3rd ed. St. Louis, Mosby, 2006.)

6. **Define the main hematologic parameters.**
   - Hematocrit
   - The ratio of RBCs to serum expressed in percentages:
     - In anemia, hematocrit is low, whereas in polycythemia it is high
     - Normal values: men, 39% to 49%; women, 33% to 43%
   - MCV of erythrocytes
     - The average calculated volume of a single RBC (hematocrit/erythrocyte count)
     - On the basis of MCV, anemias may be defined as microcytic, normocytic, or macrocytic
     - Normal values: 76 to 100 mm^3.
   - MCH
     - The average content of hemoglobin in each RBC (hemoglobin/erythrocyte count)
     - According to MCH, anemia can be defined as hypochromic or normochromic
     - Normal values: 27 to 33 pg
   - MCHC
     - The average concentration of hemoglobin in a given volume of packed RBCs (hemoglobin/hematocrit)
     - According to MCHC, anemia may be defined as hypochromic, normochromic, or hyperchromic
     - Normal values: 33 to 37 g/dL
     - In contrast to MCH, MCHC considers the size of erythrocytes, therefore diminishing the possibility of spurious results in case of low hemoglobin concentration or a decrease in erythrocyte size.

7. **Discuss how reticulocyte counts are used in clinical practice.**
   The reticulocyte is a stage of RBC maturation, normally present in both the marrow and the blood. Under normal conditions, the peripheral blood contains less than 1.5% reticulocytes, but in some anemic patients, their number may be increased. Reticulocyte count is used to assess the capacity of the bone marrow to increase RBC production in response to increased demand. On the basis of the reticulocyte count, anemias may be classified as hypoproliferative, normoproliferative, and hyperproliferative.
   - **Hypoproliferative:** Patients with anemia caused by defects in erythrocyte proliferation or maturation tend to have low reticulocyte counts. Patients suffering from pernicious anemia have low reticulocyte count, which will, however, increase after vitamin B$_{12}$ treatment.
   - **Normoproliferative or hyperproliferative:** Patients with anemia caused by decreased survival of erythrocytes with a normal bone marrow proliferative response often exhibit increased peripheral blood reticulocytes. If the degree of reticulocytosis is adequate to replace the loss of erythrocytes, the anemia is said to be compensated.

8. **List signs and symptoms common to all forms of anemia.**
   - Pale skin and mucosa (e.g., conjunctiva)
   - Easy fatigability and dyspnea on mild exertion
   - Koilonychia, a spoon-shaped concavity of the nails, associated with brittle nails; feature of prolonged anemia that is rarely seen today
   - Central nervous system hypoxia causing headaches, dim vision, and drowsiness

9. **Are there any pathologic tissue findings characteristic of anemia in general?**
   No. Most of the tissue changes caused by anemia are nonspecific. These findings include consequences of prolonged mild ischemia and hypoxia, such as fatty change of liver and heart cells. Prolonged and severe anemia leads to a loss of neurons in the brain, but such a loss cannot be readily recognized in routine histologic sections.

10. **Describe the typical hematologic changes following acute massive blood loss.**
    Massive blood loss may result in shock and even death. If the person survives, the blood volume is rapidly restored by entry of water from the interstitial spaces into the circulation. This redistribution of water results in hemodilution, which lowers the hematocrit. The RBC counts performed at this point will usually show anemia, which is typically normocytic and normochromic. Thrombocytosis and leukocytosis may be found in peripheral blood because of mobilization of these cells from the marginal pools. Reactive reticulocytosis occurs a few days later. It is mediated by erythropoietin released from the kidneys in response to low oxygen tension in the blood depleted of RBCs. Reticulocytosis will reach its peak 7 to 10 days after hemorrhage and may be as high as 10% to 15% (i.e., 10 times higher than normal).

11. **How does chronic blood loss cause anemia?**
    Chronic blood loss causes a loss of iron, but significant anemia occurs only when the rate of loss exceeds the regenerative capacity of the bone marrow or when iron reserves are markedly depleted. Anemia of chronic blood loss is common in menstruating women, who lose approximately 70 mL of blood during every menstruation. Frequent pregnancies and childbirth are other important causes of anemia. Gastrointestinal diseases are the most common cause of iron-deficiency anemia in men. Nevertheless, in all patients with iron-deficiency anemia, testing of stools and the urine for occult blood loss should be performed.

12. **List the three main features common to all forms of hemolytic anemia.**
    - Premature destruction of erythrocytes, which live less than the normal 120 days
    - Accumulation of the hemoglobin degradation products (e.g., hemosiderin) in phagocytic cells
    - A marked increase in erythropoietin stimulating compensatory erythropoiesis within the bone marrow

13. **What is the difference between intravascular and extravascular hemolysis?**
    - **Intravascular hemolysis:** Significant lysis of erythrocytes rarely occurs within the vascular spaces. In intravascular hemolysis, normal erythrocytes are damaged by:
      - Mechanical injury
        - Mechanical cardiac valves
        - Thrombi within microcirculation
      - Complement fixation to red cells
        - Transfusion of mismatched blood
      - Exogenous toxic factors or infections
        - *Falciparum* malaria
        - Clostridial sepsis
    - **Extravascular hemolysis:** Most frequently, the premature destruction of erythrocytes occurs within the mononuclear phagocyte system of the spleen and liver. In extravascular hemolysis, erythrocytes are destroyed because:
      - They are rendered "foreign" by autoantibodies that attach to them in autoimmune hemolytic anemia.
      - They become less deformable as in sickle cell anemia or hereditary spherocytosis.
      In both forms of hemolysis, there is anemia and jaundice. Hemoglobinemia and hemoglobinuria occur only in intravascular hemolysis. Hypertrophy of the mononuclear phagocyte system and consequent splenomegaly are seen only in extravascular hemolysis.

14. **What are the main features of intravascular hemolysis?**
    - **Jaundice:** It is related to the excessive formation of unconjugated bilirubin from the heme portion of hemoglobin. Unconjugated bilirubin is bound to albumin and does not appear in urine.
    - **Hemoglobinemia:** It results from the release of free hemoglobin released from RBCs. Free hemoglobin binds to haptoglobin, which prevents its excretion into urine. Hemoglobin–haptoglobin complex is rapidly cleared by the mononuclear phagocyte system. Accordingly,

the blood concentration of haptoglobin will be reduced. Decreased serum haptoglobin is a reliable sign of intravascular hemolysis.

- **Methemalbuminemia:** When the serum haptoglobin is depleted, the unbound or free hemoglobin is in part rapidly oxidized to methemoglobin, which binds to albumin forming methemalbumin.

- **Hemoglobinuria:** Hemoglobin in urine appears after the haptoglobin binding capacity has been exceeded and the free hemoglobin is filtered through the glomeruli. Both hemoglobin and methemoglobin are excreted through the kidneys, imparting a red-brown color to the urine.

- **Hemosiderinuria:** Hemosiderin in urine is derived from hemoglobin degradation in the renal tubules.

15. **What is the mechanism of erythroid hyperplasia of the bone marrow in hemolytic anemia?**
All forms of hemolytic anemia are accompanied by premature destruction of erythrocytes. The resulting anemia and lowered oxygen saturation of blood stimulate increased production of erythropoietin in the kidneys, which leads to an increase in the number of normoblasts in the bone marrow and prominent reticulocytosis in the peripheral blood.

16. **Name the common pathologic tissue findings common to all forms of chronic hemolytic anemia.**
- Increase in the number of normoblasts in the bone marrow
- Prominent reticulocytosis in the peripheral blood
- Formation of pigment gallstones (cholelithiasis) caused by elevated levels of bilirubin when it is excreted through the liver
- Hemosiderosis due to hemosiderin accumulation in the mononuclear phagocyte system in long-term anemias (Hemosiderin accumulation is due in part to hemosiderin released from damaged RBCs and in part to the transfusions of blood that such patients typically receive.)

17. **What is the difference between anemia caused by extrinsic factors (extracorpuscular defects) and anemia caused by intrinsic factors (intracorpuscular defects)?**
Because the classification of intravascular and extravascular hemolytic disorders is not entirely satisfactory, a classification based on the underlying cause of red cell destruction is proposed:
- Extracorpuscular
  - Extrinsic underlying cause
  - Acquired disorders (i.e., antibody mediated, mechanical trauma to red cells, infections, and chemical injury)
- Intracorpuscular
  - Hereditary disorders (i.e., red cell membrane disorders, red cell enzyme deficiencies, and disorders of hemoglobin synthesis)
  - Acquired disorders (i.e., paroxysmal nocturnal hemoglobinuria)

KEY POINTS: HEMATOLOGY AND RED BLOOD CELL DISORDERS ✓

1. Hematology covers diseases of red blood cells (RBCs), platelets, blood coagulation factors, leukocytes, and lymphoid cells.

2. Anemia is a decrease in the red cell mass and hemoglobin content of the blood, reducing the capacity of the blood to transport oxygen.

3. Anemia can be classified etiologically into three groups: anemia due to blood loss, hemolytic anemia, and anemia due to impaired RBC production.

4. Hemolytic anemias develop due to inherent RBC defects or due to antibodies and other extracorpuscular causes.

5. RBC production can be impaired due to deficiency of iron, vitamin B$_{12}$, and folic acid or as a consequence of bone marrow failure in aplastic anemia.

6. Polycythemia vera can occur in two forms: as polycythemia vera, which is a neoplastic disorder, and as a secondary polycythemia, which is related to excessive stimulation of RBC precursors by erythropoietin.

18. **What is hereditary spherocytosis?**
    Hereditary spherocytosis (HS) is caused by several inherited defects in the red cell membrane skeleton that render the RBCs spheroid (round) and less deformable during their passage through the splenic sinusoids. Spherical RBCs are thus more prone to splenic sequestration and destruction, which lead to intracorpuscular hemolysis.

19. **What are the exact molecular defects in HS?**
    The normal membrane cytoskeleton of RBCs is composed of several proteins, the most important of which are α and β spectrin, ankyrin, actin, and proteins known as band 4.1 and band 3 (Fig. 9-2). Together these proteins maintain the normal biconcave shape of RBCs. The mutation of ankyrin gene is the most common defect in autosomal dominant HS, and the mutations of gene encoding protein band 3 account for 20% of cases. Genes encoding other cytoskeletal proteins are less often mutated.

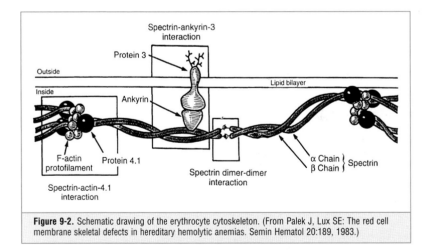

Figure 9-2. Schematic drawing of the erythrocyte cytoskeleton. (From Palek J, Lux SE: The red cell membrane skeletal defects in hereditary hemolytic anemias. Semin Hematol 20:189, 1983.)

20. **How common is HS, and how is it inherited?**
    The prevalence of HS is as high as 1 in 5000 in Caucasians of northern European origin. The autosomal dominant pattern of inheritance accounts for 75% of these cases. The autosomal recessive form of the disease is less common, but it is much more severe than the autosomal dominant form.

21. **Describe the pathologic findings in HS.**
The most prominent changes are found in the peripheral blood, the bone marrow, and the spleen:
   - **Blood smears:** Spheroid red cells appear uniformly red in routine smears (spherocytosis). Their central pallor, corresponding to the central concavity, is lacking. Although this morphology of RBCs is distinctive, it is not pathognomonic of HS and may also be seen in autoimmune hemolytic anemias.
   - **Bone marrow:** Erythroid hyperplasia with an increased number of normoblasts is seen in bone marrow biopsy.
   - **Spleen**
     - Splenomegaly of moderate extent (500–1000 g) results from marked congestion of the red pulp cords. The sinuses appear virtually empty.
     - Erythrophagocytosis can be seen within the congested cords.
     - Hemosiderosis of the splenic red pulp is prominent and typically associated with hemosiderosis of the liver.
   - **Biliary system:** Pigment gallstones are found in 40% to 50% of affected adults.

22. **How is hereditary spherocytosis diagnosed clinically?**
The diagnosis is based on:
   - Family history to document autosomal dominant or recessive inheritance
   - Laboratory findings, including spherocytosis, increased osmotic fragility of RBCs, and hyperbilirubinemia (Osmotic lysis of RBCs can be seen in two thirds of patients and is induced in vitro by immersing patients' RBCs into a hypotonic salt solution. Because the spherical RBCs cannot expand more, the influx of water leads to their early rupture.)
   - Clinical features including anemia, mild jaundice, and splenomegaly.

23. **What is the clinical course of hereditary spherocytosis?**
The severity of the disease is variable among individuals:
   - In a minority of patients, hereditary spherocytosis presents at birth with marked jaundice, requiring exchange transfusion.
   - Twenty to thirty percent of patients are largely asymptomatic because of compensatory increased erythropoiesis.
   - Most patients have a chronic anemia of mild to moderate severity. This more-or-less stable clinical course may be aggravated by intercurrent infections, either by reducing erythrocyte formation (aplastic crisis) or by increasing erythrocyte destruction (hemolytic crisis). The formation of pigmented gallstones may also cause symptoms.

24. **Explain why glucose-6-phosphate dehydrogenase (G6PD) causes hemolytic anemia.**
Exposure of RBCs to drugs or toxins that generate oxygen radicals is counteracted by reduced glutathione. To form this antioxidant, the cells must increase the breakdown of glucose through the hexose-monophosphate shunt. G6PD is an enzyme that plays a crucial role in this metabolic pathway and is essential for maintaining the glutathione in its active form. Erythrocytes deficient in G6PD are less resistant to oxidant injury, and consequently any exposure to oxidants will cause hemolysis.

25. **What should one know about G6PD deficiency?**
   - It is an X-linked disorder, comprising more than 350 variants, and exclusively affects males.
   - There is geographic variability. It is most prevalent in Mediterranean countries and western Africa and in Americans whose ancestors came from those regions.
   - Overall prevalence is 1 in 1000, but it is more common in some populations (e.g. African Americans, 15%).

- Periodic hemolysis can be induced by a variety of oxidants:
  - Oxygen free radicals generated by leukocytes in course of infections
  - Drugs (antimalarials, such as primaquine, chloroquine, sulfonamides, and nitrofurantoin)
  - Fava beans (hence the popular term for this disease, favism)
- Laboratory findings include anemia, hemoglobinemia, and occasional hemoglobinuria. Peripheral blood smear shows Heinz bodies and bite cells. Heinz bodies can be seen as dark inclusions when the smears are stained with crystal violet. When the spleen pits the Heinz bodies from RBCs, it also removes a portion of the RBC cytoplasm, leading to formation of bite cells.

26. **What is sickle cell anemia?**
Sickle cell anemia is a hereditary hemoglobinopathy caused by mutation of the b-globin gene. This mutation affects hemoglobin A (HbA), transforming it into an abnormal hemoglobin S (HbS). Aggregation and polymerization of the HbS molecules, initiated by deoxygenation, leads to the formation of HbS fibers and resultant distortion of the red cells by sickling. Initially, sickling is a reversible phenomenon, but with repeated episodes of sickling and unsickling, membrane damage ensues, and the cells become irreversibly deformed.

27. **How common is sickle cell anemia?**
Sickle cell anemia is most common in Africa, but it is also encountered in Mediterranean countries and India. In some areas of Africa, as many as 40% of inhabitants are heterozygotes for HbS. The prevalence of heterozygosity among African Americans is 10%. One in 650 of these people is monozygous and has clinical signs of sickle cell anemia. Approximately 50,000 people have sickle cell anemia in the United States.

28. **Describe the difference between the sickle cell trait and sickle cell anemia.**
The mutation that causes either sickle cell disease or sickle cell trait is a point mutation in the gene that leads to substitution of a valine for glutamic acid at the sixth position of the β-globin chain of hemoglobin:
- When an individual is homozygous for the mutant gene, all the hemoglobin is of the abnormal HbS type. Sickling and hemolysis occur in regular living circumstances, causing the spectrum of clinical signs and symptoms known as sickle cell anemia.
- In heterozygotes, only a portion (approximately 40%) of the hemoglobin is HbS, and the remainder is normal HbA. RBC sickling and possibly hemolysis occur in hypoxia and other abnormal conditions. This heterozygous state is referred to as sickle cell trait.

29. **Why do dehydration and anoxia (e.g., high altitude) potentiate sickling of RBCs in sickle cell anemia?**
The precipitation of HbS fibers has deleterious effects on the red cell membrane in irreversibly sickled cells but also in normal-appearing cells. With membrane injury, the RBCs have difficulty maintaining normal intracellular volume, and consequently intracellular hemoglobin concentration increases (MCHC is higher), with a higher concentration of the HbS within the cell. Dehydration removes the water from RBCs, bringing HbS molecules even closer to each other, thus greatly facilitating sickling.

Hypoxia, as occurs at high altitudes, increases the amount of deoxygenated HbS. Because deoxygenated HbS molecules aggregate and polymerize many times more readily than oxygenated HbS, it is obvious that hypoxia will promote sickling. Similarly, a decrease in pH lowers the affinity of hemoglobin for oxygen and therefore increases the amount of deoxygenated HbS, which will increase sickling.

30. **Name two main causes of ischemia in sickle cell anemia.**
    - **Chronic hemolytic anemia:** Anemia results from shortened life span of RBC, which survive on average only 20 days in circulation. In response to chronic hemolysis the bone marrow undergoes massive hyperplasia (Fig. 9-3).
    - **Occlusion of small blood vessels:** The altered RBC membranes favor adhesion of these cells to the endothelium. The slow down of the circulation due to increased RBC adhesion promotes hypoxia, which in turn contributes to the sickling of abnormal RBCs and finally vasoocclusion. Hypoxia affects numerous organs and may even cause death.

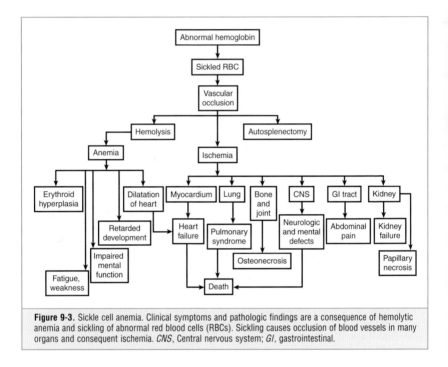

Figure 9-3. Sickle cell anemia. Clinical symptoms and pathologic findings are a consequence of hemolytic anemia and sickling of abnormal red blood cells (RBCs). Sickling causes occlusion of blood vessels in many organs and consequent ischemia. *CNS,* Central nervous system; *GI,* gastrointestinal.

31. **How does sickling of RBCs affect the spleen?**
    Irreversibly sickled cells have rigid and nondeformable membranes and have difficulty negotiating the splenic sinusoids. They become sequestered in the spleen, where they are destroyed by the mononuclear phagocytes. The spleen may become enlarged early in the disease (up to 500 g in children). There is a marked congestion of the red pulp due to the trapped sickled red cells. This erythrostasis leads to thrombosis and infarction in the spleen or at least to marked tissue hypoxia. Continued scarring causes progressive shrinkage of the spleen, resulting in autosplenectomy by adolescence or early adulthood, when only a small nubbin of fibrous tissue may be left.

32. **Why does the calvaria of sickle cell patients have a "crew-cut" appearance on x-rays?**
    The bone marrow in these patients is hyperplastic because of the compensatory expansion of normoblasts. The resorption of bone with secondary new bone formation sometimes develops as a consequence of the expansion of bone marrow. These changes on the calvaria produce the x-ray appearance of a crew cut.

33. **Discuss the most common bacteria causing infection, death, or both in children with sickle cell anemia.**
    Septicemia and meningitis caused by *Streptococcus pneumoniae* and *Haemophilus influenzae* are the most common causes of severe infection or death in these children. *Salmonella* species are a common cause of osteomyelitis.

34. **What are three types of crisis in sickle cell anemia?**
    - **Vasoocclusive (or painful) crisos:** Episodes of hypoxia and infarction are associated with severe pain in the affected area. Most commonly involved sites are bones, lungs, liver, brain, spleen, and penis.
        - In children, painful bone crises are extremely common, causing the so-called hand–foot syndrome, which can be distinguished from acute osteomyelitis with difficulty.
        - Involvement of the lungs presents with fever, cough, chest pain, and pulmonary infiltrates. Acute chest syndrome is a major cause of death in patients older than 5 years.
        - Central nervous system hypoxia may present clinically as seizures or stroke. Retarded mental development is a serious complication of these hypoxia attacks.
        - The affected spleen is initially enlarged in childhood. Following multiple infarcts, it undergoes progressive shrinkage during adolescence or early adulthood and may completely vanish (autosplenectomy).
        - Leg ulcers in adult patients develop due to ischemia of skin and the subcutaneous tissue.
    - **Aplastic crises:** Temporary cessation of bone marrow activity is usually triggered by intercurrent infections. The most common cause is a parvovirus infection that affects the erythroid progenitor cells. Such crises are marked by sudden and rapid worsening of anemia accompanied by a disappearance of reticulocytes from the peripheral blood.
    - **Sequestration crisis:** Sequestration of deformed RBCs in the spleen is accompanied by sudden splenomegaly, hypovolemia, and sometimes shock. Splenic ischemia ultimately leads to autosplenectomy.

35. **List the laboratory findings useful for diagnosing sickle cell anemia.**
    - Peripheral blood smear
        - Observation of sickle-shaped cells
    - Electrophoresis of hemoglobin
        - HbS detected on the basis of its slow mobility
    - Prenatal, molecular diagnosis
        - Analysis of mutated fetal DNA obtained by amniocentesis or chorionic biopsy

36. **What is thalassemia, and how is it classified?**
    Thalassemia is a group of disorders caused by a lack of or decreased synthesis of structurally normal hemoglobin chains. This disease is classified according to the type of chains that are missing. If the α chains are missing, it is called α-thalassemia; if the β chains are missing, it is called β-thalassemia. Low intracellular hemoglobin (hypochromia), as well as the relative excess of the other chain, accounts for the morphologic and functional disturbances seen in these diseases.

37. **What are the common features of all forms of β-thalassemia?**
    A quantitatively defective synthesis of β-globin chains is found in all β-thalassemias. The synthesis of α chains is unimpaired, leading to an excess of α chains. Free α chains tend to aggregate into insoluble inclusions within erythrocytes and their precursors, leading to:
    - Premature destruction of maturing erythroblasts within the marrow (ineffective erythropoiesis)
    - Lysis of abnormal mature red cells in the spleen (hemolysis)

38. **What are the pathologic features of β-thalassemia?**
   - Blood smear
     - Anisocytosis (variation in size)
     - Microcytic, hypochromic red cells, so MCHC is low (β-thalassemia trait is important to distinguish from iron-deficiency anemia because of opposite therapy)
     - Abnormal cell shape: target cells (so called because of the small amount of hemoglobin that precipitates in the center), stippled red cells, and fragmented red cells
     - Inclusions representing aggregates of α chains are not visible in peripheral blood (they are removed by the spleen)
     - Elevated reticulocyte count (although lower than would be expected because of ineffective erythropoiesis)
   - Bones
     - Most erythroblasts die in the bone marrow (apoptosis), resulting in ineffective erythropoiesis. This, in turn, stimulates erythropoietin secretion, which leads to severe erythroid hyperplasia in the bone marrow and often at extramedullary sites.
     - Massive erythropoiesis within the bones invades the cortex, impairs bone growth, and produces skeletal abnormalities (crew-cut appearance on x-rays).
     - If untreated, the disease often results in growth retardation.
   - Spleen
     - Sequestration and destruction of inclusion-bearing red cells is derived from precursors that escape intramedullary death.
     - Extramedullary hematopoiesis is a common compensatory change involving splenic red pulp.
     - Splenomegaly results from RBC destruction and extramedullary hematopoiesis.
   - Liver
     - Iron overload presents as hemosiderosis of Kupffer cells and hepatocytes (secondary hemochromatosis).
     - Extramedullary hematopoiesis compensates for inefficient bone marrow RBC production that may cause hepatomegaly.

39. **What are the causes of iron excess in β-thalassemia?**
   - Excessive absorption of dietary iron due to ineffective hematopoiesis
   - Iron accumulation due to repeated blood transfusions required by these patients

40. **What is the difference between the three clinical types of β-thalassemia (thalassemia major, intermedia, and minor)?**
   The clinical classification of β-thalassemias is based on:
   - Severity of the anemia
   - Type of genetic defect (βo and β+)
   - Gene dosage (homozygous or heterozygous)
   - β-Thalassemia major
     - Severe transfusion-dependent anemia that first becomes manifest 6 to 9 months after birth as hemoglobin synthesis switches from HbF to HbA
     - Either type βo or β+(βo/βo or β+/β+)
     - Homozygous
   - β-Thalassemia minor or β-thalassemia trait
     - Usually asymptomatic with a mild anemia
     - One normal gene (βo/β or β+/β+)
     - Heterozygous
   - β-Thalassemia intermedia
     - Severe anemia, but not enough so to require regular blood transfusions
     - Genetically heterogeneous

- ○ Mild variants of homozygous β+-thalassemia
- ○ Severe variants of heterozygous (βo/β or β+/β)
- ○ Some double heterozygosity for the βo or β+ genes (βo/β+)
- ○ Homozygous or heterozygous

41. **What is α-thalassemia?**
α-Thalassemias are disorders caused by reduced synthesis (α+-thalassemias) or absent synthesis (α0-thalassemias) of α-globin chains. Because there are four α-globin genes (two on each member of the chromosome pair), there are many variations. The anemia stems both from lack of adequate hemoglobin and from the effects of excess unpaired non-α chains.

42. **List the four main clinical types of α-thalassemia.**
These are classified on the basis of the number and position of the α-globin genes deleted:
- ■ Silent carrier state
  - ○ There is deletion of a single α-globin gene.
  - ○ It is asymptomatic, without anemia.
- ■ α-Thalassemia trait
  - ○ There is deletion of two α-globin genes.
  - ○ It may affect both genes of one chromosome (Asians) or one gene of each chromosome (Africans).
  - ○ There is minimal or no anemia and no physical signs; clinical findings are identical to those of β-thalassemia minor (microcytosis and hypochromia).
- ■ Hemoglobin H (HbH) disease
  - ○ There is deletion of three α-globin genes.
  - ○ Tetramers of β-globin, called HbH, are formed. These tetramers are nonfunctional in oxygen transport, so anemia is disproportionate to hemoglobin level.
  - ○ There is moderately severe anemia, resembling β-thalassemia intermedia (microcytic, hypochromic anemia with target cells and Heinz bodies in the blood smear).
- ■ Hydrops fetalis
  - ○ There is deletion of all four α-globin genes
  - ○ In the fetus, excess of γ-globin chains form tetramers (hemoglobin Bart) that are unable to deliver the oxygen to tissues. Without intrauterine transfusions, the fetus invariably dies.
  - ○ The fetus shows pallor, generalized edema, and massive hepatosplenomegaly.

43. **Discuss the cause of paroxysmal nocturnal hemoglobinuria (PNH).**
This is the only example of hemolytic anemia in which there is an acquired defect in the cell membrane. In PNH, the gene that is essential for the synthesis of the glycosyl-phosphatidyl-inositol (GPI) anchor is mutated. The absence of several GPI-linked membrane proteins renders blood cells unusually sensitive to lysis by endogenous complement. The somatic mutation affects pluripotent stem cells, and, accordingly, all their descendants (including platelets and granulocytes) are more sensitive to lysis by complement.

44. **How does PNH present clinically?**
PNH affects young people, and the average age of onset is 20 to 25 years. Patients with PNH present with intravascular hemolysis, which (despite its name) is paroxysmal and nocturnal in only 25% of cases. Hemosiderinuria with loss of iron leads to iron deficiency. Patients may also suffer from multiple episodes of venous thrombosis involving the hepatic, portal, or cerebral veins. These episodes are fatal in 50% of cases. The disease can evolve into aplastic anemia or acute leukemia. Steroid treatment may stabilize the disease in more than 50% of cases, but many patients still die within 10 years of onset.

45. **What is immunohemolytic anemia, and how is it classified?**
Immunohemolytic anemias or autoimmune hemolytic anemias are groups of hemolytic anemias caused by extracorpuscular mechanisms. The classification is based on the specific nature of the antibody:
- Warm antibody type
- Cold agglutinin type
- Cold hemolysins
    The Coombs antiglobulin test is the major tool for diagnosing this disease. It relies on the capacity of the antibodies prepared in animals against human globulins to agglutinate red cells if these globulins are present on red cell surfaces. The temperature dependence of the autoantibody also helps to specify the type of the antibody.

46. **What is the difference between warm antibody and cold antibody hemolytic anemia?**
- Warm antibody hemolytic anemia:
    - Immunoglobulin (Ig) G, or occasionally IgA antibody
    - Primary or idiopathic
    - Secondary (lymphomas, leukemias, and drugs)
    - Antibody active at 37°C
    - In many cases, antibody binds to the Rh-antigen on erythrocytes. The coated cells then bind to Fc receptors on monocytes and splenic macrophages. They undergo spheroidal transformation (intravascular hemolysis rarely occurs) and are sequestered and removed in the spleen. There is moderate splenomegaly.
- Cold antibody hemolytic anemia:
    - IgM antibodies bind to the RBC. Two distinct forms are recognized:
        - Acute (self-limited disease, rarely causes any manifestations and tends to occur during the recovery phase of certain infectious diseases)
        - Chronic (idiopathic or associated with lymphoma)
    - The clinical symptoms result from agglutination of RBC accompanied by activation of complement in distal body parts, where the temperature may decrease to below 30°C:
        - Intravascular hemolysis mediated by activated complement
        - Vascular obstruction results in pallor and cyanosis of body parts exposed to cold temperatures

47. **List the most common causes of anemia owing to mechanical injury of red blood cells.**
- Macroangiopathic hemolysis (intravascular prostheses in the heart and major arteries)
- Microangiopathic hemolysis (disseminated intravascular coagulation, malignant hypertension, systemic lupus erythematosus, thrombotic thrombocytopenic purpura, hemolytic–uremic syndrome, and disseminated cancer)
- March hemoglobinuria (vigorous exercise)
- Hypersplenism (passage of RBCs through an enlarged spleen associated with mechanical injury of RBCs; such damaged RBCs tend to fall apart in circulation)

48. **What is megaloblastic anemia, and how is it classified?**
Megaloblastic anemias are characterized by impaired DNA synthesis and distinctive morphologic changes of affected RBC precursors and their descendants in the blood and bone marrow. It is a disease of older age, most commonly diagnosed in the fifth to eighth decade of life. Two main types are:
- Pernicious anemia, the major form of vitamin B_{12} deficiency anemia
- Folate deficiency anemia
    A deficiency of vitamin B_{12} and folic acid or impairment in their use results in defective nuclear maturation due to deranged or inadequate synthesis of DNA.

49. **List the main hematologic features of megaloblastic anemia.**
Peripheral blood shows the following features:
- Pancytopenia (decreased erythrocytes, leukocytes, and platelets)
- Anisocytosis (marked variation in size and shape) and normochromic red cells (MCHC is not elevated)
- Many erythrocytes are macrocytic and oval (macroovalocytes), with MCV above 100 μm^3
- Erythrocytes are thicker than normal; consequently, most lack central pallor of normal red cells
- Reticulocyte count is lower than normal, and nucleated red cells occasionally appear in the circulating blood with severe anemia
- Neutrophils are larger than normal (macropolymorphonuclear) and are hypersegmented (five, six, or more nuclear lobules)

50. **What are the changes seen in bone marrow in megaloblastic anemia?**
Bone marrow shows the following changes:
- Hypercellularity—much or all of the normally fatty marrow may be converted to red marrow.
- The erythroid-to-myeloid ratio is increased, and there is abundant stainable iron.
- Megaloblastic change is detected in all stages of red cell development.
- As these cells differentiate, the nucleus retains its finely distributed chromatin and thus fails to undergo the chromatin clumping typical of the normoblasts.
- There are giant metamyelocytes, band forms, and hypersegmentation of the neutrophils.
- Megakaryocytes may be abnormally large and have bizarre, multilobate nuclei.

51. **How is vitamin B_{12} absorbed?**
Humans are totally dependent on dietary animal products for their vitamin B_{12} requirement. Absorption of vitamin B_{12} requires intrinsic factor (IF), which is secreted by the parietal cells of the stomach along with hydrochloric acid. The vitamin is released from its protein-bound form by action of pepsin and then binds to salivary vitamin B_{12}–binding proteins called cobalophilins, or R-binders. R–vitamin B_{12} complexes are broken down by pancreatic proteases in the duodenum. The released vitamin B_{12} then attaches to IF and goes to the ileum, where it adheres to IF-specific receptors on the ileal cells. Vitamin B_{12} enters the mucosal cells, which pass it on to transcobalamin II, a plasma transport protein.

52. **What are the most important causes of vitamin B_{12} deficiency?**
- Impaired absorption
  - ○ IF deficiency (pernicious anemia and gastrectomy)
  - ○ Malabsorption diseases affecting the small intestine
  - ○ Ileal resection and Crohn disease (ileitis)
- Decreased intake
  - ○ Inadequate diet and vegetarianism
- Increased requirement
  - ○ Pregnancy, hyperthyroidism, and disseminated cancer

53. **What is the pathogenesis of pernicious anemia?**
Pernicious anemia is believed to result from immunologically mediated, possibly autoimmune, destruction of gastric mucosa. The resultant chronic atrophic gastritis is marked by a loss of parietal cells, a prominent infiltrate of lymphocytes and plasma cells, and nuclear changes in the mucosal cells similar to those found in the erythroid precursors. It is suspected that an autoreactive T cell response initiates gastric mucosal injury, which then triggers the formation of autoantibodies. These antibodies cause further injury to the epithelium, and after the mass of IF-secreting cells is significantly depleted (together with reserves of stored vitamin B_{12}), anemia develops. Two processes aggravate anemia:

- Ineffective erythropoiesis (megaloblasts are especially prone to intramedullary destruction; premature destruction of granulocytic and platelet precursors also occurs)
- Increased hemolytic destruction of red cells

54. **What are the pathologic findings in pernicious anemia?**
    - **Bone marrow and blood:** These changes are similar to those in other forms of megaloblastic anemia (e.g., due to folate deficiency).
    - **Gastrointestinal tract:** The tongue is shiny, glazed, and "boofy rod" (atrophic glossitis) Changes in the stomach are those of diffuse chronic gastritis, and there is atrophy of the fundic glands (the parietal cells are virtually absent). The glandular lining epithelium is replaced by mucus-secreting goblet cells that resemble those of the intestine; this metaplasia is called intestinalization. Some of the cells and their nuclei may increase to double the normal size. Patients with pernicious anemia have a higher incidence of gastric cancer.
    - **Central nervous system:** Neural lesions occur in approximately three fourths of all cases of fulminant pernicious anemia. The principal alteration is myelin degeneration of the dorsal and lateral tracts of the spinal cord. These changes are sometimes followed by axonal degeneration and neuronal death. Signs and symptoms include spastic paraparesis, sensory ataxia, and severe paresthesia in the lower limbs.

55. **What are the causes of folate deficiency?**
    - Decreased intake
      - ○ Inadequate diet: chronic alcoholics, the indigent, and the elderly
      - ○ Impaired absorption: malabsorption syndromes (nontropical and tropical sprue), diffuse infiltrative disease of the small intestine (e.g., lymphoma), and certain drugs (anticonvulsants and oral contraceptives)
    - Increased loss: hemodialysis
    - Increased requirements: pregnancy, infancy, disseminated cancer, and markedly increased hematopoiesis (hemolytic anemias)
    - Impaired use: folic acid antagonists used in cancer therapy (methotrexate and cyclophosphamide)—all rapidly growing cells affected, leading to ulcerative lesions within the gastrointestinal tract as well as megaloblastic anemia

56. **What is the difference between megaloblastic anemia of vitamin B_{12} deficiency and folate deficiency?**
    - Vitamin B_{12} reserves in the body are sufficient for years, whereas the body's reserves of folate are relatively modest, and a deficiency may arise within months.
    - Megaloblastic anemia associated with vitamin B_{12} deficiency is almost always associated with absorption problems, whereas in folate deficiency it is usually caused by a nutritional deficiency.
    - Neurologic symptoms typical of the vitamin B_{12} deficiency do not occur in a folate deficiency (folic acid therapy produces prompt hematologic response heralded by the appearance of a reticulocytosis in both folate and vitamin B_{12} deficiency).

57. **How is iron absorbed, transported, and stored inside the human body?**
    - Approximately 25% of heme iron and 1% or 2% of nonheme iron is absorbable. The duodenum is the primary site of absorption.
    - Dietary heme iron enters the mucosal cells directly. In contrast, nonheme iron appears to be transported into the cell by a mechanism involving three proteins (luminal mucin, integrin-like molecule, and mobilferrin).
    - Iron is stored as ferritin or hemosiderin.
    - A fraction of the absorbed iron is rapidly delivered to plasma transferrin. Most, however, is deposited as ferritin (protein–iron complex), some to be transferred more slowly to plasma transferrin and some to be lost with exfoliation of mucosal cells.

- The most important function of plasma transferrin is to deliver iron to the cells, including erythroid precursors, which require iron for hemoglobin synthesis. Very small amounts of circulating ferritin can normally be found in plasma.
- With normal iron stores, only trace amounts of hemosiderin are found in the body. On the other hand, iron-overloaded cells contain most of the iron stored in the form of hemosiderin.

58. **How does one measure or estimate body iron stores?**
- **Serum ferritin:** Because serum ferritin is largely derived from the storage pool of iron, its level is a good indicator of the adequacy of body iron stores.
- **Total iron binding capacity (TIBC):** It depends on serum transferrin, which is approximately 33% saturated with iron.
- **Serum iron concentration:** It depends on intake and loss.

59. **What are the most important causes of iron deficiency?**
Deficiency of iron probably represents the most common nutritional disorder in the world. The most important causes of iron deficiency are:
- **Dietary deficiency:** It is a rare cause of iron deficiency in industrialized countries, affecting the elderly, the very poor, infants, and children.
- **Impaired absorption:** Typically it occurs in chronic intestinal diseases such as sprue and other intestinal malabsorption syndromes. Gastrectomy also impairs iron absorption by decreasing the secretion of hydrochloric acid and transit time through the duodenum.
- **Increased requirement:** Growing infants and children, adolescents, and pregnant women have a much greater requirement than do other adults.
- **Chronic blood loss:** External hemorrhage depletes iron reserves. In women, the most common cause of blood loss is heavy menstrual bleeding. Iron deficiency in adult men and postmenopausal women in the Western world should be considered to be caused by gastrointestinal blood loss until proven otherwise.

60. **What are the hematologic and laboratory features of iron deficiency?**
- Peripheral blood smear
  - Hypochromic, microcytic anemia (sometimes poikilocytosis)
- Bone marrow
  - Mild to moderate increase in erythropoietic activity, manifested by increased numbers of normoblasts
  - Disappearance of stainable iron from the mononuclear phagocytic cells in the bone marrow
- Laboratory results
  - Hemoglobin and hematocrit below normal levels
  - Low serum iron and serum ferritin levels
  - Transferrin saturation is low (below 15%) and the total plasma iron-binding capacity (reflecting transferrin concentration) is high

61. **What are the most important causes of anemia of chronic disease?**
Impaired red cell production associated with chronic disease is the most common cause of anemia among hospitalized patients in the United States. It is associated with impaired iron utilization and reduced erythroid proliferation. Chronic illnesses associated with this form of anemia are:
- Chronic microbial infections (e.g., osteomyelitis, bacterial endocarditis, and lung abscess)
- Chronic immune disorders (e.g., rheumatoid arthritis)
- Chronic diseases of unknown etiology (e.g., regional enteritis)
- Neoplasms (most notably Hodgkin lymphoma and carcinomas of the lung and breast)

62. **List the hematologic and laboratory features of anemia of chronic disease.**
    - Normocytic/normochromic or microcytic/hypochromic anemia
    - Low serum iron
    - Decreased or normal total iron-binding capacity
    - Increased or normal serum ferritin levels
    - Transferrin receptors level within normal range
    - Increased storage iron in marrow macrophages

63. **What is aplastic anemia?**
    Aplastic anemia is a disease characterized by a loss of multipotent myeloid stem cells, resulting from direct injury of those cells or an abnormal microenvironment that cannot support their existence. Stem-cell failure impairs the erythroid, granulocytic, and thrombocytic hematopoiesis resulting in pancytopenia.

64. **How is aplastic anemia diagnosed?**
    The diagnosis rests on examination of bone marrow biopsy and peripheral blood:
    - Peripheral blood smear
      ○ Anemia (It is normocytic and normochromic and typically there is a low reticulocyte count.)
      ○ Neutropenia
      ○ Thrombocytopenia
    - Bone marrow
      ○ Bone marrow aplasia (It is hypocellular and composed largely of empty marrow spaces populated by fat cells, fibrous stroma, and scattered or clustered foci of lymphocytes and plasma cells, whereas hematopoietic cells are very rare or absent.)

65. **List the clinical features of aplastic anemia.**
    - May occur at any age, affecting both men and women equally
    - Gradual onset of signs and symptoms, which include:
      ○ **Anemia (low RBC count):** Symptoms are nonspecific and include progressive weakness, cutaneous and conjunctival pallor, and dyspnea.
      ○ **Thrombocytopenia:** It causes petechiae, ecchymoses, and gingival hemorrhages.
      ○ **Granulocytopenia:** It is related to infections and sudden onset of chills and fever.

66. **What are the main causes of aplastic anemia?**
    - Idiopathic (65%)
    - Acquired—that is, secondary to:
      ○ Cytotoxic drugs (fluorouracil, methotrexate, and doxorubicin)
      ○ Chemicals (benzene and insecticides)
      ○ Infections (human immunodeficiency virus [HIV]; Epstein–Barr virus)
      ○ Whole body irradiation
    - Inherited (rare)
      ○ Fanconi anemia

67. **What could cause a dry tap during a bone marrow biopsy?**
    Dry tap denotes poor aspirability of the bone marrow, and it can be found in different disorders of bone marrow:
    - Aplastic anemia
    - Myelofibrosis
    - Hairy cell leukemia

68. **What is myelophthisic anemia?**
    This is an anemia in which the bone marrow is replaced or infiltrated by metastatic cancer. It also may result from progressive fibrosis of the bone marrow (myelofibrosis). The replacement of the bone marrow by tumor or fibrous tissue affects all hematopoietic lineages. Characteristically,

immature forms of erythrocytes and white blood cells appear in the peripheral blood (leukoerythroblastosis). Extramedullary hematopoiesis may reappear in the liver or the spleen.

69. **Why does chronic renal failure cause anemia?**
A normocytic, normochromic anemia occurs in almost all patients with chronic renal disease. The severity of anemia is proportional to the degree of uremia. This anemia is multifactorial and entails both decreased production and increased destruction of erythrocytes:
- Damage to the kidney results in inadequate synthesis of erythropoietin, leading to decreased production of erythrocytes.
- Uremic toxins (still unidentified) may suppress the erythroid progenitor or precursor cells and cause increased destruction of erythrocytes.

70. **What is the difference between absolute and relative erythrocytosis (polycythemia)?**
Polycythemia (erythrocytosis) denotes an increased concentration of red cells, usually with a corresponding increase in hemoglobin level. It can be classified into the following categories:
- Relative polycythemia is caused by any kind of dehydration (deprivation of water, prolonged vomiting, diarrhea, or excessive use of diuretics).
- Absolute polycythemia is an actual increase in the number of red cells and can be primary or secondary.

71. **Discuss the difference between primary and secondary polycythemia.**
- Primary polycythemia is caused by an intrinsic abnormality of myeloid stem cells. This can be a clonal proliferation of myeloid stem cells (as in the polycythemia vera) or an increased responsiveness to erythropoietin because of mutation in the erythropoietin receptor.
- Secondary polycythemia presents with normal red cell progenitors but increased amounts of erythropoietin, which causes proliferation of erythrocytes. This increased secretion may be either appropriate (high altitude and lung disease) or inappropriate (erythropoietin-secreting tumor).

72. **What are the clinical features of polycythemia vera?**
Most symptoms can be explained by hyperviscosity of blood and volume expansion and include:
- High RBC, hemoglobin, and hematocrit
- Massive splenomegaly and hepatomegaly due to pooling of blood
- Neurologic symptoms due to sluggish circulation and hypoxia (e.g., somnolence, fatigue)
- Visual symptoms due to sluggish blood flow and clogging of retinal vessels
- Auditory and vestibular symptoms due to sluggish blood flow (e.g., tinnitus, vertigo)
- Systolic hypertension
- Venous thrombosis, for example, thrombosis of hepatic veins leads to an increased incidence of Budd–Chiari syndrome

BLEEDING DISORDERS

73. **How are bleeding disorders classified on the basis of their pathogenesis?**
- Increased fragility of vessels
- Platelet deficiency or dysfunction
- Derangements in the coagulation mechanism
- Combinations of any of these

74. **What is the significance of prolonged bleeding time?**
Bleeding time is the name for a standard test performed by puncturing the skin with a needle and measuring the time it takes for the bleeding to stop. Normal values are less than

10 minutes. This test is useful for detecting abnormalities involving platelets and the integrity of blood vessels. Bleeding time is prolonged in:

- Vascular purpuras (e.g., scurvy and Marfan syndrome)
- Thrombocytopenia (idiopathic thrombocytopenic purpura [ITP], thrombotic thrombocytopenia purpura [TTP], and disseminated intravascular coagulation [DIC])
- Functional platelet defects (e.g., thrombasthenia)
- Aspirin and nonsteroidal antiinflammatory drug therapy

KEY POINTS: BLEEDING DISORDERS ✔

1. Bleeding disorders develop because of three main factors: blood vessel diseases, platelet disorders, and coagulation disorders.

2. Bleeding disorders can be congenital or acquired, acute or chronic.

3. In disseminated intravascular coagulation and other microangiopathies, bleeding may occur in association with thrombosis of small blood vessels.

75. **What is measured by prothrombin time (PT), and when is it prolonged?**
PT measures the integrity of the extrinsic and common coagulation pathways. It is prolonged in conditions characterized by a deficiency of factors V, VII, and X; prothrombin; or fibrinogen. Prolonged PT occurs when the blood concentration of these factors declines to less than 30% to 40% and is seen in:
- Cirrhosis (end-stage liver disease)
- Vitamin K deficiency
- Disseminated intravascular coagulation (DIC)
- Warfarin treatment

76. **What is measured by the activated partial thromboplastin time, and when is it prolonged?**
The test known as activated partial thromboplastin time (aPTT) measures the integrity of the intrinsic and common coagulation pathway. It is prolonged because of a deficiency of factors V, VIII, IX, X, XI, and XII; prothrombin; or fibrinogen. The normal values for aPTT are in the range of 11 to 15 seconds. Prolongation of aPTT occurs only when the levels of a coagulation factor decline to less than 30% to 40% of normal and is seen in:
- Hemophilia A and B
- von Willebrand disease
- DIC
- Cirrhosis (end-stage liver disease)
- Heparin treatment

77. **List the hematologic parameters of vascular purpura.**
Vascular purpura is a broad term including a number of diseases. Accordingly, the tests will give a variety of results, depending on the nature of the disease.
- In scurvy, vitamin C deficiency that leads to weakening of the capillary walls, the bleeding time (BT) is prolonged, but other bleeding parameters are normal.
- In hypersensitivity vasculitis caused by an allergic reaction to drugs, the vascular lesions are focal and the BT is normal.
- Microangiopathic purpuras, like DIC, are associated with thrombocytopenia and prolonged BT, aPTT, and PT because of consumption of coagulation factors.

78. **What are the most important causes of systemic bleeding caused by vessel wall abnormalities?**
    - Infections (meningococcemia, infective endocarditis, and rickettsioses)
    - Drug reactions
    - Scurvy
    - Henoch–Schönlein purpura (purpuric rash, colicky abdominal pain, polyarthralgia, and acute glomerulonephritis)
    - Hereditary hemorrhagic telangiectasia (autosomal dominant disorder characterized by dilatated, tortuous blood vessels that have thin walls and hence bleed, most commonly under the mucous membranes of the nose, tongue, mouth, and eyes)
    - Amyloid infiltration of vessels
      In most of these conditions, the hemorrhagic diathesis does not cause massive bleeding but more often is a readily visible sign of a systemic underlying disorder.

79. **Name the main mechanisms of thrombocytopenia.**
    - Decreased production of platelets (e.g., aplastic anemia, leukemias, and B_{12} and folate deficiency)
    - Decreased platelet survival (e.g., due to immunologic and nonimmunologic destruction)
    - Increased splenic sequestration (e.g., hypersplenism syndrome, but also in any splenomegaly)
    - Dilutional (e.g., massive transfusions may produce a dilutional thrombocytopenia)

80. **At what level of thrombocytopenia will a bleeding occur?**
    - Greater than $100,000/mm^3$ = thrombocytopenia (laboratory finding—usually asymptomatic)
    - $20,000$ to $50,000/mm^3$ = posttraumatic bleeding
    - Less than $20,000/mm^3$ = spontaneous bleeding

81. **What are the principal clinical subtypes of ITP?**
    Two clinical forms of ITP are recognized: acute and chronic. Both forms are caused by antibodies to platelets:
    - Acute ITP
      - It is the most common thrombocytopenia in children.
      - Self-limited disease resolves spontaneously within 6 months or with corticosteroid treatment (20% prolonged ITP).
      - Abrupt onset of epistaxis and purpura that is due to thrombocytopenia.
      - It is preceded by a viral disease.
      - Bone marrow contains increased numbers of megakaryocytes; no splenomegaly.
    - Chronic ITP (more common form)
      - A diagnosis of exclusion should be made only after all the possible known causes for platelet deficiencies have been ruled out (e.g., systemic lupus erythematosus [SLE], acquired immune deficiency syndrome, heparin, and drug related).
      - It is most common in adult women younger than 40 years (female-to-male ratio, 3:1).
      - It has an insidious onset, characterized by bleeding into the skin (petechiae and ecchymoses) and mucosal surface.
      - Usually there is a long history of easy bruising, epistaxis, bleeding gums, and extensive soft tissue hemorrhages from relatively minor trauma (may also present with melena, hematuria, or excessive menstrual flow).

82. **How are platelets destroyed in chronic ITP ?**
    - Autoantibodies (mostly IgG) against platelet membrane glycoproteins (glycoprotein [GP] IIb/IIIa) bind to platelets.
    - Opsonized platelets are phagocytosed by monocytes and macrophages, mostly in the spleen.
    - The critical role of the spleen is evident from the fact that 75% to 85% of patients respond well to splenectomy.

83. **What are the pathologic and laboratory findings in chronic ITP?**
    - **Spleen:** Macroscopically it is of normal in size without pathognomonic changes (splenomegaly and lymphadenopathy are extremely rare). Histologic changes include:
        - Hyperactivity and enlargement of the follicles with germinal centers
        - Congestion of the sinusoids
        - Megakaryocytes found within the sinuses and in the sinusoidal wall
    - **Bone marrow:** Microscopic findings are not characteristic but merely represent accelerated thrombopoiesis.
        - Increased number of megakaryocytes (a decrease virtually rules out the diagnosis)
        - Some megakaryocytes are immature with a large, nonlobulated, single nucleus
        - Peripheral blood smear
        - Absent or low platelet count; platelets may be larger than normal (megathrombocytes)
    - **Laboratory findings**
        - Bleeding time prolonged
        - PT and aPTT normal

84. **Which disorders are included under the term thrombotic microangiopathies?**
    The term thrombotic microangiopathies encompasses a spectrum of clinical syndromes, the most important being:
    - Thrombotic thrombocytopenic purpura (TTP)
    - Hemolytic-uremic syndrome (HUS)
    - Disseminated intravascular coagulation (DIC)

85. **List the pentad of findings in thrombotic thrombocytopenic purpura.**
    - Fever
    - Thrombocytopenia
    - Microangiopathic hemolytic anemia
    - Transient neurologic deficits (with fluctuating levels of consciousness)
    - Renal failure

86. **Describe the difference between TTP and HUS.**
    - Both HUS and TTP are associated with microangiopathic hemolytic anemia and thrombocytopenia.
    - HUS is distinguished from TTP by the absence of neurologic symptoms and the dominance of acute renal failure.
    - The onset of HUS is in childhood, whereas TTP mostly occurs in adult women.
    - Triggers for endothelial injury in HUS are verotoxins produced by certain strains of *Escherichia coli*, whereas the cause of TTP has not been identified.

87. **What are the features of bleeding disorders caused by the abnormalities of clotting factors?**
    - A deficiency of each of the known clotting factors can be a cause of a bleeding disorder.
    - In contrast to thrombocytopenias, in which the spontaneous appearance of petechiae or purpura is common, abnormalities in clotting factors present with bleeding in the form of large ecchymoses or hematomas after an injury or as prolonged bleeding after a laceration or surgery.
    - Common manifestations are bleeding in gastrointestinal and urinary tracts and particularly into weight-bearing joints (hemarthrosis).

88. **List common bleeding disorders caused by a deficiency of coagulation factors.**
    - Acquired disorders (characterized by multiple clotting abnormalities)
        - Vitamin K deficiency (affects factors II, VII, IX, and X and protein C)
        - Severe liver disease (liver produces almost all the clotting factors)
        - DIC
    - Hereditary deficiencies (typically involve a single clotting factor)

○ Hemophilia A (deficiency of factor VIII)
○ Hemophilia B or Christmas disease (deficiency of factor IX)
○ von Willebrand disease

89. **How does factor VIII interact with von Willebrand factor (vWF)?**
vWF is produced by endothelial cells (major source) and megakaryocytes, whereas factor VIII is mostly synthesized in the liver. They are synthesized separately but in plasma circulate as a complex that promotes the clotting as well as the platelet vessel wall interactions that are necessary to ensure hemostasis. vWF forms 99% of the complex, serving as a carrier for factor VIII, and is important for its stability; the half-life of factor VIII in the circulation is 12 hours if vWF levels are normal but only 2 to 4 hours if serum vWF is deficient or abnormal (as in patients with von Willebrand disease).

90. **What is the most common form of von Willebrand disease?**
More than 20 variants of von Willebrand disease (one of the most common hereditary bleeding disorders in humans) have been described. Type I is the most common, accounting for approximately 70% of cases, and is relatively mild. It is an autosomal dominant disorder associated with reduced quantity of circulating vWF.

91. **List the hematologic laboratory findings in von Willebrand disease.**
   - Spontaneous bleeding from mucous membranes, excessive bleeding from wounds, and menorrhagia (in contrast to hemophilia, hemarthroses are rare)
   - Prolonged BT and aPTT, normal PT, and normal platelet count
   - Plasma level of vWF is reduced, with secondary decrease in factor VIII

92. **What is the difference between the mild, moderate, and severe forms of hemophilia A?**
Hemophilia A (the most common hereditary disease with serious bleeding) is caused by a reduction in the amount or activity of factor VIII. It is inherited as an X-linked recessive trait. Three forms of disease are recognized on the basis of the severity of bleeding and the level of factor VIII activity:
   - Severe—factor VIII levels less than 1% of normal (bleeding frequent even without discernible trauma)
   - Moderate—factor VIII levels at 2% to 5% of normal activity (less frequent bleeding episodes)
   - Mild—factor VIII levels at 6% to 50% of normal (bleeding occurs usually after trauma)

93. **What are the hematologic and clinical–pathologic findings in hemophilia A?**
   - Easy bruising
   - Massive hemorrhage after trauma or operative procedures
   - Spontaneous bleeding into joints (hemarthroses)
   - Petechia are not a feature of hemophilia
   - Normal bleeding time and normal platelet count
   - Prolonged aPTT; factor VIII deficiency

94. **Describe how hemophilia B differs from hemophilia A.**
Hemophilia A and hemophilia B are clinically indistinguishable. Hemophilia A is much more common, accounting for 80% of cases. The only difference is that hemophilia A is caused by a deficiency of factor VIII and hemophilia B by a deficiency of factor IX.

95. **What is DIC, and what are its main causes?**
DIC is an acute, subacute, or chronic disorder occurring as a secondary complication in a variety of diseases, characterized by formation of microthrombi throughout the microcirculation of the body. Two major mechanisms by which DIC can be triggered are:

- Release of tissue factor (tissue thromboplastin) into the circulation, caused by:
  - Obstetrical complications (50% of all patients with DIC): abruptio placentae, retained dead fetus, septic abortus, and amniotic fluid embolism
  - Neoplasms (33% of all patients with DIC)
    - Carcinoma of pancreas, prostate, lung, and stomach
    - Acute promyelocytic leukemia
  - Infections
    - Gram-negative sepsis
  - Massive tissue injury (e.g., trauma and extensive surgery)
- Widespread injury of endothelial cells
  - Deposition of circulating antigen–antibody complexes in the vessel wall (e.g., SLE)
  - Formation of antigen–antibody complexes in the wall of blood vessels (e.g., vasculitis)
  - Temperature extremes (e.g., burns or frostbite)
  - Microorganisms that invade endothelial cells (e.g., rickettsiae)

96. **What are the laboratory, hematologic, and pathologic findings in DIC ?**
    - Laboratory findings
      - Prolongation of PT and PTT
      - Decrease in the plasma fibrinogen level
      - Elevated levels of fibrinopeptide A and D dimer (as markers of coagulation and fibrinolytic activation, respectively)
    - Hematologic findings
      - Thrombocytopenia
      - Microangiopathic hemolytic anemia (schistocytes or fragmented blood cells arising from cell trapping and damage within fibrin thrombi)
    - Pathologic findings (microthrombi with infarction and hemorrhage found in many organs: brain, heart, lungs, kidneys, adrenals, spleen, and liver):
      - Brain—microinfarcts and fresh hemorrhage
      - Lungs—microthrombi in alveolar capillaries, sometimes associated with pulmonary edema and exudation of fibrin creating hyaline membranes, reminiscent of adult respiratory distress syndrome
      - Kidney—small thrombi in renal glomeruli; microinfarcts or bilateral renal cortical necrosis in severe cases
      - Adrenal—massive hemorrhage of the Waterhouse–Friderichsen syndrome caused by meningococci
      - Placenta—widespread microthrombi cause premature atrophy of cytotrophoblast and syncytiotrophoblast

97. **Explain the pathogenesis of bleeding in DIC.**
    DIC is characterized by sequential intravascular coagulation and bleeding. Coagulation develops because of endothelial cell injury or a release of tissue factor from damaged tissue. Thrombi forming inside the small blood vessels result in a consumption of clotting factors, whereupon bleeding begins to occur in many places, resulting in purpura and oozing of blood from mucosal surfaces (consumption coagulopathy). Thrombosis in the small blood vessels is also associated with deformation and fragmentation (microangiopathic hemolysis).

98. **What is the clinical course of DIC?**
    DIC can be divided into the following categories:
    - Acute (endotoxic shock, obstetric complications, or major trauma): tends to present by bleeding diathesis
    - Chronic (carcinomatosis or retention of dead fetus): tends to present initially with thrombotic complications

Although the clinical course of DIC can vary greatly, there are some common patterns:
- Microangiopathic hemolytic anemia
- Respiratory symptoms
  - Dyspnea
  - Cyanosis
  - Extreme respiratory difficulty
- Neurologic signs and symptoms, such as convulsions and coma
- Renal changes including oliguria and acute renal failure
- Circulatory failure and shock, appearing suddenly or developing progressively

WHITE CELL DISORDERS

99. **Name the main forms of leukopenia.**
Leukopenia can be defined as a condition in which there is an abnormally reduced amount of white blood cells (normal white blood cell count is 4000–11,000/µL). It may appear as generalized leukopenia or as
- Neutropenia or granulocytopenia (normal neutrophil count is 1800–7000/µL)
- Lymphopenia (normal lymphocyte count is 1500–4000/µL)

100. **What is the pathogenesis of neutropenia (agranulocytosis)?**
The pathogenesis of neutropenia can be divided into two broad categories:
- Inadequate or ineffective production of neutrophils
  - Suppression of myeloid stem cells (aplastic anemia) and a variety of infiltrative marrow disorders (tumors and granulomatous disease)
  - Suppression of committed granulocytic precursors (after exposure to certain drugs)
  - Diseases characterized by ineffective granulopoiesis (megaloblastic anemias and myelodysplastic syndromes)
  - Rare inherited conditions characterized by impaired granulocytic differentiation caused by genetic defects in specific genes
- Accelerated removal or destruction of neutrophils
  - Immune-mediated injury of neutrophils: idiopathic, associated with a well-defined immunologic disorder (e.g., SLE), drugs (alkylating agents and antimetabolites)
- Splenic sequestration
- Overwhelming bacterial, fungal, or rickettsial infection (increased peripheral use)

KEY POINTS: WHITE CELL DISORDERS ✓

1. Reduction of leukocyte number is called leukopenia, whereas increased numbers can be seen in reactive leukocytosis or neoplastic conditions known as leukemias and myeloproliferative diseases.

2. Leukemias are clinically and pathologically classified as myelogenous or lymphoid, acute or chronic.

3. Lymphocytic and lymphoblastic leukemias are closely related to lymphomas.

4. Hodgkin lymphoma is a form of lymphoma that differs clinically and in response to therapy from non-Hodgkin lymphomas.

5. Multiple myeloma is the most important neoplasia of plasma cells.

101. **What are the bone marrow findings in neutropenia?**
Two diametrically opposite pathologic changes can be seen:
- **Marrow hypocellularity:** In this condition, the bone marrow precursors of leukocytes have been damaged or eliminated by drugs, toxins, irradiation, or other factors. In some cases, the bone marrow has been replaced by fibrous tissue (myelofibrosis) or tumor cells (myelophthisic anemia).
- **Marrow hypercellularity:** The bone marrow is packed with cells, mostly immature granulocytic precursors. This is typically seen in myelodysplastic syndromes or megaloblastic anemia.

102. **What are the clinical features of neutropenia?**
- Reduced resistance to bacterial infections
- Infections most often present as ulcerations of the oral mucosa, gingivitis, or pharyngitis (so-called agranulocytic angina)
- Local lymph nodes typically enlarged
- Pneumonias common in advanced cases
- Sepsis often found in terminal cases

103. **Describe the causes of various forms of leukocytosis.**
- Neutrophilic leukocytosis
  - Acute bacterial infection
  - Sterile inflammation, specifically tissue necrosis such as myocardial infarct or burns
- Eosinophilic leukocytosis
  - Allergies such as asthma, hay fever, and allergic skin diseases
  - Parasitic infestations
  - Drug reactions
- Basophilic leukocytosis (rare)
- Myeloproliferative disease (chronic myelogenous leukemia)
- Monocytosis
  - Chronic infections (tuberculosis, bacterial endocarditis, rickettsiosis, and malaria)
  - Autoimmune diseases (e.g., SLE)
  - Inflammatory bowel diseases (ulcerative colitis)

104. **What is a leukemoid reaction, and how does it differ from leukemia?**
Leukemoid reaction denotes pronounced neutrophilia (>40,000 cells/ml) in acute inflammatory reaction that may be mistaken for leukemia, especially chronic myeloid leukemia. Leukocytosis occurs initially because of accelerated release of cells from the bone marrow and is associated with increased count of more immature neutrophils in the blood (shift to the left). Differentiation of leukemoid reaction and neoplastic leukocytosis includes the following:
- Cells in the peripheral blood in the leukemoid reaction are usually more mature than myelocytes.
- Leukocytic alkaline phosphatase activity is high in a leukemoid reaction but low in chronic myeloid leukemia.

105. **Discuss the clinical–pathologic features of acute lymphadenitis.**
- **Macroscopic findings:** lymph nodes swollen and enlarged
- **Microscopic findings:** follicular hyperplasia and interfollicular and sinusoidal infiltrates of inflammatory cells, which include neutrophils in bacterial infections and lymphocytes in viral infections
- **Clinical findings:** palpable enlarged lymph nodes, which may be tender and covered with red skin

106. **What are the histologic findings in chronic nonspecific lymphadenitis?**
Chronic nonspecific lymphadenitis is particularly common in inguinal and axillary nodes, which drain relatively large areas of the body. Lymph nodes in chronic reactions are not tender because their capsules are not under increased pressure. Histologically, these lymph nodes show:
- **Follicular hyperplasia (mostly B cell reaction):** It is typically found in response to bacterial infections.
- **Paracortical lymphoid hyperplasia (mostly T-cell reaction):** It may represent immunologic reactions to drugs or viral infection (infectious mononucleosis) and is found after vaccination against certain viral diseases.
- **Sinus histiocytosis (response of macrophages):** This is most prominent in chronic infection or in lymph nodes draining the lymph from an area involved by cancer.

107. **Name the major groups of WBC neoplasms.**
- Lymphoid neoplasms originating from precursors of T and B lymphocytes
  - Malignant lymphomas (non-Hodgkin lymphomas [NHLs] and Hodgkin lymphoma [HL])
  - Plasmacytoma and multiple myeloma
- Myeloid neoplasms
  - Myelodysplastic syndrome
  - Myeloproliferative disorders
  - Myeloid leukemias
- Histiocytoses

108. **Discuss the difference between leukemia and lymphoma.**
- Leukemia (literally, white blood; caused by malignant WBCs in circulation) is a malignancy of hematopoietic cells arising in bone marrow and involving peripheral blood and other tissues.
- Lymphoma is a malignant solid neoplasm of the lymphoid system, developing most frequently in the lymph node. Other organs containing lymphoid tissue, such as bone marrow, spleen, tonsils, gastrointestinal tract, skin, pulmonary system, and central nervous system, may also be the primary sites of lymphoma.

109. **How do lymphomas present clinically?**
- **Painless lymph node enlargement:** Two thirds of NHLs and virtually all cases of HL present with painless nodal enlargement (often >2 cm). Lymphadenopathy may be localized or generalized. The remaining NHLs arise at extranodal sites (e.g., skin, stomach, and brain) and do not present with lymph node enlargement.
- **Nonspecific constitutional symptoms (fever, night sweats, and weight loss):** These symptoms may prompt a workup, which will ultimately lead to proper diagnosis.

110. **What is the basis for classifying NHLs according to the World Health Organization?**
The World Health Organization (WHO) classifies pathologic entities on the basis of their microscopic morphology but also takes into account the specific features of tumor cells, including their
- Immunophenotype
- Genotype whenever genetic analysis is possible

111. **List the main groups of NHLs according to WHO.**
- Precursor B-cell neoplasms (neoplasms of immature B cells)
- Peripheral B-cell neoplasms (neoplasms of mature B cells)
- Precursor T-cell neoplasms (neoplasms of immature T cells)
- Peripheral T-cell and natural killer (NK) cell neoplasms (neoplasms of mature T cells and NK cells)

112. **What is the role of histopathology, bone marrow biopsy, immunohistochemistry, cytogenetics, and molecular biology techniques in diagnosis of NHL?**
    - Histopathology
        - Provides information about pattern of tumor growth within lymph nodes (nodular or diffuse), cell type (level of differentiation), and size (small, large, or mixed small and large)
        - Essential for interpreting immunophenotypic and genotypic data
        - The gold standard for classifying lymphomas, formulating the prognosis, and deciding about treatment options
    - Bone marrow biopsy
        - Important for staging of disease, which is essential for treatment and prognosis
    - Immunohistochemistry
        - Helps establish monoclonality of a neoplastic population
        - Aids in identifying tumor cell type and the level of differentiation, which is important for the classification of lymphoid neoplasms, therapy, and prognosis
    - Cytogenetics and molecular biology
        - Specific genetic and chromosomal abnormalities are useful for classifying lymphomas into subtypes that are difficult to recognize by other techniques
        - Specific genetic and chromosomal abnormalities provide proof that a lymphoma was properly classified by other means

113. **Are all lymphomas malignant?**
    Yes. There are no benign lymphomas. Even though all lymphoid neoplasms are malignant, the degree of malignancy varies among various entities.

114. **Name the cell of origin of most NHLs.**
    The majority of lymphoid neoplasms (80%–85%) are of B-cell origin. T-cell tumors are less common, and neoplasms originating from NK cells or histiocytes are very rare.

115. **Describe which anatomic parts of the lymph nodes are occupied by neoplastic T lymphocytes and which by B lymphocytes.**
    Neoplastic B and T cells tend to home to and grow in parts of the lymph node previously occupied by their nonneoplastic counterparts. For example, follicular lymphomas proliferate in the B-cell areas of the lymph node, producing a nodular or follicular pattern of growth, whereas T-cell lymphomas typically grow in paracortical T-cell zones.

116. **Why is the staging of NHL and HL important?**
    Staging of NHLs provides useful prognostic information, but staging is even more important in the evaluation of patients with HL. The spread of HL is remarkably predictable: Nodal involvement precedes splenic disease, which usually precedes hepatic disease, and hepatic disease usually precedes marrow involvement and extranodal disease.

117. **Which four pathologic entities account for the majority of lymphoid and plasmacellular neoplasms?**
    - Follicular lymphoma
    - Diffuse large B-cell lymphoma
    - Chronic lymphocytic leukemia/small lymphocytic lymphoma
    - Multiple myeloma

118. **Name the two most common NHLs of childhood and adolescence.**
    - Acute lymphoblastic leukemia/lymphoblastic lymphoma (ALL/LBL)
    - Burkitt lymphoma

119. **List the key facts about ALL/LBL.**
   - There is neoplastic clonal proliferation of lymphoid stem cells called lymphoblasts.
   - Bone marrow, lymph nodes, and other lymphoid organs are primarily involved.
   - Extranodal spread to other nonlymphoid organs (e.g., brain and testis) often occurs.
   - Immunophenotypically classified as:
     - B cell (85%), showing rearrangement of immunoglobulin gene
     - T cell (10%)
     - Null cell (pre-B and pre-T cell; <5%)
   - Terminal deoxynucleotidyl transferase (TdT), a specialized DNA polymerase that is found in pre-T and pre-B lymphoblasts, is expressed in more than 95% of cases.
   - Chromosomal changes (numerical and structural—mostly translocations) in more than 90% of patients correlate with immunophenotype and sometimes affect prognosis.

120. **What is the peak age of incidence of ALL/LBL?**
   Most patients are younger than 15 years, and the peak incidence in children is at approximately 4 years. ALL/LBL can also occur in adults.

121. **What are the common clinical features of ALL/LBL?**
   - Abrupt, stormy onset
   - Fatigue (related to anemia)
   - Fever (related to neutropenia)
   - Bleeding (related to thrombocytopenia)
   - Bone pain and tenderness (due to marrow expansion with infiltration of the subperiosteum)
   - Generalized lymphadenopathy, splenomegaly, hepatomegaly, and testicular enlargement
   - Nervous system manifestations, such as headache, vomiting, and nerve palsies resulting from meningeal spread

122. **Discuss the prognosis of ALL/LBL.**
   Prior to the advent of modern chemotherapy, the median survival after diagnosis was only 2 months. With aggressive chemotherapy, more than 90% of children achieve complete remission, and at least two thirds are considered permanently cured.

   Overall, the most important prognostic features are age at onset, extent of disease evidenced in the peripheral blood cell count, and extent of extranodal involvement.

123. **List features of ALL/LBL associated with favorable and unfavorable prognosis.**
   See Table 9-2.

TABLE 9-2. PROGNOSTIC FEATURES ASSOCIATED WITH ACUTE LYMPHOBLASTIC LEUKEMIA/LYMPHOBLASTIC LYMPHOMA

Features	Favorable	Unfavorable
Immunophenotype	Pre-B cell	Mature B cell and T cell
Lymphocytosis	<10,000	>50,000
Chromosomal changes	Hyperdiploidy	Other translocations (>50 chromosomes), t(12,21)
Age	3–7 years	<1 or >10 years and adults
Sex	Female	Male

124. **What is chronic lymphocytic leukemia/small cell lymphocytic lymphoma?**
Chronic lymphocytic leukemia (CLL) is the most common form of leukemia in the United States (30%). Small cell lymphocytic lymphoma (SLL) is a common form of lymphoma. The male-to-female ratio is 2:1. The most important features of CLL/SLL are:
- Malignant clonal expansion of well-differentiated lymphoid cells
- Malignant cells resemble mature B lymphocytes and express typical B cell markers, such as CD20
- May present as generalized lymphadenopathy (i.e., lymphoma) or leukemia with bone marrow involvement
- Chromosomal changes seen in more than 50% of cases

125. **Describe the pathologic features of CLL/SLL.**
- **Peripheral blood:** There is increased count of small, round lymphocytes with scant cytoplasm. These cells are frequently disrupted in the process of making the smear, producing so-called smudge cells.
- **Bone marrow:** Involvement is observed in all cases of CLL and most cases of SLL, taking the form of interstitial infiltrates or nonparatrabecular aggregates of small lymphocytes.
- **Lymphoid tissues:** There is diffuse infiltration of lymph nodes by small cells with obliteration of architecture, as well as splenomegaly (white and red pulp are infiltrated by tumor cells).

126. **How does CLL/SLL present clinically?**
- It is often asymptomatic.
- Median age at presentation is 60 years. (Young people are rarely affected.)
- Initial symptoms are nonspecific and include easy fatigability, weight loss, and anorexia.
- Generalized lymphadenopathy and hepatosplenomegaly (50%–60% of cases).
- There is bone marrow involvement in CLL and also many cases of SLL.
- There is lymphocytosis.
- Thre is increased susceptibility to bacterial infections because of hypogammaglobulinemia.
- Autoimmune hemolytic anemia or thrombocytopenia is caused by antibodies directed against red blood cells or platelets.

127. **Describe the clinical course and outcome of CLL/SLL.**
The disease usually has a protracted course, but there is considerable variation from one case to another and based on the clinical stage. Mean survival is 6 years but may be 10 years or more for those with minimal tumor burden. Richter's syndrome is rare and aggressive type of acute leukemia that results from a transformation of CLL/SLL into diffuse large B cell lymphoma. Unfavorable prognosis is portended by:
- Advanced stage (stages 0–II, favorable; stages III and IV, unfavorable)
- Anemia and thrombocytopenia
- Diffuse rather than nodular involvement of bone marrow
- Multiple chromosomal abnormalities

128. **What is follicular lymphoma?**
This form of NHL is a malignant tumor composed of well-differentiated B lymphocytes. These cells form follicles, thus mimicking the maturation of normal B cells. The condition presents with painless lymphadenopathy, which is frequently generalized. In 10% of patients, the peripheral blood involvement is sufficient to produce lymphocytosis. Bone marrow involvement with paratrabecular lymphoid aggregates occurs in 85% of patients. Splenic white pulp and hepatic portal triads are frequently involved.

129. How common is follicular lymphoma?

It is the most common form of NHL, accounting for approximately 45% of all adult lymphomas. It affects men and women equally and occurs in middle age. It is less common in Europe than in the United States, and it is rare in Asia.

130. What is the role of the *bcl-2* gene in the pathogenesis of follicular lymphoma?

The hallmark of follicular lymphoma is a t(14;18) translocation, which leads to overexpression of the *bcl-2* gene. This gene encodes a protein that inhibits apoptosis. B cells with a normal follicular center do not express *bcl-2* and are programmed to die after some time. On the other hand, follicular lymphoma cells expressing *bcl-2* are long-lived and thus remain in the lymph nodes over a prolonged period.

131. What is the typical clinical course of follicular lymphoma, and why do most patients suffering from this disease die?

Patients present with painless generalized lymphadenopathy that will transform to a diffuse large B-cell lymphoma in 30% to 50% of cases. Follicular lymphoma is incurable, with a median survival of 7 to 9 years. Aggressive therapy does not improve survival, so the usual clinical approach is to palliate patients with low-dose chemotherapy or radiation when they become symptomatic.

132. Describe the main pathologic features of diffuse large B-cell lymphoma.

The common morphologic features of diffuse large B-cell lymphoma (DLBCL) are:
- Relatively large size of lymphoma cells
- Diffuse growth pattern resulting in an effacement of normal lymph node architecture
- Considerable morphologic variation from cell to cell (Some cells may even resemble Reed–Sternberg cells, from which they can be distinguished only by immunohistochemistry.)

133. What is the typical clinical course of DLBCL?

DLBCL present with a rapidly enlarging, often symptomatic mass at a single nodal or extranodal site. These sites include the gastrointestinal tract, skin, bone, brain, Waldeyer ring, liver, and spleen. Bone marrow involvement occurs late in the disease, and, rarely, a leukemic picture may occur.

Diffuse large B-cell lymphomas are aggressive tumors that are rapidly fatal if left untreated. With heavy combination chemotherapy, complete remission is achieved in 60% to 80% of patients, and approximately 50% remain free of disease. Disease limited to a single area has a better prognosis than the disease presenting with widespread involvement of lymph nodes and bulky tumor masses.

134. What is Burkitt lymphoma?

Burkitt lymphoma is a tumor of relatively mature B cells associated with translocations of the *c-myc* gene on chromosome 8. The hallmark of Burkitt lymphoma is a t(8;14) translocation. Three clinical forms are recognized:
- African (endemic) Burkitt lymphoma
- Sporadic (nonendemic) Burkitt lymphoma
- Subset of aggressive lymphomas occurring in patients infected with HIV

Burkitt lymphoma is histologically identical in all three forms, but some clinical, genotypic, and etiologic differences exist.

135. **List the principal microscopic features of Burkitt lymphoma.**
   - There is diffuse infiltration of lymph nodes by intermediate-sized lymphoid cells with round or oval nuclei, coarse chromatin, and several nucleoli.
   - Mitoses are common.
   - Numerous apoptotic tumor cells taken up by resident macrophages give the lymph node a "starry-sky" appearance.
   - Extranodal involvement is common.

136. **Does endemic Burkitt lymphoma differ from the nonendemic form of the disease?**
   Both endemic and nonendemic Burkitt lymphoma preferentially affect children and young adults. Both forms respond well to chemotherapy.
   The endemic form presents with a mass on the mandible and involvement of the abdominal viscera: kidneys, ovaries, and adrenals.
   The nonendemic form presents as an abdominal mass involving the ileocecum and peritoneum.

137. **What are the main characteristics of plasma cell neoplasms and related entities?**
   Plasma cell neoplasms and related entities are lymphoid neoplasms of terminally differentiated B cells, all of which exhibit the expansion of a single clone of Ig-secreting plasma cells. Consequently, a resultant increase in serum levels of a single homogeneous Ig or its fragments is also common to all of these disorders. Often (but not always), these clonal proliferations (also referred to as dyscrasias) show malignant behavior. The monoclonal Ig in the blood is known as an M component, in reference to myeloma. Complete M components are restricted largely to circulating plasma and extracellular fluid. They may also appear in the urine, in case of glomerular damage with heavy proteinuria.

138. **What are the main pathologic and clinical features of multiple myeloma?**
   - It is characterized by multiple tumorous masses of neoplastic plasma cells, which involve the skeletal system. (Lymph nodes and extranodal sites, such as the skin, are also sometimes involved.)
   - Incidence is higher in men and in older adults (the peak age is between 50 and 60 years).
   - Frequently the disease is located in the vertebral column, ribs, skull, clavicle, and scapula.
   - Microscopically, the marrow reveals diffuse infiltration or sheetlike masses of plasma cells (usually >30% of cells) with prominent Golgi apparatus and an eccentrically placed nucleus.
   - Clinically patients present with bone pain, pathologic fractures, or both because of bone infiltration. Hypercalcemia results from bone reabsorption, which causes confusion, weakness, lethargy, constipation, and polyuria and contributes to renal disease. Decreased production of normal Ig leads to recurrent bacterial infections. Cellular immunity is relatively unaffected. The marrow involvement gives rise to a normocytic, normochromic anemia, and sometimes leukopenia and thrombocytopenia.
   - Solitary myeloma or solitary plasmacytoma is an infrequent variant consisting of a plasma cell neoplasm presenting as a solitary lesion of either bone or soft tissue.
   See Fig. 9-4.

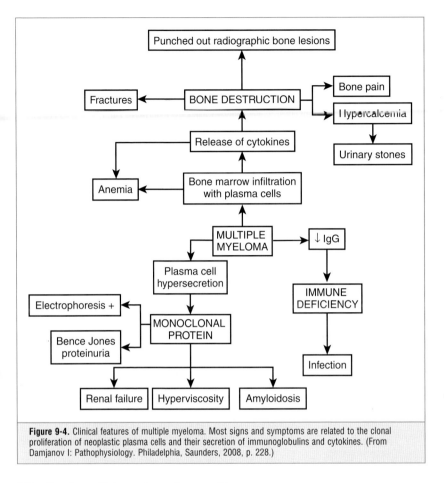

Figure 9-4. Clinical features of multiple myeloma. Most signs and symptoms are related to the clonal proliferation of neoplastic plasma cells and their secretion of immunoglobulins and cytokines. (From Damjanov I: Pathophysiology. Philadelphia, Saunders, 2008, p. 228.)

139. **How is multiple myeloma diagnosed?**
   - The clinicopathologic diagnosis of multiple myeloma is based on radiographic and laboratory findings.
   - Radiographically, the bone lesions appear as sharply punched-out defects having a rounded soap-bubble appearance, but generalized osteoporosis may also be seen.
   - With electrophoretic analysis, 99% of patients with multiple myeloma will have increased levels of IgG (or IgA) in the blood, light chains (Bence Jones proteins) in the urine, or both.
   - Marrow examination sometimes shows increased interstitial plasma cells or sheets of aggregated tumor cells that completely replace the normal elements.
   - Bence Jones proteinuria and a serum M protein are both observed in 60% to 70% of all myeloma patients. In approximately 20% of patients, Bence Jones proteinuria is present as an isolated finding. However, 1% of myelomas are nonsecretory and thus occur in the absence of detectable serum or urine M proteins.

140. **What is Bence Jones proteinuria?**
Normal plasma cells are characterized by tightly balanced production and coupling of heavy and light chains. This balance is frequently lost in neoplastic plasma cells, resulting in production of excess light or heavy chains along with complete Ig. Only light chains or heavy chains can be produced without complete Ig. The free light chains, known as Bence Jones proteins, are small enough to be rapidly excreted in the urine. Therefore they are often completely cleared from the blood or present at very low levels. However, in case of renal failure or massive synthesis, Bence Jones proteins may appear in the blood in significant concentrations.

141. **Name the most common complications and the most common causes of death in patients with multiple myeloma.**
The most common complications are:
- Bone pain due to increased osteoclastic activity
- Microfractures
- Anemia due to the crowding of bone marrow by the proliferating plasma cells
- Renal failure resulting from Bence Jones proteinuria or amyloidosis is the most common cause of death
- Normal IgG synthesis is suppressed and infections are common because of the hypogammaglobinemia

142. **What is the prognosis of multiple myeloma?**
Prognosis is generally poor. Multiple lytic lesions portend a survival of 6 to 12 months, whereas indolent myeloma can last for years. Chemotherapy induces remission in 50% to 70% of cases, with median survival of 3 years. Autologous bone marrow transplant somewhat improves survival but it is not curative.

143. **What are the main pathologic and clinical features of lymphoplasmacytic lymphoma?**
This diffuse B-cell lymphoma is characterized by diffuse infiltrate in the bone marrow of lymphocytes, plasma cells, and intermediate plasmacytoid lymphocytes. PAS-positive inclusions containing Ig are sometimes present in the cytoplasm (Russell bodies) or nucleus (Dutcher bodies).
Patients present with nonspecific symptoms (weakness, fatigue, and weight loss), generalized lymphadenopathy, hepatosplenomegaly, and sometimes hyperviscosity syndrome.

144. **What is Waldenström macroglobulinemia?**
- It is a specific syndrome most commonly seen in middle-aged and elderly patients with lymphoplasmacytic lymphoma that shows substantial fraction of the tumor cells terminally differentiated into plasma cells.
- Neoplastic plasma cells secrete monoclonal IgM, often in amounts sufficient to cause a hyperviscosity syndrome. It presents with:
  ○ Visual impairment due to tortuous, distended veins as well as retinal hemorrhage and exudates
  ○ Neurologic problems, such as headaches, dizziness, deafness, and stupor
  ○ Bleeding related to the formation of complexes between IgM and clotting factors, along with altered platelet function
  ○ Cryoglobulinemia due to precipitation of IgM at low temperatures, producing symptoms such as Raynaud phenomenon and cold urticaria

145. **List the main characteristics of peripheral T cell lymphoma, unspecified.**
- No morphologic feature is pathognomonic of peripheral T cell lymphoma, and as a group, these lymphomas are heterogeneous and not easily categorized.

- The architecture of involved lymph nodes is diffusely effaced by the tumors that are typically composed of a plemorphic mixture of small, intermediate, and large malignant T lymphocytes.
- Only immunophenotyping definitely confirms the diagnosis.
- Patients present most frequently with generalized lymphadenopathy, sometimes accompanied by eosinophilia, pruritus, fever, and weight loss.
- The incidence of relapse appears to be higher than that observed with aggressive mature B-cell neoplasms.

146. **Which form of lymphoma occurs in Human T-Cell Leukemia Virus (HTLV)-1-infected people?**
- Patients infected by HTLV-1 (an oncogenic virus) present with adult T cell leukemia/lymphoma, a neoplasm of CD4+ T cells.
- The disease is characterized by skin lesions, generalized lymphadenopathy, hepatosplenomegaly, peripheral blood lymphocytosis, and hypercalcemia.
- In most cases, the disease is rapidly progressive and fatal within months to 1 year, and it is unresponsive to aggressive chemotherapy.

147. **What are the common features and differences between mycosis fungoides and Sézary syndrome?**
- Mycosis fungoides and Sézary syndrome are different manifestations of a single neoplastic entity. Mycosis fungoides is an indolent disorder of peripheral CD4+ T cells characterized by the involvement of skin. Thus it belongs to the group of cutaneous T-cell lymphoid neoplasms.
- Mycosis fungoides presents with an inflammatory premycotic phase and progresses through a plaque phase to a tumor phase. It is histologically characterized by infiltration of the epidermis and upper dermis by neoplastic T cells. These cells have a "cerebriform nucleus" seen by electron microscopy as extensive infolding of the nuclear membrane. Disease usually spreads extracutaneously, most commonly to lymph nodes and bone marrow.
- Sézary syndrome is a variant in which skin involvement characteristically presents as a generalized exfoliative erythroderma. In contrast to mycosis fungoides, the skin lesions rarely result in evident tumefactions. In addition, patients often develop an associated leukemia of Sézary cells that have the same cerebriform appearance noted in the tissue infiltrates of mycosis fungoides. Circulating tumor cells can also be identified in peripheral smears in up to 25% of cases of mycosis fungoides in the plaque or tumor phase, emphasizing the overlap between mycosis fungoides and Sézary syndrome.
- The median survival rate in patients who have mycosis fungoides or Sézary syndrome is usually 8 or 9 years. Transformation into large-cell lymphoma of T-cell type sometimes develops as a terminal event.

148. **What is Hodgkin lymphoma (HL)?**
HL is a form of lymphoma arising in a single node or chain of nodes and spreading characteristically to the anatomically contiguous nodes. It is characterized morphologically by the presence of neoplastic giant cells, Reed–Sternberg (RS) cells, which induce the accumulation of reactive lymphocytes, histiocytes, and granulocytes. The neoplastic cells comprise a minor fraction (1%–5%) of the total tumor cell mass. HL is one of the most common forms of malignancy in young adults, with an average age at diagnosis of 32 years. The disease is curable in most cases.

149. **List the main subtypes of Hodgkin lymphoma.**
Five subtypes of HL are recognized. The first four are grouped into the so-called classical HL, whereas the last form (lymphocyte predominance) is considered to be a separate entity:
- HL, nodular sclerosis type (65%–75% of cases)
- HL, mixed cellularity type (20%–25% of cases)
- HL, lymphocyte rich (rare)
- HL, lymphocyte depletion type (a rare and somewhat controversial form of disease)
- HL, lymphocyte predominance type (6%)

150. **What are RS and lacunar cells?**
    - RS cells are large and binucleate or bilobed, with the two halves often appearing as mirror images of each other. There may also be multiple nuclei or multilobulate single nuclei variants. The nucleus is enclosed within an abundant amphophilic cytoplasm. Large, inclusion-like, owl-eyed nucleoli are generally surrounded by a clear halo.
    - Lacunar cells, seen predominantly in the nodular sclerosis subtype, are RS cell variants that have more delicate folded or solitary nuclei surrounded by abundant pale cytoplasm that can retract during processing.

151. **Discuss how HL spreads and how the extent of spread is used for staging the disease.**
    HL spreads in a contiguous, predictable fashion, with nodal disease preceding splenic disease, preceding hepatic disease, preceding bone marrow involvement and extranodal disease. Therefore patients with limited disease can be cured with radiotherapy, and the staging of HL predicts prognosis and guides therapy choice. There are four stages based on spread of tumor cells:
    - I: Involvement of single lymph node, most often on the neck
    - II: Involvement of two or more lymph nodes on the same side of the diaphragm
    - III: Involvement of lymph node regions on both sides of the diaphragm and can include the spleen
    - IV: Multiple or disseminated foci of involvement of one or more extralymphatic organs with or without lymph node involvement

152. **Describe the typical presentation, clinical course, and prognosis of HL.**
    HL presents with an enlargement of localized lymph node groups. The lymph nodes are usually firm, freely movable, and nontender, although they may become tender on ingestion of alcohol.
    Localized nodal enlargement spreads to contiguous lymphoid structures and ultimately to nonlymphoid tissue. Growth can be variable, with some nodes remaining stable for long periods and others spontaneously regressing.
    Prognosis is primarily based on tumor burden (i.e., stage) rather than histologic subtype. Other good prognostic features are young age and the absence of B symptoms. Treatment usually consists of radiation for early presentation and multidrug chemotherapy for later stages of disease. Long-term complications of treatment include secondary malignancies and nonneoplastic complications of radiation. The leading secondary neoplasms are myelodysplastic syndromes and acute myelogenous leukemia (AML; attributable to alkylating agents), as well as lung cancer (attributable to radiation).

153. **What are the clinical features that distinguish HL from NHL?**
    See Table 9-3.

TABLE 9-3. CLINICAL FEATURES THAT DISTINGUISH HODGKIN LYMPHOMA FROM NON-HODGKIN LYMPHOMA	
Hodgkin Lymphoma	**Non-Hodgkin Lymphoma**
Localized to single axial group of nodes	Involvement of multiple peripheral nodes
Contiguous spread	Noncontiguous spread
Rarely involves mesenteric nodes and Waldeyer ring	Usually involves mesenteric nodes and Waldeyer ring
Rare extranodal involvement	Common extranodal involvement

154. **What is the common progenitor cell of all myeloid neoplasms?**
The common progenitor is a myeloid precursor that normally gives rise to terminally differentiated cells of the myeloid line (i.e., erythrocytes, granulocytes, monocytes, and platelets).

155. **What are the three broad categories of myeloid neoplasia?**
Myeloid neoplasms almost always primarily involve the bone marrow and, to a lesser degree, the secondary hematopoietic organs (spleen, liver, and lymph nodes) and present with altered hematopoiesis. There are three broad categories of myeloid neoplasia:
   - AML, characterized by accumulation of immature myeloid cells in the bone marrow
   - Myelodysplastic syndromes (MDSs), associated with ineffective hematopoiesis and associated cytopenias
   - Chronic myeloproliferative disorders (MPDs), usually associated with an increased production of terminally differentiated myeloid cells

156. **Define acute myelogenous leukemia.**
AML is a neoplastic disease that results in the replacement of normal bone marrow with more than 20% blasts being of early (i.e., undifferentiated) myeloid lineage. One or several types of cells may be present. The most common consequence is crowding of the marrow with suppression of normal hematopoiesis, resulting in anemia, neutropenia, and thrombocytopenia. Thus complications besides anemia are infection and uncontrolled bleeding.

157. **How common is AML, and whom does it affect most often?**
AML constitutes 20% of all the leukemias in Western countries. It primarily affects adults between ages 15 and 39 years but is also observed in children and older adults. It represents 20% of childhood leukemias.

158. **How is AML classified?**
AML is classified according to WHO on the basis of chromosomal and other genetic data and immunophenotypic markers of differentiation. This classification includes also the previous French–American–British (FAB) classification based on bone marrow morphology. The most common FAB subtypes of acute myelogenous leukemia are:
   - M2: AML with maturation
   - M1: AML without maturation
   - M4: Acute myelomonocytic leukemia

159. **How is AML diagnosed?**
   - Clinical features are considered.
   - Bone marrow biopsy must contain at least 20% myeloid blasts.
   - Cytogenetics are an essential part of diagnosis.
   - Chromosomal translocations, deletions, or monosomies are typical.
   - Peripheral blood smears typically contain blast cells.
   - The peripheral smear of some leukemic patients may contain no blasts at all (aleukemic leukemia).
   - Secondary hematopoietic organ involvement may be present (spleen, liver, and lymph nodes)

160. **How does AML present clinically? List the most common complications.**
   - AML most commonly presents with signs of fatigue, fever, and spontaneous mucosal (gingival and urinary tract) and cutaneous bleeding (petechiae and ecchymoses).
   - Procoagulants released by leukemic cells may produce disseminated intravascular coagulation.

- Infections of the oral cavity, skin, lungs, kidneys, urinary bladder, and colon.
- Mild lymphadenopathy and organomegaly.
- In tumors with monocytic differentiation, infiltration of the skin and the gingiva (sometimes).
- Central nervous system involvement may occur but is less common than in ALL.
- Uncommonly, patients present with localized masses composed of myeloblasts in the absence of marrow or peripheral blood involvement (myeloblastomas, granulocytic sarcomas, or chloromas).
- Treatment-related complications include venoocclusive liver disease, graft versus host disease, and infections.

161. **Define myelodysplastic syndromes.**
MDS refers to a group of clonal stem-cell disorders characterized by defects in cell maturation. The consequence is ineffective hematopoiesis and an increased risk of transformation to AML. The bone marrow of patients with MDS is partly or wholly replaced by the clonal progeny of a mutant multipotent stem cell. Although the stem cell retains the capacity to differentiate into red cells, granulocytes, and platelets, the differentiation is ineffective and disordered. Therefore the bone marrow is usually hypercellular or normocellular, but the peripheral blood shows pancytopenia.

162. **What are the two main forms of MDS?**
Idiopathic or primary MDS usually affects people older than age 50 years and often develops insidiously.
Therapy-related MDS (t-MDS) appears as a complication of previous myelosuppressive drug or radiation therapy, usually 2 to 8 years after exposure.

163. **What is the clinical course of a typical MDS?**
When patients present with MDS, they may be asymptomatic, or they may present with weakness, infections, and hemorrhages (due to pancytopenia). Depending on a subtype of primary MDS, median survival varies from 9 to 29 months. Patients with t-MDS have a poor prognosis, with overall median survival of only 4 to 8 months. Progression to AML occurs in 10% to 40% of patients, and some die of bleeding (thrombocytopenia) or infection (neutropenia). There is no effective treatment for MDS in adults, although children may receive allogenic bone marrow transplantation.

164. **Name four entities included under the name chronic MPDs?**
- Chronic myelogenous leukemia (CML)
- Polycythemia vera (PCV)
- Essential thrombocytosis (ET)
- Chronic idiopathic myelofibrosis (CIM)

165. **What are the main characteristics of chronic MPDs?**
The target of neoplastic transformation in most chronic MPDs is a multipotent progenitor cell that gives rise to mature erythrocytes, platelets, granulocytes, and monocytes. CML is an exception because it seems to affect the pluripotent stem cell that can give rise to lymphoid and myeloid cells.
The neoplastic cells and their offspring flood the bone marrow and suppress residual normal progenitor cells, as in AML. The main difference is terminal cell differentiation, which is initially unaffected in chronic MPDs. It results in marrow hypercellularity and increased hematopoiesis, often accompanied by elevated peripheral blood counts.
In all chronic MPDs, the neoplastic stem cells have the capacity to circulate and home to secondary hematopoietic organs, particularly the spleen, in which they give rise to extramedullary hematopoiesis. Therefore all chronic MPDs cause varying degrees of

splenomegaly. They also share the propensity to terminate in a spent phase, which includes marrow fibrosis and peripheral blood cytopenias. All MPDs can progress over time to acute leukemia, but only CML does so invariably.

In contrast to the lymphoid neoplasms and AML, the pathologic findings in the chronic MPDs are not specific. They share a considerable degree of overlap with one another and also with some reactive conditions that produce marrow hyperplasia. Diagnosis and classification are based on correlation of morphologic findings with other clinical and laboratory findings.

166. **What is CML?**

CML is a chronic MPD, primarily seen in adults between 25 and 60 years of age, that contains the *BCR-ABL* fusion gene. In more than 90% of CML cases, karyotyping reveals t(9:22) translocation, producing the Philadelphia chromosome (oncogene resulting in increased tyrosine kinase activity):

- Bone marrow is usually 100% cellular (normally, it is 50% fat) and characterized histologically by predominantly maturing granulocytic precursors and increased numbers of megakaryocytes (often including small dysplastic forms).
- Peripheral blood shows marked leukocytosis, with many neutrophils, metamyelocytes, and myelocytes, and less than 10% myeloblasts.
- Neoplastic extramedullary hematopoiesis causes splenomegaly (expansion of red pulp), with possible hepatomegaly and lymphadenopathy.
- Neoplastic leukocytes lack leukocyte alkaline phosphatase.

167. **What is the clinical course of CML?**

CML patients present with nonspecific symptoms: weight loss, fatigue, malaise, fever, and sweating. These symptoms result from mild to moderate anemia and hypermetabolism. Left upper quadrant pain results from splenomegaly or splenic infarcts, and bleeding abnormalities result from platelet defects. There are three phases in CML:

- The stable phase is characterized by slow course of disease (50% of patients will progress to an accelerated phase).
- The accelerated phase is characterized by gradual failure of response to treatment accompanied by increasing anemia and thrombocytopenia.
- Blast crisis is characterized by a large increase of blast cells in the marrow and blood. Treatment is bone marrow transplantation during the stable phase. Without treatment, median survival is 3 years.

168. **Define PCV.**

PCV is a neoplasm arising from multipotent myeloid stem cell, characterized by increased proliferation and production of erythroid, granulocytic, and megakaryocytic elements. Increased marrow production is reflected in the peripheral blood by erythrocytosis (polycythemia), granulocytosis, and thrombocytosis, but the absolute increase in red cell mass is responsible for most of the clinical symptoms.

169. **What are the morphologic characteristics, clinical course, and laboratory findings in PCV?**

- Pathology
  - The bone marrow is hypercellular. The increase in erythroid progenitors is usually accompanied by increased numbers of maturing granulocytic precursors and megakaryocytes. Mild organomegaly is common as a result of congestion that appears early in the course of PCV. Extramedullary hematopoiesis is minimal at this point. The peripheral blood smear contains giant platelets and megakaryocytic fragments.
  - Occasionally, late in the course of disease, the marrow may progress to a spent phase. In this phase, fibrosis fills the intertrabecular space and displaces hematopoietic cells, so extramedullary hematopoiesis increases in the spleen and liver, producing more prominent organomegaly.

- Clinical course
  - Median age of onset is 60 years.
  - Patients are typically plethoric and somewhat cyanotic.
  - Headache, dizziness, pruritus, and peptic ulceration are described.
  - Seventy percent of patients are hypertensive, and 5% to 10% show hyperuricemia and gout.
  - There is increased risk of major hemorrhage and thrombotic episodes (deep venous thrombosis, hepatic veins, the portal and mesenteric veins, and venous sinuses of the brain), which can cause myocardial infarction, stroke, and bowel infarction
  - There may be minor hemorrhages (epistaxis and bleeding gums).
  - With treatment, median survival is approximately 10 years.
- Laboratory findings
  - MCHC is lower than normal, whereas hematocrit values are 60%.
  - Occasionally, chronic bleeding may lead to iron deficiency.
  - Elevated white cell count.
  - Platelet count is often greater than 500,000 cells/mm^3.
  - Philadelphia chromosome is absent.
  - Elevated leukocyte alkaline phosphatase.

170. **How is essential thrombocytosis diagnosed?**

Essential thrombocytosis is a hematopoietic stem-cell disorder characterized by increased proliferation and production of megakaryocytic elements, with most patients having platelet counts exceeding 600,000 cells/mm^3. It is a diagnosis of exclusion.

- Bone marrow (most helpful in excluding other chronic MPDs)
  - Mild to moderate increase in the marrow cellularity
  - Often significantly increased number of megakaryocytes and the presence of abnormally large cell forms
  - Possible deposition of delicate reticulin fibrils but does not resemble the overt fibrosis characteristic of CIM
- Peripheral blood smear
  - Abnormally large platelets, often accompanied by mild leukocytosis
- Clinical manifestations
  - Thrombosis and hemorrhage

171. **Describe the pathologic features of myelofibrosis and how the changes in the bone marrow are reflected in the peripheral blood.**

CIM is caused by neoplastic transformation of a multipotent myeloid stem cell. The hallmark of this disease is early progression to marrow fibrosis (myelofibrosis) that is histologically identical to the spent phase of the other chronic MPDs. The pathologic features stem from extensive collagen deposition by nonneoplastic fibroblasts, which displace hematopoietic elements from the marrow, causing stem cells to circulate in peripheral blood and eventually seed the spleen, liver, and lymph nodes, leading to extramedullary hematopoiesis (the spleen is markedly enlarged, the liver is moderately enlarged, and significant lymphadenopathy is uncommon).

- Bone marrow
  - In the early stages, the marrow is often hypercellular and the number of maturing cells of all lineages is increased.
  - In time, the marrow changes include hypocellularity and diffuse fibrosis.
  - Late in the disease course, the fibrotic marrow space may be largely converted to bone (osteosclerosis).
- Peripheral blood
  - The presence of erythroid and granulocytic precursors (leukoerythroblastosis), along with numerous teardrop erythrocytes (dacryocytes), is observed.
  - Abnormally large platelets and basophilia are seen.

- Laboratory findings
  - There is moderate to severe normochromic normocytic anemia accompanied by leukoerythroblastosis.
  - There is usually normal to reduced WBC, which may be significantly elevated during the early cellular phase.
  - The platelet count is usually normal or elevated at the time of diagnosis, but later in the course of the disease thrombocytopenia is a common finding.

SPLEEN

172. **What are the main causes of splenomegaly?**
   - Nonspecific splenitis caused by infectious mononucleosis, tuberculosis, typhoid fever, malaria, cytomegalovirus, histoplasmosis, toxoplasmosis, leishmaniasis, echinococcosis, and autoimmune disorders
   - Congestive states related to portal hypertension: liver cirrhosis, portal or splenic vein thrombosis, and cardiac failure
   - Lymphohematogenous disorders lymphoma, leukemia, multiple myeloma, MPDs, hemolytic anemias, and thrombocytopenic purpura
     A useful mnemonic for remembering the causes of splenomegaly is *splenic*:
   - **S**plenitis due to infection, especially sepsis
   - **P**ortal hypertension (e.g., cirrhosis of the liver)
   - **L**eukemia/lymphoma
   - **E**rythrocyte disorders (e.g., hereditary spherocytosis)
   - **N**eonatal disorders (inborn errors of metabolism such as Gaucher disease)
   - **I**mmune disorders (e.g., rheumatoid arthritis, Felty syndrome, SLE, and ITP)
   - **C**ardiac failure (congestive splenomegaly)

173. **What is hypersplenism?**
   Hypersplenism is a syndrome characterized by the triad of:
   - Splenomegaly
   - A reduction of one or more types of blood cells, leading to anemia, leukopenia, thrombocytopenia, or any combination of these, accompanied by hyperplasia of the marrow precursors of the deficient cell type
   - Correction of the cytopenia(s) in the blood after splenectomy

THYMUS

174. **What is DiGeorge syndrome?**
   DiGeorge syndrome represents thymic hypoplasia or aplasia with resultant T-cell immunodeficiency that derives from a failure of development of the third and fourth pharyngeal pouches. In addition to loss of T-cell-mediated immunity and poor defense against fungal and viral infections (lack of thymus), patients also suffer from tetany due to hypoparathyroidism (lack of parathyroid glands causing hypocalcemia) and congenital defects of the heart and great arteries.

175. **What is thymoma?**
   - Thymoma is a neoplasm derived from cortical or medullary thymic epithelial cells.
   - These tumors occur mostly in adults, equally in both sexes.
   - It is located in the anterosuperior mediastinum.
   - Most thymomas (75%) are benign.
   - Malignant thymomas are less common and are divided into two groups:
     - Locally invasive thymomas
     - Thymic carcinomas, which may metastasize

KEY POINTS: SPLEEN AND THYMUS ✓

1. Enlargement of the spleen, called splenomegaly, can occur in response to infections, as a complication of portal hypertension, or in the course of leukemia and lymphoma.

2. Thymic diseases are associated with immune disturbances.

3. Enlargement of the thymus can occur because of hyperplasia or tumors (thymomas and lymphomas).

176. **List the main clinical features of thymomas.**
    - Approximately 60% to 70% of thymomas are discovered accidentally as a radiologically visible but asymptomatic mediastinal mass. Some of these tumors cause local pressure symptoms.
    - The remaining thymomas present in association with myasthenia gravis and other paraneoplastic syndromes which include:
      - Acquired hypogammaglobinemia
      - Pure red cell aplasia
      - Graves disease
      - Pernicious anemia
      - Dermatomyositis–polymyositis
      - Cushing syndrome

WEBSITES 🌐

1. http://www.ncbi.nlm.nih.gov/entrez/query.fcgi?db=PubMed

2. http://www-medlib.med.utah.edu/WebPath/webpath.html#MENU

3. http://image.bloodline.net/bd1

4. http://www.leukemia.org

5. http://pathologyoutlines.com/leukemia.html

6. http://pathologyoutlines.com/lymphoma.html

7. http://pleiad.umdnj.edu/hemepath/default.html

BIBLIOGRAPHY

1. Arber DA: Realistic classification of acute myeloid leukemias. Am J Clin Pathol 115:552–560, 2001.
2. Brodsky RA, Jones RJ: Aplastic anaemia. Lancet 365:1647–1656, 2005.
3. Esteve FR, Roodman GD: Pathophysiology of myeloma bone disease. Best Pract Res Clin Haematol 20:613–624, 2007.
4. Hunt KE, Reichard KK: Diffuse large B-cell lymphoma. Arch Pathol Lab Med 132:118–124, 2008.
5. Matutes E: Adult T-cell leukaemia/lymphoma. J Clin Pathol 60:1373–1377, 2007.
6. Olivieri NF: The beta-thalassemias. N Engl J Med 341:99–109, 1999.
7. Sawyers CL: Chronic myeloid leukemia. N Engl J Med 340:1330–1340, 1999.
8. Stuart MJ, Nagel RL: Sickle-cell disease. Lancet 364:1343–1360, 2004.

CHAPTER 10

THE RESPIRATORY SYSTEM

Marin Nola, MD, PhD, and Snježana Dotlić, MD

1. **What are the most important diseases of the respiratory system?**
   - Collapse of the alveoli (atelectasis) and pneumothorax
   - Circulatory disturbances, such as pulmonary edema and chronic passive congestion, and adult respiratory distress syndrome
   - Infections such as rhinitis, laryngitis, bronchitis, and pneumonia
   - Immunologically mediated diseases, such as asthma
   - Environmentally induced diseases, such as pneumoconioses, asbestosis, and silicosis
   - Tumors

2. **Define atelectasis.**
   Atelectasis refers to incomplete expansion of the lungs or the collapse of previously inflated lung substance (Fig. 10-1). It is a pathologic condition that produces areas of relatively airless pulmonary parenchyma. Severe atelectasis significantly reduces oxygenation and predisposes to infection. Acquired atelectasis is generally encountered in adults and may be divided into the following categories:
   - Obstruction (or resorption) atelectasis
   - Compression atelectasis
   - Patchy atelectasis
   - Contraction atelectasis

   Atelectasis is a reversible disorder (except that caused by contraction).

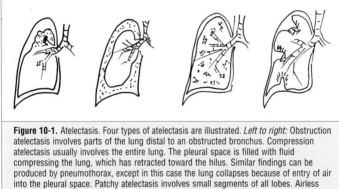

Figure 10-1. Atelectasis. Four types of atelectasis are illustrated. *Left to right:* Obstruction atelectasis involves parts of the lung distal to an obstructed bronchus. Compression atelectasis usually involves the entire lung. The pleural space is filled with fluid compressing the lung, which has retracted toward the hilus. Similar findings can be produced by pneumothorax, except in this case the lung collapses because of entry of air into the pleural space. Patchy atelectasis involves small segments of all lobes. Airless patches of lung parenchyma, which have collapsed because of a deficiency of surfactant, are distributed irregularly and usually are found in both lungs. Contraction atelectasis usually occurs in subpleural areas and is typically caused by interstitial fibrosis, which prevents the expansion of the parenchyma.

3. **What are the main characteristics of obstruction atelectasis?**
   Obstruction (or resorption) atelectasis results from complete obstruction of an airway and, in time, it causes resorption of the oxygen trapped in the dependent alveoli.
   The mediastinum may shift toward the atelectatic lung.
   It is most often found in bronchial asthma, chronic bronchitis, bronchiectasis, postoperative states, and with aspiration of foreign bodies; bronchial neoplasms may also cause it.

4. **What are the main characteristics of compression, patchy, and contraction atelectasis?**
   - Compression atelectasis ensues whenever the pleural cavity is partially (or completely) filled by fluid exudate, tumor, blood, or air (pneumothorax) or, in the case of tension pneumothorax, when the entry of air into the pleural cavity causes pulmonary collapse. It is most commonly found in patients with cardiac failure who develop pleural effusions as well as in patients experiencing malignant effusions within the pleural cavities; abnormal elevation of the diaphragm (peritonitis and subdiaphragmatic abscesses) induces basal atelectasis. With compression atelectasis, the mediastinum shifts away from the affected lung.
   - Patchy atelectasis develops when there is loss of pulmonary surfactant, as in neonatal and adult respiratory distress syndrome.
   - Contraction atelectasis occurs when local or generalized fibrotic changes in the lung or pleura prevent full expansion of the lung.

5. **What are the main causes of pulmonary edema?**
   - Hemodynamic disturbances
     ○ The most common mechanism is the one attributable to increased hydrostatic pressure, as occurs in left-sided congestive heart failure.
     ○ It can also occur as a consequence of decreased plasma oncotic pressure.
   - Direct increase in capillary permeability
     ○ The most common causes are infectious agents, inhaled gases, liquid aspiration, and drugs.
     ○ The edema results from primary injury to the vascular endothelium or damage to alveolar epithelial cells (with secondary microvascular injury).
   - Lymphatic insufficiency
     ○ Lymphangitic carcinomatosis
     ○ Fibrosing lymphangitis (e.g., silicosis)

6. **What are the pathologic features of pulmonary congestion and edema?**
   - Macroscopic features
     ○ Pulmonary congestion and edema are macroscopically characterized by heavy, wet lungs.
     ○ Long-standing pulmonary congestion causes brown induration of the lungs (the lungs are firm and brown), which predisposes to infection.
   - Histologic features
     ○ The alveolar capillaries are engorged.
     ○ Proteinaceous material is located within the alveoli; it appears pink in the hematoxylin and eosin-stained specimens.
     ○ In long-standing cases of pulmonary congestion, numerous heart failure cells, as well as fibrosis and thickening of the alveolar walls, appear.

7. **What is adult respiratory distress syndrome (ARDS)?**
   - ARDS has many synonyms, such as diffuse alveolar damage, adult respiratory failure, shock lungs, acute alveolar injury, and traumatic wet lungs.
   - Its clinical features are the rapid onset of life-threatening respiratory insufficiency, cyanosis, and severe arterial hypoxemia that is refractory to oxygen therapy and sometimes progresses to extrapulmonary multisystem organ failure.
   - It is almost always associated with evidence of severe pulmonary edema (often called noncardiogenic, low-pressure, or high-permeability pulmonary edema).

8. **Which conditions are associated with the development of ARDS?**
   - Direct lung injuries
     - ○ Diffuse pulmonary infections
     - ○ Oxygen toxicity
     - ○ Inhalation of toxins and other irritants
     - ○ Aspiration of gastric contents
   - Systemic conditions
     - ○ Septic shock
     - ○ Shock associated with trauma
     - ○ Hemorrhagic pancreatitis
     - ○ Burns
     - ○ Complicated abdominal surgery
     - ○ Narcotic overdose and other drug reactions

9. **What are the pathologic features of ARDS?**
   - **Macroscopic findings:** The lungs are heavy, filled with fluid, firm, red, and boggy.
   - **Microscopic findings in acute stage:** There is congestion, interstitial and intraalveolar edema, inflammation, and fibrin deposition along the inside of alveoli in form of hyaline membranes.
   - **Healing stage:** It is characterized by the organization of fibrin exudate, with resultant intraalveolar fibrosis and marked thickening of the alveolar septa.
   - **Fatal cases:** These often exhibit superimposed bronchopneumonia.

10. **Describe the pathogenesis of ARDS.**
    - ARDS is the end result of acute alveolar injury caused by a variety of insults, whereas the respiratory distress syndrome of newborns is caused by deficiency in pulmonary surfactant.
    - In ARDS, the initial injury affects capillary endothelium (most frequently) or alveolar epithelium (occasionally), but in the end both are clearly affected.
    - Increased capillary permeability is caused by an action of leukocytes on the endothelium.
    - Increased capillary permeability is followed by interstitial and then intraalveolar edema, fibrin exudation, and formation of hyaline membranes.
    - The exudates and diffuse tissue destruction cannot be easily resolved, and the result is organization with scarring, in contrast to the transudate of cardiogenic pulmonary edema, which usually resolves.

11. **What is the clinical course of ARDS?**
    Initially, patients may have no pulmonary symptoms. ARDS is heralded by profound dyspnea and tachypnea, but the chest radiograph is initially normal. Subsequently, progressive cyanosis and hypoxemia develop, followed by respiratory failure and the appearance of diffuse bilateral infiltrates on x-ray examination. Hypoxemia can then become unresponsive to oxygen therapy, sometimes resulting in respiratory acidosis. Patients' lungs can be divided into areas that are infiltrated, consolidated, or collapsed (and thus poorly aerated and poorly compliant) and regions that have almost normal levels of compliance and ventilation.

    Therapy of ARDS is extremely demanding, and the disorder is frequently fatal (60%). High concentrations of oxygen, required in therapy for ARDS, can contribute to perpetuation of the damage (oxygen toxicity).

CHRONIC OBSTRUCTIVE AND RESTRICTIVE LUNG DISEASES

12. **What are the main differences between obstructive and restrictive lung diseases?**
    Obstructive diseases (or airway diseases) are characterized by an increase in resistance to airflow due to partial or complete obstruction from the trachea and larger bronchi to the terminal

and respiratory bronchioles. Pulmonary function tests in patients with obstructive lung disease always show a decrease in expiratory flow rates. The major obstructive disorders (excluding tumor or inhalation of a foreign body) are:

- Emphysema
- Chronic bronchitis
- Bronchiectasis
- Asthma

Restrictive diseases are characterized by reduced expansion of lung parenchyma with decreased total lung capacity. The hallmark of the restrictive pattern of disease is a decrease in lung volumes. Restrictive diseases occur in the following conditions:

- Chest wall disorders in the presence of normal lungs
- Neuromuscular diseases (poliomyelitis)
- Severe obesity
- Pleural diseases
- Kyphoscoliosis
- Interstitial and infiltrative lung disease
  - Acute ARDS
  - Chronic pneumoconiosis and most of the infiltrative conditions

13. **Define chronic obstructive pulmonary disease (COPD).**
    The term COPD includes a group of conditions that share one major symptom—dyspnea—and are accompanied by chronic or recurrent obstruction to airflow within the lung.

    The incidence of COPD has increased dramatically in the past few decades (largely because of cigarette smoking and environmental pollutants) and currently represents a major cause of activity-restricting or bed-confining disability in the United States.

14. **What are the main differences between various types of COPD?**
    See Table 10-1.

TABLE 10-1. MAJOR DIFFERENCES IN VARIOUS TYPES OF CHRONIC OBSTRUCTIVE PULMONARY DISEASE

	Chronic Bronchitis	Bronchiectasis	Asthma	Emphysema	Bronchiolitis
Anatomic site	Bronchus	Bronchus	Bronchus	Acinus	Bronchiole
Pathology	Mucous gland hyperplasia, hypersecretion	Airway dilatation, scarring	Smooth muscle hyperplasia, excess mucus, inflammation	Airspace enlargement, wall destruction	Inflammatory scarring, obliteration
Etiology	Tobacco smoke, air pollutants	Persistent or severe infections	Immunologic or undefined causes	Tobacco smoke	Tobacco smoke, air pollutants, miscellaneous
Main symptoms	Cough, sputum production	Cough, purulent sputum, fever	Episodic wheezing, cough, dyspnea	Dyspnea	Cough, dyspnea

15. **What is emphysema?**

Emphysema is a condition of the lung in which abnormal permanent enlargement of the airspaces distal to the terminal bronchiole is accompanied by destruction of their walls, without obvious fibrosis. There are four main types of emphysema:

- Centriacinar (centrilobular)
- Panacinar (panlobular)
- Paraseptal (distal acinar)
- Irregular

Only the first two types cause clinically significant airflow obstruction. Centriacinar emphysema accounts for 95% of all cases and is far more common than the panacinar form or other rare forms of emphysema.

16. **What are the main characteristics of different types of emphysema?**

- Centriacinar (centrilobular)
  - The central or proximal parts of acini, formed by respiratory bronchioles, are affected, whereas distal alveoli are spared.
  - The lesions are often localized and usually more severe in the upper lobes, particularly in the apical segments.
  - The walls of the emphysematous spaces often contain abundant black pigment.
  - It tends to occur in heavy smokers.
- Panacinar (panlobular)
  - The acini are uniformly enlarged because the process affects all of the structures, from the respiratory bronchiole to the alveoli (the prefix pan refers to the entire acinus but not to the entire lung).
  - It tends to occur in the lower zones and in the anterior margins of the lung and is associated with a1-antitrypsin deficiency.
- Paraseptal (distal acinar)
  - The proximal part of the acinus is normal, and the distal acinar portion is dominantly involved (more severe in the upper half of the lungs).
- Irregular
  - It is almost invariably associated with scarring.
  - The acinus is irregularly involved.

17. **Describe the main clinical symptoms of emphysema.**

The clinical manifestations of emphysema do not appear until at least one third of the functioning pulmonary parenchyma is incapacitated. Dyspnea is usually the first symptom, but in some patients the main complaints are cough or wheezing. Weight loss is common, and patients are barrel-chested and dyspneic, with an obviously prolonged expiration. Classically, patients sit bending forward in a hunched-over position, attempting to squeeze the air out of the lungs with each expiratory effort. Patients have a pinched face and breathe through pursed lips.

18. **What is the difference in clinical presentation between patients with emphysema and those with chronic bronchitis?**

In patients with severe emphysema, cough is often slight, but overdistention is severe. They exhibit low diffusing capacity, and blood gas values are relatively normal. Overventilation helps them remain well oxygenated (pink puffers).

Patients with chronic bronchitis often have a history of recurrent infection and abundant purulent sputum, followed by hypercapnia and severe hypoxemia (blue bloaters). The important complication in severe bronchitis, in addition to the respiratory difficulties, is the development of cor pulmonale and eventual congestive heart failure, associated with secondary pulmonary hypertension.

19. **List the most frequent causes of death in patients with COPD.**
    - Respiratory insufficiency causing severe hypoxia, respiratory acidosis, and coma
    - Right-sided heart failure
    - Massive collapse of the lungs secondary to pneumothorax from ruptured bullae

20. **What is chronic bronchitis?**
    Chronic bronchitis is defined clinically as persistent cough with sputum production for at least 3 months of the year, in at least 2 consecutive years. Clinically there are several forms of chronic bronchitis:
    - **Simple chronic bronchitis:** Patients experience a productive cough but have no evidence of airflow obstruction.
    - **Chronic asthmatic bronchitis:** Some patients may demonstrate severe dyspnea and wheezing in association with inhaled irritants or during respiratory infections due to hyperreactive airways.
    - **Chronic obstructive bronchitis:** Some patients, especially heavy smokers, develop chronic airflow obstruction, usually accompanied by emphysema.

21. **List the factors important for the pathogenesis of chronic bronchitis.**
    - Chronic irritation by inhaled substances (cigarette smoking)
    - Infections

22. **Discuss the pathologic characteristics of chronic bronchitis.**
    Hyperemia, swelling, and bogginess of the mucous membranes are the main macroscopic features. They are frequently accompanied by excessive mucinous to mucopurulent secretions covering the epithelial surfaces. Heavy casts of secretions and pus occasionally fill the bronchi and bronchioles.
    The typical histologic feature of chronic bronchitis is enlargement of the mucus-secreting glands of the trachea and bronchi. Increase in the size of the mucous glands is assessed by the ratio of the thickness of the mucous gland layer to the thickness of the wall between the epithelium and the cartilage (Reid index). The Reid index is normally 0.4. Marked narrowing of bronchioles caused by goblet cell metaplasia also occurs, as do mucous plugging, inflammation, and fibrosis. In the most severe cases, obliteration of lumens (bronchiolitis obliterans) further aggravates the patient's condition.

23. **What are the clinical features of chronic bronchitis?**
    - There is a persistent cough productive of copious sputum.
    - When persistent for years, eventually dyspnea on exertion develops.
    - In time, and usually with continued smoking, hypercapnia, hypoxemia, and mild cyanosis with other elements of COPD may appear.
    - Long-standing severe chronic bronchitis often results in cor pulmonale with cardiac failure.

24. **Define bronchial asthma and status asthmaticus.**
    Bronchial asthma is a chronic relapsing inflammatory disorder presenting with hyperreactive airways that cause episodic, reversible bronchoconstriction. The reaction is the consequence of increased responsiveness of the tracheobronchial tree to various stimuli. Patients experience unpredictable disabling attacks of severe dyspnea, coughing, and wheezing triggered by sudden episodes of bronchospasm. Between the attacks, virtually no symptoms occur, but in some people, chronic bronchitis or cor pulmonale supervenes. In the most severe form of asthma, status asthmaticus, the severe acute paroxysm persists for days and even weeks, threatening the ventilatory function enough to cause severe cyanosis and even death.

25. **What are the main differences between extrinsic and intrinsic asthma?**
The extrinsic type is induced by exposure to an extrinsic antigen (type I hypersensitivity reaction). It comprises:
- Atopic (allergic) asthma (the most common type)
- Occupational asthma (fumes, organic and chemical dusts, gases, and other chemicals)
- Allergic bronchopulmonary aspergillosis
The intrinsic (idiosyncratic) type is initiated by diverse, nonimmune mechanisms, including:
- Ingestion of aspirin (drug-induced asthma)
- Pulmonary infection, especially viral (most frequent cause of nonatopic asthma)
- Cold
- Inhaled irritants
- Stress
- Exercise

26. **What is the pathogenesis of atopic asthma?**
Atopic asthma usually begins in childhood, when it is triggered by environmental antigens, such as dusts, pollens, animal dander, and foods. Patients with this condition usually have a positive family history of atopy, and asthmatic attacks are often preceded by allergic rhinitis, urticaria, or eczema. It is a classic example of type I immunoglobulin E (IgE)-mediated hypersensitivity reaction. In the airways, inhaled antigens (allergens) initiate reactions, which eventually promote IgE production by B cells, growth of mast cells, and growth and activation of eosinophils.

KEY POINTS: CHRONIC OBSTRUCTIVE AND RESTRICTIVE DISEASES

1. Dyspnea (i.e., difficulty in breathing) can be caused by several pathologic conditions, such as atelectasis, edema, diffuse alveolar damage (adult respiratory distress syndrome), pneumonia, and chronic obstructive pulmonary disease.

2. Clinically and pathologically, the lung diseases can be classified as obstructive or restrictive.

3. Asthma, a disease that has an immunologic basis, is the most common childhood respiratory disease encountered in the emergency room setting.

4. Chronic bronchitis and emphysema are most often caused by cigarette smoking.

27. **Describe the main differences between acute and late-phase reactions in patients with bronchial asthma.**
Acute (immediate) response is caused by exposure of presensitized IgE-coated mast cells to the same or cross-reacting antigen and occurs within minutes after stimulation. Either directly or via neuronal reflexes, the mediators induce bronchoconstriction and increase vascular permeability (edema), mucus production, and, in extreme instances, hypotension. Mast cells also release cytokines that cause the influx of other leukocytes (particularly eosinophils).
Late-phase response is mediated by mediators released from leukocytes (neutrophils, monocytes, lymphocytes, basophils, and eosinophils), endothelium, and epithelial cells. It occurs 4 to 8 hours after exposure and may persist for 12 to 24 hour or more.

28. **What are the major mediators responsible for bronchospasm in patients with bronchial asthma?**
- Leukotrienes C4, D4, and E4 cause prolonged bronchoconstriction, increased vascular permeability, and increased mucus secretion.
- Acetylcholine causes smooth muscle constriction in the walls of airways.

- Histamine is a potent bronchoconstrictive agent.
- Prostaglandin D2 causes bronchoconstriction and vasodilatation.
- Platelet-activating factor causes aggregation of platelets and release of histamine and serotonin from their granules.

29. **What are the main pathologic characteristics of bronchial asthma?**
Grossly, the lungs are overdistended because of overinflation, although small areas of atelectasis are sometimes evident as well. The most striking macroscopic finding is bronchial and bronchiolar occlusion by thick, tenacious mucous plugs.

Histologically, the mucous plugs contain whorls of shed respiratory epithelium, forming the well-known Curschmann spirals. Numerous eosinophils and Charcot–Leyden crystals (collections of crystalloids) are present. The basement membrane of the bronchial epithelium is thickened, the bronchial walls show edema, and an inflammatory infiltrate is present. Submucosal glands are increased in size, whereas bronchial wall muscle is hypertrophic because of prolonged bronchoconstriction.

30. **Discuss the clinical characteristics and prognosis of patients with bronchial asthma.**
The classic asthmatic attack can last up to several hours. It is followed by prolonged coughing, and the raising of copious mucous secretions provides considerable relief. The clinical diagnosis is confirmed by the demonstration of an elevated peripheral eosinophil count and the presence of eosinophils, Curschmann spirals, and Charcot–Leyden crystals in the sputum.

Appropriate therapy relieves the attacks, so that patients are able to maintain productive lives. Emphysema sometimes occurs, predisposing to chronic bacterial infections and sometimes chronic bronchitis, bronchiectasis, or pneumonia. In some patients, cor pulmonale and heart failure eventually develop.

31. **What is bronchiectasis, and how does it manifest clinically?**
Bronchiectasis is defined as an abnormal dilatation of bronchi and bronchioles usually associated with chronic infection. Patients present with cough, fever, and expectoration of copious amounts of foul-smelling, purulent sputum. The dilatation should be permanent to be considered bronchiectasis. (Reversible bronchial dilatation is often found with viral and bacterial pneumonia.)

32. **What are the most frequent causes of bronchiectasis?**
- Localized obstruction of bronchus by tumor, foreign bodies, and mucous impaction
- Diffuse obstructive airway diseases such as asthma and chronic bronchitis
- Congenital and hereditary conditions such as cystic fibrosis, immunodeficiency states, immotile cilia syndrome, and Kartagener syndrome
- Necrotizing pneumonia caused by *Mycobacterium tuberculosis,* staphylococci, and mixed infections

33. **What is the triad of Kartagener syndrome?**
Kartagener syndrome is characterized by bronchiectasis, sinusitis, and situs inversus, which are caused by a defect in ciliary motility, associated with structural abnormalities of cilia. It is inherited as an autosomal recessive trait. Males with this condition tend to be infertile because of ineffective motility of the sperm tail.

34. **Describe the major morphologic characteristics of bronchiectasis on gross inspection.**
Bronchiectasis usually affects the lower lobes bilaterally and is most severe in the more distal bronchi and bronchioles (Fig. 10-2). When tumors or aspiration of a foreign body lead to bronchiectasis, the pathologic changes may be sharply localized to a single segment of the

lungs. The airways are significantly dilatated (sometimes up to 4 times normal size). According to shape, bronchiectasis can be divided into the following categories:
- Cylindroid bronchiectasis
- Fusiform bronchiectasis
- Saccular bronchiectasis

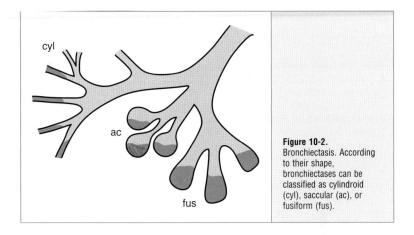

Figure 10-2.
Bronchiectasis. According to their shape, bronchiectases can be classified as cylindroid (cyl), saccular (ac), or fusiform (fus).

PNEUMONIA

35. **What is the difference between bronchopneumonia and lobar pneumonia?**
Bacterial pneumonia is characterized by exudative solidification (consolidation) of the pulmonary tissue, which is caused by bacterial invasion of the lung parenchyma. According to gross anatomic distribution, it can be classified into the following categories:
- Lobular pneumonia (bronchopneumonia) is a patchy consolidation of the lung (areas of acute suppurative inflammation). This infection is usually an extension of a preexisting bronchitis or bronchiolitis. It tends to occur more frequently in infancy and old age. The consolidation is more often multilobar and frequently bilateral and basal.
- Lobar pneumonia is an acute bacterial infection involving a large portion of one lobe or an entire lobe. It is infrequent today because of the effectiveness with which antibiotics abort these infections and prevent the development of full-blown lobar consolidation.

36. **List the defense mechanisms that protect the lung against bacterial infection**
- Nasal clearance (sneezing, blowing, and swallowing)
- Tracheobronchial clearance (mucociliary action)
- Alveolar clearance (alveolar macrophages)
  Whenever these defense mechanisms are impaired or whenever the resistance of the host is generally lowered (chronic disease, immunologic deficiency, treatment with immunosuppressive agents, leukopenia, and unusually virulent infections), the end result may be pneumonia.

37. **Which agents most commonly cause bacterial pneumonia?**
Bronchopneumonia is caused by staphylococci, streptococci, pneumococci, *Haemophilus influenzae, Pseudomonas aeruginosa,* and the coliform bacteria.
  Lobar pneumonia is most frequently (90%–95%) caused by pneumococci (*Streptococcus pneumoniae*).

KEY POINTS: PNEUMONIA ✔

1. Pneumonia is most often caused by infections and is most often localized to a lobule (lobular bronchopneumonia) rather than involving the entire lobe of the lung (lobar).

2. Acute pneumonias are caused by viruses and bacteria, whereas chronic pneumonia is a feature of tuberculosis or fungal infections.

38. **Name the four classical stages of lobar pneumonia.**
    - Congestion is characterized by heavy, boggy, and red lung. Histologic characteristics are vascular engorgement, intraalveolar fluid with few neutrophils, and often the presence of numerous bacteria.
    - Red hepatization is characterized by consolidation of the airspaces of the lungs. On cross-section the lungs appear brown-red, firm, and airless, and they resemble the liver. Histologically, the alveolar capillaries are congested, and the alveolar spaces are filled with erythrocytes, neutrophils, and fibrin.
    - Gray hepatization is characterized by persistent consolidation. The exudate inside the alveoli compresses the capillaries and reduces the pulmonary blood flow. On cross-section the lung parenchyma appears airless, consolidated and pale, and grayish-yellow. Histologically, the alveoli are filled with a fibrinopurulent exudate, and the capillaries in the alveolar walls appear compressed and contain less blood than in the previous stage.
    - Resolution is the final stage, characterized by granular, semifluid debris that is resorbed, ingested by macrophages, or coughed up.

39. **List the most important complications of bacterial pneumonia.**
    - **Pleuritis:** It is so common that some authorities consider it a feature of pneumonia and not a separate complication.
    - **Abscess:** It results from the lytic action of neutrophils and is most often found in pneumonia caused by *Staphylococcus aureus*.
    - **Empyema:** Intrapleural fibrinosuppurative reaction.
    - **Chronic pneumonia:** Caused by organization of exudate and persistence of infection.
    - **Bacteremia with hematogenous dissemination:** May cause metastatic abscesses, endocarditis, meningitis, or suppurative arthritis.

40. **What are the clinical features of bacterial pneumonia?**
    - The major symptoms of pneumonia include malaise, fever, and cough productive of sputum. If fibrinosuppurative pleuritis develops, it manifests with pleuritic pain and pleural friction rub.
    - The typical radiologic appearance of lobar pneumonia is that of a radiopaque infiltrate involving the entire lobe. Bronchopneumonia shows focal opacities.
    - The identification of the causative microorganism and the subsequent determination of its antibiotic sensitivity are the keystones to appropriate therapy. The clinical findings are dramatically modified by the administration of antibiotics.

41. **What is primary atypical pneumonia, and what are its most common causes?**
    Primary atypical pneumonia is an acute febrile respiratory disease characterized by patchy inflammatory changes in the lungs, largely confined to the alveolar septa and pulmonary

interstitium. The term *atypical* emphasizes the lack of alveolar exudates, although a much more accurate designation is interstitial pneumonitis.

The most common etiologic agent is *Mycoplasma pneumoniae*. Other etiologic agents are viruses, *Chlamydia* spp., and *Coxiella burneti* (Q-fever). In many cases, the cause cannot be identified.

42. **What are the most frequent conditions that predispose to the formation of pulmonary abscess?**

Pulmonary abscess is a local suppurative process within the lung characterized by necrosis of lung tissue. The causative organisms (e.g., aerobic and anaerobic streptococci, *S. aureus,* and gram-negative organisms) are introduced by the following mechanisms:

- Aspiration of infective material is the most common cause, particularly in conditions in which the cough reflexes are depressed (e.g., acute alcoholism, coma, anesthesia, sinusitis, gingivodental sepsis, and debilitation)
- Antecedent primary bacterial infection of the lungs
- Septic embolism
- Neoplasia (postobstructive pneumonia)
- Direct traumatic penetration of the lungs, spread of infections from a neighboring organ, and hematogenous seeding of the lung by pyogenic organisms

43. **Discuss the main pathologic characteristics of primary tuberculosis.**

The lungs are the usual location of primary infection with *M. tuberculosis* (Fig. 10-3). Most frequently, disease is a result of inhaling infected aerosols produced by coughing on the part of a person with cavitary tuberculosis. The initial focus of primary infection, called the Ghon complex, consists of:

- A parenchymal subpleural lesion, usually just above or just below the interlobar fissure
- Enlarged lymph nodes (often caseous) draining the parenchymal focus

Most frequently, patients with this initial infection are asymptomatic, and the lesions undergo fibrosis and calcification. In some instances, self-limited extension to the pleura with secondary pleural effusion occurs. Less commonly, progressive spread with cavitation, tuberculous bronchopneumonia, or miliary tuberculosis may follow a primary infection.

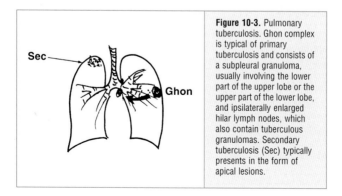

Figure 10-3. Pulmonary tuberculosis. Ghon complex is typical of primary tuberculosis and consists of a subpleural granuloma, usually involving the lower part of the upper lobe or the upper part of the lower lobe, and ipsilaterally enlarged hilar lymph nodes, which also contain tuberculous granulomas. Secondary tuberculosis (Sec) typically presents in the form of apical lesions.

44. **What are the main pathologic characteristics of secondary (reactivation) pulmonary tuberculosis?**

Secondary pulmonary tuberculosis in most cases represents reactivation of an old, possibly subclinical infection and tends to produce more damage to the lungs than does primary tuberculosis. The lesion is located in sites with high oxygen tension, particularly in the lung apices. A diffuse, fibrotic, poorly defined lesion develops, with focal areas of caseous necrosis. Most commonly, these foci heal and calcify, but some erode into a bronchus, after which drainage of infectious material creates a tuberculous cavity. A yellow grayish caseous material fills the cavity, which is more or less surrounded by fibrous tissue. The most important complications of secondary tuberculosis are:

- Miliary tuberculosis in the lungs due to hematogenous dissemination
- Hematogenous miliary spread to other internal organs
- Spread of infection through expectorated sputum (laryngitis); sputum may be swallowed, resulting in gastrointestinal (GI) infection

45. **Define miliary tuberculosis and tuberculous bronchopneumonia.**

Miliary tuberculosis refers to the presence of multiple, small tuberculous granulomas in many organs, which result from the hematogenous dissemination of bacteria. Favored targets for miliary seeding are the bone marrow, liver, spleen, kidney, and retina.

Highly susceptible, highly sensitized individuals may exhibit the spread of the tuberculous infection that rapidly involves large areas of lung parenchyma and produces diffuse bronchopneumonia or lobar exudative consolidation (galloping consumption).

46. **Which histologic and laboratory methods are useful in diagnosis of tuberculosis?**

If tuberculosis is suspected in certain tissue changes, the diagnosis is confirmed by histologic staining, smears, and cultures of acid-fast organisms.

Mycobacterium tuberculosis can be demonstrated in the early exudative and caseous phases, but it is usually impossible to find the bacteria in the late fibrocalcific stages. Lesions with sparse organisms can be highly infective, and their absence in histologic sections cannot be assumed as a sign of total microbial destruction.

Histologically, granulomas are composed of epithelioid cells surrounded by a zone of fibroblasts, lymphocytes, and Langhans giant cells. Some necrosis (caseation) is usually present in the centers of these tubercles.

INTERSTITIAL LUNG DISEASES

47. **Describe the main pathologic characteristics of diffuse interstitial (infiltrative and restrictive) diseases of the lung.**

Diffuse interstitial diseases are a heterogeneous group of diseases that share diffuse and usually chronic changes of the pulmonary connective tissue, principally the interstitium in the alveolar walls. The clinical and pulmonary functional changes are usually those of restrictive lung disease. Patients experience dyspnea, tachypnea, and eventual cyanosis, without wheezing or other evidence of airway obstruction. In time, secondary pulmonary hypertension and right-sided heart failure with cor pulmonale occasionally develop. The entities can be distinguished in the early stages, but the advanced forms are difficult to differentiate because the result is always scarring and gross destruction of the lung, often referred to as end-stage lung or honeycomb lung.

48. **How can diffuse interstitial diseases be classified according to etiology?**

- Known etiology
  - Environmental agents—asbestos, silica, and beryllium (25% of all cases)
  - Ionizing radiation

- ○ Following ARDS
- ○ Hypersensitivity pneumonitis
- Unknown etiology
  - ○ Collagen vascular diseases (10%)
  - ○ Sarcoidosis (20%)
  - ○ Idiopathic pulmonary fibrosis (15%)
  - ○ Wegener granulomatosis

49. **What are the morphologic manifestations of diffuse interstitial diseases of the lung?**

Regardless of the type of interstitial disease or specific cause, the earliest common manifestation of most of the interstitial diseases is alveolitis—accumulation of inflammatory macrophages, lymphocytes, neutrophils, eosinophils, and immune effector cells within the alveolar walls and spaces. The accumulation of leukocytes distorts the normal alveolar structures and results in the release of mediators that can injure parenchymal cells and stimulate fibrosis. The consequence is an end-stage fibrotic lung in which the alveoli are replaced by cystic spaces, with thick bands of connective tissue infiltrated by inflammatory cells. In diseases such as sarcoidosis, cell-mediated immune reactions cause the accumulation of monocytes and T cells as well as the formation of granulomas.

KEY POINTS: INTERSTITIAL LUNG DISEASES ✓

1. Interstitial lung diseases are caused by inhaled substances from the environment or have an unknown etiology.

2. Pneumoconioses result from exposure to inorganic dust particles and include diseases such as coal workers lung disease, silicosis, and asbestosis.

3. Sarcoidosis is the most common interstitial lung disease of unknown etiology, presenting with granulomas in lungs and mediastinal lymph nodes.

50. **List the main pneumoconioses.**

In the past, the pneumoconioses were defined as pulmonary diseases caused by the inhalation of inorganic dusts. Currently, the use of the term pneumoconiosis is broadened to include diseases induced by organic as well as inorganic particulates and chemical fumes and vapors. The major categories of pneumoconioses are:

- Anthracosis (coal dust)
- Silicosis (silica)
- Asbestosis (asbestos)
- Berylliosis (beryllium)
- Siderosis (iron dust)
- Stannosis (tin dust)
- Baritosis (barium dust)
- Talcosis (talc dust)

51. **Which factors are associated with the development of pneumoconioses?**

- The amount of dust accumulated in the lung and airways
- The size, shape, and buoyancy of the particles (the diameter of most dangerous particles is 1–5 mm)
- Solubility and physiochemical reactivity of the particles
- Additional effects of other irritants (e.g., concomitant tobacco smoking)

52. **How is pneumoconiosis of coal workers classified according to lung findings?**
    - Asymptomatic anthracosis, in which pigment accumulates, without a perceptible cellular reaction, in the connective tissue along the lymphatics or in organized lymphoid tissue along the bronchi or in the lung hilus.
    - Simple pneumoconiosis of coal workers is characterized by coal macules (1–2 mm in diameter) and the somewhat larger coal nodules with little to no pulmonary dysfunction.
    - Complicated pneumoconiosis of coal workers, or progressive massive fibrosis, is characterized by compromised lung function, which is caused by extensive fibrosis and intensely blackened scars larger than 2 cm.

53. **What is Caplan syndrome?**
    Caplan syndrome represents the coexistence of rheumatoid arthritis with pneumoconiosis of coal workers, asbestosis, or silicosis. The syndrome is characterized by formation of distinctive nodular lesions, with a central necrosis surrounded by fibroblasts, macrophages, and collagen.

54. **How does pneumoconiosis of coal workers present?**
    Pneumoconiosis of coal workers is usually a benign disease with little abnormality of lung function. Only rarely does progressive massive fibrosis develop, leading to increasing pulmonary dysfunction, pulmonary hypertension, and cor pulmonale.

55. **Describe the main characteristics of silicosis.**
    Silicosis is the most prevalent chronic occupational lung disease in the world and is caused by inhalation of crystalline silicon dioxide (silica). It is more common in mine workers and workers employed in sandblasting. It is characterized by the insidious development of fibrotic pulmonary nodules (simple nodular silicosis) containing quartz crystals in the upper zones of the lungs. As the disease progresses, these nodules may coalesce into hard collagenous scars (progressive massive fibrosis), and sometimes a honeycomb pattern develops. The disease may be asymptomatic for prolonged periods or cause only mild to moderate dyspnea. Heavy exposure over months to a few years occasionally results in acute silicosis. This lesion is characterized by the generalized accumulation of a lipoproteinaceous material within alveoli.

56. **What are the main consequences of occupational exposure to asbestos?**
    - Localized fibrous plaques or, rarely, diffuse pleural fibrosis
    - Pleural effusion
    - Parenchymal interstitial fibrosis (asbestosis)
    - Bronchogenic carcinoma
    - Mesothelioma

57. **Define asbestos bodies and pleural plaques.**
    Asbestosis is marked by diffuse pulmonary interstitial fibrosis, which starts in the lower lobes and subpleurally. These findings are indistinguishable from those resulting from other causes of diffuse interstitial fibrosis, except for the presence of asbestos bodies. Asbestos bodies stain golden brown, assuming the shape of fusiform or beaded rods with a translucent center. They represent asbestos fibers coated with an iron-containing proteinaceous material.

    Pleural plaques are the most common feature of asbestos exposure. They appear as well-circumscribed plaques of dense collagen, often containing calcium. Pleural plaques are usually found on the anterior and posterolateral aspects of the parietal pleura and over the domes of the diaphragm. They do not contain asbestos bodies.

58. **Which organs are most frequently involved in sarcoidosis?**
Sarcoidosis is a systemic disease of unknown cause that presents with noncaseating granulomas in many tissues and organs. Bilateral lymphadenopathy (specifically, hilar and mediastinal nodes) or lung involvement is diagnosed in 90% of cases, followed by eye and skin lesions. The spleen, liver, and bone marrow are also frequently involved. Bilateral sarcoidosis of the parotid, submaxillary, and sublingual glands is the feature of the combined uveoparotid involvement designated as Mikulicz syndrome. Sarcoid granulomas can appear in the heart, kidney, central nervous system, and endocrine glands as well.

59. **How is the diagnosis of sarcoidosis established?**
Because mycobacterial, fungal infections, and berylliosis can also produce noncaseating granulomas, the histologic diagnosis of sarcoidosis is made by exclusion.

60. **Discuss the most frequent clinical symptoms in patients with sarcoidosis.**
In the majority of cases, patients have respiratory abnormalities (shortness of breath, cough, chest pain, and hemoptysis) or constitutional signs and symptoms (fever, fatigue, weight loss, anorexia, and night sweats). Sometimes, sarcoidosis may be discovered because of peripheral lymphadenopathy, cutaneous lesions, eye involvement, splenomegaly, or hepatomegaly.

61. **What is the clinical course of sarcoidosis?**
  - Complete recovery (65%–70%)
  - Permanent injury resulting in partial loss of lung function (20%)
  - Progressive lung disease (10%), lethal because of progressive pulmonary fibrosis and resultant cor pulmonale.

62. **Describe the difference between usual interstitial pneumonia (UIP) and desquamative interstitial pneumonia (DIP).**
  - UIP (synonyms are idiopathic pulmonary fibrosis, Hamman–Rich syndrome, and idiopathic fibrosing alveolitis) is a pulmonary disease of unknown etiology characterized clinically by severe hypoxemia and cyanosis. The hallmark is the presence of chronic inflammation in the interstitial spaces. There is also widespread fibrosis of alveolar septa. Because the end stage of the disease (honeycomb lung) occurs in many disorders, it is necessary to exclude the known causes of interstitial fibrosis. Average survival is less than 5 years.
  - DIP is characterized by interstitial inflammation and a striking accumulation of macrophages in the alveoli, originally thought to be desquamated epithelial cells from the alveolar walls. Patients with this disorder usually present with slow development of cough and dyspnea. Steroid therapy is successful in most patients, often leading to clearing of the lungs. A minority of patients have or subsequently develop significant interstitial fibrosis.

63. **Define hypersensitivity pneumonitis.**
Hypersensitivity pneumonitis refers to a group of immunologically mediated conditions caused by intense, often prolonged exposure to organic dusts. It is important to recognize these diseases early because progression to chronic fibrotic lung disease can be prevented by removal of the environmental agent. Histologic alterations include:
  - Interstitial pneumonitis
  - Interstitial fibrosis

- Obliterative bronchiolitis
- Granuloma formation

Examples of hypersensitivity pneumonitis include:
- Farmer's lung
- Pigeon breeder's lung
- Humidifier or air-conditioner lung
- Mushroom picker's lung
- Byssinosis (in textile workers)

64. **Which diseases belong to pulmonary hemorrhage syndromes?**
   - Goodpasture's syndrome is characterized by the simultaneous appearance of proliferative, usually rapidly progressive glomerulonephritis and necrotizing hemorrhagic interstitial pneumonitis. Both the lung hemorrhage and the glomerulonephritis improve with intensive plasma exchange. Otherwise, the prognosis is unfavorable.
   - Idiopathic pulmonary hemosiderosis.
   - Vasculitis-associated hemorrhage (hypersensitivity angiitis, Wegener's granulomatosis, and lupus erythematosus).

65. **List the most common therapy-related pulmonary complications.**
   - Drug-induced lung disease
     - Drugs—can cause bronchospasm, pulmonary edema, chronic pneumonitis with fibrosis, and hypersensitivity pneumonitis
   - Radiation-induced lung disease
     - Acute radiation pneumonitis, morphologically characterized by diffuse alveolar damage
     - Chronic radiation pneumonitis, characterized by interstitial fibrosis
   - Lung transplantation may cause two major complications:
     - Pulmonary infections
     - Acute or chronic rejection

TUMORS

66. **What are the main characteristics of bronchogenic carcinomas?**
   - The vast majority (90%–95%) of lung cancers are bronchogenic carcinomas. Others are bronchial carcinoids, mesenchymal, and other miscellaneous neoplasms. The term *bronchogenic* refers to the origin of the bronchial (and sometimes bronchiolar) epithelium.
   - It is the second most frequent malignancy in Western countries.
   - It is the most frequent fatal malignancy.
   - It occurs most often between ages 40 and 70 years, with a peak incidence in the 50s and 60s.

67. **Which etiologic agents have been known to promote lung cancers?**
   - Tobacco smoking
     - An invariable statistical association between the frequency of lung cancer and the amount of daily smoking, the tendency to inhale, and the duration of the smoking habit is well documented.
     - Eighty percent of lung cancers occur in smokers.
   - Industrial hazards
     - All types of radiation may be carcinogenic, such as an atomic bomb blast and uranium (particularly in smokers).
     - The risk is increased with exposure to asbestos (particularly in smokers) and among people who work with nickel, chromates, coal, mustard gas, arsenic, beryllium, and iron, as well as newspaper workers and African gold miners.

- Air pollution
  - ○ Radon

68. **List the main histologic types of bronchogenic carcinomas.**
    - **Squamous cell (epidermoid) carcinoma:** Composed of groups of squamous cells, often with central keratinization.
    - **Adenocarcinoma:** Composed of glands lined by mucin producing columnar cells. A variant of peripheral adenocarcinoma lining the alveolar spaces is called bronchioloalveolar carcinoma.
    - **Small cell carcinoma:** Composed of "small blue cells" that have some neuroendocrine feature, recognizable by electron microscopy or immunohistochemistry (e.g., staining with antibodies to chromogranin or synaptophysin).
    - **Large cell carcinoma:** Composed of anaplastic undifferentiated cells growing without any distinct pattern.

KEY POINTS: TUMORS ✔

1. Lung tumors are the most common cancer-related cause of death in the United States.

2. Most lung tumors originate from bronchial epithelium and are related to cigarette smoking.

3. Lung tumors occur in several histologic forms, but all have a poor prognosis.

69. **How are lung cancers divided according to their response to chemotherapy?**
    For clinical purposes lung cancers are divided into two groups: small cell carcinoma and non–small cell carcinoma, including squamous cell carcinoma, adenocarcinoma, and large cell carcinoma.
    - Small cell carcinomas show an excellent initial response to chemotherapy.
    - Non–small cell carcinomas are less responsive to chemotherapy and are treated surgically plus radiation

70. **Which types of carcinomas are most closely related to smoking?**
    - Squamous cell carcinoma in the central (hilar) location
    - Small cell carcinoma (only 1% of cases occur in nonsmokers) of main bronchi

71. **In which parts of the lung do most of the bronchogenic carcinomas arise?**
    Bronchogenic carcinomas usually arise in and about the hilus of the lung. The minority of primary carcinomas arise in the periphery of the lung parenchyma, originating from bronchioles.

72. **Describe the most common pathways of lung cancer spread.**
    Extension to the pleural surface is common, sometimes followed by dissemination to the pleural cavity or into the pericardium (Fig. 10-4). Most patients experience spread to the tracheal, bronchial, and mediastinal lymph nodes. The frequency of nodal involvement is greater than 50%. Distant spread of bronchogenic carcinoma results from both lymphatic and hematogenous dissemination. The most common sites of metastases are adrenals, liver, brain, and bones.

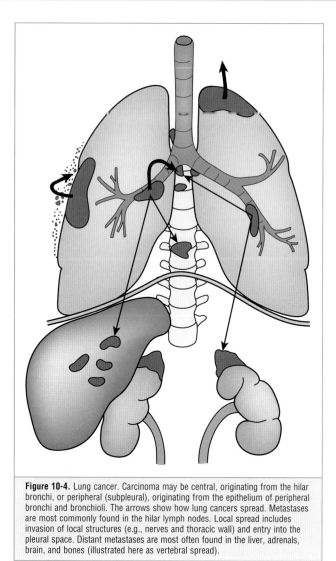

Figure 10-4. Lung cancer. Carcinoma may be central, originating from the hilar bronchi, or peripheral (subpleural), originating from the epithelium of peripheral bronchi and bronchioli. The arrows show how lung cancers spread. Metastases are most commonly found in the hilar lymph nodes. Local spread includes invasion of local structures (e.g., nerves and thoracic wall) and entry into the pleural space. Distant metastases are most often found in the liver, adrenals, brain, and bones (illustrated here as vertebral spread).

73. **How does lung carcinoma present clinically, and how is it diagnosed?**
   - Peak age at the time of diagnosis is 50 to 60 years.
   - The major symptoms are cough (average duration 7 months), weight loss, chest pain, and dyspnea.
   - There are x-ray findings of a tumor mass in the lung.
   - Cytologic diagnosis: expectorated sputum of these patients, or they can be obtained with fine needle aspiration.
   - Biopsy is essential for diagnosis. It may be obtained by bronchoscopy, transthoracic needle biopsy, or surgically.

74. **What are the most common local effects and complications of lung cancer?**
The most common local effects of lung tumor spread are:
- Pneumonia, abscess, and lobar collapse due to the obstruction of the bronchus
- Lipid pneumonia
- Pleural effusion
- Hoarseness (recurrent laryngeal nerve invasion by tumor in the apical portion of the lung)
- Dysphagia (esophageal invasion)
- Diaphragm paralysis (phrenic nerve invasion)
- Rib destruction (chest wall invasion)
- Superior vena cava syndrome (venous congestion, dusky head and arm edema, and circulatory compromise)
- Horner syndrome (enophthalmos, ptosis, miosis, and anhidrosis)
- Pericarditis and tamponade

75. **What is the treatment and prognosis of lung cancer?**
- The overall 5-year survival rate for all lung cancers is approximately 10%.
- Peripheral adenocarcinomas tend to remain localized longer and have a slightly better prognosis than centrally located cancers of other histologic types.
- Surgical resection of small cell carcinoma is so ineffective that the diagnosis essentially precludes surgery. Most patients have distant metastases on diagnosis. This cancer is particularly sensitive to radiation and chemotherapy, but even with treatment, mean survival after diagnosis is approximately 1 year.
- In the rare localized solitary tumors less than 4 cm in diameter, surgical resection results in a 5-year survival rate of up to 40% for patients with squamous cell carcinoma. The same procedure results in a 5-year survival rate of 30% for patients with adenocarcinoma and large cell carcinoma.

76. **What are the most frequent paraneoplastic syndromes in patients with lung cancer?**
Bronchogenic carcinoma can be associated with a number of paraneoplastic syndromes. These syndromes, often caused by tumor-derived hormones (given in parentheses), include:
- Hyponatremia (antidiuretic hormone [ADH])
- Cushing syndrome (adrenocorticotropic hormone [ACTH])
- Hypercalcemia (parathormone and parathyroid hormone–related peptide)
- Hypocalcemia (calcitonin)
- Gynecomastia (gonadotropins)
- Carcinoid syndrome (serotonin)
- Lambert–Eaton myasthenic syndrome
- Peripheral neuropathy
- Dermatologic abnormalities, including acanthosis nigricans
- Hematologic abnormalities, such as leukemoid reactions
- Hypertrophic pulmonary osteoarthropathy with clubbing of the fingers

The incidence of clinically significant syndromes related to these hormones or hormone-like factors ranges from 1% to 10%. Tumors producing ACTH and ADH are predominantly small cell carcinomas, whereas those producing hypercalcemia are mostly squamous cell tumors. The carcinoid syndrome is associated rarely with small cell carcinoma but is more common with the bronchial carcinoids.

77. **What are the main clinical and pathologic characteristics of bronchial carcinoids?**
Carcinoids are low-grade malignant tumors composed of well-differentiated neuroendocrine cells.
- **Macroscopic findings:** Most tumors are usually small (3–4 cm in diameter) and found in the wall of bronchi. They may grow into the bronchial lumen and protrude as spherical polypoid masses covered by mucosa.

- **Microscopic findings:** Tumors are composed of nests, cords, and masses of cells, separated by a scant fibrous stroma. The individual cells are usually quite regular, with uniform round nuclei, and show infrequent mitosis. Tumor cells show neuroendocrine differentiation and are thus considered to be low-grade equivalents of small cell lung carcinoma.
- **Epidemiology:** Most patients are younger than 40 years. Unrelated to cigarette smoking.
- **Biology of tumor:** Tumors may secrete hormonally active polypeptides and cause the carcinoid syndrome. It is characterized by intermittent attacks of diarrhea, flushing, and cyanosis
- **Tumor growth and metastasis:** Many tumors have infiltrative growth or spread to local lymph nodes at the time of resection. This local spread has no adverse effect on postsurgery prognosis. Distant metastases occur rarely, but such cases have less favorable prognosis.
- **Survival rate:** Following surgical resection, it is greater than 90%.

78. **List the usual features of metastatic tumors in the lungs.**
    Usually, multiple discrete nodules are scattered throughout all lobes, mostly on the periphery of the lung parenchyma (primary bronchogenic carcinoma tends to occur in the central locations as solitary lesions).
    Alternatively, metastatic growth may be confined to peribronchiolar and perivascular tissue spaces, where lung septa and connective tissue are diffusely infiltrated with the gray-white tumor.
    The tumor cells may form multiple emboli or remain in the pulmonary vessels, permeate the pulmonary lymphatics (lymphangitis carcinomatosa), or both. Such tumors may not be visible radiologically and are diagnosed only on histologic examination.

PLEURAL DISEASES

79. **What is the pathogenesis of pleural effusion?**
    Several pathogenetic mechanisms may be responsible for pleural effusion:
    - Increased hydrostatic pressure, as in congestive heart failure
    - Increased vascular permeability, as in pneumonia
    - Decreased oncotic pressure, as in nephrotic syndrome
    - Increased intrapleural negative pressure, as in atelectasis
    - Decreased lymphatic drainage, as in mediastinal carcinomatosis

80. **What are the main forms of pleuritis?**
    - Serofibrinous pleuritis may be caused by tuberculosis, pneumonia, lung infarcts, lung abscess, bronchiectasis, rheumatoid arthritis, disseminated lupus erythematosus, uremia, diffuse systemic infections, other systemic disorders, metastatic involvement of the pleura, or radiation.
    - Suppurative pleuritis (empyema) usually results from bacterial or mycotic seeding of the pleural space.
    - Hemorrhagic pleuritis is manifested by sanguineous inflammatory exudates, and it is found in hemorrhagic diathesis, rickettsial diseases, and neoplastic involvement of the pleural cavity.

81. **What are the main types of noninflammatory pleural effusions?**
    - Hydrothorax is a noninflammatory collection of serous fluid within the pleural cavities. The effusion is clear and straw colored. Hydrothorax is unilateral or bilateral. The most common cause of hydrothorax is cardiac failure, but it is also frequently the result of renal failure and cirrhosis of the liver.
    - Hemothorax represents escape of blood into the pleural cavity and may represent a fatal complication of a ruptured aortic aneurysm or vascular trauma.
    - Chylothorax is an accumulation of milky fluid (lymphatic in origin) within the pleural cavity. It is generally caused by thoracic duct trauma or obstruction, resulting in rupture of major lymphatic ducts. Most frequently, it is caused by malignant conditions in the mediastinum.

KEY POINTS: PLEURA ✔

1. The main pleural diseases include hydrothorax related to circulatory disturbances; pleuritis, an inflammatory disease; and tumors.

2. Pleural tumors include primary neoplasms, such as mesotheliomas, and more often metastases from tumors of the lungs or other organs.

82. **What is pleural empyema?**
Empyema represents a collection of pus that may be yellow-green, creamy, or semifluid. Histologically, it is composed of dead and dying neutrophils, proteinaceous material, and cell debris. Empyema sometimes resolves, but this outcome is less common than organization of the exudate. In that case, the formation of dense, tough fibrous adhesions occurs and frequently obliterates the pleural space or envelops the lungs.

83. **Describe the main types of pneumothorax.**
Pneumothorax refers to accumulation of air or gas in the pleural cavity and is classified as follows:
- Spontaneous pneumothorax is a possible complication of any form of pulmonary disease that causes rupture of an alveolus, such as the following:
  - Emphysema
  - Asthma
  - Tuberculosis
- Traumatic pneumothorax is usually caused by some perforating injury to the chest wall.
- Therapeutic pneumothorax was once commonly used in the treatment of tuberculosis.
Pneumothorax may cause compression, collapse, and atelectasis of the lung and may be responsible for marked respiratory distress.

84. **What are the most frequent pleural tumors?**
Secondary metastatic tumors are far more common than primary tumors. Primary pleural tumors are rare and include a benign tumor called solitary fibrous tumor and malignant mesothelioma.

85. **Which etiologic agents are associated with malignant mesothelioma?**
The incidence of malignant mesothelioma is increased after long exposure to asbestos in the work place. A period of 25 to 45 years is sometimes necessary for the development of asbestos-related mesothelioma. Smoking does not increase the risk of mesothelioma in asbestos workers, in contrast to the 50 to 60 times higher risk for bronchogenic carcinoma in smoking asbestos workers.

86. **What are the morphologic characteristics of malignant mesothelioma?**
- Malignant mesothelioma is a diffuse lesion that spreads widely in the pleural space. Extensive pleural effusion and direct invasion of thoracic structures usually accompany this tumor. The affected lung is surrounded by a thick layer of soft, gelatinous, grayish-pink neoplasm.
- Microscopically, malignant mesotheliomas may be divided into three histologic subtypes:
  - Sarcomatoid type-composed of spindle cells
  - Epithelial type-composed of cuboidal cells lining gland like or tubular spaces
  - Mixed type-composed of epithelial and sarcomatous cells

87. **What is the clinical course of disease in patients with malignant mesothelioma?**
   - The most frequent symptoms are chest pain, dyspnea, and pleural effusions.
   - The lung is invaded directly, and there is often metastatic spread to the hilar lymph nodes and eventually to the liver and other distant organs.
   - Half of those with pleural disease die within 12 months of diagnosis, and few survive longer than 2 years.
   - Aggressive therapy (extrapleural pneumonectomy, chemotherapy, and radiation therapy) appears to improve this poor prognosis in some patients.

WEGSITES

1. http://www.nlm.nih.gov/medlineplus/lungdiseases.html
2. http://www-medlib.med.utah.edu/WebPath/webpath.html#MENU
3. http://www.emedicine.com
4. http://www.pathologyoutlines.com/lung.html
5. http://www.pathologyoutlines.com/lungtumor.html
6. http://www.pathologyoutlines.com/mediastinum.html
7. http://www.cancer.gov/cancertopics/types/lung

BIBLIOGRAPHY

1. Bush A, Thomson AH: Acute bronchiolitis. BMJ 335:1037–1041, 2007.
2. Chroneou A, Zias N, Beamis JF Jr, Craven DE: Healthcare-associated pneumonia: principles and emerging concepts on management. Expert Opin Pharmacother 8:3117–3131, 2007.
3. Goldhaber SZ: Pulmonary embolism. N Engl J Med 339:93–104, 1998.
4. Gonzales R, Sande MA: Uncomplicated acute bronchitis. Ann Intern Med 133:981–991, 2000.
5. Hasleton PS, Roberts TE: Review: adult respiratory distress syndrome—an update. Histopathology 34:285–294, 1999.
6. Hill A, Gompertz S, Stockley R: Factors influencing airway inflammation in chronic obstructive pulmonary disease. Thorax 55:970–977, 2000.
7. Hirsch FR, Franklin WA, Gazdar AF, Bunn PA Jr: Early detection of lung cancer: clinical perspectives of recent advances in biology and radiology. Clin Cancer Res 7:5–22, 2001.
8. Leslie KO, Colby TV: Pathology of lung cancer. Curr Opin Pulmonary Med 3:252–256, 1997.
9. Mauad T, Dolhnikoff M: Pathologic similarities and differences between asthma and chronic obstructive pulmonary disease. Curr Opin Pulm Med 14:31–38, 2008.
10. Peters-Golden M, Henderson WR Jr: Leukotrienes. N Engl J Med 357:1841–1854, 2007.
11. Steinert HC. Lung cancer. Recent Results Cancer Res 170:81–92, 2008.
12. Ware LB, Matthay MA: The acute respiratory distress syndrome. N Engl J Med 342:1334–1349, 2000.
13. Wistuba II, Gazdar AF: Lung cancer preneoplasia. Annu Rev Pathol 1:331–348, 2006.

CHAPTER 11

HEAD AND NECK

Ivan Damjanov, MD, PhD, and Anamarija Morović, MD

1. **What are the normal structures included in the category of "head and neck?"**
   Head and neck is the colloquial term used for the face and underlying structures of the upper respiratory and alimentary tracts, the ears, and the neck organs. The diseases of this area are usually treated by dentists and oral surgeons and otorhinolaryngologists (ear, nose, and throat specialists).

2. **What are the main diseases of the head and neck?**
   - Dental disease, including caries and periodontal disease
   - Infections of the mouth, salivary glands, nose, throat, and inner ear
   - Tumors

INFLAMMATORY LESIONS

3. **What is caries?**
   Caries is a dental disease characterized by decay of enamel and dentin caused by bacteria. The most important pathogen is the acid-producing *Streptococcus mutans*, which thrives in saliva that contains residual sugar from the food. The attachment of bacteria to teeth is promoted by the formation of plaques (i.e., masses of calcified debris and desquamated epithelium that are seen on the surface of enamel).

4. **What are the complications of caries?**
   Destruction of enamel and dentin will allow the bacteria to enter the pulp and extend into the bone at the tip of the tooth (Fig. 11-1). Typical complications are as follows:
   - **Acute pulpitis:** Infection in the central cavity of the tooth is associated with pain.
   - **Apical abscess:** Bacteria extend from the pulp into the bone surrounding the root of the tooth. The pain is severe and usually throbbing. Pus may drain into the mouth along the lateral sides of the infected tooth.
   - **Periapical granuloma:** This term, a misnomer, is used to describe the granulation tissue that develops inside the healing periapical abscess.
   - **Radicular cyst:** If the pus from an abscess is resorbed, a cavity remains. This initial pseudocyst (no epithelial lining) may be partially covered by ingrowths of gingival epithelium.

5. **What is periodontitis?**
   Periodontitis is the inflammation of the periodontal recesses, involving the gingiva, periodontal membrane, and alveolar bone of the tooth socket. It may be associated with gingivitis, pyorrhea (pus oozing from the tooth socket), resorption of the peridental bone, and loosening and loss of teeth. Periodontal disease is the most common cause of tooth loss in the United States.

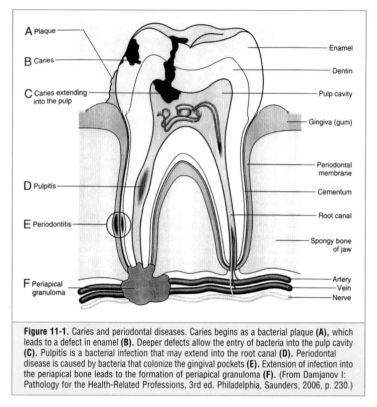

Figure 11-1. Caries and periodontal diseases. Caries begins as a bacterial plaque **(A)**, which leads to a defect in enamel **(B)**. Deeper defects allow the entry of bacteria into the pulp cavity **(C)**. Pulpitis is a bacterial infection that may extend into the root canal **(D)**. Periodontal disease is caused by bacteria that colonize the gingival pockets **(E)**. Extension of infection into the periapical bone leads to the formation of periapical granuloma **(F)**. (From Damjanov I: Pathology for the Health-Related Professions, 3rd ed. Philadelphia, Saunders, 2006, p. 230.)

6. **What is stomatitis?**
   Stomatitis is an inflammation of the mouth. It can be caused by infection or immunologic mechanisms. Infections are caused most often by viruses, bacteria, and fungi.

KEY POINTS: INFLAMMATORY LESIONS ✓

1. The main diseases of the head and neck are inflammatory diseases and tumors.

2. The most important diseases of the teeth and gingiva are caries and periodontitis.

3. Stomatitis, an infection of the mouth mucosa, can be caused by viruses, bacteria, and fungi.

4. Otitis media is an inflammation of the middle ear that may occur in an infectious and noninfectious form.

7. **List the most common infectious diseases affecting the mouth and oropharynx.**
   See Table 11-1.

TABLE 11-1. MOST COMMON INFECTIOUS DISEASES AFFECTING THE MOUTH AND OROPHARYNX
Disease/microbe
Lesion
Herpes simplex virus (HSV-1), herpes labialis (cold sores), ulcerative gingivostomatitis
Coxsackie A virus
Herpangina
Measles Koplik spots (around parotid duct orifice)
Infectious mononucleosis (Epstein–Barr virus)
Exudative pharyngitis with swollen lymph nodes, hairy leukoplakia in acquired immune deficiency disease
Strep throat (*Streptococcus pyogenes*)
Exudative pharyngitis/tonsillitis
Diphtheria (*Corynebacterium diphtheriae*)
Pseudomembranous pharyngitis
Candidiasis (*C. albicans*) thrush
Syphilis (*Treponema pallidum*)
Chancre of primary syphilis
Vincent angina (*Spirocheta vincenti*)
Gingivitis and pharyngitis and bleeding from the gingivae and Fusobacteria
Ludwig angina (multiple bacteria)
Spreading cellulitis of the throat
Aphthous stomatitis
Ulcers of unknown etiology

8. **Describe how herpes simplex virus (HSV) affects the mouth.**
HSV-1 infection often involves the mouth. Most often, it causes clusters of small vesicles on the lips (herpes labialis), but it may also cause widespread gingivostomatitis. Blisters tend to rupture and transform into ulcers, which form a crust and heal spontaneously.

9. **Why does herpes labialis recur?**
Following the initial HSV-1 infection, the virus migrates along the facial nerves into the trigeminal ganglion, where it may remain in a dormant form indefinitely. Various other infections and even stressful conditions may activate the virus in the trigeminal ganglion. Activated viruses migrate along the nerves into the labial mucosa or skin, and thus herpetic vesicles reappear. Most often, reactivation of HSV-1 occurs after the common cold, which is why the herpetic vesicles are often called cold sores or fever blisters.

10. **Define herpangina.**
Herpangina is an acute vesicoulcerative mucosal infection caused by Coxsackie A virus. It tends to occur in epidemics and affects small children. It begins in the form of vesiculopapular red lesions on the tonsils, soft palate, and uvula. These lesions are painful and ulcerate but heal spontaneously over a period of 2 to 5 days.

11. **What is aphthous stomatitis?**
Aphthae are shallow ulcers that occur on the oral mucosa. The cause of these lesions is not known, but in some people they tend to recur months or years after the initial occurrence. Minor aphthae (<5 mm) last a few days and heal without scarring. Major aphthae (>1 cm) may persist for longer periods and may evoke scarring. Aphthae tend to involve movable parts of the mouth (inner surface of the lips and buccal mucosa or the tongue), in contrast to herpetic infections, which also affect the gingivae.

12. **Define strep throat.**
Exudative pharyngitis and tonsillitis caused by *Streptococcus pyogenes* are colloquially called strep throat. Infection with group A β-hemolytic *S. pyogenes* accounts for less than one third of all conditions suspected clinically to be strep throat. The most common causes of exudative pharyngitis are viruses, which account for more than 50% of all such infections.

13. **Describe the features of strep throat.**
Infection with *S. pyogenes* is accompanied by fever, swelling of the neck, and pain on swallowing. The pharynx appears beefy red and moist, and a fibrinous grayish-yellow exudate appears on the tonsils. The cervical and submaxillary lymph nodes may become enlarged and painful. Definitive diagnosis depends on demonstrating streptococci in throat swab cultures. Antibodies to streptolysin O appear in the blood of 80% of reconvalescents after 2 weeks or later. It is important to follow the rise of the titer of these antibodies because they may be high from a previous infection.

14. **What is thrush?**
Thrush is the common name for oral infection caused by *Candida albicans*. It presents in the form of white pseudo-membranes covering the mucosal surface of the tongue, buccal mucosa, or anywhere else in the oropharynx. These mucosal plaques can be easily scraped away, revealing an inflamed oral mucosa.

15. **Who develops oral candidiasis?**
C. albicans is a common fungal saprophyte, found in approximately 40% of all healthy adults. Overgrowth of fungi is encountered in people suffering from diabetes, debilitating diseases, and immunodeficiency states and in cancer patients treated with cytotoxic drugs. Oral candidiasis is also encountered in some bottle-fed infants and older children treated with broad-spectrum antibiotics.

16. **List the oral manifestations of acquired immune deficiency syndrome (AIDS).**
    - Gingivitis (in the form of gingival erythema or necrotizing ulcerative periodontitis; a common early sign of AIDS)
    - Candidiasis
    - Persistent aphthous stomatitis
    - Hairy leukoplakia (Epstein–Barr virus [EBV] related lesion, typically located on the lateral sides of the tongue but sometimes occurring in the form of white plaques. May occur anywhere in the mouth.)
    - Kaposi sarcoma (Heroes virus 8–related vascular tumor. Red patches appear most often on the hard palate.)

17. **Which skin or systemic diseases may present with oral manifestations?**
Important vesiculobullous and ulcerating diseases include the following:
- Bullous pemphigoid (bullae with linear deposits of immunoglobulin G (IgG) along the basal membrane between the epithelium and the connective tissue)
- Pemphigus vulgaris (bullae with deposits of IgG along the cell membrane of epithelial cells)
- Erythema multiforme (complex hypersensitivity reaction to infectious agents and drugs presenting with bullae and "multiforme" lesions)
- Stevens–Johnson syndrome (severe erythema multiforme, often lethal)
- Lichen planus (T-cell-mediated hypersensitivity)

18. **List oral manifestations of some deficiency states.**
- Vitamin B_2: Angular cheilitis
- Vitamin B_{12}: Glossitis ("burning of the tongue")
- Vitamin C: Bleeding from gums
- Iron: Atrophic glossitis (Plummer–Vinson syndrome)

19. **What is sialadenitis?**
Sialadenitis is inflammation of the salivary glands. The parotid gland, the largest of all salivary glands, is most often affected. The inflammation can be acute or chronic. The salivary gland is typically enlarged and sensitive to palpation. Inflammation may affect the production of saliva and result in sialorrhea (excess of saliva) or xerostomia (dry mouth due to the cessation of salivation).

20. **What are the main causes of parotitis?**
Inflammation can be caused by viruses, bacteria, or immunologic mechanisms:
- **Viral parotitis:** The best-known cause of infectious parotitis in children is the mumps virus. Other viruses that can cause parotitis are parainfluenza and influenza virus, cytomegalovirus, EBV, and human immunodeficiency virus.
- **Suppurative parotitis:** Ascending bacterial infection through the parotid duct occurs in elderly people who have dry mouth from debilitating diseases, poor oral hygiene, drugs (anticholinergic drugs stop salivation), and following general anesthesia. The most common cause is *Staphylococcus aureus*.
- **Autoimmune parotitis:** Salivary and lacrimal glands are involved in Sjögren syndrome. This autoimmune disease may occur in a primary form involving only the salivary and lacrimal glands or in a secondary form, in the course of another autoimmune disease such as systemic lupus erythematosus.

21. **What is Mikulicz syndrome?**
The term Mikulicz syndrome is used in clinics to describe chronic painful swelling of salivary and lacrimal glands. It may be a manifestation of Sjögren syndrome or another autoimmune disease, sarcoidosis, or tuberculosis. Biopsy must be performed to determine the exact cause of chronic salivary and lacrimal gland swelling and to exclude an underlying lymphoma or tumor.

22. **What are the most common causes of rhinitis?**
Rhinitis (i.e., inflammation of the nasal mucosa) may be caused by infections or allergies.
- Acute infectious rhinitis is most often caused by viruses and is a typical manifestation of the common cold.
- Allergic rhinitis is usually chronic and is a typical feature of hay fever (i.e., allergy to pollen and other airborne allergens).

23. **What are the most common causes of sinusitis?**
Typically sinusitis is a consequence of bacterial superinfection that follows other upper respiratory tract inflammatory diseases. It is most often caused by *Streptococcus pneumoniae*

and other streptococci, as well as *Haemophilus influenzae*. Most often, it is a suppurative infection: Pus accumulates in the sinuses, causing pain, fever, and purulent discharge.

In contrast to rhinitis, which is a common manifestation of acute respiratory tract infections, inflammation of paranasal sinuses occurs rarely in acute viral infections.

24. **What is otitis media?**

Otitis media is an inflammation of the middle ear. It may present in several forms:

- **Acute serous otitis media:** The cavity of the middle ear is filled with a transudate that accumulates because of the difference between the high ambient air pressure and the pressure in the middle ear (aerootitis or barotitis media). Under such conditions, as during the descent of an airplane or deep-sea diving, the air must enter the middle ear through the Eustachian tube to equalize the pressure. If the Eustachian tube is occluded because of infection or allergies, serous transudate is formed, and if the pressure gradient persists or is increased, this may be accompanied by bleeding.
- **Infectious myringitis:** The inflammation involves the tympanic membrane, causing hearing loss. Typically, it is caused by viruses, mycoplasma, or *S. pneumoniae*.
- **Acute suppurative otitis media:** This infection is caused by pyogenic bacteria, most often *S. pneumoniae*. Pus accumulates in the middle ear, causing bulging and perforation of the tympanic membrane. Incompletely healed suppurative otitis media may transform into a chronic serous otitis media. Under such conditions, pus resorbs but is replaced by serous fluid. It is almost always associated with the obstruction of the Eustachian tube.
- **Chronic suppurative otitis media and mastoiditis:** Persistent bacterial infection leads to chronic drainage through the ruptured tympanic membrane. The destruction of auditory ossicles leads to loss of hearing. The infection also spreads into the mastoid, causing destruction of mastoid air cells.
- **Chronic otitis media:** Lingering inflammation may persist following an acute infection and is usually associated with perforation of the tympanic membrane. Granulation tissue may protrude through the hole in the membrane in the form of aural inflammatory polyps.

25. **Describe the most important complications and consequences of otitis media.**

- **Loss of hearing:** A consequence of perforation of the tympanic membrane, auditory ossicles, or the auditory nerve.
- **Cholesteatoma:** This expansile lesion results from ingrowths of squamous epithelium into the middle ear through the perforated eardrum. The epithelial cells produce keratin, which elicits a foreign body giant cell reaction. Cholesteatomas are frequently infected by bacteria. The main danger from cholesteatomas is that they tend to erode bone.
- **Intracranial spread of infection:** Severe otitis media may spread and cause meningitis and epidural, subdural, or intracerebral abscesses.

26. **What is otosclerosis?**

Otosclerosis is an autosomal dominant disease characterized by immobilization of the stapes to the oval window in the middle ear. It is the most common cause of conductive hearing loss in young and middle-aged adults in the United States. It is more common in women and typically affects both ears.

27. **What is Ménière disease?**

Ménière disease is a disease of unknown etiology characterized by recurrent attacks of vertigo, sensory hearing loss, tinnitus, and a feeling of fullness in the inner ear. It is associated with distention of the cochlear endolymphatic system, leaking of endolymphatic fluid into the perilymph, and possible rupture of the membranous wall. Symptoms of vertigo are accompanied by nausea, which lasts a few hours and disappears spontaneously. Hearing loss may become permanent. Treatment with salt-losing diuretics may improve the condition.

28. **What are the most common causes of acute labyrinthitis?**
Labyrinthitis is usually caused by viruses. In children, it is caused by rubella or mumps. In immunosuppressed people, it is most often caused by cytomegalovirus.

NEOPLASMS AND RELATED CONDITIONS

29. **What is the difference between leukoplakia and erythroplakia?**
Leukoplakia is a clinical term for a persistent white patch on the mucosa. Erythroplakia is a similar patch of red color. Such plaques may be caused by a variety of conditions, such as smoking, tobacco chewing, local mechanical irritation, and heavy use of alcohol. It should always be considered as potentially precancerous and biopsied whenever indicated. Some of these biopsies will reveal invasive squamous cell carcinoma.

30. **What are the histologic features of leukoplakia?**
Leukoplakia appears as a white patch because of accumulation of keratin over a variety of epithelial changes that may be classified as benign and reactive, preneoplastic, or frankly neoplastic:
   - **Acanthosis, parakeratosis, and keratosis (85%):** In this benign lesion caused by irritation, the epithelium is thickened (acanthosis) and covered with a keratinized cell layer. If the nuclei are preserved in the keratotic squames, the change is called parakeratosis; if the nuclei are not seen, the thick keratin layer is called keratosis.
   - **Squamous cell dysplasia (10%):** This lesion is associated with cytoplasmic atypia similar to the changes seen in squamous cell cancer. The dysplasia may be graded as mild or severe. Severe dysplasia has a tendency to progress to invasive carcinoma.
   - **Squamous cell carcinoma (5%):** Histologically, this cancer does not differ from squamous cell carcinomas in other locations.

31. **List the essential facts about oral cancer.**
   - Squamous cell carcinoma accounts for more than 95% of all oral malignant tumors.
   - Peak age is 50 to 60 years; men are more often affected than women.
   - Risk factors include smoking and alcohol abuse.
   - Tumors may present as leukoplakia, ulceration, or exophytic induration.
   - The most common location is the anterior two thirds of the tongue and lower lip.
   - Metastases involve submandibular, superficial, and deep neck lymph nodes.
   - With surgical and radiation treatment, the 5-year survival rate is 40% to 50%.

KEY POINTS: NEOPLASMS AND RELATED CONDITIONS ✔

1. Leukoplakia and erythroplakia may be signs of neoplasia but may also be caused by chronic irritation, smoking, or inflammation.

2. Squamous cell carcinoma, the most common form of oral cancer, may originate from any part of the mouth, but most often it originates from the anterior two thirds of the tongue and lower lip.

3. Pleomorphic adenoma, the most common tumor of the salivary glands, is a benign mixed tumor composed of epithelial, myoepithelial, and stromal cells.

4. Nasopharyngeal carcinoma may be related to infection with the Epstein–Barr virus.

32. **What is ameloblastoma?**
Ameloblastoma is a tumor originating from the cells forming the enamel organ during odontogenesis. It is the most common benign odontogenic tumor, usually located in the mandible. It is locally invasive but does not metastasize.

33. **List the main facts about salivary gland tumors.**
   - The parotid gland (the largest salivary gland) is most often affected, but the tumors may occur in other major and minor salivary glands as well.
   - Most tumors are benign, but the ratio of benign to malignant tumor decreases proportionately with the decreasing size of the glands (parotid > submaxillary > sublingual > minor salivary glands).
   - The most common tumor is pleomorphic adenoma (mixed tumor of salivary glands). It may recur if not excised adequately. Malignant transformation occurs in 2% or 3% of tumors (carcinoma ex pleomorphic adenoma).
   - The most common malignant tumor is mucoepidermoid carcinoma. It is a low-grade malignancy (5-year survival >90%).

34. **List the most common salivary gland tumors.**
See Table 11-2.

TABLE 11-2. MOST COMMON SALIVARY GLAND TUMORS	
Tumor (Incidence)	Clinical Behavior
Pleomorphic adenoma (60%)	Benign, may recur locally
Carcinoma ex pleomorphic adenoma (2%)	Malignant
Warthin tumor (10%)	Benign
Monomorphic adenoma (3%)	Benign
Mucoepidermoid carcinoma (5%)	Low-grade malignant, but may be high grade
Acinic cell carcinoma (3%)	Low-grade malignant
Adenoid cystic carcinoma (3%)	Malignant and invasive
Adenocarcinoma of ductal origin (2%)	Highly malignant

35. **Name the main facts about nasopharyngeal carcinoma.**
   - It is the most common malignant nasopharyngeal tumor, usually located on the roof of the pharynx.
   - Males are affected more often than females.
   - It is associated with EBV infection, especially in China and areas of Africa, where it has a high incidence.
   - Microscopic features include squamous epithelial cells intermixed with lymphocytes.
   - Metastases to external cervical lymph nodes occur early and may be the first symptoms of the tumor.
   - Radiation therapy and surgery offer good results, and the 5-year survival rate is 60%.

36. **List the main facts about carcinoma of the larynx.**
   - Squamous cell carcinoma accounts for more than 95% of cases.
   - Risk factors include smoking and alcohol abuse; the male-to-female ratio is 7:1.

- Location:
  - ○ Supraglottic (epiglottis and aryepiglottic folds): 50%
  - ○ Glottic (involving the vocal cords): 35%
  - ○ Infraglottic (below the vocal cords): 15%
- Metastases found in local neck lymph nodes; distal metastases in later stages.
- Symptoms include hoarseness and coughing.
- Five-year survival rate with surgery and radiation therapy is greater than 60%.

37. **What are nasal polyps?**

Polyps are inflammatory or neoplastic lesions protruding from the nasal mucosa into the lumen of airspaces. The most important forms are:

- **Inflammatory polyps:** This is the most common form, and it represents swollen parts of the inflamed nasal mucosa protruding into the lumen of the nose. It is typically a complication of chronic or recurrent allergic rhinitis or chronic infection involving nasal sinuses. In children younger than 10 years of age, nasal polyps may be a feature of cystic fibrosis.
- **Squamous papilloma:** These epithelial tumors are usually benign but may be locally invasive, especially if histologically classified as inverted papillomas.
- **Juvenile angiofibroma:** These benign tumors are composed of thin blood vessels enclosed in loose fibroblastic stroma. Angiofibromas occur in young men and tend to bleed if traumatized.

38. **Can lymphomas occur in the nasopharynx?**

Waldeyer's ring is a common site of extranodal lymphoma. Most of these tumors are of B-cell origin and are most often classified as large cell, high-grade lymphomas. Hodgkin lymphoma usually does not involve the nasopharyngeal lymphoid tissue.

39. **Can tumors occur in the ear?**

Tumors may originate in the external ear as well as in the middle and inner ear. The external ear is covered by squamous epithelium, and the tumors originating in it are similar to those found elsewhere on the skin. Ceruminous glands can give rise to adenomas or adenocarcinomas. The epithelium of the endolymphatic sacs may give rise to rare adenomas. The most common tumors of the inner ear are schwannomas arising from the VIII cranial nerve.

WEBSITES

1. http://www.ncbi.nlm.nih.gov/entrez/query.fcgi?db=PubMed

2. http://www-medlib.med.utah.edu/WebPath/webpath.html#MENU

3. http://www.uiowa.edu/~oprm/AtlasHome.html

BIBLIOGRAPHY

1. Batsakis JG, Suarez P: Schneiderian papillomas and carcinomas: a review. Adv Anat Pathol 8:53–64, 2001.
2. Berger WE, Schonfeld JE: Nonallergic rhinitis in children. Clin Allergy Immunol 19:197–207, 2007.
3. Bisno AL: Acute pharyngitis. N Engl J Med 344:205–211, 2001.
4. Choong N, Vokes E: Expanding role of the medical oncologist in the management of head and neck cancer. CA Cancer J Clin 58:32–53, 2008.

5. Hamilos DL. Approach to the evaluation and medical management of chronic rhinosinusitis. Clin Allergy Immunol 20:299–320, 2007.

6. Koufman JA, Burke AJ: The etiology and pathogenesis of laryngeal carcinoma. Otolaryngol Clin North Am 30:1–15, 1997.

7. Kutok JL, Wang F: Spectrum of Epstein–Barr virus–associated diseases. Annu Rev Pathol 1:375–404, 2006.

8. Rinia AB, Kostamo K, Ebbens FA, et al: Nasal polyposis: a cellular-based approach to answering questions. Allergy 62:348–358, 2007.

CHAPTER 12

THE GASTROINTESTINAL SYSTEM

Ivan Damjanov, MD, PhD, and Anamarija Morović, MD

1. **What is the basic structure of the gastrointestinal (GI) system?**
   The entire GI tract has a relatively uniform structure and consists of four layers:
   - Mucosa composed of epithelium lining the lumen of the cavity
   - Submucosa composed of loose connective tissue, blood vessels, and nerves
   - Muscle layer (muscularis propria) composed predominantly of smooth muscle cells responsible for the peristaltic movement of these hollow organs
   - Adventitia or serosa forming the outer layer (In the esophagus, the adventitia is a connective tissue structure linking it with other thoracic organs. The external surface of the stomach and small and large intestines is covered with serosa, a layer of peritoneum continuous with the peritoneum covering the other parts of the abdominal cavity and other organs, such as the liver and the spleen.)

2. **What are the main diseases of the GI system?**
   - Developmental disorders
   - Inflammatory diseases, usually caused by infections but often of unknown etiology (e.g., inflammatory bowel disease)
   - Functional disorders affecting the digestion, absorption of nutrients, or motility of the intestines
   - Circulatory disturbances
   - Tumors

3. **Discuss the possible consequences of abnormal development of the GI system.**
   - Atresia (absence of lumen; The normal GI system is a tube that develops from cords of embryonic cells. The cells forming the central part of these cords undergo apoptosis, and a lumen is thus formed. If the centrally located cells do not undergo apoptosis, the lumen never forms, and the affected part of the GI system will be atretic, i.e., unpassable.)
   - Stenosis (narrowing)
   - Diverticulosis (formation of outpouchings)
   - Fistula (a connection between the lumen of the GI tract and another tubular system; e.g., an esophageal–tracheal fistula)

KEY POINTS: MOST IMPORTANT SYMPTOMS AND SIGNS PERTAINING TO THE GI SYSTEM ✓

1. Dysphagia

2. Vomiting

3. Hematemesis

4. Hematochezia and melena

5. Colics, diarrhea, and constipation

ESOPHAGUS

4. **What are the main clinical symptoms and signs of esophageal disease?**
   - **Dysphagia:** Difficulty in swallowing. It may be caused by anatomic lesions (e.g., stricture, webs, and rings), cancer, or functional disorders (e.g., achalasia and paralysis).
   - **Odynophagia:** Pain on swallowing. It is a sign of esophageal lesions, such as gastroesophageal reflux disease (GERD) and infectious esophagitis caused by viruses or fungi.
   - **Heartburn:** A burning sensation behind the sternum. It is usually caused by GERD.
   - **Acid regurgitation:** Reflux of gastric contents into the mouth is a sign of GERD.

5. **What is the most common developmental abnormality of the esophagus?**
   Esophageal atresia with tracheoesophageal fistula is the most common developmental abnormality. Several anatomic variants are recognized. Food cannot pass into the stomach because the lumen of the esophagus ends in a blind pouch. Food passing through the fistula enters the trachea, causing choking and coughing. Symptoms appear soon after birth, requiring immediate surgical correction.

6. **What are esophageal diverticula?**
   Diverticula are outpouchings of the wall of the esophagus. These outpouchings are classified on the basis of the following (Fig. 12.1):
   - Stricture
     - True diverticula (composed of all four layers of the normal esophageal wall)
     - False diverticula (representing outpouchings of the mucosa and submucosa only)

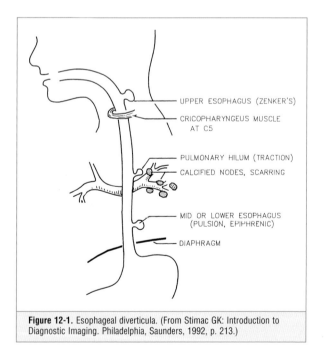

Figure 12-1. Esophageal diverticula. (From Stimac GK: Introduction to Diagnostic Imaging. Philadelphia, Saunders, 1992, p. 213.)

- Pathogenesis
  - ○ Traction diverticula (pull from outside; e.g., fibrous adhesions)
  - ○ Pulsion diverticula (push from inside; e.g., increased intraluminal pressure)
- Location
  - ○ Upper esophageal diverticula (also known as Zenker pulsion diverticula)
  - ○ Diverticula of the midportion of esophagus (traction diverticula due to mediastinal and bronchial lesions; e.g., scarring of lymph nodes in tuberculosis)
  - ○ Epiphrenic (lower esophageal) diverticula (pulsion diverticula associated with diaphragmatic hernia and GERD)

7. **Define achalasia.**

   Achalasia is a functional disorder characterized by a loss of normal esophageal peristalsis and incomplete or abnormal relaxation of the lower esophageal sphincter (LES). The LES must relax during swallowing, but if it does not and remains contracted, it will act as a barrier to the food destined to enter the stomach. Secondary dilatation of the aperistaltic esophagus proximal to the constriction occurs.

   The cause of primary achalasia, a rare disease (1:100,000), is not known. Histologic studies show, however, that the spasm of the LES is associated with a loss of ganglion cells from the lower esophagus. Secondary achalasia may occur in Chagas disease because of the destruction of ganglion cells infected with *Trypanosoma cruzi*.

8. **What are esophageal webs and rings?**

   Webs are mucosal folds causing narrowing of the lumen. Dysphagia caused by webs in the upper esophagus may be associated with glossitis and iron deficiency anemia (Plummer–Vinson syndrome). The disease is common in Scandinavian countries but rare in the United States.

   Schatzki ring is a subepithelial semicircular fibrous strand in the wall of the esophagus. It narrows the lumen at the gastroesophageal junction. It may cause dysphagia and is best demonstrated by esophagoscopy.

9. **What is hiatal hernia?**

   Hiatal hernia is a protrusion of the stomach above the diaphragm through a widened diaphragmatic hiatus. Hiatal hernias are quite common. Two forms are recognized (Fig. 12-2):

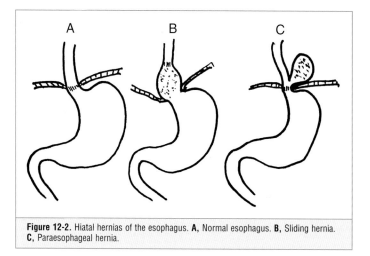

Figure 12-2. Hiatal hernias of the esophagus. **A,** Normal esophagus. **B,** Sliding hernia. **C,** Paraesophageal hernia.

- **Sliding hernia (90%):** The gastroesophageal junction is pulled into the thorax and is found above the diaphragm. In most instances, it is asymptomatic and diagnosed accidentally during the workup of the patient for some other disease. It may be associated with GERD, heartburn, and dysphagia.
- **Paraesophageal hernia (10%):** The gastroesophageal junction is in the normal location, but a portion of the stomach rolls up beside it into the thorax. In most instances, it is asymptomatic, but the invaginated gastric mucosa may become strangulated by the diaphragm.

10. **What is congenital diaphragmatic hernia?**
    Congenital diaphragmatic hernia is a severe developmental defect in which the diaphragm is defective or incompletely developed. Abdominal organs dislocate through the defect into the thoracic cavity, compressing the lung and the heart. The condition is often associated with other developmental abnormalities and is usually lethal. Minor diaphragmatic defects may be repaired surgically.

11. **What is GERD?**
    Reflux of gastric contents into the esophagus is a common disorder, typically associated with incompetence of the LES. It presents with odynophagia and dysphagia and may even cause hemorrhage. The diagnosis is suspected on the basis of typical clinical presentation and is confirmed by esophagoscopy. Esophageal biopsy may be performed during endoscopy to document the extent of inflammation or ulceration and to determine whether Barrett esophagus (with or without dysplasia) has developed.

12. **Discuss the causes of GERD.**
    GERD develops because of malfunction of the LES, which in normal circumstances prevents the entry of the gastric contents into the esophagus. Reflux may be caused by:
    - Temporary increase in intraabdominal pressure (e.g., after overeating or drinking carbonated drinks)
    - Prolonged intraabdominal pressure in pregnancy or obesity
    - Protracted LES relaxation and uncoordinated contraction due to the action of alcohol, fatty food, cigarettes, and drugs (e.g., morphine and diazepam)
    - Hiatal hernia
    - Scleroderma (Fibrous tissue replacing smooth muscle cells weakens the sphincter; the esophagus is involved in 70% of patients with scleroderma.)

13. **List the most common complications of GERD.**
    Complications of long-lasting GERD are:
    - Esophagitis
    - Barrett esophagus
    - Esophageal bleeding (with melena or hematemesis)
    - Peptic ulceration (ulcers may develop in gastric or intestinal metaplasia of Barrett esophagus)
    - Esophageal strictures (due to healing with scarring)
    - Esophageal perforation (rare; preceded by ulceration)

14. **What is the etiology of esophagitis?**
    Three major etiologic groups are recognized:
    - Infectious esophagitis
    - Chemical esophagitis (the most common form of esophagitis)

- Esophagitis as a manifestation of other diseases
  - ○ Skin diseases (e.g., pemphigus and erythema multiforme)
  - ○ Crohn disease of the ileum and colon
  - ○ Graft versus host disease (after bone marrow transplantation)

15. **What are the causes of infectious esophagitis?**
    The esophagus is covered by squamous epithelium, which is relatively resistant to infections. Most infections occur in people with poor health, systemic disease, or those with reduced immune response. A breach in the mucosal barrier (e.g., in GERD) may allow infection to take place. The most common infections are:
    - **Fungal infection:** *Candida albicans* and other fungi may grow on the surface of the squamous epithelium, such as in the mouth or the vagina.
    - **Viral infections:** Herpes simplex virus or cytomegalovirus (CMV) infection typically occurs in immunosuppressed people.
    - **Bacterial infections:** Bacteria do not penetrate the intact squamous epithelium but may invade ulcerated mucosa damaged by GERD. Bacterial infections account for 15% to 20% of all cases of infectious esophagitis.

16. **What are the most common forms of chemical esophagitis?**
    - **Hydrochloric acid:** HCl regurgitated from the stomach is the most common cause of esophagitis in GERD.
    - **Strong acids or lye:** These chemicals cause erosive esophagitis. Children sometimes ingest these substances accidentally, and adults may drink them intentionally while trying to commit suicide.
    - **Cytotoxic drugs:** Such drugs inhibit the proliferation of the esophageal epithelium and prevent or delay the repair of small ulcerations that develop during feeding. These ulcerations provide a route of entry for bacteria.

KEY POINTS: ESOPHAGUS ✓

1. The most common diseases of the esophagus are reflux esophagitis and hiatal hernia, resulting in gastroesophageal reflux disease.

2. Carcinomas of the esophagus are of two histologic types: (1) squamous cell carcinoma originating from the squamous epithelium normally covering the esophagus and (2) adenocarcinomas arising from the metaplastic glandular epithelium in Barrett esophagus.

17. **What is Barrett esophagus ?**
    Barrett esophagus is a form of metaplasia of the esophagus. Typically, it involves the lower segment of the esophagus and is thought to be most often caused by GERD. It can be recognized on endoscopy and biopsy:
    - **Endoscopy:** Salmon-red patches replace the normal white squamous lining of the esophagus.
    - **Microscopy:** Columnar epithelium similar to gastric or intestinal columnar epithelium is found replacing the normal squamous esophageal epithelium. The underlying connective tissue usually shows signs of chronic inflammation.

18. **What is the significance of Barrett esophagus?**
    Barrett esophagus is associated with a variety of clinical symptoms, most often odynophagia. The esophagus may ulcerate and bleed. The most important complication of Barrett esophagus is adenocarcinoma of the esophagus, which develops in a significant number of cases (10%).

19. **Which pathologic changes precede adenocarcinoma in Barrett esophagus?**
    Adenocarcinoma developing in Barrett esophagus is typically preceded by histologically recognizable dysplasia. Pathologists classify such dysplasia as mild or severe. Severe dysplasia must be followed up clinically in every case, and partial resection of the esophagus is recommended in some instances because such dysplasia has a propensity to progress to invasive adenocarcinoma.

20. **What is Mallory–Weiss syndrome?**
    Mallory–Weiss syndrome is characterized by bleeding from esophageal lacerations that develop because of violent retching. It is typically encountered in chronic alcoholics.

21. **List key facts about esophageal varices.**
    - Dilatation of submucosal veins of the esophagus may occur.
    - Dilatated veins bulge underneath the epithelium of the esophagus and can be recognized through esophagoscopy.
    - One cause is portal hypertension.
    - Cirrhosis is the most common cause; thrombosis of portal vein and hepatocellular carcinoma are less common causes.
    - Rupture of varices is an important cause of hematemesis.
    - Hematemesis is accompanied by high mortality.

22. **How common is esophageal cancer?**
    Esophageal cancer is not common in the United States, but it is a disproportionately high cause of cancer-related deaths. The incidence of esophageal cancer is increasing in the United States:
    - Six percent of all GI cancers (incidence: 6:100,000 in the United States)
    - Peak age, 50 to 60 years
    - More common in men than in women (4:1)
    - More common in African Americans than in others (4:1)
    - More common in areas of Asia (e.g., Iran and China) and Africa than in the United States and Europe
    - Poor prognosis (25% 5-year survival rate)

23. **List the risk factors for esophageal cancer.**
    - Environmental factors that could account for the higher incidence of esophageal cancer in areas of Asia and Africa (e.g., soil, tea, or food) have not been identified.
    - Tobacco smoking is the major risk factor in the United States (increased risk: 10–20 times).
    - Chronic alcohol abuse increases risk by 5 times.
    - Barrett esophagus is a definite risk factor for adenocarcinoma (10–20 times).
    - Preexisting esophageal disease increases the risk, but these diseases (e.g., achalasia) are rare.

24. **Which part of the esophagus is most often affected by carcinoma?**
    Most esophageal carcinomas develop in the midportion or the lower third of the esophagus. The upper third of the esophagus is least commonly involved.

25. **Describe the gross appearance of esophageal carcinoma.**
Esophageal carcinoma typically narrows the lumen of the esophagus or affects peristalsis, thus causing dysphagia. On gross examination, tumors may present as:
- Ulceration (most common)
- Polypoid outgrowth protruding into the lumen
- Induration of the wall, with concentric or excentric narrowing of the lumen
Tumor cells spread early through the lymphatics into adjacent mediastinal organs. Metastases are first found in the local lymph nodes

26. **How are esophageal carcinomas classified histologically?**
- **Squamous cell carcinoma:** It accounts for 60% of all esophageal tumors in the United States, 90% in Africa and Asia.
- **Adenocarcinoma:** It accounts for 40% of all esophageal tumors in the United States. Adenocarcinomas develop in Barrett esophagus and are typically located in the lower segment of the esophagus and at the gastroesophageal junction.

STOMACH

27. **What is the most important developmental disorder of the stomach?**
Congenital hypertrophic pyloric stenosis affects 1 in 400 to 600 infants. The disease shows a multifactorial pattern of inheritance, but it may also be associated with chromosomal developmental disorders (e.g., Turner syndrome). Typically, it presents with projectile vomiting. It is caused by hypertrophy of the smooth muscle in the pyloric portion of the stomach, which may be palpated through the abdominal wall. Surgical incision provides relief and is routinely performed with excellent results.

28. **What is gastritis?**
Gastritis is an inflammation of the mucosa of the stomach. It is a common disease that may occur in an acute or a chronic form. Morphologically, acute gastritis typically presents with shallow erosions of the mucosa (erosive gastritis). Chronic gastritis may be erosive or nonerosive.

29. **What are the most common causes of acute gastritis?**
Acute erosive gastritis is a self-limited inflammation of the gastric mucosa. Clinically, it presents with epigastric burning, pain, nausea, and vomiting. Variable amounts of blood may be found in the vomitus. Pathologically it is characterized by shallow blood-suffused mucosal erosions surrounded by acute inflammatory cells. These mucosal changes may be caused by:
- Aspirin and nonsteroidal antiinflammatory drugs (NSAIDs)
- Alcohol
- Acid and alkali (e.g., suicidal ingestion)
- Stress
- Shock-related mucosal ischemia (e.g., in burns, brain trauma, and surgery)
- Sepsis (This is most often streptococcal sepsis, but other systemic infections may affect the stomach as well. Viral gastritis is found in immunosuppressed people.)
A mnemonic for the previous list is "3A + 3S": aaacute ssstress)

30. **Discuss why gastric erosions develop in acute gastritis.**
Erosions may develop because of the direct effects of a potentially toxic substance (e.g., alcohol), oversecretion or back-diffusion of hydrochloric acid, or a breakdown of the local mucosal defense system against the corrosive action of gastric juice. For example, hypoperfusion of the gastric mucosa in shock makes the mucosal cells more susceptible to the action of pepsin and hydrochloric acid. Aspirin and NSAIDs inhibit the local synthesis of prostaglandins and weaken the mucosal defense system.

KEY POINTS: STOMACH ✅

1. Acute gastritis is caused by irritants and nonsteroidal antiinflammatory drugs, whereas chronic gastritis is most often caused by *Helicobacter pylori*.

2. Peptic ulcer, a multifactorial disease associated with *H. pylori* infection, is the most common cause of hematemesis.

3. Gastric carcinoma is an adenocarcinoma that occurs in several forms but always has a poor prognosis.

31. **What are Cushing and Curling ulcers?**
These eponyms are used for gastric stress ulcers. Such ulcers are deeper than erosions and may extend all the way to the muscularis mucosae. Cushing (who was a famous neurosurgeon) gave his name to ulcers caused by brain injury. Curling ulcers are found in burn patients. (An easy way to remember which is which is to think "things curl in fire.")

32. **Describe the main forms of chronic nonerosive gastritis.**
Chronic nonerosive gastritis is inflammation of the mucosa of the stomach that may be caused by immunologic mechanisms, infection, and prolonged ingestion of drugs or alcohol or cigarette smoking. Several clinicopathologic forms of chronic gastritis are recognized:
    - Chronic type A gastritis (autoimmune gastritis)
    - Chronic type B gastritis (*Helicobacter pylori* gastritis)
    - Hypertrophic gastritis (Menetrier disease; in this rare form of gastritis, the gastric mucosa has giant folds.)
    - Uncommon forms of gastritis (e.g., eosinophilic, lymphocytic, and granulomatous gastritis; these are rare, and diagnosis is made histologically.)

33. **Is it possible to distinguish type A and type B chronic gastritis in biopsy material examined microscopically?**
Type A is an autoimmune disease, whereas type B is an infectious disease caused by *H. pylori*. In early stages of the disease, it is possible to distinguish type A from type B gastritis histologically, but in advanced stages, such a distinction is not always possible.
    In the early stages of autoimmune gastritis, the mucosa of the fundus and body is infiltrated with lymphocytes and plasma cells. Acute stages of *H. pylori* infection are associated with infiltrates of neutrophils in the glands and the lamina propria. *H. pylori* can be seen in the gastric glands, mostly in the pyloric antrum. As the diseases progress, both forms of chronic gastritis are accompanied by:
    - Atrophy of gastric glands
    - Intestinal metaplasia
    - Lymphocytic follicles in the atrophic mucosa
    In this advanced stage of the disease, it is difficult to find *H. pylori*, which does not survive in the metaplastic intestinal glands. Reliable histopathologic distinction of type A from type B chronic gastritis becomes impossible in the disease's later stages.

34. **Is it possible to clinically distinguish type A from type B chronic gastritis?**
As stated previously, the histologic diagnosis of type B chronic gastritis depends primarily on finding *H. pylori* in the gastric biopsies. Because the gastroscopic findings are similar in both forms of gastritis and *H. pylori* cannot always be found in advanced stages of the disease, other tests (e.g., urea breath test or antibody test for *H. pylori*) must be performed. The most important aspects of type A and type B gastritis useful for distinguishing one form of gastritis from the other are listed in Table 12-1.

TABLE 12-1. MAJOR ASPECTS OF TYPE A AND TYPE B GASTRITIS

Feature	Type A Gastritis*	Type B Gastritis
Distribution of lesions	Fundus, diffuse	Pyloric antrum, focal
Gastric secretion	Reduced	Normal, +, or −
Antibodies to parietal cells	Yes	No
Other autoimmune diseases	Yes	No
Vitamin B_{12} (in serum)	Low	Normal
Pernicious anemia	+	−
Gastrin (in serum)	Increased	Normal
Antibodies to *Helicobacter pylori*	−	+
Incidence	Less common	More common
Age dependence	Yes	Yes
Cancer risk	Increased	Increased

*Type A gastritis is associated with four As: autoimmune disease, antibodies to pyloric cells, anemia (pernicious), and achlorhydria (reduced hydrochloric acid secretion).

35. **Which form of chronic gastritis is associated with a higher risk of cancer?**
    Type A gastritis is associated with a higher relative risk of gastric adenocarcinoma. However, because type B chronic gastritis is much more prevalent, it is thought to be the cause of many more cancers than type A gastritis. In this context, it is worth noting that the World Health Organization has designated *H. pylori* as a potential human carcinogen. Epidemiologic data link *H. pylori* to an increased incidence of gastric adenocarcinoma and lymphoma in many areas of the world, especially southern Europe, South America, and Asia.

36. **Explain the pathogenesis of peptic ulcer.**
    The pathogenesis of peptic ulcers is not fully understood. It is, however, generally accepted that the mucosal ulcerations are chemically mediated and develop because of the action of HCl and pepsin on a "weakened" or "susceptible" gastric or duodenal mucosa. Because the gastric acid of ulcer patients does not contain unusually high quantities of HCl or pepsin, it is postulated that the glands are damaged by a back-diffusion of hydrogen ions.

37. **Which factors play a role in the development of peptic ulcers?**
    Peptic ulcer is a multifactorial disease, and several factors contribute to its pathogenesis:
    - **Infection:** *H. pylori* is found in 90% of duodenal and 65% of gastric ulcer patients. *H. pylori* secretes urease, protease, and phospholipases that may cause mucosal injury and may serve as "barrier breakers," facilitating the chemical injury of mucosal cells. Eradication of *H. pylori* infections contributes to the healing of peptic ulcers.
    - **Neuroendocrine factors:** The secretion of gastric juices is under neuroendocrine control, which becomes dysregulated in peptic ulcer patients. Stress, nervous tension (type A personality), and endocrine disorders have been implicated in the pathogenesis of peptic ulcers, but the exact role of these putative insults is not known. For example, the hypersecretion of hormones such as corticosteroids and gastrin is associated with peptic ulcers in hormonal hypersecretion syndromes such as Cushing and Zollinger–Ellison syndromes, respectively. However, there is no definitive evidence that these hormones play

a role in the pathogenesis of "garden variety" solitary peptic ulcers. Vagotomy (excision of the vagus nerve) is used only in the treatment of complicated persistent ulcers resistant to other treatment modalities.

- **Local mucosal factors:** Drugs such as NSAIDs reduce the secretion of prostaglandins and damage the mucosal barrier. Alcohol, spicy food, and substances that stimulate acid secretion may play a pathogenetic role. Antacid treatment and suppression of gastric acid with histamine-2 blockers promote healing of ulcers. There is no evidence that dietary modification is helpful in the treatment of peptic ulcer disease.

38. **Where are peptic ulcers most often located?**
    - Ninety-eight percent of all peptic ulcers are located in the duodenum and stomach.
    - Duodenal ulcers are more common than gastric ones (4:1) and are located in the proximal area just beyond the pylorus.
    - Gastric ulcers are located on the lesser curvature, most often at the junction of the body and pyloric antrum.
    - Most ulcers are solitary.
    - In approximately 20% of cases, the ulcers are multiple, and both duodenum and stomach are involved.
    - Rare locations for ulcers include the esophagus, the small intestine, and the Meckel diverticulum.
    - Peptic ulcers in unusual locations, multiple ulcers, and ulcers that do not respond to the usual therapy are found in association with gastrin-secreting tumors (Zollinger–Ellison syndrome).

39. **Describe the gross pathology of peptic ulcers.**
    - On gross examination or gastroscopy, peptic ulcers present as a sharply demarcated round or oval defect of the mucosa.
    - Most ulcers are small (1 or 2 cm in diameter); those greater than 4 cm are rare.
    - The bottom is smooth (because of the action of HCl and pepsin, which keep it "clean"), but it may be covered with blood.
    - Borders are sharp, but around the long-lasting lesions, the adjacent mucosa may show some puckering due to fibrosis.

40. **Describe the histologic layers found in a typical chronic peptic ulcer.**
    Histologically, there are four layers (from top to bottom; Fig. 12-3):
    - Superficial zone of necrosis composed of amorphous debris
    - Acute inflammatory exudate full of neutrophils

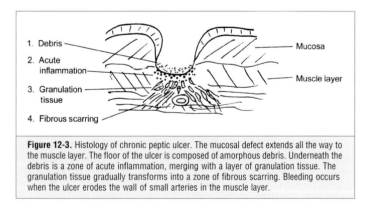

Figure 12-3. Histology of chronic peptic ulcer. The mucosal defect extends all the way to the muscle layer. The floor of the ulcer is composed of amorphous debris. Underneath the debris is a zone of acute inflammation, merging with a layer of granulation tissue. The granulation tissue gradually transforms into a zone of fibrous scarring. Bleeding occurs when the ulcer erodes the wall of small arteries in the muscle layer.

- Granulation tissue rich in blood vessels and macrophages
- Scarring at the bottom (If the ulcer extends into the muscle layer, it may erode blood vessels and cause bleeding.)

41. **What are the most common complications of peptic ulcers?**
    - **Hemorrhage:** This is the most common complication. Minor hemorrhage may present with melena and cause iron deficiency anemia. Major hemorrhage is found in 10% to 20% of patients and may be associated with hematemesis.
    - **Perforation:** It is found in approximately 10% of patients and is typically associated with peritonitis and paralytic ileus. Air may be seen by x-ray under the diaphragm.
    - **Stenosis:** It may cause narrowing or obstruction of the duodenum or gastric outlet due to fibrosis that develops around the ulcers in approximately 5% of patients.
    - **Penetration:** It includes extension of granulation tissue into the pancreas, typically as a complication of posterior wall duodenal ulcers. It is accompanied by dull pain and elevated serum amylase.
      See Fig. 12-4.

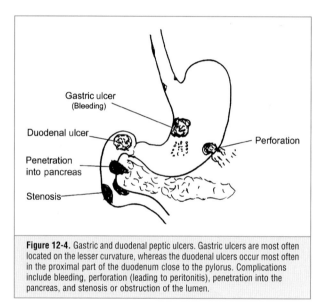

Figure 12-4. Gastric and duodenal peptic ulcers. Gastric ulcers are most often located on the lesser curvature, whereas the duodenal ulcers occur most often in the proximal part of the duodenum close to the pylorus. Complications include bleeding, perforation (leading to peritonitis), penetration into the pancreas, and stenosis or obstruction of the lumen.

42. **List the most common malignant tumors of the stomach.**
    - Adenocarcinoma (95%)
    - Lymphoma (3%)
    - Carcinoids and neuroendocrine carcinomas (1%)
    - Stromal tumors (GI stromal tumors [GISTs] and leiomyomas, 1%)

43. **List key facts about gastric carcinoma.**
    - Epidemiology: It is the third most common GI cancer in the United States, accounting for 2% to 3% of all cancer death.
    - The high incidence of gastric cancer in maritime countries (Japan, Iceland, and Chile) may be related to high consumption of smoked fish containing nitrosamines.

- Its incidence has decreased in the United States during the past 80 years (from 38:100,000 to 7:100,00).
- It affects older people—75% are older than 50 years of age.
- Histologically it is an adenocarcinoma.
- Prognosis is poor for most cases with a 5-year survival rate of 20%.

44. **Which diseases predispose to gastric cancer?**
   - *H. pylori* infection (The World Health Organization has designated this bacterium as a Grade I carcinogen.)
   - Chronic atrophic gastritis with intestinal metaplasia
   - Postgastrectomy states (Three percent of people undergoing gastrectomy develop cancer over a period of 20 years.)
   - Gastric adenomatous polyps (These rare tumors may undergo malignant transformation. Tumors >2 cm give rise to adenocarcinoma in 50% of cases.)

45. **How does gastric carcinoma appear on gross examination?**
   - **Flat mucosal lesions:** Early intramucosal carcinoma may present in the form of mucosal patches or a loss of rugae. Such early cancers are often not visible on macroscopic examination or endoscopy. Japanese physicians have pioneered early diagnosis of such tumors, which are discovered by screening high-risk people yearly with endoscopy and with cytologic examination of gastric brushings. Early intramucosal carcinoma has good prognosis.
   - **Exophytic tumors:** These tumors protruding into the lumen of the stomach are usually described as polypoid or fungating (cauliflower-like).
   - **Ulcerating tumors:** These tumors must be distinguished from benign peptic ulcers. Benign peptic ulcers have sharp regular margins, whereas ulcerated cancer has irregular margins and is not clearly demarcated from the normal mucosa. Ulcerated gastric carcinomas often have raised borders and are described as craterlike.
   - **Diffusely infiltrating tumors:** Tumors that invade all layers of the gastric wall give the stomach a "leather-bottle" appearance and are called linitis plastica. Histologically, these infiltrating tumors often contain signet ring tumor cells filled with mucus.
   See Fig. 12-5.

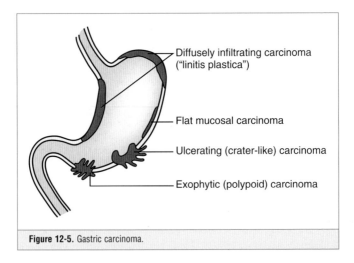

Figure 12-5. Gastric carcinoma.

46. **Where do gastric carcinomas metastasize?**
    - They may metastasize to local lymph nodes.
    - They may metastasize to the Virchow node. This supraclavicular lymph node filters the lymph from the thoracic duct prior to its entry into the systemic veins.
    - Liver and lung may be involved by hematogenous metastases.

47. **How important is gastric lymphoma?**
    The GI tract is the most common site of extranodal malignant lymphoma, and the stomach is involved in 60% of cases. Like other gastrointestinal lymphomas, gastric lymphoma may be primary (i.e., isolated lymphoma of the stomach without lymph node or bone marrow involvement) or secondary due to the spread of lymphoma from lymphoid organs.

48. **What is GIST?**
    GIST is an acronym for gastrointestinal stromal tumor. These tumors originate from stromal stem cells that are precursors of smooth muscle cells or GI fibroblasts. If a stromal tumor shows histologic signs of smooth muscle differentiation, it is called leiomyoma or leiomyosarcoma. If the cells retain the phenotype of undifferentiated stromal cells, the tumor is called GIST. It may be benign or malignant. Benign GISTs are small (2–5 cm) and have few dividing cells. Malignant GISTs are spindle cell sarcomas measuring more than 6 cm and showing the usual signs of malignancy (necrosis, hemorrhage, high mitotic activity, and anaplasia).

INTESTINES

49. **Name the most important developmental disorders of the intestines.**
    Developmental disorders involving the intestines are either rare or relatively unimportant:
    - **Meckel diverticulum** is known as the "left-sided" appendix. It represents the remnant of the omphalomesenteric (vitelline) duct presenting as an outpouching of the ileum. A useful mnemonic is *four 2s*:
      ○ Present in 2% of normal people
      ○ 2 feet from the ileocolic junction (80–90 cm)
      ○ 2% may become symptomatic and cause symptoms similar to appendicitis or volvulus
      ○ Site of 2% of ectopic ulcers
    - **Hirschsprung disease** is also known as congenital megacolon or megacolon with congenital agangliosis.
      ○ Incidence is 1 in 5000 infants.
      ○ Male infants are more often affected (male-to-female ratio is 4:1).
      ○ Multifactorial inheritance is suggested by higher incidence in some families.
      ○ Dilatation of the colon is proximal to an aganglionic segment of the rectum.
      ○ The defect in innervation results from faulty migration of precursors of intestinal ganglionic cells. These cells develop from the neural crest and migrate into fetal intestine. Normally, these cells populate the entire colon, but if they do not reach the terminal part of the rectum, this segment remains aganglionic.
      ○ The diagnosis is made clinically (chronic constipation in a young child) but must be confirmed by biopsy, which typically shows an absence of ganglion cells.
      ○ The part of the intestine that does not contain ganglion cells must be resected.

50. **What are the possible causes of intestinal obstruction?**
    Intestinal obstructions are of three kinds (Fig. 12-6):
    - Intraluminal causes
      ○ Tumors (most often carcinoma of the large intestine)
      ○ Foreign bodies
      ○ Intussusception of the intestinal loops (invagination of one loop into another)

- Intramural causes
  - ○ Chronic inflammation and fibrosis
  - ○ Hematomas
  - ○ Complications of surgery
- Extraintestinal causes
  - ○ Hernia
  - ○ Adhesions
  - ○ Volvulus (rotation of the intestinal loops at the mesentery)
  - ○ Metastases on the serosa or mesentery

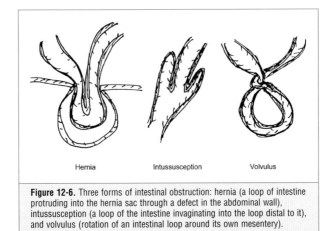

Figure 12-6. Three forms of intestinal obstruction: hernia (a loop of intestine protruding into the hernia sac through a defect in the abdominal wall), intussusception (a loop of the intestine invaginating into the loop distal to it), and volvulus (rotation of an intestinal loop around its own mesentery).

51. **How does intussusception develop?**
    Intussusception develops most often under two conditions:
    - **In small children with very active peristalsis:** In these children, one small intestinal loop invaginates into another, like the finger of an inverted glove. The loop is said to be "telescoped into another loop" (because the loops resemble the old navigators' telescopes), and intussusceptum is strangulated by the out-sided intussuscipient. The inner loop may become necrotic unless the invagination is everted surgically (or spontaneously, as may sometimes occur).
    - **In the presence of tumors:** Small pedunculated tumors carried by peristalsis may pull forward the loop to which such a tumor is attached.

KEY POINTS: INTESTINES ✓

1. Intestinal disease may present with obstruction, diarrhea, malabsorption, and bleeding.

2. Diarrhea can be classified as osmotic, secretory, exudative, malabsorptive, or mixed.

3. Malabsorption syndromes characterized by steatorrhea may result from small intestinal diseases, such as celiac disease, Whipple disease, or lactase deficiency.

4. Crohn disease and ulcerative colitis share some features but also differ in many respects, allowing doctors to diagnose them as two separate forms of the inflammatory bowel disease.

5. Colonic polyps, which can be inflammatory and neoplastic, and colonic carcinoma are important causes of occult bleeding and hematochezia.

52. Where does volvulus occur most often?
Volvulus is a rotation of a mobile loop of the intestine around its own mesenteric root. This occurs most often in the sigmoid colon but is also found in the small intestines.

53. What is paralytic ileus?
Paralytic (adynamic) ileus is a lack of intestinal peristalsis associated with stagnation of intestinal contents. The most common causes are:
- Abdominal surgery (usually transient ileus, lasting not more than 2 or 3 days)
- Peritonitis (bacterial or chemical as in acute pancreatitis)
- Shock and vascular collapse

54. What is diarrhea?
Diarrhea is an increased frequency or volume of stools (>250 g per day). It can be classified as acute or chronic. From the etiologic/pathogenetic standpoint, diarrhea can be classified as:
- Osmotic (due to decreased absorption time)
- Secretory
- Mixed
- Exudative

55. Explain the pathogenesis of osmotic diarrhea.
It is caused by nonabsorbable osmotic substances in the intestinal lumen. Such substances (e.g., mannitol or sorbitol in people who chew large amounts of sugar-free gum or magnesium sulfate from Epsom salt) stimulate an osmotic influx of water and electrolytes into the intestinal lumen. Osmotic diarrhea stops on its own as soon as the patient stops taking the substance that caused it.

The best example of osmotic diarrhea related to endogenous pathology is diarrhea caused by milk in people with genetic lactase deficiency. Such people cannot absorb lactose and develop diarrhea after eating cheese or drinking milk. Lactose found in milk products cannot be absorbed and remains in the intestine, acting as an osmotic stimulus.

56. What is secretory diarrhea?
In this form of diarrhea, the intestinal cells secrete more water than they can absorb. This form of diarrhea can be caused by:
- **Cholera toxin:** *Vibrio cholerae* ingested by mouth remains in the intestine and does not invade the intestinal mucosa. It secretes a toxin that activates the adenyl cyclase cyclic adenosine 3′,5′-monophosphate (cAMP)-dependent water pump in the cell membrane. Intestinal cells secrete into the lumen chloride accompanied by water, and a watery diarrhea develops. Similar toxins are secreted by enterotoxigenic strains of *Escherichia coli* and *Salmonella* spp.
- **E. coli toxin:** The heat-stable *E. coli* toxin stimulates water influx through mechanisms that are not cAMP dependent.
- **Enteropathogenic viruses**: Rotavirus and Norwalk virus account for most infections.
- **Vasoactive polypeptides:** Vasoactive intestinal polypeptide (VIP), serotonin, and other polypeptides secreted by neuroendocrine tumors (carcinoids and pancreatic islet cell tumors) stimulate the influx of water through complex mechanisms. These substances account for the diarrhea of carcinoid syndrome and the so-called pancreatic cholera in people who have pancreatic VIPoma.

57. How does exudative diarrhea develop?
Exudative diarrhea develops in the course of diseases that disrupt the intestinal layer or damage the mucosa:

- Infections of the small and large intestine (e.g., *E. coli*, *Clostridium difficile*, and *Shigella* species)
- Inflammatory bowel disease (ulcerative colitis and Crohn disease)
- Tumors (e.g., lymphoma and carcinoma)

58. **List the most important infectious causes of diarrhea.**
See Table 12-2.

TABLE 12-2. MAJOR INFECTIOUS CAUSES OF DIARRHEA			
Virus	**Bacteria**	**Ingested Bacterial Toxin**	**Protozoa**
Rotavirus	*Escherichia coli*	*Staphylococcus aureus*	*Giardia* species
Norwalk virus	*Campylobacter jejuni*	*Bacillus cereus*	*Entamoeba* species
Cytomegalovirus	*Vibrio cholerae*	*E. coli*	
	Clostridium difficile		
	Shigella species		
	Salmonella species		
	Yersinia jejuni		

59. **Explain the differences between inflammatory and noninflammatory diarrhea.**
Noninflammatory diarrhea is typically a consequence of small intestinal disease. Typical features are:
- Watery diarrhea of sudden onset
- Nausea and vomiting, cramps, and upper abdominal pain suggesting small bowel enteritis
- Copious excrement not containing inflammatory cells or blood
  Typical food poisoning and travelers' diarrhea present in this form. Epidemics of cholera are another example.
  Inflammatory diarrhea typically has the following features:
- Bloody diarrhea with pus and necrotic tissue debris (dysentery)
- Leukocytes and red blood cells (easily found in the feces on microscopic examination)
- A smaller volume of excrement that contains more formed elements than the watery noninflammatory diarrhea (Feces associated with tenesmus, lower left quadrant pain, and urgency suggest large intestinal disease.)

60. **What is enteric fever?**
Enteric fever is a form of diarrhea that is of protracted duration and is associated with signs of systemic disease, such as high fever, rash, and respiratory or neurologic symptoms. *Salmonella typhimurium* and *Salmonella paratyphi* are the most common causes.

61. **Define malabsorption syndrome.**
Malabsorption syndrome is characterized by abnormal intestinal absorption of nutrients and other substances from the intestine. Consequences include nutritional deficiencies (e.g., fat and protein or vitamin deficiencies), weight loss, retarded growth in children, and osmotic diarrhea, often combined with steatorrhea (fat in the stool).
  Three main causes of malabsorption are:
- **Maldigestion:** Intraluminal phase of digestion may be disturbed by a deficiency of:
  ○ Gastric juices (e.g., postgastrectomy states)
  ○ Pancreatic juices (e.g., chronic pancreatitis)
  ○ Bile salts (e.g., biliary obstruction; excessive deconjugation of bile salt by bacterial overgrowth [e.g., in surgically created blind loops] has the same effect)

- **Intrinsic bowel disease:** Absorption of nutrients may be blocked at the surface of enterocytes in the mucosa. Diseases that destroy the mucosa cause malabsorption as well. The best examples are:
  - Abetalipoproteinemia (genetic enzyme deficiency in enterocytes)
  - Celiac disease
  - Whipple disease
  - Crohn disease
- **Obstruction of lymphatics:** Diseases that block the passage of absorbed nutrients include:
  - Intestinal lymphoma
  - Scleroderma

62. **What are the laboratory and clinical findings in malabsorption syndrome?**
    See Table 12-3.

TABLE 12-3. LABORATORY AND CLINICAL FINDINGS IN MALABSORPTION SYNDROME

Laboratory Finding (Deficiency)	Clinical Findings
Protein	Growth retardation, muscle wasting, edema
Iron	Microcytic, hypochromic anemia
Folic acid/vitamin B_{12}	Macrocytic, megaloblastic anemia
Vitamin A	Night blindness, keratomalacia
Vitamin D	Osteomalacia
Vitamin K	Bleeding tendency
Calcium	Tetany, paresthesia, secondary hyperparathyroidism

63. **What is celiac disease?**
    Celiac disease (also known as celiac sprue or nontropical sprue) is a gluten-sensitive enteropathy presenting in the form of a malabsorption syndrome. The exact pathogenesis of celiac disease is not fully understood. Essential facts about celiac disease are the following:
    - The disease has a genetic basis.
      - There is familial occurrence: 15% of first-degree relatives may be affected.
      - HLA-B6 is found in 80% of affected people.
      - Similar intestinal pathology is seen in unaffected siblings.
    - Gluten sensitivity plays a pathogenetic role.
      - Ninety percent of patients have antibodies to gliadin.
      - A gluten-free diet relieves symptoms.
    - The immune system is involved and may play a pathogenetic role.
      - Association with immunoglobulin A–mediated dermatitis herpetiformis is common.
      - Autoantibodies: endomysial antibodies (90%) are used for screening; antibody to tissue transglutaminase is often present.
      - Intestinal lymphoma is a late complication in 10% of patients.
    - Intestinal biopsy is essential for diagnosis. It reveals typical mucosal changes, which can be reversed with a gluten-free diet.
    - There is a biphasic peak age curve. Symptoms usually appear in childhood, then disappear but may reappear in the fifth and sixth decades.

64. **List the typical pathologic features of celiac disease.**
   Pathologic changes seen in small intestinal mucosal biopsy include (Fig. 12-7):
   - Shortening or subtotal atrophy of the villi
   - Elongation of crypts containing proliferating enterocytes
   - An increase in lymphocytes and plasma cells in the lamina propria and invading the crypts

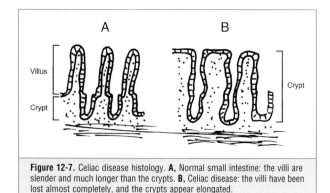

Figure 12-7. Celiac disease histology. **A,** Normal small intestine: the villi are slender and much longer than the crypts. **B,** Celiac disease: the villi have been lost almost completely, and the crypts appear elongated.

65. **List the main clinical features of celiac disease.**
   Clinical features include:
   - Diarrhea or steatorrhea
   - Weight loss or retarded growth in children
   - Deficiency of fat-soluble vitamins (A, D, E, and K)
   - Iron deficiency anemia
   - Abnormal d-xylose absorption test
   - Good response to gluten-free diet

66. **What is tropical sprue?**
   Tropical sprue is an infectious disease presenting with malabsorption syndrome. It may resemble celiac sprue, but often folic acid deficiency and megaloblastic anemia dominate the clinical picture. Symptoms typically develop following a visit to the tropics (e.g., Caribbean islands, South America, and Southeast Asia). Intestinal biopsy shows only partial villous atrophy. Tropical sprue responds well to tetracycline.

67. **Define Whipple disease.**
   Whipple disease is a systemic disease caused by the bacterium *Tropheryma whippelii*. It usually affects men in the 30- to 60-year age group. Chronic diarrhea is almost always present and may be associated with abdominal pain, pleural effusions, arthralgia, skin pigmentation, and anemia. The diagnosis is made by small intestinal biopsy, which shows typical accumulation of bacteria containing foamy macrophages in the lamina propria. Lymph node enlargement and cardiac and cerebral symptoms may also be present in disseminated disease.

68. **What is lactase deficiency?**
   Lactase is an enzyme in the apical cell membrane of intestinal villi, and it may be missing in some people who have a congenital deficiency. More often the deficiency is acquired at the time of puberty. Some degree of acquired lactase deficiency is found in most adults, but it is as high as 75% in African Americans and 100% in the Chinese. Intolerance to dairy products is associated with osmotic diarrhea and malabsorption. Diagnosis may be suggested by typical occurrence of diarrhea after ingesting milk or cheese and is confirmed by a lactose tolerance test.

69. **What is the pathogenesis of appendicitis?**
    - Appendicitis is an acute bacterial infection of the appendix precipitated by the obstruction of the lumen. The causes of the obstruction include:
      ○ Fecaliths and inspissated fecal material
      ○ Submucosal lymphoid tissue hyperplasia in the course of viral infections
      ○ Pinworms, carcinoid, and barium from x-ray studies (and other less common causes)
    - Inflammation causing mucosal ulceration, allowing bacteria to penetrate through the wall of the appendix to the peritoneal surface
    - Transmural inflammation or rupture of the appendix due to necrotizing inflammation that is accompanied by entry of pus into the peritoneal cavity
    - Periappendiceal abscess capsule formation, limiting further spread of infection
    - Infection may spread and cause diffuse peritonitis (rare today)

70. **Discuss how appendicitis presents clinically.**
    Symptoms are typical in most cases. Atypical presentation is encountered if the appendix is in a retroperitoneal or intrapelvic location. Small children and the elderly may show less typical signs of the disease. In a classical form, appendicitis presents as follows.
    - **Pain:** It is most prominent in the right lower quadrant but may be periumbilical and even epigastric, depending on the extent of inflammation.
    - **Rebound tenderness:** Typically, it can be elicited by pushing the abdominal wall at McBurney's point.
    - **Systemic symptoms:** Typically, there is fever, nausea, and vomiting.
    - **Laboratory findings:** These typically include leukocytosis (10,000–20,000/mL).
    - **A mass in the right lower quadrant:** Such a mass may be palpated following rupture of the appendix and the formation of a periappendiceal abscess. It can be visualized by ultrasound or computed tomography if the diagnosis is questionable.

71. **What is pseudomembranous colitis?**
    It is an acute inflammation of the colon presenting with the formation of plaquelike fibrinous exudate (pseudomembranes) covering parts of the large intestinal mucosa. It is caused by a toxin produced by an overgrowth of *C. difficile,* replacing the normal intestinal flora. It typically develops in patients treated with broad-spectrum antibiotics. Clinically it presents with diarrhea, fever and lower abdominal tenderness. *C. difficile* toxin can be detected in the stool. Treatment includes discontinuation of the antibiotic treatment that has allowed the overgrowth of *C. difficile* combined with hydration and specific antibacterial therapy (vancomycin or metronidazole) to eradicate *C. difficile,* which provides good results. Relapse occurs in 20% of cases cured by such an approach.

72. **What are pseudomembranes?**
    They are patches of fibrinous exudate forming on the surface of colonic mucosa injured by *C. difficile* toxin. Necrosis of the surface epithelium and mucosal blood vessel injury lead to an exudation of fibrinogen, which is polymerized into fibrin. Fibrin mixed with the mucus from the colonic glands and necrotic tissue forms the pseudomembranes attached loosely to the remnants of mucosa beneath it. These plaques are called pseudomembranes to distinguish them from true anatomic membranes lining the surface of internal organs. They are grayish-white but soon acquire a yellow, brown, or greenish color from the fecal material in the lumen. If removed by force, pseudomembranes leave behind bleeding ulcerations.

73. **Define inflammatory bowel disease (IBD).**
    IBD is a term encompassing two diseases of unknown etiology: ulcerative colitis (UC) and Crohn disease (CD). UC and CD share many features but also differ so that in typical cases, each can be diagnosed with ease. In approximately 15% to 20% of cases, the disease cannot be classified as UC or CD and is called indeterminate colitis.

74. **Describe the common features shared by UC and CD.**
    - Unknown etiology and pathogenesis
    - Basic pathology is inflammation of the colon
    - Peak incidence in the same age group (15–25 years)
    - Genetic predisposition
        - Close blood relatives of affected persons have increased incidence of either UC or CD in approximately 20% of cases
        - Can occur in the same family
    - Extraintestinal manifestations
        - Arthritis
        - Eye lesions (iritis and episcleritis)
        - Primary sclerosing cholangitis
        - Skin lesions such as pyoderma gangrenosum and erythema nodosum

75. **What are the differences between UC and CD?**
    See Table 12-4.

TABLE 12-4. MAJOR DIFFERENCES BETWEEN ULCERATIVE COLITIS AND CROHN DISEASE		
Feature	Ulcerative Colitis	Crohn Disease
Distribution	Predominantly left-sided colon	Right-sided colon
	Diffuse	Patchy, with skipped areas
Involvement of ileum	Rare (backwash ileitis, 10%)	Common (80%)
Intestinal wall	Thin	Thickened, rigid
Lumen	Dilatated megacolon	Stenosis ("string sign" rare complication)
Mucosa	Friable, surface ulceration	Deep linear ulceration; cobblestone-like
Inflammation	Limited to mucosa	Transmural
Granulomas	No	Yes (50%)
Serosa	Smooth, unaffected	Inflamed
Adhesions	No	Yes
Intestinal fistulas	No	Yes
Perianal abscess and fistula	No	Yes (50%)
Gastrointestinal ulceration (e.g., mouth and stomach)	No	May occur in 1%–5%
Carcinoma	10%	<1%

76. **Can one distinguish UC from CD by intestinal biopsy?**
    The diagnosis of UC and CD is made by exclusion and by correlating all the clinical, endoscopic, radiologic, and pathologic findings. Negative bacteriologic and confirmatory biopsy findings are of paramount importance for such an exclusion diagnosis. Histologic

findings are useful to confirm active inflammation. However, biopsy findings do not allow a clear distinction between UC and CD. Finding of granulomas (50% of cases) is typical of CD. Involvement of the ileum also favors CD over UC.

77. **What are crypt abscesses?**
Crypt abscesses are diagnosed microscopically as an accumulation of neutrophils inside the colonic crypts. They are a sign of active inflammation and are found in both UC and CD.

78. **What are pseudopolyps?**
Pseudopolyps are remnants of normal or regenerating colonic mucosa surrounded by ulcerations. Because the ulcerated surface is thinner than normal, the remaining normal mucosal patches protrude and resemble polyps. Some of the pseudopolyps represent hyperplastic granulation tissue intermixed with regenerating colonic epithelium. The regenerating epithelium may acquire atypia and change into dysplasia and even give rise to colonic adenocarcinoma. Pseudopolyps are easier recognized endoscopically in UC than in CD, which has a "cobblestone," lumpy appearance. Dysplasia and adenocarcinomas develop more often in UC than in CD. Carcinomas are also easier to recognize by endoscopy in UC than in CD because in UC they protrude from the ulcerated mucosa, forming a typical dysplasia-associated lesion or mass.

79. **What is toxic megacolon?**
Megacolon is massive dilatation of the entire large intestine. It is a severe, life-threatening complication of UC but is rarely found today. It is called toxic to distinguish it from congenital megacolon of Hirschsprung disease and acute nontoxic megacolon (Ogilvie syndrome). Nontoxic megacolon is also called colonic pseudoobstruction. It may be caused by various drugs, anesthesia, metabolic disorders (uremia), severe infection, or shock.

80. **What is fistula?**
A fistula is an abnormal channel between the loops of two hollow organs or a hollow organ and a skin surface. Fistulas develop because of the destruction of tissue by pus that breaks through the wall of the juxtaposed intestinal loops held together by an inflammatory exudate or granulation tissue. Enteroenteric fistulas are typical of CD.

81. **Are fistulas found in both UC and CD?**
No. Fistulas are found in CD but not in UC. CD is typically a transmural inflammation, and serosal inflammation regularly occurs. This leads to adhesions between intestinal loops and formation of channels that break through the granulation tissue, linking one intestinal loop to another. In addition to these enteroenteric fistulas, approximately 20% of CD patients develop perianal fistulas, draining to the skin and perianal abscesses. Enterovaginal or enterovesical fistulas are less common.

82. **What is diverticulosis?**
Diverticulosis is a disease of old age characterized by the appearance of pulsion diverticula in the colon. These outpouchings of the mucosa and submucosa through the muscular layer of the intestine occur presumably because of increased pressure in the large intestine related to straining during defecation. Typically, such diverticula are:
- Multiple, usually located at the point of entry of arteries through the muscularis
- More common in the United States and Western Europe than in underdeveloped countries of Africa and Asia (presumably because of constipation related to low-fiber food)
- Age related (in Western countries, 30% of 50 year olds and 60% of 80 year olds have diverticulosis)
- Located in the sigmoid colon (85%)

83. **What is diverticulitis?**

Diverticulitis is an inflammation of the intestinal wall altered by diverticula. It results from entry of bacteria through the ulceration of the herniated mucosa caused by fecaliths, or circulatory disturbances. Symptoms include pain, changes in bowel movement, and hemorrhage. There are also signs of inflammation, such as fever and leukocytosis. The area is sensitive to palpation.

84. **List the complications of diverticulitis.**
   - Pericolonic abscess, resulting from an extension of inflammation into the pericolonic fat
   - Pericolonic fibrosis, developing as a reaction to pericolonic inflammation
   - Peritonitis, resulting from rupture of diverticula on the free surface of the sigmoid colon
   - Colonic stenosis or obstruction, resulting from fibrosis encircling the intestine

85. **List key facts about intestinal ischemia.**
   - Ischemia causes pathologic changes when the perfusion of the intestines declines below 50% of normal.
   - The small intestinal blood is supplied by the superior mesenteric artery, the branches of which form anastomosing arcades. Ischemia develops only if more than one of the major branches is narrowed by atherosclerosis or occluded by thrombi, or if the entire field is hypoperfused.
   - The parts of the colon that are the most susceptible to ischemia are the watershed border zones between the perfusion superior and inferior mesenteric arteries (splenic flexure) and the left colic and sigmoid-superior rectal branches of the inferior mesenteric artery (rectosigmoid junction).

86. **What is the difference between occlusive and nonocclusive small intestinal ischemia?**

Occlusive ischemia results from thrombi or emboli occluding the main trunk or several branches of the superior mesenteric artery. Thrombi account for most of such occlusions. These thrombi usually develop over ruptured atheromas. Ischemic lesions are usually transmural (i.e., the necrosis involves the entire thickness of the intestinal wall).

Nonocclusive ischemia develops in the course of hypotension caused by any kind of shock. Ischemia may be mild (involving only the tips of the intestinal villi), moderate, or severe (transmural).

87. **What is the most common cause of chronic colonic ischemia ?**

Chronic ischemia of the large intestine (also called chronic ischemic colitis) is caused by atherosclerotic narrowing of the branches of the mesenteric arteries. It may present in the form of ischemic infarcts or progressive ischemic ulceration and atrophy of mucosa.

88. **Can intestinal ischemia cause hematochezia?**

Yes. Ischemic necrosis of intestinal mucosa results in hemorrhagic infarcts. The necrotic area is usually reperfused by the blood coming from numerous anastomoses in the intestines. Blood oozes into the lumen from the surface of such hemorrhagic infarcts and may present as rectal bleeding.

89. **List the most common causes of intestinal bleeding.**
   - Hemorrhoids—dilatated hemorrhoidal veins, classified as internal or external
   - Angiodysplasia, a localized dilatation of thin-walled vessels typically found in the mucosa of the intestine of the elderly (It may occur in any part of the intestines, but most often it is located in the cecum. It is best diagnosed by angiography.)
   - Polyps and carcinoma
   - Colitis due to infection or idiopathic IBD
   - Ischemic colitis

90. **What are intestinal polyps?**
Polyps are benign tumors or tumor-like protrusions of the intestinal mucosa. Polyps are classified as neoplastic and nonneoplastic. See Table 12-5.

TABLE 12-5. NEOPLASTIC AND NONNEOPLASTIC POLYPS	
Neoplastic Polyps	**Nonneoplastic Polyps**
Tubular adenoma	Hyperplastic polyp
Villous adenoma	Hamartomatous polyp (Peutz–Jeghers syndrome)
Carcinoid	Juvenile (retention) polyp
Benign connective tissue tumors (e.g., leiomyoma and lipoma)	Lymphoid polyp
	Inflammatory polyp

91. **What are hyperplastic polyps?**
   - The most common intestinal polyps
   - Small, dewlike, glistening nodules (most are <0.5 cm)
   - Most often found in the rectum
   - Nonneoplastic hyperplasia of colonic epithelium leads to the formation of elongated glands with sawtooth appearance on cross-section
   - Clinically innocuous; do not progress to cancer

92. **What are juvenile (retention) polyps?**
These polyps are hamartomas typically found in the rectum of children aged younger than 10 years. They are pedunculated, round, and have a smooth surface. Histologically, they are composed of mucus-filled cystic glands and edematous, usually inflamed stroma.

93. **What is Peutz–Jeghers syndrome?**
An autosomal dominant syndrome characterized by:
   - Multiple hamartomatous intestinal polyps (Polyps may be found in any part of the intestine but are most numerous in the small intestine.)
   - Pigmented macules on the lips and the perioral skin
   - Increased risk of cancer in the lungs, breast, uterus, and pancreas
   - Intestinal polyps composed of irregularly arranged glands surrounded by strands of smooth muscles (These polyps are not precancerous and only exceptionally progress to adenocarcinoma.)

94. **List key facts about tubular adenomas.**
   - The most common neoplastic intestinal polyp (90%)
   - Equally distributed throughout the entire large intestine
   - Often multiple, usually small (<1 cm) and pedunculated
   - Composed of tubular glands lined by dysplastic columnar epithelium
   - Adenocarcinomas arise in 1% to 3% of polyps
   - Risk of cancer proportional to the increasing size and number of polyps
   - Most (99%) are cured by polypectomy through the endoscope
     See Fig. 12-8.

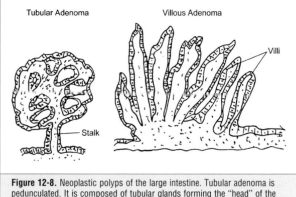

Figure 12-8. Neoplastic polyps of the large intestine. Tubular adenoma is pedunculated. It is composed of tubular glands forming the "head" of the polyp, which is attached to the intestine by a stalk. Villous adenoma is sessile and has a broad base. Fingerlike projections (villi) protrude from the base of the polyp into the lumen of the intestine.

95. **List key facts about villous adenomas.**
   - Account for 10% of neoplastic polyps
   - Solitary, sessile, and broad based, most often located in the rectum
   - Larger than tubular adenomas (1–5 cm or larger)
   - Composed of villi (i.e., fingerlike protrusions lined with columnar epithelium)
   - Adenocarcinomas arise in approximately 50% of all villous adenomas
   - Endoscopic removal often not possible

96. **What are tubulovillous adenomas?**
   Some tubular adenomas contain villous parts, and if such components comprise more than 40% of the total, the tumor is called a tubulovillous adenoma. These tumors represent an intermediate step between tubular and villous adenomas in all respects.

97. **What is familial adenomatous polyposis (FAP) coli?**
   - It is an autosomal dominant hereditary tumor syndrome.
   - It is linked to deletion of the tumor suppressor gene called adenomatous polyposis coli (APC) on chromosome region 5q21.
   - The colon contains numerous (>100) tubular adenomas.
   - Tumors are not present at birth but appear in childhood and become clinically evident in the second decade of life
   - Adenocarcinoma develops in all patients. By age 40 years, cancer is found in 100% of patients.
   - Prophylactic colectomy must be performed in midlife.

98. **Discuss the other hereditary colonic cancer syndromes.**
   - **Gardner syndrome:** A variant of FAP, it also shows autosomal dominant inheritance of numerous colonic tubular adenomas. In addition, patients have multiple osteomas, fibromatosis, and epidermal inclusion cysts.
   - **Turcot syndrome:** In this rare syndrome, adenomatous polyposis coli is associated with brain tumors (gliomas).

- **Hereditary nonpolyposis colorectal cancer (HNPCC):** Also known as Lynch's syndrome, it shows autosomal dominant inheritance of a mutator gene encoding a DNA mismatch repair enzyme. It is characterized by an increased incidence of colonic adenocarcinoma, endometrial, and ovarian cancer. Adenomas of the colon may be present, but most adenocarcinomas develop unrelated to these benign tumors. Colonic adenocarcinomas are often multiple.

99. **List key facts about the epidemiology of carcinoma of the large intestine.**
    - The third most common malignant tumor in the United States
    - The third most common cancer-related cause of death in the United States
    - Equally affects men and women
    - Higher incidence in the United States and Western Europe than in the rest of the world
    - Peak incidence in the 60- to 80-year age group
    - Uncommon in individuals aged under 40 years in the absences of a predisposing condition (e.g., FAP and ulcerative colitis)
    - Risk factors not fully understood, but mostly thought to be related to food:
      - High intake of calories, leading to obesity
      - Low-fiber food associated with constipation
      - High content of fat and refined sugars (potential carcinogens)

100. **How are risk factors for colonic cancer used in clinical practice?**
    Three groups of people are recognized, according to a scheme developed by the American Cancer Society:
    - **Individuals at average risk:** Most colonic carcinomas (70%–80%) occur among people who do not have any familial history of cancer or any other evidence of increased predisposition to cancer.
    - **Individuals at increased risk:** Approximately 15% to 20% of colorectal cancers develop in people who have some risk factors, such as adenomatous polyps and family history of colorectal cancer or adenomas, especially if such tumors were diagnosed before age 60 years.
    - **Individuals at high risk:** Approximately 5% to 10% of colorectal carcinomas develop in people with a well-defined predisposing condition, such as ulcerative colitis, HNPCC, or FAP. Genetic factors play a major role in this group.

101. **Which genes are involved in the evolution of cancer from adenomatous polyps?**
    The so-called adenoma-carcinoma sequence involves several well-defined cancer genes:
    - The APC tumor suppressor gene and MSH2 mutator gene involved in DNA mismatch repair set the background for the development of tubular adenomas.
    - The k-ras oncogene plays a role in the formation of tubular adenomas.
    - The p53 gene is involved in the growth of adenomas and the onset of early malignancy.
    - Invasive cancer develops because of the complex interaction of several genes.

102. **In which part of the large intestine do most carcinomas develop?**
    - Rectosigmoid, 40%
    - Descending colon, 15%
    - Cecum and ascending colon, 35%
    - Transverse colon, 10%
      See Fig. 12-9.

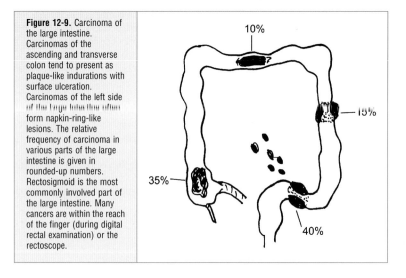

Figure 12-9. Carcinoma of the large intestine. Carcinomas of the ascending and transverse colon tend to present as plaque-like indurations with surface ulceration. Carcinomas of the left side of the large intestine often form napkin-ring-like lesions. The relative frequency of carcinoma in various parts of the large intestine is given in rounded-up numbers. Rectosigmoid is the most commonly involved part of the large intestine. Many cancers are within the reach of the finger (during digital rectal examination) or the rectoscope.

103. **What are the differences between carcinomas of the right and left colon ?**
   - Histologically, most colorectal carcinomas are adenocarcinomas.
   - Carcinomas of the right colon protrude into the lumen and are described as exophytic, polypoid, or craterlike ulcerations with raised margins.
   - Carcinomas of the sigmoid are circumferential, napkin-ring-like lesions causing narrowing of the lumen. In barium enema studies, these tumors are described as apple-core-like lesions.

104. **How do colorectal cancers metastasize?**
   - Lymphatic spread to mesenteric lymph nodes
   - Hematogenous spread through the portal vein to the liver
   - Distant hematogenous metastases to the lungs and, later, the brain

105. **How are colorectal carcinomas staged for prognostic purposes?**
   The most widely used staging system is the Astler–Coller modification of the original Dukes system. See Table 12-6.

TABLE 12-6.	ASTLER–COLLER MODIFICATION OF DUKES SYSTEM	
Stage	Extent of Cancer	5-Year Survival (%)
A	Limited to mucosa/submucosa	~100
B1	Extends into muscularis	67
B2	Penetrates through muscularis (no lymph node metastases)	55
C1	Partial invasion of muscularis with lymph node metastasis	40
C2	Extends beyond muscularis	20
D	Distant metastases	<10

106. **How common are adenocarcinomas in the small intestine?**
Adenocarcinomas of the small intestine are rare, accounting for less than 2% of all intestinal cancers.

107. **What is carcinoembryonic antigen (CEA)?**
CEA is a glycoprotein secreted by fetal intestinal cells into the meconium. It is also secreted by adenocarcinoma cells and may be found in the blood of patients with colorectal cancer. The CEA test lacks specificity and cannot be used for screening of persons at risk of developing colon cancer. It is useful for monitoring tumor burden and recurrence of cancer following surgical resection of the primary colon cancer.

108. **Which conditions are associated with elevated blood CEA?**
   - Adenocarcinoma of colon (60%–80%)
   - Adenocarcinoma in other sites (e.g., pancreas, gallbladder, and lung)
   - UC and CD (regenerating mucosal cells)
   - Alcoholic cirrhosis
   - Smoking

109. **What are intestinal carcinoid tumors?**
   - They are low-grade malignant tumors.
   - They are composed of neuroendocrine cells.
   - Cells with round, uniform nuclei form solid nests or rosettes around blood vessels (and secrete hormones into blood vessels).
   - Electron microscopy shows cytoplasmic granules.
   - Neuroendocrine hormones are demonstrable by immunohistochemistry.
   - Most cases present as small intramucosal or submucosal nodules (95% are <2 cm).
   - They are locally invasive, but not metastatic in most instances.
   - Only larger tumors (usually >2 cm) metastasize to the liver and other sites.
   - May produce carcinoid syndrome (diarrhea, facial flushing, bronchospasm, and right heart failure).
   - Urinary 5-hydroxyindolacetic acid may be elevated.

110. **Where are most carcinoids located?**
   - Appendix, 40%
   - Small intestine, 25%
   - Colon, 30%
   - Stomach, 5%

111. **Do malignant lymphomas involve the GI tract?**
Several types of GI lymphomas are recognized:
   - MALTomas (These primary GI tumors are low-grade malignant B-cell lymphomas originating from the mucosa-associated lymphoid tissue.)
   - Primary diffuse large B-cell lymphomas
   - Primary T-cell lymphomas
   - Secondary lymphomas (These B- or T-cell tumors represent extranodal spread of primary nodal or bone marrow–derived lymphomas.)

112. **List conditions predisposing to primary GI lymphoma.**
   - Gastric *H. pylori* infection
   - Celiac disease
   - Acquired immune deficiency syndrome
   - Mediterranean α-heavy chain disease

WEBSITES

1. http://www.gastroresource.com

2. http://www.gastromd.com/education

3. http://www.ncbi.nlm.nih.gov/entrez/query.fcgi?db=PubMed

4. http://www-medlib.med.utah.edu/WebPath/webpath.html#MENU

5. http://www.merck.com/mmpe/sec02.html

BIBLIOGRAPHY

1. Andrew PG, Friedman LS: Epidemiology and the natural course of inflammatory bowel disease. Gastroenterol Clin North Am 28:255–281, 1999.

2. Atherton JC: The pathogenesis of *Helicobacter pylori*–induced gastro-duodenal diseases. Annu Rev Pathol 1:63–96, 2006.

3. Cuvelier C, Demetter P, Mielants H, et al: The interpretation of ileal biopsies: morphological features in normal and diseased mucosa. Histopathology 38:1–12, 2001.

4. Grizzle WE, Manne U, Jhala NC, Weiss HL: Molecular characterization of colorectal neoplasia in translational research. Arch Pathol Lab Med 125:91–98, 2001.

5. Kulke MH: Clinical presentation and management of carcinoid tumors. Hematol Oncol Clin North Am 21:433–455, 2007.

6. Shamir R: Advances in celiac disease. Gastroenterol Clin North Am 32:931–947, 2003.

7. Shanahan F, O'Sullivan GC, O'Leary C: Colorectal cancer: still a major killer despite progress on many fronts. Q J Med 93:131–134, 2000.

CHAPTER 13

THE HEPATOBILIARY SYSTEM

Ivan Damjanov, MD, PhD

1. **What are the main diseases of the liver and the biliary system?**
   - Disorders of bilirubin metabolism and excretion resulting in jaundice
   - Acute and chronic hepatitis caused by viruses, bacteria, and other pathogens
   - Diseases caused by drugs, toxins, and alcohol
   - Metabolic and genetic diseases
   - Autoimmune diseases
   - Cholelithiasis
   - Tumors

2. **What are the most common morphologic signs of liver injury?**
   Hepatocytes are the main target of liver injury. Morphologically, liver injury can manifest in several forms:
   - **Vacuolar change:** Affected hepatocytes are enlarged and have a swollen, clear cytoplasm. This hydropic swelling of hepatocytes is a common response to injury. It is reversible, but if intensified or prolonged, it may lead to liver cell necrosis.
   - **Apoptosis:** The hepatocytes undergoing apoptosis appear rounded and detach from the other liver cells. They have a pyknotic nucleus, which ultimately disappears, leaving the remaining cytoplasm as a "round red body," also known as acidophilic body. Apoptosis of single hepatocytes is a typical feature of viral hepatitis, but it may be induced by other liver diseases as well.
   - **Necrosis:** Irreversible injury of hepatocytes induced by ischemia, toxins, and viruses typically involves portions of the liver acinus. It is customary to describe necrosis as either focal (random) or zonal, if limited to one of the three zones of the liver acinus. Zone 3 necrosis (also known as centrolobular necrosis) is the most common form of necrosis and is found in ischemic liver injury (e.g., in hypotensive shock) but also in many forms of toxic liver injury.

KEY POINTS: THE HEPATOBILIARY SYSTEM ✔

1. The liver is a central metabolic organ involved in all metabolic pathways; thus it is affected by most systemic diseases and is a common site of adverse drug reactions.

2. The liver is the source of bile and thus a cause of biliary diseases and jaundice.

3. End-stage liver disease, called cirrhosis, is a fatal disease that can be treated only by liver transplantation.

3. **How does the liver respond to injury?**
   - **Inflammation:** Injured liver cells must be removed. To this end, the body sends in inflammatory cells that react with injured hepatocytes. For example, hepatocytes infected with hepatitis virus elicit a T-cell response. These lymphocytes enter the liver and kill the infected hepatocytes, which are thereafter removed by macrophages.

- **Regeneration:** Liver cells are stable facultative mitotic cells that can enter into the mitotic cycle on demand and by dividing replace the damaged cells. Regeneration of the liver is a major response of the liver to injury. In experimental animals, it has been shown that the liver can regenerate even after two thirds of it has been removed. Massive necrosis induced by toxins and viruses typically elicits a major regeneration wave, but in many instances, this is not sufficient to save the patient's life. However, focal necrosis and apoptosis are easily repaired.
- **Fibrosis:** Extensive necrosis, especially if accompanied by persistent inflammation or toxic influences, cannot be repaired by regeneration. Portions of the liver are replaced by connective tissue scars. Fibrosis associated with nodular regeneration of the remaining hepatocytes is typical of end-stage liver disease, known as cirrhosis.

4. **How is liver function evaluated clinically?**
   Liver function is evaluated with laboratory tests colloquially known as liver function tests (LFTs). These tests were designed to monitor the following:
   - Liver cell integrity (known as necroinflammatory indices)
   - Hepatic secretory function
   - Biliary excretory function
   - Hepatic catabolic function

5. **Discuss the necroinflammatory indices, that is, the laboratory tests used to monitor the integrity of liver cells.**
   The most widely used tests are those measuring the blood concentration of aspartate aminotransferase (AST) and alanine aminotransferase (ALT). In massive liver necrosis (e.g., after acetaminophen intoxication), blood levels of AST and ALT increase 50 times over the normal values. In viral hepatitis, levels of AST and ALT are 4 to 6 times above the normal values.

6. **Which tests are used to measure hepatic secretory function?**
   - **Albumin:** Normally, the blood contains 3.5 to 5.0 g/dL (35–50 g/L) albumin, the most copious plasma protein. Chronic liver injury will reduce blood concentration of albumin to less than 3 g/dL.
   - **Coagulation proteins:** The easiest way to estimate the concentration of the coagulation factors is by measuring the prothrombin time (PT), which is normally 10 to 13 seconds. Prolonged PT is a sensitive index of liver function loss.

7. **Discuss the tests used to measure biliary excretion.**
   - **Bilirubin:** Bilirubin that has been conjugated in the liver to be excreted into the intestine may accumulate in the blood of patients who have bile duct obstruction.
   - **Alkaline phosphatase:** This enzyme is found along the liver cell membrane lining the intercellular canaliculi. Obstructive jaundice interferes with the normal biliary elimination of this enzyme, which then appears in the blood. Elevated levels of alkaline phosphatase in blood are typical of obstructive jaundice.
   - **Gamma-glutamyltransferase (GGT):** In contrast to alkaline phosphatase, which is found in many other organs, GGT is primarily a hepatic enzyme. Elevation of GGT is a reliable sign of biliary obstruction. However, GGT is also induced in liver cells by alcohol or phenobarbital and some other drugs that stimulate the P450 system. GGT is thus a marker of liver cell injury (especially alcohol-induced injury).

8. **Which tests are used for estimating liver catabolic functions?**
   Catabolic functions of the liver include the detoxification of many metabolites. However, it is impractical to measure these functions and, in practice, the only function that is monitored is the capacity of the liver to remove ammonia. Elevation of blood ammonia is a good marker of severe liver injury.

JAUNDICE

9. **Define jaundice.**
   Jaundice, or icterus, is a yellow discoloration of the skin, sclerae, and mucous membranes due to increased levels of bilirubin in circulation. Normally, blood contains 0.5 to 1.2 mg/dL of bilirubin. Jaundice becomes apparent when the blood levels of bilirubin reach the concentration of 2.5 to 3.0 mg/dL.

10. **Describe how bilirubin is formed.**
    Bilirubin is produced at a constant rate of approximately 4 mg/kg body weight per day. Accordingly, 200 to 300 mg of bilirubin is produced daily in the body. Bilirubin stems from the following:
    - Normal hemolysis of senescent red blood cells (85%)
    - Inefficient hematopoiesis (i.e., heme not utilized for the synthesis of hemoglobin in nascent red blood cells in the bone marrow; 10%)
    - Release of hemoproteins (e.g., cytochrome P450) from senescent hepatocytes and other somatic cells (5%)

11. **How is bilirubin processed?**
    The major steps in the processing and excretion of bilirubin derived from senescent red blood cells are as follows:
    - Release of heme, a tetrapyrrole component of hemoglobin
    - Transformation of heme into biliverdin in the fixed macrophages of the spleen and the liver
    - Reduction of biliverdin to bilirubin, which is released into the circulation
    - Binding of bilirubin to albumin (Bilirubin bound to albumin is not water soluble and does not appear in urine. In clinical laboratories, it is measured as indirect bilirubin.)
    - Transport of albumin-bound bilirubin to the liver (It is worth remembering that this bilirubin is called unconjugated or indirect bilirubin.)
    - Uptake of bilirubin by hepatocytes
    - Conjugation of bilirubin to glucuronic acid (This is accomplished by a microsomal hepatic enzyme, bilirubin–uridine diphosphate–glucuronyltransferase [UGT]. The bilirubin glucuronidating isoform of this enzyme is called UGT1A1.)
    - Excretion of water-soluble bilirubin glucuronides in bile (This bilirubin is called conjugated or direct bilirubin.)
    - Deconjugation of some bilirubin glucuronides by bacteria in the intestine (This process leads to the formation of colorless urobilinogen, 80% of which is excreted in feces together with the remaining conjugated bilirubin.)
    - Recirculation of urobilinogen in an enterohepatic cycle (Approximately 20% of urobilinogen is recirculated and returned to the liver. A small amount of urobilinogen is excreted in urine.)

12. **Why is it important to fractionate bilirubin in the serum?**
    Fractionation of bilirubin is used for elucidating the causes and pathogenesis of jaundice. Pathologists can fractionate total serum bilirubin and determine the ratio of unconjugated bilirubin, also known as indirect bilirubin, to conjugated bilirubin (CB), also known as direct bilirubin. Normally, blood contains less than 1.2 mg/dL (20 μmol/L) of bilirubin, most of it in an unconjugated form (95%).
    According to laboratory analysis, hyperbilirubinemia can be classified as follows:
    - Predominantly unconjugated (CB < 20%)
    - Mixed (CB 20%–50%)
    - Predominantly conjugated (CB > 50%)

KEY POINTS: JAUNDICE ✔

1. There are three forms of jaundice: hemolytic, hepatic, and obstructive jaundice.

2. Jaundice can be caused by inborn errors of metabolism.

3. Hepatic jaundice, characterized by elevation of conjugated and unconjugated bilirubin, is most often caused by viral or drug-induced hepatitis.

4. Obstructive jaundice can be caused by hepatic and extrahepatic lesions, primarily those affecting the common bile duct.

13. **Describe the main forms of jaundice.**
    Three pathogenetic forms of jaundice are recognized clinically (Fig. 13-1):
    - **Prehepatic hemolytic jaundice:** Bilirubin is predominantly in an unconjugated form.
    - **Hepatic jaundice:** Bilirubin is partially in a conjugated and partially in an unconjugated form.
    - **Posthepatic obstructive jaundice:** Bilirubin is mostly in a conjugated form.

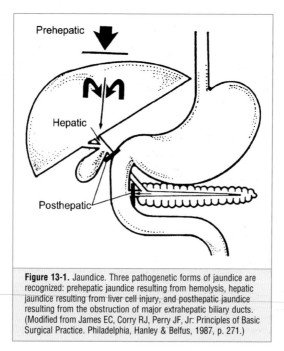

Figure 13-1. Jaundice. Three pathogenetic forms of jaundice are recognized: prehepatic jaundice resulting from hemolysis, hepatic jaundice resulting from liver cell injury, and posthepatic jaundice resulting from the obstruction of major extrahepatic biliary ducts. (Modified from James EC, Corry RJ, Perry JF, Jr: Principles of Basic Surgical Practice. Philadelphia, Hanley & Belfus, 1987, p. 271.)

14. **Is bilirubin present in urine in all forms of jaundice?**
    Unconjugated bilirubin, typically found in hemolytic jaundice, circulates bound to albumin. This bilirubin–albumin complex does not pass into the urine. On the other hand, conjugated bilirubin typically found in the blood of patients suffering from hepatocellular or obstructive jaundice is water soluble and will readily pass into urine.

15. **What are the main causes of predominantly unconjugated hyperbilirubinemia?**
Unconjugated bilirubinemia is most often caused by hemolysis. The most important clinical conditions in this category are as follows:
- Autoimmune hemolytic anemia
- Transfusion reaction due to the hemolysis of donor red blood cells (RBCs) by recipient's natural anti-AB antibodies
- Malaria (infestation of RBCs with parasites, leading to hemolysis)
- Erythroblastosis fetalis (transplacental immunization of the mother to fetal RBC antigens, reacting with RBCs of the second baby and causing severe hemolysis in the fetus or neonate. This results in kernicterus, i.e., deposition of bilirubin in basal ganglia of the baby's brain.)
- Resorption of bilirubin from internal hemorrhages (e.g., massive hematoma and intestinal hemorrhage)
- Inefficient hematopoiesis in the bone marrow (e.g., pernicious anemia and thalassemia)

16. **Can unconjugated hyperbilirubinemia be caused by liver disease?**
Yes. This typically occurs because of impaired uptake of bilirubin or impaired conjugation of bilirubin taken up by the liver cells.
   Impaired uptake by damaged hepatocytes is seen in viral hepatitis or drug-induced liver injury (e.g., probenecid-related jaundice).
   Defect of conjugation of bilirubin is the cause of unconjugated hyperbilirubinemia in some genetic disorders, such as Crigler–Najjar syndrome or Gilbert syndrome.

17. **What is the cause of jaundice in genetic diseases characterized by unconjugated hyperbilirubinemia?**
Crigler–Najjar syndrome, which occurs in two forms (severe, fatal Type I and a milder Type II), and Gilbert syndrome are caused by defective function of UGT and present with unconjugated hyperbilirubinemia.

18. **Name the most common genetic form of jaundice.**
Gilbert's syndrome is the most common form of hereditary jaundice, affecting approximately 5% of the population at large. This autosomal dominant disorder has been linked to a mutation of the gene encoding UGT1A1. This mutation is associated with reduced enzymatic activity of UGT1A1, resulting in fluctuating hyperbilirubinemia.

19. **How does Gilbert syndrome present clinically?**
Gilbert syndrome presents as mild jaundice unrelated to any other symptoms. It is typically diagnosed during the investigation of jaundice that has appeared in the course of some common disease (e.g., flu) that usually does not affect the liver. Jaundice may also be precipitated by minor stress (e.g., medical school examinations), exercise, or fasting. Jaundice is not accompanied by any other symptoms and subsides on its own. Patients should be assured that the disease is not progressive and that no treatment is required.

20. **Could genetic diseases present as benign isolated conjugated hyperbilirubinemia?**
Rare genetic disease related to abnormal processing and biliary excretion of bilirubin from liver cells may cause conjugated hyperbilirubinemia. The most important diseases in this category are Dubin–Johnson syndrome, a jaundice caused by the mutation of the multidrug resistance protein 2 (MRP2) and Rotor syndrome, a disease of unknown genetics.

21. **List common causes of mixed hyperbilirubinemia.**
Mixed hyperbilirubinemia is a sign of "hepatic jaundice" and it is typically seen in:
- Viral hepatitis
- Alcoholic hepatitis
- Drug-induced hepatitis
- Cirrhosis (usually mild)

22. **What is the difference between intrahepatic and extrahepatic biliary obstruction?**
Intrahepatic and extrahepatic biliary obstruction cause elevation of conjugated bilirubin. In both conditions, hyperbilirubinemia is associated with an elevation of alkaline phosphatase in blood. However, because the intrahepatic cholestasis may cause or even result from liver cell or bile ductular injury, it is usually accompanied by additional laboratory abnormalities (e.g., elevation of LFTs), immunologic abnormalities (such as antimitochondrial antibodies in primary biliary cirrhosis), or virologic data (e.g., hepatitis B virus antibodies). Extrahepatic biliary obstruction often presents with progressively worsening jaundice and pale ("acholic") stools and few other symptoms. Prolonged jaundice of any type is associated with itching.

23. **What are the most important causes of intrahepatic cholestasis?**
- Viral hepatitis
- Drug-induced hepatitis
- Sepsis
- Postsurgical jaundice
- Benign cholestasis of pregnancy
- Primary biliary cirrhosis
- Autoimmune hepatitis
- Primary sclerosing cholangitis

24. **List the most important causes of extrahepatic biliary obstruction in adults.**
- Stones in the common bile duct
- Carcinoma of the pancreas
- Carcinoma of the common bile duct and ampulla of Vater
- Postsurgical stenosis of bile ducts

25. **What are the most common causes of biliary obstruction in infants and children?**
- Congenital atresia of bile ducts, which is usually idiopathic
- Cystic fibrosis
  A mnemonic for remembering the causes of obstructive jaundice is *gallstone*:
  Gallstones
  Adenocarcinoma (of pancreas or common bile duct)
  Liver diseases (primary biliary cirrhosis and primary sclerosing cholangitis)
  Lymph node enlargement in the hilus
  Surgery (postsurgical scarring)
  Treatment related (drugs and cholangiography)
  Outside invasion (e.g., ascaris and other worms)
  Neonatal atresia of bile ducts
  Extraneous compression (e.g., cysts and adhesions)

HEPATIC FAILURE

26. **Compare acute and chronic liver failure.**
Acute liver failure is a disease of sudden onset that may cause death in a few days or weeks. Typically, it is associated with massive hepatic necrosis following viral infection, adverse drug reaction, or ingestion of toxins. Chronic liver failure develops over a period of years and is typically associated with cirrhosis. Cirrhosis is used as a synonym for end-stage chronic liver disease and, as such, it may be caused by a number of preexisting diseases.

27. **What are the features of acute liver failure?**
- Jaundice of sudden onset
- Shrinkage of the liver best seen on ultrasound examination
- Massive elevation of AST, ALT, and lactate dehydrogenase

- Hypoglycemia
- Bleeding tendency with prolongation of PT
- Hepatic encephalopathy and hyperammonemia
- Electrolyte disturbances, water retention, and renal failure

28. **What are the clinical features of chronic liver failure?**
    - Cirrhosis with changes in the shape and size of the liver best visible by computed axial tomography (CAT) scan
    - Portal hypertension
    - Splenomegaly
    - Hypoalbuminemia
    - Ascites
    - Bleeding tendency and prolonged PT, low plasma fibrinogen
    - Hepatorenal syndrome resulting in water and sodium retention
    - Hepatopulmonary syndrome resulting in dyspnea
    - Endocrine changes associated with gynecomastia, palmar erythema, and spider nevi
    - Hepatic encephalopathy with fetor hepaticus and asterixis
    - Increased incidence of infections (e.g., peritonitis due to infection of ascites)
    A mnemonic for the consequences of liver failure is *jaundice*:
    Jaundice
    Ascites
    Urinary failure (i.e., hepatorenal syndrome)
    Neurologic (i.e., hepatic encephalopathy)
    Dyspnea (i.e., hepatopulmonary syndrome)
    Infections (increased incidence)
    Coagulopathy (prolonged PT and bleeding esophageal varices)
    Endocrine (gynecomastia, spider angiomas, and testicular atrophy)

KEY POINTS: HEPATIC FAILURE ✔

1. Hepatic failure may develop suddenly or slowly over a period of time.
2. The main signs and symptoms of liver failure are consequences of metabolic disturbances and portal hypertension.

29. **Define portal hypertension.**
    The portal system drains the venous blood from the gastrointestinal system into the liver. It comprises the portal vein and its tributaries—the splenic vein, the mesenteric veins, and the gastric veins. In normal circumstances, the blood flows through the portal system under low pressure (7 mmHg). Portal hypertension is elevation of the portal venous blood pressure over the normal value of 12 mmHg.

30. **What are the main forms of portal hypertension?**
    Three forms of portal hypertension are recognized depending on the site of obstruction:
    - **Presinusoidal:** This is due to obstruction of the portal vein or its major intrahepatic branches. Typically, this occurs in portal vein thrombosis or fibrosis of bile ducts (e.g., schistosomiasis) that affects the adjacent blood vessels in the liver.
    - **Sinusoidal:** This is due to intrahepatic obstruction of blood flow through the sinusoids. It accounts for 90% of all cases of portal hypertension and is typically a feature of cirrhosis.
    - **Postsinusoidal:** This is due to obstruction of the hepatic vein and its tributaries by thrombi (e.g., Budd–Chiari syndrome) or tumors.

31. **What are the consequences of portal hypertension?**
    - Ascites
    - Splenomegaly
    - Anastomoses between the portal and systemic veins

32. **Where do portal–systemic anastomoses develop in portal hypertension?**
    Shunting of portal venous blood into the systemic circulation occurs at three anatomic sites:
    - **Eoophageal and gastric veins:** Esophageal varices are the most common site of massive bleeding in patients with chronic liver disease. Exsanguination from ruptured esophageal varices is a major cause of death in cirrhosis.
    - **Hemorrhoidal venous plexus:** Hemorrhoids are a common cause of hematochezia.
    - **Periumbilical veins:** Varices develop rarely in this location but can be seen on physical examination as whorls of dilatated veins (caput medusae).

33. **Discuss the pathogenesis of ascites in cirrhosis.**
    The pathogenesis of ascites is not fully understood, but it appears to be a consequence of several disturbances found in patients with cirrhosis (Fig. 13-2):
    - **Portal hypertension:** Increased hydrostatic pressure leads to transudation of fluid into the abdominal cavity.
    - **Hypoalbuminemia:** Cirrhotic livers cannot produce albumin in adequate amounts, and hypoalbuminemia is a common finding in these patients. Hypoalbuminemia is associated with reduced oncotic pressure of the plasma and reduced reentry of fluid into the blood vessels at the venular side of the microcirculation.
    - **Lymphatic overflow:** The lymph flow through the thoracic duct in patients with cirrhosis exceeds the capacity of this duct to drain the lymph from the portal area, and it "overflows" into the abdominal cavity.
    - **Hyperaldosteronism:** The escape of fluids from blood vessels into the abdominal cavity is recognized by the volume regulatory sensors as "depletions" of circulating fluid mass, which triggers a release of aldosterone. Aldosterone acts at the level of renal tubules, conserving sodium and water, which then flows over into the abdominal cavity, further contributing to the formation of ascites.

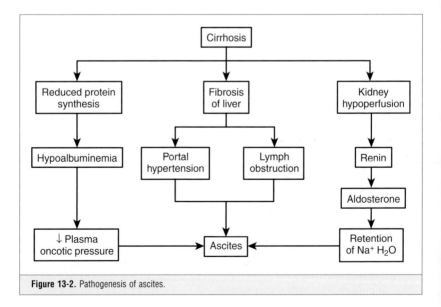

Figure 13-2. Pathogenesis of ascites.

34. **What is the pathogenesis of hepatorenal syndrome?**
    Hepatorenal syndrome is defined as sudden functional renal failure (i.e., without an underlying kidney disease) in a patient with end-stage liver failure. The exact pathogenesis of this complication of cirrhosis is not known, but all data indicate that the renal failure is caused by hypoperfusion of kidneys. It presents with oliguria and retention of water and sodium. If the patient dies, his or her kidneys can be transplanted into another person and will function normally.

35. **Explain the pathogenesis of palmar erythema, gynecomastia, and spider angiomas in patients with cirrhosis.**
    These signs of end-stage liver disease are related to hyperestrinism. Hyperestrinism results from decreased degradation of steroid hormones in the diseased liver. Weak estrogens normally produced in all men are then converted in peripheral fat tissues into more potent estrogens, which in turn act on the breast to produce gynecomastia or on the blood vessels of the skin to induce palmar erythema and spider angiomas.

36. **Explain the bleeding tendency commonly found in patients with cirrhosis.**
    - **Reduced concentration of coagulation factors in blood:** One should remember that most of the plasma coagulation factors are produced in the liver. Loss of synthetic activity of hepatocytes results in hypofibrinogenemia and reduced levels of all other coagulation proteins. Typically PT and activated partial thromboplastin time are prolonged.
    - **Thrombocytopenia:** The low platelet count is caused by splenomegaly, which leads to a sequestration of platelets and their destruction in the spleen.
    - **Disseminated intravascular coagulation (DIC):** Irregular blood flow through the liver makes the hepatocytes prone to ischemia and necrosis. Necrosis, typically precipitated by sudden onset of hepatic hypoperfusion (e.g., after massive bleeding from the esophageal varices), will result in a release of thromboplastin and activation of the coagulation cascade. Patients with cirrhosis are also prone to infections, which may potentiate DIC. Massive uncontrollable bleeding is a major cause of death in patients with cirrhosis.

INFECTIOUS DISEASES

37. **Discuss the most important infectious diseases affecting the liver.**
    - **Viral diseases:** These diseases are most often caused by hepatotropic viruses (e.g., hepatitis virus A, B, and C) but also may occur in the course of other viral infections (e.g., herpes simplex and cytomegalovirus [CMV]).
    - **Bacterial diseases:** These diseases are caused by ascending infection from the intestine or by hematogenous dissemination of bacteria from other organs.
    - **Parasitic diseases:** These diseases occur most often in the tropics and include a variety of intestinal infestations (e.g., amebiasis and schistosomiasis).

38. **What is viral hepatitis?**
    Although hepatitis may be caused by many viruses, the term *viral hepatitis* is reserved in clinical practice for infections caused by the hepatotropic viruses. Only six viruses have been definitively identified (A–E and G). One of these is a DNA virus (hepatitis B virus [HBV]), one is an incomplete RNA virus (hepatitis virus type D [HDV]), and the remaining four are RNA viruses.

39. **Do all hepatitis viruses belong to the same group, and do they share the same structural properties?**
    Hepatitis viruses do not belong to the same group: Hepatitis A virus (HAV) is a picornavirus, HBV is a hepadna virus, hepatitis C virus (HCV) is a flavivirus, and hepatitis E virus (HEV) is a calicivirus. Accordingly, immunity against one virus will not protect against other viruses.

KEY POINTS: INFECTIOUS DISEASES ✔

1. Infection by hepatotropic viruses is the most important form of infectious hepatitis.

2. Viral hepatitis can occur in an acute and chronic form, and in some instances it can progress to cirrhosis or even predispose to liver cancer.

40. **Is liver biopsy useful for diagnosing acute viral hepatitis?**

Liver biopsy is rarely used in the diagnostic workup of a patient suspected of having acute viral hepatitis. The main reasons for the uncommon use of liver biopsy for diagnosing acute viral hepatitis are as follows:

- The changes caused by various hepatotropic viruses are nonspecific. Microscopically, acute HAV cannot be distinguished from HBV or other hepatitides of this type.
- Serologic tests for hepatitis viruses, which are much more specific and less expensive, are the diagnostic method of choice for diagnosing viral hepatitides.
- Liver biopsy is an invasive procedure. It is used only after all other approaches have found negative results. It is performed by highly trained specialists and requires hospitalization of the patient. It carries a small risk for potentially serious complications (e.g., bleeding).

41. **Which viral diseases are best diagnosed by liver biopsy?**

When a patient develops acute viral hepatitis, serologic tests will usually identify the causative pathogen. However, if the serologic tests for viral hepatitides are negative, liver biopsy may provide insight into the clinical problem. For example, if the disease is caused by herpes virus or CMV, the liver biopsy may disclose intranuclear viral particles. However, because many drugs may produce "virus hepatitis-like changes," even this approach will not yield absolutely diagnostic results. Accordingly, liver biopsy is used in clinical practice as the last resort for evaluating acute liver diseases. It is useful for estimating the extent of liver injury and is widely used for estimating the extent and degree of chronic hepatitis and for documenting cirrhosis. Liver biopsy is also used for evaluating liver transplant rejection.

42. **How is acute viral hepatitis diagnosed?**

Symptoms of acute viral hepatitis are usually nonspecific and include loss of appetite, nausea, fatigue, and mild fever. Jaundice, dark urine, or light yellow ("clay-colored") stools are more specific and point to the liver as a source of clinical problems. The suspected diagnosis is confirmed by laboratory tests, showing abnormal LFTs and hyperbilirubinemia. Final diagnosis of viral hepatitis requires serologic confirmation of viral infection.

43. **Describe the biochemical abnormalities in acute viral hepatitis.**

- Elevation of serum aminotransferases (ALT and AST) 3 to 5 times above normal (Elevation of serum aminotransferases over 1000 IU/L is not uncommon in severe hepatitis. Transaminases return to normal level over a period of several months.)
- Modest increase of alkaline phosphatase and GGT.
- Hyperbilirubinemia and bilirubinuria, although many cases may be anicteric and have no bilirubin disturbances

44. **How is viral hepatitis A transmitted?**

- **Fecal–oral route:** Dirty hands and food or water contaminated by human sewage account for 80% of all infections. Travelers to underdeveloped countries are at high risk. Shellfish is an important source of infection in the United States.

- Anal intercourse is a risk factor for male homosexuals.
- Blood transmission can occur but is uncommon because the viremic phase of the infection is short lived. This mode of transmission is nevertheless common among people addicted to intravenous drugs. Blood for transfusions is screened for HAV and is not a source of infections.

45. **How widespread is viral HAV?**
HAV is endemic worldwide. Approximately 30% of the entire U.S. population has antibodies to HAV, indicating that many Americans have had an HAV infection (usually unrecognized) sometime during their lives. The prevalence of positivity increases with age, and 50% of all 50-year-old Americans are positive for HAV. This indicates that most infections occur in childhood but that many additional infections occur later in life.

46. **What should one remember about HAV?**
    - There is a short incubation period (2–6 weeks).
    - Children are most often affected. In adults, disease usually occurs after travel abroad.
    - The virus is shed in feces 2 or 3 weeks before and 1 week after onset of jaundice.
    - Symptoms are mild, and complete recovery is to be expected in most patients.
    - No chronic hepatitis or carrier state results.
    - There is minimal mortality (1 per 1000 of clinically apparent infections).
    - The vaccine against HAV is highly efficient.

47. **How is HBV transmitted?**
    - Blood and blood products (blood transfusion, sharing needles among addicts, and needlestick in health care workers)
    - Sexual contact (virus is present in semen)
    - Close contact (virus is present in saliva, tears, and breast milk)
    - Transplacental infection of the fetus
    - The source of infection is not established in approximately 30% of cases.

48. **How widespread is HBV?**
HBV is endemic in areas of Southeast Asia and Africa. There are more than 300 million carriers worldwide. Approximately 300,000 cases are diagnosed annually in the United States.

49. **What are the clinical features and possible outcomes of acute hepatitis caused by HBV?**
    - **Acute hepatitis:** It may be icteric or unicteric and even subclinical (asymptomatic).
    - **Complete recovery:** In the population at large, for each person diagnosed with acute icteric HBV, there are at least three infected people who are asymptomatic. Most of these people (i.e., 85%–90% of all people infected with acute HBV) will recover completely.
    - **Fulminant acute hepatitis:** It presents with massive hepatic necrosis that develops in less than 1% of clinically diagnosed HBV infections. These patients die unless an emergency liver transplantation is performed.
    - **Chronic asymptomatic carriers:** People with persistent infection (10%–15%) who are otherwise healthy, are infectious to others and can transmit infection sexually or by blood.
    - **Chronic hepatitis:** It is found in approximately 5% of all those who were ever infected with HBV.
    - **Cirrhosis:** End-stage liver disease develops in only 1.5% of those initially infected with HBV or 30% of those who have chronic hepatitis.
    - **Hepatocellular carcinoma:** Malignant tumors develop in 0.15% of those initially infected with HBV, that is, 10% of those who have cirrhosis.

50. **What should one remember about HBV?**
    - Infection is parenteral and transmitted by blood and body fluids.
    - The incubation period is longer than for HAV: 2 to 26 weeks, on average 8 weeks.

- Viremia and virus surviving in body fluids account for the infectivity.
- Serologic tests are essential for diagnosis and can identify those who have persistent infections or are infectious.
- Antibodies form complexes with the virus and can cause symptoms, such as serum sickness–like disease (skin rash, glomerulonephritis, and arthritis) or polyarteritis nodosa.
- Chronic disease and carrier states are encountered in a significant number of cases.
- Serious forms of disease (massive necrosis of the liver and cirrhosis) are uncommon but important complications
- HBV is a potential carcinogen: chronic hepatitis → cirrhosis → hepatocellular carcinoma.
- Vaccine is efficient in preventing disease.

51. **How is HCV transmitted?**
    - **Blood transfusion:** Because blood is screened for HCV, chances are low (1:600,000 units transfused).
    - **Medical accidents:** Needlesticks or intraoperative cuts of surgeons carry a low risk of infection (1:300).
    - **Intravenous drug abuse and sharing of needles:** This are the most common mode of transmission.
    - Mode of transmission is unknown in 40% patients.

52. **How widespread is HCV?**
    HCV is endemic worldwide. Approximately 1.8% of U.S. citizens (5.5 million) have antibodies to HCV; 70% of these people have histologic signs of mild chronic hepatitis, but most have no clinical signs.

53. **Is HCV hepatotoxic?**
    HCV is not directly hepatotoxic (i.e., the virus does not kill liver cells directly). Many chronically infected people do not show any signs of liver cell injury. Cytopathic effects cannot be induced in cultured human liver cells. The killing of liver cells in a living patient is apparently mediated by activated T lymphocytes.

54. **What is the outcome of HCV infection?**
    Exactly what happens following most acute HCV infections is unknown. Authorities estimate that most patients recover and show no clinical or laboratory signs of hepatitis. HCV persists in most of those who have been infected, and at least 85% of these people are considered to have chronic HCV. Complete elimination of the virus occurs in a minority of infected people. Likewise, fulminant hepatitis is rare.

55. **What are the manifestations of chronic HCV?**
    Chronic HCV is in most instances a subclinical disease, and the only evidence of infection are the positive serologic tests. In some patients, LFTs are elevated, but even these people have no clinical signs of infection. Histologic signs of chronic hepatitis may be found by liver biopsy, but the inflammatory infiltrates are usually limited to portal areas, and such hepatitis is classified as mild. Severe chronic hepatitis is found in a minority of cases. Cirrhosis develops in some of these patients, and a small number of patients with cirrhosis will develop hepatocellular carcinoma.

56. **What should one remember about HCV?**
    - Infection is parenteral.
    - The incubation period is 2–26 weeks (similar to HBV).
    - Persistent infection is a rule (>85%).
    - Chronic hepatitis is common, but clinically it is usually mild.
    - There is no vaccine.

- Cirrhosis occurs in a minority of cases. Nevertheless, HCV is still a major cause of cirrhosis in the United States and worldwide.
- Hepatocellular carcinoma occurs in a minority of patients with cirrhosis (10%; same risk as in HBV caused cirrhosis).

57. **Which coexistent conditions aggravate the adverse effects of HCV?**
    - Hepatitis virus B infection
    - Alcoholism (Note: 70% of chronic alcoholics who have clinical signs of liver disease have antibodies to HCV.)
    - Hemochromatosis
    - α1-Antitrypsin deficiency

58. **Does HCV cause extrahepatic symptoms?**
    HCV evokes an immune response that may cause a number of extrahepatic lesions:
    - **Cryoglobulinemia:** Cryoglobulins (immunoglobulin M [IgM]) precipitate at 4°C and dissolve again at 37°C and are found in 35% of patients. Mixed cryoglobulinemia (IgG and IgM) is found in some patients with HCV infection.
    - **Membranoproliferative glomerulonephritis:** It is also mediated by deposits of cryoglobulins.
    - **Vasculitis:** Deposits of cryoglobulins in the vessel wall may be associated with purpura or Raynaud phenomenon.

59. **How does HDV cause infection?**
    HDV is a replication-defective RNA virus dependent on HBV. Human infection occurs under two conditions:
    - **Acute coinfection:** Typically it occurs following infection with blood that contains both HBV and HDV viruses. Clinically such infection varies from mild to severe. Coinfection increases the rate of fulminant hepatitis from 1% in regular HBV to 4% in patients coinfected with HBV and HDV. Chronic hepatitis is rare.
    - **Superinfection of an HBV carrier by HDV:** Clinically such an infection will progress to chronic hepatitis in 80% of cases.

60. **What kind of liver disease is caused by HEV?**
    HEV is a RNA virus transmitted by the fecal–oral route, causing periodic epidemics in underdeveloped countries. It causes mild hepatitis that lasts approximately 6 weeks. Generally, this infection resembles HAV, but it is more common in adults than in children. HEV does not cause chronic hepatitis.

61. **How high is the mortality of HEV?**
    HEV is a self-limited disease with low mortality (1%). For unknown reasons, infection during pregnancy is associated with high mortality (20%).

62. **What is viral hepatitis G (HGV)?**
    HGV is a Flavivirus transmitted parenterally by blood. HGV is found in 1% or 2% of blood donors and at a much higher rate among intravenous drug abusers. There is no definitive evidence that this virus causes hepatitis.

63. **List the clinical syndromes caused by viral hepatitides.**
    - Asymptomatic infection (This subclinical infection is typically discovered serologically during the workup of the patient for insurance or other reasons.)
    - Acute hepatitis (It may present as jaundice or an unicteric systemic disease recognized as hepatitis only following a serologic workup.)
    - Chronic hepatitis
    - Carrier state
    - Cirrhosis
    - Hepatocellular carcinoma

64. **Describe the typical phases of acute icteric viral hepatitis.**
   - **Incubation period:** This is from the time of infection until the first symptoms appear.
   - **Preicteric phase:** During this phase, the patient may have fever, malaise, lassitude, and loss of appetite. In 10% of HBV-infected patients, there are signs of serum sickness (e.g., skin rash, arthralgia, or mild proteinuria).
   - **Icteric phase:** The appearance of jaundice is associated with elevation of LFT and bilirubin in blood, darkening of urine, and acholic stools. Jaundice is usually accompanied by improvement of constitutional symptoms.
   - **Convalescence:** The duration of this recovery phase varies.
   - **Persistent viral infection:** This phase occurs only in HBV and HCV infection.

65. **What are the pathologic features of acute viral hepatitis?**
   Two major features of acute viral hepatitis are lobular disarray and hypercellularity, both of which are related to the following:
   - **Liver cell injury:** Injured liver cells appear ballooned, and there are scattered apoptotic hepatocytes (acidophilic bodies). Scattered mitotic liver cells and several-cell-thick liver cords are signs of regeneration. Bile accumulates inside the hepatocytes, causing feathery degeneration, or in the intercellular canaliculi.
   - **Inflammatory response:** The liver parenchyma contains an increased number of inflammatory cells, including Kupffer cells and macrophages, as well as lymphocytes. Lymphocytes and macrophages also accumulate in the portal tracts.

66. **What are the pathologic features of chronic hepatitis?**
   Chronic hepatitis is pathologically classified as mild, moderate, or severe depending on the extent of liver cell injury, inflammation, and repair:
   - **Liver cell injury:** Injured liver cells resemble those seen in acute hepatitis. There are also scattered apoptotic cells or groups of necrotic liver cells. In many instances, however, lobules contain no obviously damaged cells.
   - **Inflammation:** Infiltrates of lymphocytes, macrophages, and plasma cells are most prominent in portal tracts. These cells spill over across the limiting plate into the lobules. This interface hepatitis is also known as "piecemeal necrosis." Kupffer cells are also prominent and increased in number.
   - **Repair:** Connective tissue septa are laid down to replace damaged liver cells. Fibrosis may be limited to expanded portal, or it may extend into the lobules. Bridging fibrosis connecting adjacent portal tracts or portal tracts with terminal hepatic venules is a sign of severe necrosis of hepatocytes. Coalescence of fibrous strands, associated with regeneration of hepatocytes, may lead to cirrhosis.

67. **Is it possible to make histologically the diagnosis of chronic viral hepatitis?**
   Chronic hepatitis can be diagnosed histologically by liver biopsy. Unfortunately, there are no histologic findings diagnostic of viral hepatitis, and accordingly, microscopy is not a reliable approach to distinguishing chronic viral hepatitis from other nonviral causes of chronic hepatitis (e.g., autoimmune hepatitis and primary biliary cirrhosis).

68. **How can the bacteria reach the liver?**
   Bacterial infection presents in the form of hepatic abscesses (Fig. 13-3). Bacteria may reach the liver hematogenously, through the bile ducts, or by direct invasion or inoculation through the Glisson capsule.

- **Arterial route of infection:** Bacteria reach the liver through the hepatic artery during sepsis or in septic thromboemboli found in bacterial endocarditis. These infections may be caused by a variety of bacteria, such as *Streptococcus*, *Staphylococcus*, and gram-negative bacteria.
- **Portal vein infection:** Bacteria may originate in infected diverticula or mucosal abscesses. In the preantibiotic era, bacterial appendicitis was a common cause of liver abscesses; today it is uncommon in the United States.
- **Ascending biliary infection:** Bacteria ascending into the liver from the duodenum are most often gram negative. Such infections usually occur in patients who have bile stones or other diseases of the biliary tract.
- **Direct invasion of the liver:** Bacterial infection of the gallbladder may extend to the liver. Transdiaphragmatic infection or direct entry of bacteria into the liver from the infected peritoneum is a rare complication of severe infection and is usually found in terminally ill patients or those who have had extensive surgery.
- **Direct inoculation of bacteria:** This type of infection is typically found following penetrating abdominal wounds involving the liver (e.g., knife or bullet).

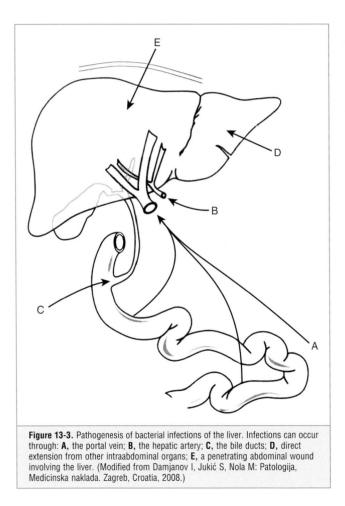

Figure 13-3. Pathogenesis of bacterial infections of the liver. Infections can occur through: **A,** the portal vein; **B,** the hepatic artery; **C,** the bile ducts; **D,** direct extension from other intraabdominal organs; **E,** a penetrating abdominal wound involving the liver. (Modified from Damjanov I, Jukić S, Nola M: Patologija, Medicinska naklada. Zagreb, Croatia, 2008.)

69. **List the most important parasitic and helminthic infections of the liver.**
Parasitic and helminthic infections are rare in the United States but are still important in tropical countries. Such infections include the following:
- Malaria
- Amebiasis
- Leishmaniasis
- Liver fluke infections (*Fasciola hepatica* and *Clonorchis sinensis*)
- *Echinooocous* infection

IMMUNOLOGIC DISEASES OF THE LIVER

70. **What are the most important immunologic diseases of the liver?**
An immunologic pathogenesis has been proposed for several liver diseases, the most important of which are the following:
- Autoimmune hepatitis
- Primary biliary cirrhosis
- Primary sclerosing cholangitis

71. **Define autoimmune hepatitis.**
Autoimmune hepatitis is a form of chronic hepatitis associated with a number of phenomena typically found in systemic autoimmune diseases, such as systemic lupus erythematosus. Hence it is also called lupoid hepatitis. Pathologically, it resembles other forms of chronic hepatitis. In typical cases, the portal tract infiltrates contain prominent plasma cells. However, in many other cases, plasma cells are not so prominent, and the disease cannot be distinguished from other forms of chronic hepatitis.

72. **What are the main features of autoimmune hepatitis?**
- It accounts for 20% of chronic hepatitis cases in the United States.
- It preferentially affects young women (20–30 years). The female-to-male ratio is 4:1.
- Immunoglobulin is elevated in the plasma (IgG > 2.5 g/dL).
- Antibodies to specific autoantigens are found in more than 80% of patients.
- There are two most common clinical forms:
  - Type I (classical) with antibodies to nuclear antigen (ANA), smooth muscle antigen (SMA), and some other antigens
  - Type II with antibodies to liver–kidney microsomes (LKM) and liver cytosolic proteins
- It is often associated with other autoimmune diseases (e.g., rheumatoid arthritis, thyroiditis, Sjögren syndrome).
- Favorable response to corticosteroids (initial response of 80%).

Viral hepatitis must be excluded serologically in all patients suspected of having autoimmune hepatitis. One should note that 10% of HCV-infected patients have the same serologic features typically found in autoimmune hepatitis. Furthermore, 5% of patients with autoimmune hepatitis have false-positive tests for HCV.

KEY POINTS: IMMUNOLOGIC DISEASES OF THE LIVER ✔

1. Autoimmune hepatitis, primary biliary cirrhosis, and primary sclerosing cholangitis are associated with systemic immunologic disorders and other extrahepatic diseases.

2. They are also associated with autoantibodies in blood.

73. **What is primary biliary cirrhosis?**

Primary biliary cirrhosis (PBC) is a disease of unknown origin, characterized by destruction of small intrahepatic bile ducts, progressing over time to cirrhosis. It accounts for 2% of all deaths due to cirrhosis.

Bile duct destruction by T lymphocytes suggests that PBC is caused by a type IV hypersensitivity reaction to autoantigens expressed on bile ductular cells. The presence of antimitochondrial antibodies, found in the blood of most patients, and the coexistence of other autoimmune diseases are more proof of the immunologic nature of PBC. It appears that both cell-mediated and humoral immunity play a role in the pathogenesis of liver injury.

74. **List the main features of PBC.**

- It is an autoimmune disease preferentially affecting women 30 to 60 years old (i.e., older than those with autoimmune hepatitis).
- It has insidious onset (the initial symptoms may be nonspecific), ultimately leading to progressive jaundice associated with pruritus and progressing to liver failure.
- Antibodies to mitochondria are found in 95% of patients.
- Hyperlipidemia (mostly in the form of ↑ high-density lipoprotein) is associated with the formation of dermal xanthomas (aggregates of lipid-laden macrophages).
- Steatorrhea and malabsorption of fat-soluble vitamins may occur. If not corrected, this may cause deficiency of essential nutrients (e.g., osteomalacia due to D-avitaminosis, night blindness due to A-avitaminosis).
- Cirrhosis develops over a period of 10 to 15 years.
- The condition is not curable; liver transplant is the only available treatment for patients with cirrhosis.

75. **What is primary sclerosing cholangitis?**

Primary sclerosing cholangitis (PSC) is a chronic liver disease characterized by chronic inflammation and fibrosis around major intrahepatic and extrahepatic bile ducts. Inflammation is presumed to be of immune origin. Focal fibrosis leads to segmental obliteration of bile ducts. Biliary obstruction leads to secondary biliary cirrhosis.

76. **What are the features of primary sclerosing cholangitis?**

- It is a disease of unknown origin affecting medium sized and large intrahepatic and large extrahepatic bile ducts.
- It predominantly affects males younger than 40 years old (M:F = 2:1).
- Ulcerative colitis is found in 70% of patients.
- It is associated with other fibrosing conditions, such as retroperitoneal fibrosis or Riedel's struma.
- Autoantibodies (e.g., antineutrophil cytoplasmic antibodies and antimitochondrial antibodies) are found in a nondiagnostic pattern and found in only 10% of patients.
- Cholangiography shows typical "beading" due to segmental fibrotic narrowing and subsequent dilatation of intrahepatic bile ducts.
- Cirrhosis develops 5 or 6 years after the onset of the first symptoms.
- The incidence of cholangiocarcinoma is 10%.
- The only treatment available is liver transplantation.

77. **What is the difference between primary and secondary biliary cirrhosis?**

Primary biliary cirrhosis is an autoimmune disease. Cirrhosis develops because of autoimmune destruction of intrahepatic bile ducts and fibrous repair of these lesions.

Secondary biliary cirrhosis develops in response to chronic bile duct obstruction. The causes of secondary biliary cirrhosis are PSC, cholelithiasis, bile duct atresia, and other causes of extrahepatic biliary obstruction. Biliary stasis leads to the destruction of bile ducts and fibrous repair, which ultimately subdivides the liver into small nodules typical of cirrhosis.

78. **Can one distinguish primary biliary cirrhosis from secondary biliary cirrhosis or classic portal cirrhosis?**

    Not really. In most instances, the end-stage liver disease has the same morphologic features, and accordingly, stage III primary biliary cirrhosis cannot be confidently distinguished from secondary biliary cirrhosis or other forms of cirrhosis. Pathologists used to state that biliary cirrhosis typically leads to greenish-yellow discoloration of the liver due to bile stasis, but similar changes can occur in other forms of cirrhosis as well. The diagnosis is based on clinical data and the knowledge of the preexisting disease.

LIVER INJURY BY DRUGS, ALCOHOL, TOXINS, AND METABOLITES

79. **How do drugs affect the liver?**

    Drug-induced liver injury may result from:
    - Direct toxicity
    - Indirect toxicity caused by metabolites and free radicals formed from the metabolized drug
    - Immune reaction against the drug or its metabolites (Some drugs may also combine with tissue proteins and act as haptens, forming "neoantigens" that evoke an autoimmune reaction.)

80. **List two main forms of drug reactions.**

    - **Predictable:** It is typically dose related. For example, acetaminophen taken in small amounts is innocuous but in large doses will always cause liver necrosis.
    - **Unpredictable:** These reactions, also called idiosyncratic, occur for unknown reasons in some patients.

81. **List the drug-related changes that can be recognized microscopically in liver biopsy.**

    - **Cholestasis:** Bile accumulation inside the hepatocytes and in the intercellular canaliculi represents the most common drug-related injury. It may be caused by chlorpromazine, oral contraceptives, or antibiotics.
    - **Fatty change:** Small lipid droplets in liver cells (microvesicular steatosis) are typically found in almost all patients treated with tetracycline.
    - **Hepatitis-like changes:** Changes resembling acute or chronic hepatitis are found in some patients treated with methyldopa, isoniazid, nitrofurantoin, or other drugs.
    - **Granuloma:** Noncaseating granulomas are seen in some patients treated with sulfonamides, hydralazine, allopurinol, and other drugs.
    - **Necrosis:** Acetaminophen, the most common cause of intoxication in the United States, typically causes a dose-related necrosis of liver cells.
    - **Fibrosis:** Fibrosis develops in some patients treated with methotrexate or amiodarone.

KEY POINTS: LIVER INJURY BY DRUGS ✓

1. Drug-induced liver injury can be predictable and dose related or unpredictable and most often related to the formation of toxic metabolites or hypersensitivity to drugs.

2. Alcohol is the most common cause of liver injury in the United States, and it is known to induce fatty change, alcoholic hepatitis, or cirrhosis.

82. **List three liver diseases caused by alcohol.**

    Three pathologic changes are linked to alcohol abuse:
    - **Fatty change:** Essentially all chronic alcoholics have fatty livers (steatosis). The liver is enlarged, fatty, and yellow, but patients usually have no significant clinical symptoms.

- **Alcoholic hepatitis:** Acute inflammation with fibrosis is found in approximately 15% of chronic alcoholics. Fever, leukocytosis, and abnormal laboratory findings are typically found during the acute phase of the disease. The disease is still reversible, but many patients who continue drinking develop cirrhosis.
- **Alcoholic cirrhosis:** Cirrhosis develops in approximately 10% to 15% of all chronic alcoholics.

83. **Are any histologic features found in liver biopsy diagnostic of alcoholic hepatitis?**
    None of the histologic changes seen in liver biopsies are pathognomonic of alcohol abuse. Nevertheless, if found in a chronic alcoholic who shows clinical signs of acute inflammatory disease, such changes are supportive of the diagnosis of alcoholic hepatitis. Liver biopsy is used to confirm the clinical suspicion of alcoholic hepatitis. Furthermore, the biopsy is used to establish whether the liver disease is progressing to cirrhosis or is still reversible.

84. **What is hemochromatosis and how does it affect the liver?**
    Hemochromatosis is characterized by iron accumulation in the body. It occurs in two forms: genetic (primary or hereditary) and secondary. The liver is a major iron storage site and is often affected.

85. **What is hereditary hemochromatosis?**
    Hereditary hemochromatosis is an autosomal recessive disease caused by a mutation of a gene encoding the protein that regulates the absorption of iron in the intestine. Mutations of this gene are found at a rate of 1:9; accordingly, homozygotes are found in the general population at a rate of 1:220. The incidence of hemochromatosis is 1:400, indicating that not all homozygotes will develop the disease.

86. **What are the clinical features of hereditary hemochromatosis?**
    In the classical form it is known as "bronze diabetes with cirrhosis." Clinical findings resulting from the accumulation of iron in various organs include:
    - Cirrhosis of the liver (The liver is dark brown ["pigmentary cirrhosis"] because of the accumulation of hemosiderin in liver cells, bile ducts, and Kupffer cells.)
    - Diabetes mellitus
    - Hyperpigmentation of the skin
    - Arthritis
    - Cardiomyopathy (Together with cirrhosis, it is the most common cause of death in these patients.)
    - Endocrine gland atrophy (Atrophy occurs at a variable rate and involves the thyroid, testes, pituitary.)

87. **What is Wilson disease?**
    Also known as hepatolenticular degeneration, it is an autosomal recessive disorder of copper excretion in the bile. It has a prevalence of 3 per 100,000. Clinical pathologic features are related to the deposition of excessive amounts of copper in various organs and include the following:
    - **Liver disease:** It begins as fatty liver, progressing to acute and chronic hepatitis and ultimately terminating in cirrhosis. Increased amounts of copper in liver biopsy are typically found; accordingly, the liver biopsy is important for the diagnosis of this disease.
    - **Neurologic symptoms:** These include motor disturbances (resembling Parkinson disease) and behavioral changes requiring psychiatric treatment. Copper accumulates in the basal ganglia, leading to neurotoxic changes, which are most prominent in the putamen.

- **Eye lesions:** Deposits of iron in the Descemet membrane lead to the formation of a green or brown Kayser–Fleischer ring.
- **Kidney changes:** These lead to proteinuria, aminoaciduria, and phosphaturia and are evidence of renal tubular injury. Renal changes are related to osteomalacia.
- **Hemolytic episodes:** These occur in 15% of patients and are related to copper toxicity.

88. **How is Wilson disease diagnosed?**
    The diagnosis of Wilson disease is based on correlating clinical and laboratory findings. Typical laboratory findings include the following:
    - Increased concentration of copper in liver tissue, usually obtained by biopsy
    - Decreased serum ceruloplasmin
    - Increased urinary copper excretion

89. **How does α1-antitrypsin (AAT) deficiency affect the liver?**
    The gene encoding AAT is polymorphic, and its mutations may result in several genotypes. Most dangerous is the PiZZ genotype. This mutation is accompanied by 90% inhibition of hepatic secretion of AAT. Although AAT accumulates in the liver cells of all those who have this genotype, only 10% of affected people develop cirrhosis. The pathogenesis of cirrhosis is not fully understood.

90. **What are the liver diseases caused by AAT deficiency?**
    Major deleterious genotypes of mutated AAT are found in 1 in 2000 people. Most of these people will have no major liver disease. Liver disease may present in several forms:
    - **Neonatal hepatitis:** Severe jaundice develops in approximately 15% of infants born with this disease. The outcome of such a jaundice is unpredictable; it may subside or progress to liver failure and cirrhosis. AAT deficiency accounts for 30% of all conjugated hyperbilirubinemias of infancy.
    - **Cirrhosis:** This develops in approximately 10% of adults carrying the mutated gene.
    - **Hepatocellular carcinoma:** This develops in 2% of those who carry the AAT mutation. Most liver cancers arise in the context of cirrhosis, but in some cases the liver shows no evidence of cirrhosis.

91. **Can one recognize histologically the accumulation of AAT in hepatocytes?**
    AAT accumulates in the rough endoplasmic reticulum of liver cells. Over time, it aggregates into eosinophilic droplets that are readily seen in liver cells. These cytoplasmic droplets stain red with PAS. Immunohistochemical staining with antibodies to AAT provides the definitive proof that the droplets are AAT and not some other protein.

CIRRHOSIS

92. **What is cirrhosis?**
    Cirrhosis, a term derived from the Greek word for "yellow" (*kirrhos*), is a synonym for chronic end-stage liver disease. It is characterized by:
    - Loss of normal acinar organization of the liver parenchyma
    - Replacement of normal liver acini by liver cell nodules that can be seen on macroscopic or microscopic examination of the liver
    - Irregular fibrosis forming septa between the nodules of liver cells

93. **Are cirrhotic livers typically small or large?**
    The size of cirrhotic livers varies: Some are enlarged, whereas others are much smaller than normal. In alcoholic cirrhosis, the liver is usually fatty and enlarged. If the alcoholic patient stops drinking, the fat will disappear, and the liver will shrink in size. In cirrhosis following chronic viral hepatitis, the liver is usually of normal size or smaller than normal.

KEY POINTS: CIRRHOSIS ✔

1. Cirrhosis, another name for chronic liver disease, can have many causes but is most often a consequence of viral hepatitis and alcoholism.

2. There are several pathologic types of cirrhosis, but all are fatal unless treated by liver homotransplantation.

94. **What is the difference between portal and biliary cirrhosis?**
Portal cirrhosis, also known as Laennec cirrhosis, is the term used to describe the "classical" micronodular cirrhosis caused by alcohol abuse or viral hepatitis. It was assumed that the initial lesions in such livers are septa forming between portal tracts across the terminal hepatic venule (i.e., across the entire acinus). Biliary cirrhosis, found in conditions accompanied by prolonged biliary obstruction, was thought to result from bridging fibrosis connecting the adjacent portal tract. In typical cases, such septa appear to form "arcade-like arches" and are accompanied by yellow or greenish discoloration of liver parenchyma by bile. Although the terms portal and biliary cirrhosis are widely used, in practice it is difficult to classify each specific case into one or the other category.

95. **What is cardiac cirrhosis?**
Cardiac cirrhosis develops because of prolonged chronic passive congestion of the liver. Accumulation of blood in the terminal hepatic venule (THV) and adjacent sinusoids leads to atrophy of hepatocytes in zone 3. These hepatocytes are replaced by fibrous tissue forming bridges between THV and THV in adjacent acini. Cardiac cirrhosis is not accompanied by clinical and laboratory findings typical of "true" cirrhosis. The diagnosis is usually made at autopsy, most often in patients who had constrictive pericarditis.

96. **List the most common causes of cirrhosis in the United States.**
   - Alcohol abuse
   - Viral hepatitis (HBV and HCV)
   - Autoimmune diseases (PBC, autoimmune hepatitis, and PSC)
   - Biliary diseases
   - Metabolic and hereditary diseases (e.g., hereditary hemochromatosis, AAT deficiency, Wilson disease, and cystic fibrosis)
   - Cryptogenic (unknown etiology; 15%–20%)
   Alcohol abuse and viral hepatitis C infection, often combined one with the other, account for most cases of cirrhosis.

97. **Is cirrhosis reversible?**
Fibrosis of the liver, the most prominent feature of cirrhosis, is irreversible. There is no medical treatment for this end-stage liver disease. The only treatment for this invariably lethal disease is liver transplantation.

LIVER TUMORS

98. **How are primary liver tumors classified?**
Tumors are classified clinically as benign or malignant. According to their cell of origin, liver tumors are classified into three groups:
   - Liver cell tumors (liver cell adenoma, hepatoblastoma, and hepatocellular carcinoma)
   - Bile ductal tumors (cholangiocarcinoma)
   - Vascular tumors (hemangioma and angiosarcoma)

99. **What is the most common benign tumor of the liver?**

It is hemangioma. These small tumors, composed of blood vessels, are found incidentally in 7% of livers. Usually, they are asymptomatic and of no clinical significance. Larger tumors are visible on computed tomography (CT) scans and are included in the differential diagnosis of hepatic nodular lesions, such as adenomas and focal nodular hyperplasia.

100. **What is the clinical significance of liver cell adenomas?**

Liver cell adenomas are benign tumors composed of well differentiated hepatocytes. Tumor cells resemble normal liver cells. Most tumors cause no symptoms and are diagnosed incidentally (e.g., by CT scan).

Large tumors discovered by CT scan may be confused with hepatocellular carcinoma. Although malignant transformation of these adenomas is rare, it is advisable to resect all liver tumors that measure more than a few centimeters in diameter.

Subcapsular adenomas may be vascular and are prone to rupture. Massive bleeding may cause hematoperitoneum and hypovolemic shock.

Liver cell adenomas occur more often in women than in men and are thought to be induced by estrogen. Tumors found in women taking oral contraceptives may regress on discontinuation of contraceptives.

101. **What is focal nodular hyperplasia (FNH)?**

FNH is a circumscribed nodule found in an otherwise normal liver. It represents a hamartoma composed of liver cells arranged around a central fibrotic scar containing thick-walled vessels. The scar and the fibrous septa radiating from it contain infiltrates of lymphocytes and proliferating bile ducts. These findings are similar to those encountered in cirrhosis. Hence, FNH is also known as localized cirrhosis.

FNH is usually diagnosed incidentally during surgery or CT scan. It should be distinguished from other nodular lesions. FNHs do not undergo malignant transformation.

KEY POINTS: LIVER TUMORS ✅

1. Benign tumors and tumor-like conditions, such as hemangioma (the most common liver tumor), liver cell adenoma, and focal nodular hyperplasia, are of limited clinical significance.

2. Primary malignant tumors, such as hepatocellular carcinoma and cholangiocarcinoma, are lethal but uncommon in the United States.

3. Metastases to the liver are much more common than primary malignant liver tumors.

4. α-fetoprotein (AFP) is a good serologic marker for liver cell carcinoma.

102. **List key facts about the epidemiology of hepatocellular carcinoma (HCC).**

HCC, also known as malignant hepatoma, is the most common liver tumor worldwide. Important facts about the epidemiology of this tumor are as follows:

- Incidence shows broad geographic variation. In the United States, the incidence is 3 per 100,000. In areas of Africa (e.g., Mozambique) and Asia (e.g., Korea, Taiwan, and south China), the incidence is 50 times higher (i.e., 150:100,000)
- High incidence of HCC in areas of the world correlates with the prevalence of HBV and virus-related cirrhosis in these countries.
- HBV and HCV play a role in the carcinogenesis of HCC.

- Aflatoxins, fungus-derived carcinogens that are widespread in some underdeveloped countries, probably play a pathogenetic role as well.
- Men are more often affected, but the male-to-female ratio also shows geographic variability, from 4:1 in the United States to 9:1 in endemic areas of Asia and Africa.

103. **Do all hepatocellular carcinomas develop in cirrhotic livers?**
No. Most (80%) cases of HCC develop in the background of cirrhosis. The remaining 20% of HCC cases arise in normal livers or from preexisting adenomas. Fibrolamellar HCC, a tumor with a better prognosis than classical HCC, typically occurs in otherwise normal livers of young people.

104. **Describe the macroscopic features of hepatocellular carcinoma.**
HCC appear in three forms:
- **Unifocal:** The tumor may present as a large mass replacing part of the liver or a nodule of a different color and consistency in a cirrhotic liver.
- **Multifocal:** These tumors present as nodules involving parts of the liver. The nodules may be grouped or widely scattered.
- **Diffusely infiltrative:** These tumors permeate and diffusely enlarge the liver. Tumor cells penetrate the cirrhotic liver, becoming imperceptibly intermixed with the remaining liver cells.

105. **Describe the typical histologic features of hepatocellular carcinoma.**
HCCs present histologically as well differentiated, moderately well differentiated, and poorly differentiated carcinomas. In well-differentiated tumors, the tumor cells resemble normal liver cells. For example, tumor cells may secrete bile, which accumulates in the intercellular canaliculi. In undifferentiated tumors, the cells are anaplastic, retaining only a vague resemblance to hepatocytes. Such cells may be small with a high nuclear-to-cytoplasmic ratio or large and even multinucleated.
Tumor cells grow in several histologic patterns described as trabecular, pseudoglandular, acinar, or otherwise. Recognition of these patterns is useful for the histologic diagnosis of HCC but is of no clinical significance.

106. **Do all histologic forms of HCC have the same prognosis?**
No. HCCs generally have an abysmal prognosis, and in most instances death occurs within 1 year of diagnosis. Those with small, resectable tumors, accounting for 20% to 30% of cases, have a better survival. In that group, the best prognosis is assigned to fibrolamellar carcinomas. These tumors are composed of large cells with well-developed cytoplasm. Strands of tumor cells are enclosed in dense connective tissue. Surgical resection of fibrolamellar hepatocellular carcinomas is associated with a 60% 5-year survival rate.

107. **What is the significance of alpha-fetoprotein (AFP) in the diagnosis of hepatocellular carcinoma?**
AFP, a protein normally secreted by fetal hepatocytes, is found only in minute amounts in adult blood (<40 ng/dL). Serum levels of AFP are markedly elevated in most patients (85%) harboring an HCC. Accordingly, AFP is a useful serologic marker of HCC.

108. **List common symptoms and signs of hepatocellular carcinoma.**
- Abdominal pain (stretching of liver capsule) and fever (cytokines, tumor necrosis)
- Weight loss and weakness (tumor acts as parasite)
- Enlarged liver may be palpated
- Ascites may increase in size (portal vein occlusion by tumor) and become hemorrhagic
- Liver failure (tumor replacing normal liver)
- Bleeding from esophageal varices or tumor ruptured into abdominal cavity

- AFP elevated in blood 10 to 100 times above normal
- CT and ultrasound may demonstrate masses in the liver
- Radiologically guided or open surgical biopsy essential for definitive histologic typing of the tumor

109. **How do hepatocellular carcinomas metastasize?**
HCCs have a tendency to invade vascular spaces and metastasize via blood. Hematogenous metastases are most often found in the lungs. Local extension to hilar lymph nodes is also common. Intraabdominal spread is usually found in advanced cases.

110. **List important facts about cholangiocarcinoma.**
    - It is an adenocarcinoma arising from bile ducts.
    - It is a rare tumor in the United States, affecting mostly the elderly (>60 years old).
    - Risk factors include PSC; in China, it is related to infestation with *Clonorchis sinensis*.
    - It originates either from intrahepatic or extrahepatic bile ducts.
    - Symptoms are usually nonspecific.
    - Extrahepatic tumors may present with early biliary obstruction.
    - Prognosis is poor (20%–30% 5-year survival).

111. **Are there any serologic markers for cholangiocarcinoma?**
Cholangiocarcinomas are adenocarcinomas, and like adenocarcinomas in other sites, they secrete carcinoembryonic antigen. However, this serologic marker has low sensitivity and specificity and is of limited value in the diagnosis of cholangiocarcinomas, or for distinguishing it from other adenocarcinomas that have metastasized to the liver.

112. **Is liver biopsy essential for the definitive diagnosis of cholangiocarcinoma?**
Yes. Liver biopsy must be performed to determine the nature of the clinically identified liver mass. Cholangiocarcinomas present histologically as adenocarcinomas and are readily distinguished from hepatocellular carcinomas. Unfortunately, cholangiocarcinoma cannot always be distinguished from other adenocarcinomas (e.g., carcinoma of the pancreas or colon) that may have metastasized to the liver. Because metastatic adenocarcinomas are more common than primary hepatic adenocarcinomas, a search for another possible primary tumor should always be undertaken.

113. **How common are metastases to the liver?**
Metastatic tumors are much more common than primary liver tumors, and in the United States metastases are overall the most common malignant tumor of the liver. The reasons for this high incidence of metastasis are not fully known, but some appear self-evident:
    - **Blood flow:** The liver is highly vascularized, receiving blood from the portal vein and the aorta. Thus many tumors circulating in the blood will readily reach it.
    - **Sinusoids:** Fenestration of sinusoids allows tumor cells to exit from circulation easier than through the continuous wall of the capillaries.
    - **Favorable soil:** The liver provides the nutrients and a generally "friendly" environment for the growth of tumor cells.

114. **How do metastases to the liver differ from primary liver tumors?**
Metastases typically have the following characteristics:
    - Multiple rather than solitary
    - Spherical rather than irregularly shaped
    - Centrally indented because of ischemic necrosis of the central part ("umbilication" of the tumor nodules seen on gross examination)
    - Solitary metastases from adenocarcinoma of the GI system or pancreas not readily distinguished from primary cholangiocarcinoma of the liver

BILIARY TRACT

115. **What are the most important diseases of the biliary tract?**
     - Gallstones
     - Inflammation (acute and chronic cholecystitis and cholangitis)
     - Malignant tumors

116. **List the most important facts about gallstones.**
     - It is the most common biliary tract disease: high prevalence: 10% to 20% of adult males and 30% to 40% of adult females are affected.
     - Two types can be recognized macroscopically and by biochemical analysis:
       ○ Cholesterol stones (80%)
       ○ Pigmentary bilirubin stones (20%)
     - It shows geographic variation and is more common in Native Americans than other ethnic groups.

KEY POINTS: BILIARY TRACT ✔

1. Gallstones and gallstone-related inflammation are the most important diseases of the gallbladder and extrahepatic bile ducts.

2. Malignant tumors of the biliary system are rare, occur in older people, and have a poor prognosis.

117. **What are the risk factors for cholesterol gallstones?**
     Risk factors include the six Fs:
     - Female
     - Forty and above
     - Fertile (multiparous)
     - Fat
     - Flatulent (intestinal disease or malabsorption)
     - Familial, including high prevalence in some ethnic groups (e.g., Native Americans)

118. **What are the features of cholesterol stones?**
     Cholesterol stones by definition contain more than 50% cholesterol. These are the typical stones found in obese people. Their incidence increases with age. They occur in two forms:
     - Pure cholesterol stones are rare. They are usually large, solitary, and spherical, resembling a bird's egg. They are hard, and if cracked into pieces, they show a yellow crystalline internal structure.
     - Mixed cholesterol stones, accounting for the majority of stones found clinically, are composed predominantly of cholesterol but also contain variable amounts of bilirubin and calcium salts. Most often, these stones are multiple, and 85% of them are radiolucent and cannot be seen on regular x-ray films.

119. **Describe the features of pigmentary stones.**
     Pigmentary stones are either black or brown:
     - Black stones are composed of calcium bilirubinate, phosphate, carbonate, and very little cholesterol. They are usually multiple, small, and friable. These stones form in the course of chronic hemolytic anemias, such as sickle cell anemia or thalassemia.

- Brown stones are composed of calcium bilirubinate, fatty acids, and cholesterol but do not contain calcium phosphate or carbonate. These stones form in the course of bacterial infections causing deconjugation of bilirubin and in prolonged biliary stasis.

120. **What are the features of acute cholecystitis?**

Acute cholecystitis is a common disease. Typically, it has the following characteristics:

- Females are affected more often than males.
- It is associated with gallstones in 90% cases, but they may be acalculous (10%).
- Secondary bacterial infection follows the obstruction in some cases; *Escherichia coli* is the most common pathogen.
- Typical symptoms include acute onset of pain in the right upper quadrant, fever, and leukocytosis, usually after a heavy meal.
- Mild jaundice is present in 20% of cases because of the impaction of small stones in the common bile duct.
- Pathologically, the gallbladder is dilatated because of cystic duct obstruction; its wall is swollen, and there may be fibrinous exudates on the serosa (if the inflammation is transmural).
- There are microscopic signs of purulent inflammation (neutrophils) in the mucosa or deeper layers of the wall
- Recovery is 90% if the obstruction of bile flow is relieved.

121. **What is chronic cholecystitis?**

This common inflammatory disease affects females more than males. It is the result of repeated attacks of acute cholecystitis or chronic irritation with gallstones. Clinically it presents with indistinct pain in the right upper quadrant 1 or 2 hours after meals.

It is associated with gallstones in 90% of cases. Bacteria (usually *E. coli*) are found in 30% of cases but are considered to be a form of secondary infection of previously damaged gallbladder.

Pathologic features include the following:

- Gallstones in the lumen
- Biliary gravel (thick viscous bile with microconcretions)
- Edematous mucosa, focally ulcerated or indurated
- Wall of gallbladder may be thickened and fibrotic (firm)
- Microscopic examination reveals chronic inflammatory infiltrates and extension of mucosal sinuses into the muscularis (so-called Rokitansky-Aschoff sinuses)

122. **What are the complications of acute and chronic cholecystitis and cholelithiasis?**

Complications result from the spread of bacteria or rupture of the gallbladder and include the following:

- Bacterial superinfection leading to local spread (cholangitis)
- Bacterial dissemination by blood (sepsis)
- Perforation leading to subhepatic abscess or bacterial peritonitis
- Empyema (i.e., accumulation of pus in an obstructed gallbladder)
- Fistula formation between the gallbladder and the intestine (cholecystoenteric fistula)
- Bile stone ileus following the impaction of a gallstone in the intestine; such stones are usually large and enter the intestines through an cholecystoenteric fistula (the common bile duct is too narrow to allow the passage of such large stones)

123. **Describe the "porcelain gallbladder."**

This term is used for gallbladders that have a thick, calcium-encrusted wall. Typically such gallbladders are expanded and have a rigid, thick, white wall. This pathologic change is a consequence of transmural chronic inflammation, evoking extensive fibrosis during the repair phase of the disease. Scarring of the wall, combined with dystrophic calcification, transforms the gallbladder into a porcelain-like vessel. The calcium-encrusted gallbladder can be seen on standard x-ray films.

124. **List the features of gallbladder carcinoma.**
   - Uncommon form of cancer (It accounts for only 5% of all gastrointestinal cancers.)
   - More common in females than in males
   - Affects older persons (average age, 65 years)
   - Associated with gallstones in 90% of cases
   - Porcelain gallbladder (encrusted fibrotic chronic cholecystitis) is a high-risk condition
   - Ethnic distribution (the same as for gallbladder stones): More common in some Native Americans, such as the Pima Indians
   - Adenocarcinoma (90%) and squamous cell carcinoma (10%) (Squamous cell carcinoma arises from squamous metaplasia in chronic cholecystitis and cholelithiasis.)
   - Poor prognosis (5% 5-year survival rate)

125. **List the features of carcinoma of the common bile duct.**
   - Uncommon form of cancer
   - Male-to-female ratio is 1:1
   - No comorbidity with gallstones
   - Jaundice is an early sign of disease (even small tumors cause obstruction)
   - Adenocarcinomas in 100% of cases
   - Poor prognosis (35% 5-year survival rate)

WEBSITES ⊕

1. http://www.nlm.nih.gov/medlineplus/liverdiseases.html

2. http://library.med.utah.edu/WebPath/LIVEHTML/LIVERIDX.html

3. http://www.hepatitis-central.com/hcv/

4. http://www.mayoclinic.com/health/liver-cancer/DS00399

BIBLIOGRAPHY

1. Batts KP, Ludwig J: Chronic hepatitis. An update on terminology and reporting. Am J Surg Pathol 19:1409–1417, 1995.
2. Czaja AJ: Autoimmune liver disease. Curr Opin Gastroenterol 23:255–262, 2007.
3. Czaja AJ, Carpenter HA. Optimizing diagnosis from the medical liver biopsy. Clin Gastroenterol Hepatol 5: 898–907, 2007.
4. De Grien PC, Gores GJ, LaRusso NF, et al: Biliary tract cancer. N Engl J Med 341:1368–1378, 1999.
5. Guidotti LG, Chisari FV: Immunobiology and pathogenesis of viral hepatitis. Annu Rev Pathol 1:23–61, 2006.
6. Pang RW, Poon RT: From molecular biology to targeted therapies for hepatocellular carcinoma: the future is now. Oncology 72(Suppl 1):30–44, 2007.
7. Tilg H, Diehl AM: Cytokines in alcoholic and nonalcoholic steatohepatitis. N Engl J Med 343:1467–1476, 2000.
8. Walsh K, Alexander G: Alcoholic liver disease. Postgrad Med J 76:280–286, 2000.

CHAPTER 14

THE PANCREAS

Ivan Damjanov, MD, PhD

1. **List the most important diseases of the enzymes produced by the exocrine pancreas.**
   Pancreatic acini secrete more than 20 digestive enzymes. These enzymes are released in response to stimulation, which may be neurogenic or hormonal with polypeptide hormones such as cholecystokinin. The most important enzyme disorders are:
   - Developmental disorders
   - Acute and chronic pancreatitis
   - Tumors
   - Diabetes

KEY POINTS: THE PANCREAS ✔

1. The pancreas is an exocrine gland attached to the duodenum that also contains endocrine cells producing insulin, glucagon, and several other polypeptide hormones.

2. The three most important diseases of the pancreas are pancreatitis, pancreatic carcinoma, and diabetes.

DEVELOPMENTAL DISORDERS

2. **Describe annular pancreas.**
   In this anomaly, the head of the pancreas encircles the duodenum. An abnormally shaped pancreas may narrow the duodenum and interfere with the passage of food.

3. **What is pancreas divisum?**
   In this anomaly, there are two separate pancreases, each of which is attached to the duodenum by a separate duct. This anomaly results from incomplete fusion of the two fetal pancreatic anlagen.

4. **Where is aberrant pancreatic tissue most often found?**
   Pancreatic acini and islets may be found anywhere in the other parts of the gastrointestinal tract in 2% of normal people. Most often, such choristomas are found in the duodenum and the stomach. These lesions are usually accidentally discovered during histologic examination of gastrointestinal organs resected or biopsied for an unrelated reason. Larger masses may be mistaken for tumors.

INFLAMMATION

5. **What is acute pancreatitis?**
    Acute pancreatitis is in most instances a sterile (noninfectious) chemically mediated inflammation of the pancreas resulting from injury of the exocrine pancreas. It occurs in two forms:
    - **Interstitial or edematous pancreatitis:** This mild inflammation is characterized by edema and widening of interstitial spaces that contain scattered inflammatory cells. There is no or only minor necrosis of acinar cells. Interstitial pancreatitis occurs relatively often in severely sick people, in various forms of shock, and after prolonged operations. It may be recognized by mild elevation of pancreatic enzymes in blood. It requires no treatment and heals spontaneously.
    - **Acute hemorrhagic pancreatitis:** This is a severe and life-threatening condition, which is not common.

6. **Describe the pathogenesis of acute hemorrhagic pancreatitis.**
    Acute hemorrhagic pancreatitis is an acute inflammatory process caused by enzyme-mediated destruction of pancreatic and peripancreatic tissue. The key event is the inappropriate activation of pancreatic digestive enzymes inside the ducts and acini of the exocrine pancreas. Activated enzymes act on the pancreatic cells, which leads to additional release of digestive enzymes into the interstitial and peripancreatic tissues and blood vessels.

7. **Describe the sequence of a hypothetical event leading to acute pancreatitis.**
    The inappropriate activation of enzymes inside the pancreas leading to autodigestion is thought to occur in the following sequence (Fig. 14-1):

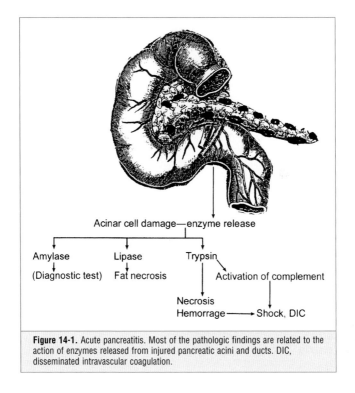

Figure 14-1. Acute pancreatitis. Most of the pathologic findings are related to the action of enzymes released from injured pancreatic acini and ducts. DIC, disseminated intravascular coagulation.

- Obstruction of the terminal portions of the choledochopancreatic duct
- Reflux of bile into the pancreatic ducts
- Increased pressure inside the excretory portion of the pancreas that reverses the flow of bicarbonate-rich pancreatic juices backward into the acini
- Activation of pancreatic lytic enzymes in the small ducts and acini
- Rupture of damaged acinar cells leading to a release of digestive enzymes into the interstitial spaces and peripancreatic tissue
- Autodigestion of proteins, lipids, and carbohydrate moieties of cells forming the pancreas, peripancreatic fat tissue, and blood vessels

8. **List the most common causes of acute pancreatitis.**
Most cases of acute hemorrhagic pancreatitis (>80%) are related to biliary tract disease and alcohol abuse. Bile stones are known to obstruct the common choledochopancreatic duct and thus cause reflux of bile into the pancreas. Alcohol is thought to cause a spasm of the sphincter of Oddi that may also lead to reflux.

9. **List other exogenous causes of acute pancreatitis.**
   - Drugs (More than 100 drugs are known to cause pancreatitis, but most often it occurs in patients taking azathioprine and mercaptopurine (2% of patients may have mild pancreatitis). Corticosteroids and high doses of estrogens are also associated with higher incidence of pancreatitis.)
   - Trauma (e.g., seatbelt injury)
   - Surgery (Surgeons refrain from operating on or palpating the pancreas unless it is essential for the treatment.)
   - Diagnostic procedures (Endoscopic retrograde cholangiopancreatography [ERCP] used to visualize pancreatic ducts and obtain cytologic samples may damage the pancreas. Note that it is not advisable to perform diagnostic fine needle aspiration biopsies of the pancreas.)
   - Sepsis
   - Hypotension (e.g., shock following massive bleeding)
   - Viruses (mumps virus, cytomegalovirus—especially in acquired immune deficiency syndrome [AIDS])

10. **List endogenous causes of acute pancreatitis.**
   - **Hyperlipidemia:** Obesity is a known risk factor, but the exact mechanism of pancreatic injury is not completely understood. It is thought that fatty acids may injure acinar cells. Endogenous hyperlipidemia (especially type V) is also associated with an increased incidence of acute pancreatitis.
   - **Hypercalcemia:** Calcium is thought to activate trypsin in the pancreas.
   - **Familial pancreatitis:** The cause of this disease is not known.
   - **Idiopathic pancreatitis:** This can occur without any obvious cause and accounts for 10% of cases; it is the most common cause of pancreatitis (after alcohol and biliary disease).

11. **What are the gross pathologic features of acute hemorrhagic pancreatitis?**
   - Enlargement of the pancreas that is focally hemorrhagic or necrotic is seen.
   - Necrosis of fat tissue around the pancreas or omentum: Fat necrosis leads to the formation of fat soaps. These foci appear white, resembling chalk.
   - Ascites is found in severe cases. The fluid is turbid, brownish yellow, or blood tinged.

12. **Describe the histologic findings in acute pancreatitis.**
   - **Necrosis of pancreatic acini, ducts, and blood vessels:** In these anatomic sites, the component cells lose their outlines and nuclei.
   - **Fat necrosis:** Fat cells become indistinct and lose their internal structure. The entire field appears bluish because of the deposition of calcium salts. Specks of calcium soaps appear like dark blue aggregates or amorphous material.

- **Hemorrhage:** Blood infiltrates the tissues.
- **Acute inflammation:** Neutrophils invade the necrotic tissue. In later stages, neutrophils are replaced by macrophages and the entire area undergoes fibrosis.

13. **What are the most important local complications of acute hemorrhagic pancreatitis?**
    - **Pseudocyst:** Massive necrosis leads to liquefactive necrosis of the tissue, which becomes enclosed by granulation tissue. The granulation tissue transforms into a fibrous scar that contains the fluid full of pancreatic enzymes.
    - **Abscess:** Infection superimposed on pancreatic necrosis leads to abscess formation. It is associated with high mortality.
    - **Hemorrhagic ascites:** Bleeding occurs from enzymatically damaged blood vessels.

14. **What are the systemic (distant) complications of acute hemorrhagic pancreatitis?**
    - **Shock:** It is multifactorial but mostly due to increased vascular permeability caused by the action of pancreatic enzyme.
    - **Disseminated intravascular coagulation:** Endothelial injury caused by pancreatic enzymes in circulation leads to the formation of platelet and fibrin thrombi in small vessels.
    - **Adult respiratory distress syndrome:** It is a manifestation of shock, but it also evolves because of enzymatic injury of the alveolar–capillary units in the lungs. Alveolar–capillary injury is accompanied by facilitated passage of fluids into the alveoli (pulmonary edema) and the formation of hyaline membranes.
    - **Renal failure:** It is mostly a consequence of shock and other complications.
    - **Subcutaneous fat necrosis:** Foci of fat necrosis develop unpredictably and are related to the action of lipolytic enzymes that have entered the circulation.

15. **What are typical symptoms and signs of acute hemorrhagic pancreatitis?**
    - Sudden onset of severe abdominal pain
    - Pain more prominent in the left upper quadrant of the abdomen; may radiate into the back
    - Nausea and vomiting, aggravated by eating
    - General distress with fever, sweating, tachypnea, and tachycardia

16. **Which enzymes appear in high concentration in blood during an attack of acute hemorrhagic pancreatitis?**
    - **Amylase:** It is a sensitive marker of acute pancreatitis, especially if the elevation is 4 times above normal values. Amylase appears in blood within hours of the onset of pancreatic injury. However, hyperamylasemia is not specific for acute pancreatitis, and it may be of extrapancreatic origin. For example, after cardiac surgery 30% of patients have hyperamylasemia, 50% of which is of salivary gland origin. The fallopian tubes also contain amylase, and it may be elevated in extrauterine pregnancy.
    - **Lipase:** It appears slightly later in blood, but it is more specific than amylase.
    - **Trypsin:** This enzyme has the highest specificity and sensitivity for pancreatic injury, but the measurement requires the use of a radioimmunoassay, which is not available in all hospitals.

17. **Which other tests give abnormal results in acute pancreatitis?**
    - **Leukocytosis:** This is self-evident because pancreatitis is associated with a mobilization of neutrophils that infiltrate the necrotic tissue.
    - **Hypocalcemia:** Fat necrosis leads to local formation of calcium soaps, and this process consumes calcium from the blood, typically leading to hypocalcemia 2 to 4 days after the onset of acute pancreatitis.
    - **Urinary amylase:** Amylase is excreted in urine, which leads to a decrease in serum amylase concentration 2 to 4 days after the onset of acute pancreatitis. Amylase levels in

urine become elevated from the second day on and may remain elevated for 7 to 10 days. This test has little specificity and sensitivity.

- **Aspartate aminotransferase, alanine aminotransferase, and alkaline phosphatase:** Elevation of these enzymes reflects liver injury and cholestasis, especially in patients who have cholelithiasis.

18. **Which other tests and examinations should be performed in patients suspected of having acute hemorrhagic pancreatitis?**
    - **X-rays:** Plain x-rays are important to exclude rupture of an ulcer (air visible), but computed tomography (CT) scan must be used for demonstrating the enlargement of the pancreas suffused with blood.
    - **Ascites:** The fluid should be analyzed biochemically because it may contain increased amounts of pancreatic enzymes. The tapped fluid should also be cultured for bacteria because infection has a bad prognosis and must be treated immediately.

KEY POINTS: PANCREATIC INFLAMMATION ✔

1. In 80% of cases, acute pancreatitis is related to alcohol intake and biliary diseases.

2. Pancreatic pseudocyst is a consequence of massive necrosis in acute pancreatitis.

3. Chronic pancreatitis is associated with pancreatic insufficiency and malabsorption, characterized by steatorrhea.

19. **What is the outcome of acute hemorrhagic pancreatitis?**
    Most patients recover if treated appropriately. Mortality is 10%, but in children it may be high (25%). Unfavorable prognostic factors are old age, severe leukocytosis (>16,000), decrease in the hematocrit, elevation of blood glucose, and elevated liver function tests. Decreased serum calcium and PaO_2 and elevated blood urea nitrogen are also signs of severe disease.

20. **What is chronic pancreatitis?**
    Chronic pancreatitis is a chronic inflammation with fibrosis leading to a progressive loss of pancreatic function. The pancreas is reduced in size, firm, and often shows calcifications. Histologically, there is:
    - Persistent chronic inflammation composed of infiltrates of lymphocytes, macrophages, and plasma cells
    - Fibrosis, calcification, and intraductal concretions
    - Loss and atrophy of acini, with partial preservation of ducts and islets of Langerhans
    - Cystic dilatation of ducts distal to narrowing by fibrous tissue

21. **What are the causes of chronic pancreatitis?**
    Chronic pancreatitis is usually the outcome of recurrent attacks of acute pancreatitis. The most common cause is chronic alcohol abuse. In patients who do not drink, the cause usually remains unknown, and the disease is considered to be idiopathic. Less common causes include cystic fibrosis of the pancreas, familial chronic pancreatitis, and "tropical chronic pancreatitis."

22. **What are the clinical features of chronic pancreatitis?**
    - Persistent upper abdominal pain radiating into the back, often precipitated by alcohol (These symptoms are related to the involvement of nerves by fibrosis.)
    - Malabsorption due to pancreatic insufficiency—steatorrhea and vitamins A, D, E, and K deficiency

- Diabetes mellitus (Secondary diabetes develops in 30%–40% of patients.)
- X-ray finding of calcifications and distorted ducts by ERCP

23. **What is the usual outcome of chronic pancreatitis?**
Chronic pancreatitis is an incurable, debilitating disease. Patients suffer from relentless pain, malabsorption, wasting, and diabetes but may live for a long time. Overall there is a 3% yearly cumulative mortality. Most patients die of intercurrent infections or other complications of chronic alcoholism.

TUMORS

24. **How are pancreatic tumors classified on the basis of their cell of origin?**
    - Ductal tumors (90%)
    - Islet cell tumors (5%)
    - Acinar tumors (2%)
    - Others (e.g., connective tissue tumors)

25. **How common is pancreatic cancer?**
    - The incidence is 10:100,000 and is increasing.
    - It is the second most common cancer of the gastrointestinal system and the fifth most frequent cause of cancer death.
    - Approximately 25,000 people die of carcinoma of the pancreas annually, which accounts for 6% of all cancer deaths.
    - It is the fourth most common cause of cancer-related deaths in the United States in men and the fifth among women.

26. **Who is affected by carcinoma of the pancreas?**
    - Most patients are older (>60 years old); tumor is rare before age 50 years.
    - Males and females are almost equally affected (male:female ratio, 1.3:1).
    - No definite cause identified.
    - Cigarette smoking has a risk of 2.5 times.
    - Chronic pancreatitis has a risk of 9 times, but because it is a rare disease, it accounts for only a small number of cancers.
    - Diet high in fat and low in vegetables has a risk of 1.4 times.

27. **What are the pathologic features of carcinoma of the pancreas?**
    - Indurated white mass enlarging parts of the pancreas (may be confused with chronic pancreatitis)
    - Head is involved most often (60%), but may occur in any part of the pancreas
    - Histologically, adenocarcinoma with desmoplastic stroma

KEY POINTS: TUMORS ✓

1. Adenocarcinomas arising from the ducts account for 90% of pancreatic neoplasms.

2. Carcinoma of the pancreas is an incurable disease of old age.

3. Islet cell tumors cause endocrine symptoms.

28. **What are the clinical features of carcinoma of the pancreas?**
    - Pain is usually the first symptom. It may be vague but persistent and usually progressive.
    - Weight loss, anorexia, and fatigue occur.
    - Jaundice is seen.
    - Migratory superficial thrombophlebitis (Trousseau sign) is seen.

29. **What are the best diagnostic tests for carcinoma of the pancreas?**
    - Ultrasonography and CT scan usually provide evidence of the mass.
    - ERCP is used to visualize the ducts and obtain cells for cytopathology.
    - Surgical exploration is used to obtain tissues for the final diagnosis and determine whether the tumor is operable.
    - There are no good serologic markers. Carcinoembryonic antigen is elevated in blood but not useful for diagnosis (too nonspecific).

30. **What is the prognosis of carcinoma of the pancreas?**
    Prognosis is extremely poor, and only 10% of patients survive 2 years.

31. **Are there any benign pancreatic tumors?**
    Yes, but they are rare. Tumors of this kind include mucinous and serous cystadenomas.

32. **List the most important features of endocrine tumors of the pancreas.**
    - Endocrine tumors are rare. The incidence is 1:1 million.
    - Histology includes cords and nests of uniform cells with round nuclei and a moderate amount of cytoplasm (identical to intestinal or bronchial carcinoids).
    - Histologically, benign tumors cannot be distinguished from malignant ones. Metastasis is the only definitive sign that a tumor is malignant.
    - Most (75%) are low-grade malignant tumors (except insulinomas, which are 90% benign).
    - They secrete hormones that produce typical syndromes.
    - Tumors are classified according to the secretory function of their cells:
      - Insulinomas (beta cell tumors)
      - Glucagonomas (alpha cell tumors)
      - Gastrinomas
      - Somatostatinomas
      - VIPomas (vasoactive polypeptide secreting tumors)
      - PPomas (pancreatic polypeptide secreting tumors)

33. **What are the features of insulinoma?**
    - The most common endocrine tumor of the pancreas
    - Most are small (<3 cm)
    - Benign (90%), only rarely malignant (10%)
    - Secrete insulin into the blood and cause episodes of hypoglycemia
    - Stroma of the tumor may contain amyloid (from precursor amylin)

34. **What are the symptoms of insulinoma?**
    Sudden onset of hypoglycemia recognized by the following symptoms (Whipple triad):
    - Sweating
    - Fainting, blurry vision, and loss of consciousness
    - Recovery upon intake of sugar

35. **What are the features of gastrinoma?**
    - Second most common endocrine tumor of the pancreas
    - Most (80%) are low-grade malignant
    - Originates from endocrine stem cells (normal islets do not contain gastrin-secreting cells)

- Similar tumors may develop in the duodenum
- Hypergastrinemia is associated with hypersecretion of HCl in stomach
- Zollinger–Ellison syndrome is the typical clinical presentation

36. **What are the features of Zollinger–Ellison syndrome?**
    - Gastrin-secreting tumor (80% in the pancreas, 15% in the duodenum, and 5% in other sites)
    - Hypergastrinemia (demonstrable in blood)
    - Peptic ulcers, solitary or multiple. Diagnosis of Zollinger–Ellison syndrome suspected if ulcers are:
      o Multiple
      o Unusual site (e.g., jejunum and Meckel diverticulum)
      o Resistant to standard ulcer therapy
      o Occur in the setting of multiple endocrine neoplasia

37. **What are the features of glucagonoma syndrome?**
    - Increased levels of glucagons in blood
    - Mild diabetes and hyperglycemia
    - Necrotizing migratory erythema (characteristic)
    - Venous thrombosis or anemia of unknown etiology

38. **What are the symptoms caused by VIPoma?**
    Increased levels of vasoactive intestinal polypeptide (VIP) in blood are associated with clinical symptoms typical of the Verner–Morrison syndrome, also known as WDHA syndrome (watery diarrhea, hypokalemia, and achlorhydria).

39. **What are the symptoms caused by somatostatinoma?**
    Increased blood levels of somatostatin are associated with inhibition of the function of other islet cells. Symptoms and signs include:
    - Mild diabetes
    - Gastric hypochlorhydria
    - Steatorrhea
    - Gallstone formation

40. **What are the features of multiple endocrine neoplasia-1 (MEN-1)?**
    - Pituitary tumor
    - Parathyroid tumor or hyperplasia
    - Gastrinoma of pancreas (Zollinger–Ellison syndrome)

41. **What are the features of MEN-2A?**
    - Medullary carcinoma of the thyroid
    - Pheochromocytoma
    - Parathyroid adenoma

42. **What are the features of MEN-2B?**
    In addition to all the features of MEN-2A, there are also mucocutaneous neuromas (e.g., on the tongue).

DIABETES MELLITUS

43. **What is diabetes mellitus?**
    Diabetes mellitus is a complex metabolic disturbance characterized by hyperglycemia due to insulin deficiency or tissue resistance to the action of insulin. It must be distinguished

from diabetes insipidus, a posterior pituitary/hypothalamic disease caused by a deficiency of antidiuretic hormone (ADH). In common parlance, the term *diabetes* means diabetes mellitus.

44. **How common is diabetes?**
   - Diabetes is one of the most common chronic metabolic diseases.
     - ○ It affects 2% of the U.S. population (5 million people).
     - ○ Incidence increases with age (10% of those >70 years old).

45. **What is the difference between primary and secondary diabetes?**
   - Primary diabetes has no obvious cause.
     - ○ It accounts for 95% of all cases.
     - ○ Two clinical types are recognized: type 1 (insulin dependent) and type 2 (noninsulin dependent).
   - Secondary diabetes (5%) is caused by:
     - ○ Destructive lesions of the pancreas (e.g., chronic pancreatitis)
     - ○ Endocrine diseases (e.g., Cushing syndrome, glucagonoma syndrome, and acromegaly)
     - ○ Drugs (e.g., diuretics such as thiazides)
     - ○ Genetic syndromes (e.g., Turner syndrome and Down syndrome)

KEY POINTS: DIABETES MELLITUS ✔

1. Diabetes is characterized by hyperglycemia and glucosuria and complex metabolic disturbances.

2. Type 2 diabetes is the most common form of this disease.

3. Diabetes affects the blood vessels and thus the entire body, but most often the complications involve the heart, kidneys, eyes, and peripheral nerves.

46. **Compare type 1 and type 2 diabetes.**
   See Table 14-1.

TABLE 14-1. FEATURES OF TYPE 1 AND TYPE 2 DIABETES		
Feature	Type 1	Type 2
Prevalence	Less common (15%)	More common (85%)
Onset: age and mode	<20 years/sudden onset	>30 years/gradual onset
Genetics	HLA related	HLA unrelated
Twins (monozygotic)	50% discordant	90% concordant
Ketoacidosis	Common	Rare
Beta cells in islets	Decreased	Normal
Insulin in blood	Decreased	Normal or increased
Antibodies to insulin	Yes	No
Treatment	Insulin	Diet, other hypoglycemic drugs

47. **Do immune mechanisms play a role in the pathogenesis of diabetes?**
Immune mechanisms have been implicated in the pathogenesis of type 1 diabetes. It is assumed that the cytotoxic T cells destroy the islets of Langerhans, thus causing an absolute deficiency of insulin. Type 1 diabetes is associated with a number of autoimmune diseases. These patients also have antibodies to insulin and beta cells of the islets. The exact role of the immune mechanisms in the pathogenesis of the disease and the nature of the event that stimulates or initiates the autoimmune phenomena are not known.

48. **Are all diabetics obese?**
No. Patients suffering from type 1 diabetes are not obese, but most (80%) of those who have type 2 diabetes are obese. Obesity aggravates diabetes. It is assumed that obesity downregulates insulin receptors to adipocytes and skeletal muscle cells, thus decreasing insulin binding. However, not all patients with type 2 diabetes are obese, which indicates that the obesity is not the cause of diabetes; it only enhances the likelihood of it developing in genetically susceptible people.

49. **List the main complications of diabetes.**
Diabetes affects basement membranes, most notably in the small and large blood vessels. The most important complications of this disorder are:
- Atherosclerosis
- Arterial hypertension
- Diabetic nephropathy
- Diabetic retinopathy
- Peripheral neuropathy
- Cataracts

50. **Why is diabetes associated with an increased susceptibility to infections?**
- Increased glucose in tissues and body fluids provides favorable growth conditions for bacteria.
- Diabetes impairs the function of neutrophils.
- Angiopathy caused by diabetes leads to tissue ischemia, and such ischemic tissues are more prone to infection.

51. **What are the clinical features of diabetes mellitus?**
- Hyperglycemia
- Glycosuria and osmotic polyuria
- Polydipsia (increased water intake due to thirst)
- Increased incidence of infections (e.g., skin and urinary infections)
- Blurred vision
- Paresthesias

52. **How is diabetes diagnosed?**
- Urinalysis: glucose in urine
- Hyperglycemia: greater than 140 mg/dL (fasting) on two separate occasions
- Glucose tolerance test
- Insulin concentration in blood (low in type 1)

WEBSITES

1. http://www.ncbi.nlm.nih.gov/entrez/query.fcgi?db=PubMed

2. http://www-medlib.med.utah.edu/WebPath/webpath.html#MENU

3. http://www.pathguy.com

BIBLIOGRAPHY

1. Apte MV, Wilson JS: Alcohol-induced pancreatic injury. Best Pract Res Clin Gastroenterol 17:593–612, 2003.
2. Atkinson MA, Maclaren NK: The pathogenesis of insulin-independent diabetes mellitus. N Engl J Med 331:1428–1436, 1994.
3. Clark CM Jr, Lee DA: Prevention and treatment of the complications of diabetes mellitus. N Engl J Med 332:1210–1217, 1995.
4. Fogel EL, Sherman O: Acute biliary pancreatitis: When should the endoscopist intervene? Gastroenterology 125:229–235, 2003.
5. Kim HJ, Kim MH, Bae JS, et al: Idiopathic acute pancreatitis. J Clin Gastroenterol 37:238–250, 2003.
6. Roy PK, Venzon DJ, Shojamanesh H, et al: Zollinger–Ellison syndrome. Medicine 79:379–411, 2000.
7. Steer ML, Waxman I, Freedman S: Chronic pancreatitis. N Engl J Med 332:1482–1490, 1995.
8. Steinberg W, Tenner S: Acute pancreatitis. N Engl J Med 330:1198–1210, 1994.
9. Werner J, Uhl W, Hartwig W, et al: Modern phase-specific management of acute pancreatitis. Dig Dis 21:38–45, 2003.

CHAPTER 15

THE KIDNEYS AND THE URINARY SYSTEM

Ivan Damjanov, MD, PhD

1. **List the most important kidney diseases.**
   - Developmental disorders
   - Glomerular diseases
   - Tubulointerstitial diseases (One percent of all people in the United States will develop renal stones during their life span.)
   - Vascular and circulatory disorders
   - Tumors

2. **Name the main clinical renal syndromes.**
   - Acute nephritic syndrome
   - Nephrotic syndrome
   - Asymptomatic hematuria, proteinuria, or both
   - Acute renal failure
   - Chronic renal failure
   - Renal tubular defects
   - Urinary infections
   - Obstructive uropathy
   - Urinary stones
   - Tumors

3. **What are the principal laboratory findings in uremia?**
   Uremia is a set of clinical and laboratory findings encountered in patients with end-stage kidney disease. Key laboratory features reflect inadequate excretion of degradation products and minerals and include:
   - Azotemia (increased blood urea nitrogen [BUN] and creatinine [Cr] due to decreased renal excretion)
   - Electrolyte abnormalities (retention of sodium, potassium, and phosphate, with secondary changes in the concentration of calcium, which is initially low but also may be high)
   - Acidosis
   - Anemia (normocytic anemia resulting from a deficiency of erythropoietin)
   - Prolonged bleeding time (because of functional defects of platelets)

KEY POINTS: TYPES OF RENAL DISEASES ✔

1. The main types of renal disease are developmental, immunologic, metabolic, infectious, circulatory, and neoplastic.

2. Autosomal dominant polycystic kidney disease is the most common clinically significant developmental renal disease.

4. **What are the common clinical features of uremia?**

Clinical features of uremia may be found in essentially all major organs and include:

- Cardiopulmonary disorders
  - ○ Hypertension
  - ○ Congestive heart failure
  - ○ Uremic pericarditis
- Gastrointestinal disturbances
  - ○ Nausea and loss of appetite
  - ○ Chronic esophagitis, gastritis, and enteritis
- Neuromuscular disorders
  - ○ Muscle weakness
  - ○ Functional peripheral nerve disease
  - ○ Encephalopathy
- Skin
  - ○ "Uremic frost"
  - ○ Chronic dermatitis and pruritus
  - ○ Sallow color (urochrome)
- Bones
  - ○ Renal osteodystrophy
  - ○ Osteomalacia or osteoporosis

5. **What are the features of acute nephritic syndrome?**

Acute nephritic syndrome classically presents 1 or 2 weeks after an upper respiratory tract infection caused by streptococci. Clinically, it is characterized by:

- **Oliguria:** It is a consequence of a reduced glomerular filtration rate (GFR).
- **Hematuria:** It results from rupture or increased porosity of damaged glomerular basement membrane (GBM). Glomerular hematuria presents with brownish-red urine ("bouillon soup–like"). Red blood cells (RBCs) may be found in the urine sediment examined by microscopy. The sediment also contains fragmented and distorted RBCs and RBC casts.
- **Proteinuria:** It reflects the increased permeability of the GBM. The amount of protein found in urine varies from mild to severe.
- **Generalized edema:** It is a complication of hypoalbuminemia. Typically it is most prominent on the face ("puffy eyes") because of periorbital edema but may involve body cavities and internal organs. Somnolence of affected children is in part related to brain edema.
- **Hypertension:** It results from the reduced GFR and a consequent release of renin.
- **Low complement levels in blood:** This laboratory findings reflect the consumption of complement, which is bound to immune complexes deposited in the glomeruli.
- **Azotemia:** Elevated BUN and Cr in blood and electrolyte disturbances (e.g., hypernatremia) result from the reduced excretion of these substances in urine.

6. **List the features of nephrotic syndrome.**

- **Proteinuria:** It is massive and typically in the "nephrotic range" (i.e., >3.5 g/day).
- There is hypoalbuminemia (<3 g/dL).
- **Generalized edema:** It results from hypoalbuminemia and reduced plasm oncotic pressure.
- **Hyperlipidemia:** It is mostly due to an increased amount of low density lipoproteins (LDLs) and lipiduria (lipid casts in urine).
- Affected patients are prone to infection and thrombotic events because of increased urinary loss of serum proteins involved in immunity and coagulation.

7. **What are the features of acute renal failure?**

Acute renal failure has a rapid onset and develops over a period of several days or weeks. Most often it is characterized by a reversible deterioration of renal function, oliguria (or anuria), azotemia, and electrolyte disturbances. Most patients recover, but in some patients, the injury is irreversible. Such patients may die or require dialysis ("artificial kidneys") to survive.

8. **What are the causes of acute renal failure?**
Three types of renal failure are recognized: prerenal, renal, and postrenal. See Table 15-1.

TABLE 15-1. CAUSE OF ACUTE RENAL FAILURE		
Type of Renal Failure	**Pathogenesis**	**Clinical Condition**
Prerenal	Decreased renal perfusion	Congestive heart failure
Loss of blood	Massive bleeding	
Renal	Glomerular disease	Acute glomerulonephritis
Tubulointerstitial nephritis	Drug reaction	
Vasculitis	Wegener granulomatosis	
Toxic tubular necrosis	Mercury poisoning	
Postrenal	Intratubular obstruction	Acute urate nephropathy
Renal–pelvic obstruction	Nephrolithiasis	
Ureteric obstruction	Urinary stones	
Bladder/urethral obstruction	Prostatic hyperplasia	

9. **How does chronic renal failure develop?**
Chronic renal failure develops insidiously. It results from a gradual but progressive loss of normal renal function. In most instances, it occurs in four sequential steps:
- **Diminished renal reserve:** These patients do not have clinical or laboratory signs of renal disease (BUN and Cr are normal). Additional testing will reveal that GFR is significantly reduced, and azotemia may develop during intercurrent diseases.
- **Renal insufficiency:** These patients have reduced GFR (20%–50% of normal) and show signs of reduced tubular function. Laboratory findings include azotemia, anemia, and polyuria.
- **Renal failure:** These patients have markedly reduced GFR (<20% of normal), edema, metabolic acidosis, hypocalcemia, and multisystemic signs of uremia.
- **End-stage renal failure:** These patients have almost no measurable GFR (<5% of normal) and show clinical signs of uremia.

10. **Define derangements of urine volume.**
- **Anuria:** It is characterized by reduced urine output (<100 mL urine per day), reflecting renal injury.
- **Oliguria:** It is defined as reduced urine output below 400 mL/day. Such urinary volume is insufficient to excrete the daily osmolar load. It occurs often in the clinical setting and may be caused by prerenal, renal, or postrenal renal failure.
- **Polyuria:** It is defined as increased volume of urine (>3 L of urine per day). It may result from excessive fluid intake (e.g., beer), osmotic diuresis (e.g., diabetes mellitus), inappropriate fluid loss (e.g., diabetes insipidus), or impaired tubular concentration (e.g., tubular necrosis). Polyuria is typically found during the recovery phase of renal tubular necrosis. (Note: Regenerating renal tubules cannot concentrate urine.)

11. **What are the features of urinary tract infection (UTI)?**
UTI is characterized by bacteriuria and pyuria (bacteria and leukocytes in the urine). Bacteriuria is defined for clinical purposes as the presence of more than 100,000 bacteria per milliliter of cultured urine. Leukocytes are counted in the urinary sediment examined microscopically. The diagnosis of urinary bacterial infection affecting either the kidneys or the lower urinary tract is made if the patient has signs of urinary irritation, urgency, or pain and the urinalysis shows more than 100,000 colonies per milliliter. If the urine contains more

than 100,000 bacterial colonies per milliliter but the patient has no clinical symptoms, the diagnosis of asymptomatic bacteriuria is made.

DEVELOPMENTAL DISORDERS

12. **Describe the most common congenital kidney disease.**
    Autosomal dominant polycystic kidney disease (ADPKD) is the most common congenital kidney disease. It has an incidence of 1 in 800 and accounts for approximately 10% of patients on maintenance renal dialysis. ADPKD, also known as adult polycystic renal disease, is usually asymptomatic in childhood. Although it is congenital, it is diagnosed only during adult life. Renal dysplasia is the most common renal congenital anomaly diagnosed during infancy and childhood.

13. **What are the pathologic features of cystic renal dysplasia?**
    This developmental abnormality may be unilateral or bilateral. It results from irregular differentiation and morphogenesis of the metanephros, the primordium of the fetal kidneys. Histologically, the parenchyma of these abnormal kidneys consists of immature nephrons, often showing signs of cystic dilatation. The tubules and glomeruli are surrounded by immature mesenchyma and heterologous cells (e.g., cartilage or striated muscle). On gross examination, the abnormal kidneys appear enlarged and cystic. It may be associated with ureteropelvic obstruction and other anomalies of the lower urinary tract.

14. **Describe how cystic renal dysplasia presents clinically.**
    Unilateral cystic dysplasia, which is more common than bilateral dysplasia, usually is discovered on abdominal palpation as an abnormal mass. With nephroblastoma (Wilms tumor) and neuroblastoma of the adrenal, it is one of the three most common abdominal masses diagnosed in infants and young children.
    Bilateral cystic dysplasia, which is often associated with other urinary tract abnormalities, presents with early onset of renal failure in the neonatal period or early childhood.

15. **What are the differences between autosomal dominant and autosomal recessive kidney disease?**
    Comparisons of autosomal dominant and autosomal recessive polycystic kidney disease are illustrated in Fig. 15-1 and listed in Table 15-2.

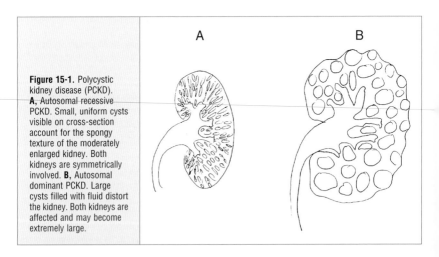

A   B

Figure 15-1. Polycystic kidney disease (PCKD). **A,** Autosomal recessive PCKD. Small, uniform cysts visible on cross-section account for the spongy texture of the moderately enlarged kidney. Both kidneys are symmetrically involved. **B,** Autosomal dominant PCKD. Large cysts filled with fluid distort the kidney. Both kidneys are affected and may become extremely large.

TABLE 15-2. AUTOSOMAL DOMINANT AND AUTOSOMAL RECESSIVE POLYCYSTIC KIDNEY DISEASE (PCKD)

Feature	Autosomal Dominant PCKD	Autosomal Recessive PCKD
Incidence	Common (1:800)	Rare (1:15,000)
Inheritance	Autosomal dominant	Autosomal recessive
Gene	Polycystin genes (PKD1 – 05%)	Fibrocystin, PKHD1
Bilateral	Yes	Yes
Gross appearance	Large cystic kidneys (>1000 g)	Spongelike symmetrically enlarged (100–200 g)
Cysts	Large (from any tubule)	Small (collecting duct derived)
Symptoms	Infancy, childhood	Adulthood (>35 years)
Associated anomalies	Polycystic liver disease (20%) Berry aneurysms of cerebral arteries	Small bile duct cysts, liver fibrosis

GLOMERULAR DISEASES

16. **What is the difference between primary and secondary glomerular diseases?**
The traditional distinction of glomerular diseases into primary and secondary glomerulopathies is arbitrary and not always convincing. Those diseases that selectively affect glomeruli or most prominently damage glomeruli are called primary.
    Primary glomerular diseases are, for example:
    - Minimal change glomerulopathy (lipoid nephrosis)
    - Primary membranous nephropathy
    - Acute poststreptococcal glomerulonephritis
    Secondary glomerular diseases occur in the course of systemic diseases such as:
    - Immunologic diseases (e.g., systemic lupus erythematosus)
    - Metabolic disorders (e.g., diabetes mellitus)
    - Hereditary diseases (e.g., Fabry's disease)
    - Acquired immune deficiency syndrome (AIDS)

17. **List the five main glomerular syndromes.**
    - Acute nephritic syndrome
    - Rapidly progressive glomerulonephritis
    - Nephrotic syndrome
    - Chronic renal failure
    - Asymptomatic hematuria/proteinuria

18. **Which cells contribute to glomerular hypercellularity in glomerulonephritis?**
Glomerular hypercellularity can be caused by proliferation of endogenous cells or exudation of inflammatory cells carried by blood. Morphologically, such hypercellularity can be intracapillary (i.e., the cells are found inside the capillaries and the mesangial areas) or extracapillary (i.e., the cells are found in the urinary space enclosed by the Bowman capsule). Such extracapillary cell aggregates are called crescents. From the pathogenetic standpoint, glomerular hypercellularity can be due to:
    - **Cellular proliferation:** Mesangial, endothelial, and sometimes parietal epithelial cells
    - **Exudation:** Neutrophils, monocytes (macrophages), and sometimes lymphocytes

- **Crescent formation:** Accumulation of proliferating epithelial cells lining the Bowman capsule and exudates composed of macrophages (Fibroblasts can grow into the urinary spaces from outside through the ruptured Bowman capsule.)

19. **What is the difference between global and segmental, diffuse and focal glomerulopathy?**
Because many of the primary glomerulonephritides are of unknown cause, they are often classified by their histology. Histologic changes can be subdivided into:
- **Global:** Involving the entire glomerulus
- **Segmental:** Affecting a part of a glomerulus
- **Diffuse:** Involving all glomeruli
- **Focal:** Involving only a certain proportion of the glomeruli
According to this nomenclature, mild nephritis of systemic lupus erythematosus (SLE) is classified as focal and segmental. This means that some and not all glomeruli are affected. In the affected glomeruli, only some loops show pathologic changes, whereas others are normal.

20. **Describe two forms of antibody-associated forms of glomerular injury.**
- **Antibodies to endogenous antigens of the GBM:** This mechanism accounts for the renal injury in Goodpasture syndrome, a disease caused by antibodies to collagen type IV.
- **Antibodies to nonglomerular antigens:** Antigen–antibody complexes found in the glomeruli may result from two pathogenetic mechanisms: in situ formation or intraglomerular deposition of circulating immune complexes.
  - In situ immune complex formation results from the binding of circulating antibodies and the "implanted" antigen fixed to the basement membrane of the glomerulus. This mechanism accounts for the formation of glomerular lesions in poststreptococcal glomerulonephritis. It is assumed that the streptococcal antigens are implanted into the GBM during the infection, and when the antibodies are formed, they reach the implanted antigens in the glomeruli, thus forming immune complexes.
  - Circulating immune complexes are antigen–antibody complexes formed from soluble antigens and corresponding antibodies in the circulating blood. The bloodstream carries these immune complexes to the glomeruli, where the blood is normally filtered. Because the preformed immune complexes represent large protein aggregates that cannot pass through the GBM, they are "caught" on the subepithelial, subendothelial side of the GBM or the lamina rara or densa of the GBM. This type of immune complex deposition typically occurs in SLE.

21. **What pattern of staining of glomeruli is seen by immunofluorescence microscopy in anti-GBM nephritis?**
Immunofluorescence microscopy tests are performed with fluoresceinated rabbit or mouse antibodies that recognize human antigens. Using these antibodies to human immunoglobulin (Ig) G, one can demonstrate where the immunoglobulins are deposited. In typical anti-GBM glomerulonephritis, such as Goodpasture syndrome, IgG is bound diffusely to all collagen type IV molecules in the GBM. Staining with antihuman IgG will produce a linear pattern (i.e., the fluoresceinated antibodies outline the GBMs).

22. **What pattern of staining of glomeruli is seen by immunofluorescence microscopy in circulating immune complex nephritis?**
Circulating immune complexes form granular deposits along the basement membrane. Typically this is seen in SLE. Depending on the size, solubility, and electric charge of the immune complexes, they may get "stuck" on the endothelial, intramembranous, or subepithelial region of the GBM or in the mesangial areas.

23. **Describe where immune complexes found in the glomeruli are affected by membranous nephropathy.**
Membranous glomerulopathy is an immunologic disease in which immune complexes appear on the GBM in a uniform granular manner (usually referred to as "lumpy-bumpy"). The subepithelial (epimembranous) location of these antigens indicates that they may be formed locally through the action of antibodies and a local foot-process antigen (megalin or gp-330) or by the implantation of preformed circulating immune complexes.

24. **In which parts of the glomeruli may the antigen–antibody complexes be seen by electron microscopy in various forms of glomerulonephritis?**
Depending on their location, immune complexes are classified as follows:
- Subepithelial "humps" (e.g., acute glomerulonephritis)
- Epimembranous granular deposits (e.g., membranous nephropathy or the membranous form of SLE nephritis)
- Subendothelial (e.g., SLE and membranoproliferative glomerulonephritis)
- Intramembranous (e.g., SLE)
- Mesangial (e.g., IgA nephropathy and SLE)
  See Fig. 15-2.

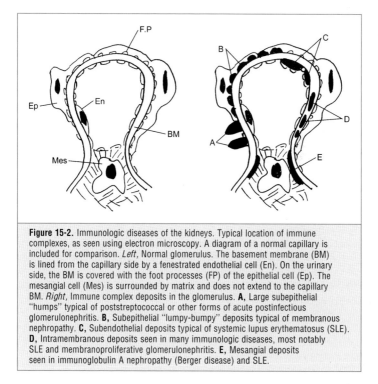

Figure 15-2. Immunologic diseases of the kidneys. Typical location of immune complexes, as seen using electron microscopy. A diagram of a normal capillary is included for comparison. *Left,* Normal glomerulus. The basement membrane (BM) is lined from the capillary side by a fenestrated endothelial cell (En). On the urinary side, the BM is covered with the foot processes (FP) of the epithelial cell (Ep). The mesangial cell (Mes) is surrounded by matrix and does not extend to the capillary BM. *Right,* Immune complex deposits in the glomerulus. **A,** Large subepithelial "humps" typical of poststreptococcal or other forms of acute postinfectious glomerulonephritis. **B,** Subepithelial "lumpy-bumpy" deposits typical of membranous nephropathy. **C,** Subendothelial deposits typical of systemic lupus erythematosus (SLE). **D,** Intramembranous deposits seen in many immunologic diseases, most notably SLE and membranoproliferative glomerulonephritis. **E,** Mesangial deposits seen in immunoglobulin A nephropathy (Berger disease) and SLE.

25. **Why does the immunologic injury of the GBM cause proteinuria?**
Proteinuria results from:
- **Increased permeability of the GBM without interruption of the filtration barrier:** It results from complex physicochemical changes caused by the action of activated complement, enzymes, and cytokines. These changes involve the biochemical composition and electric charges of the GBM and the size of internal pores that serve as normal channels for the passage of proteins.
- **Rupture of the GBM:** It is usually associated with a passage of large plasma proteins (e.g., fibrinogen) and red blood cells into the urinary space. Clinically, such proteinuria is associated with hematuria. Polymerization of fibrinogen into fibrin inside the urinary space of the glomeruli can be recognized as fibrinoid necrosis of capillary loops or the early formation of crescents for which this fibrin forms the scaffold.

26. **Which cells participate in the antibody-induced glomerular injury?**
Polymorphonuclear neutrophils, lymphocytes (including T cells and natural killer cells), platelets, and resident glomerular cells (especially the mesangial cells).

27. **List the soluble mediators of inflammation that contribute to the antibody-mediated glomerular injury.**
Most mediators of inflammation mentioned in the chapter on inflammation have been identified in the inflamed glomeruli:
- Activated complement components act as chemotactic fragments and mediate the influx of neutrophils and macrophages. Complement may also increase the permeability of the GBM and cause mechanical lesions through the action of membrane attack (C5–C9 terminal complex).
- Cytokines (especially interleukin-1 and tumor necrosis factor) and chemokines participate in the recruitment of inflammatory cells and their activation and also directly contribute to the injury of the GBM. Transforming growth factor-beta promotes extracellular matrix synthesis and contributes to glomerulosclerosis in later stages of the disease.
- Growth factors, such as platelet-derived growth factor, promote mesangial cell proliferation.
- In the coagulation system, fibrin and thrombin may activate platelets and other blood cells and local glomerular cells, as well as damage the GBM.
- Prostaglandins, nitrous oxide, and endothelin act on endothelial, mesangial, and epithelial cells and may have an important role in regulating the blood flow through the inflamed glomerulus.

28. **What are the histologic signs of chronic progression of glomerular disease?**
- **Focal segmental glomerulosclerosis:** This is a secondary change that occurs in the relatively unaffected glomeruli of a diseased kidney that has lost many nephrons. Normal glomeruli receive increased amounts of blood and undergo hypertrophy. The hemodynamic changes in the overburdened and enlarged glomeruli lead to segmental hyalinization of capillary loops and progressive narrowing of their lumen by sclerosis.
- **Tubulointerstitial damage:** Tubular damage results in hyalinization of tubular basement membranes and atrophy of tubular cells associated with a loss of their specific functions. The peritubular interstitial spaces increase in size and change their biochemical composition. Chronic inflammatory cells, predominantly lymphocytes, appear in the interstitial spaces. The factors leading to tubulointerstitial injury include ischemia distal to sclerotic glomeruli, concomitant immune reactions to shared antigens, and biochemical injury by retention of metabolites or minerals (e.g., phosphate, calcium, or ammonia).

29. Discuss the histologic features of acute glomerulonephritis.

Acute glomerulonephritis is an endocapillary exudative and proliferative glomerulonephritis. By light microscopy, one may see:

- Hypercellularity of glomeruli, which is in part due to exudation of inflammatory cells (neutrophils and macrophages) and in part due to proliferation of endogenous glomerular cells
- Widening of mesangial areas by an increased number of mesangial cells
- Narrowing of capillary spaces and reduced blood flow through the glomeruli (few RBCs in the glomerular capillaries)
- RBCs in the urinary space and the lumen of tubules (a definitive sign of glomerular hematuria)
- Proteinaceous and RBC casts in the lumen of tubules (result from combined effects of glomerular proteinuria and hematuria)
- Interstitial edema and inflammation may be present (indicates that the entire kidney is reacting to the immunologic injury of the glomeruli)

30. Describe the most common cause of postinfectious glomerulonephritis.

Group A beta-hemolytic streptococci (*Streptococcus pyogenes*) account for 90% of all glomerulonephritis cases. Glomerulonephritis typically occurs 1 to 4 weeks after a strep throat or skin infection (impetigo) caused by one of the nephritogenic strains of this microbe. Occasionally the same clinical and pathologic findings may follow staphylococcal infection and even some viral diseases, such as hepatitis B or C or hepatitis caused by human immunodeficiency virus (HIV). See Fig. 15-3.

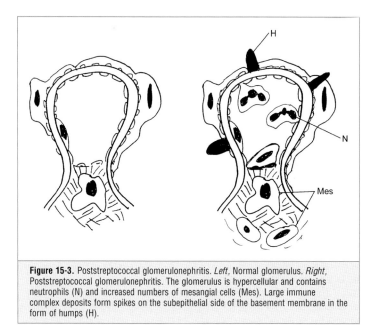

Figure 15-3. Poststreptococcal glomerulonephritis. *Left,* Normal glomerulus. *Right,* Poststreptococcal glomerulonephritis. The glomerulus is hypercellular and contains neutrophils (N) and increased numbers of mesangial cells (Mes). Large immune complex deposits form spikes on the subepithelial side of the basement membrane in the form of humps (H).

31. **What are "subepithelial humps" in acute glomerulonephritis, and how can they be seen?**
Subepithelial humps represent epimembranous deposits of immune complexes on the GBM in postinfectious glomerulonephritis. They can be seen using electron microscopy. These humps represent only the "tip of the iceberg"—that is, they are the only ultrastructurally visible immune complexes. Immunofluorescence microscopy shows that the glomeruli contain many other immune complexes, which probably are not dense enough to be seen by electron microscopy. These smaller immune complexes are found in the mesangial areas and in the basement membrane and are distributed without any regularity.

32. **What are the symptoms and signs of acute poststreptococcal glomerulonephritis?**
Classic acute glomerulonephritis is a childhood disease. It usually presents with fever, nausea, oliguria, hematuria, RBC casts in urine, mild proteinuria (usually <1 g/day), periorbital edema, and mild to moderate hypertension.
   Atypical glomerulonephritis is the term used for the disease occurring in adults. The onset may be insidious, or the disease may present with a sudden appearance of hypertension or edema and biochemical signs of azotemia.

33. **Why is the concentration of serum complement C3 low in acute poststreptococcal glomerulonephritis?**
As immune complex deposits are formed in the glomeruli, they activate complement through the classical pathway, leading to a depletion of serum complement. C3 is the complement protein consumed in both the classical and the alternate complement pathways and is therefore used for monitoring the serum concentration of the entire complement system. Other complement proteins are also depleted, but there is no need to measure all of them at the same time. When the disease wanes, C3 levels return to normal.

34. **What is the typical outcome and what are the possible long-term consequences of acute poststreptococcal glomerulonephritis?**
The disease has a better prognosis in children than in adults:
   - Children
     - Ninety percent recover within 2 or 3 months with conservative therapy aimed at maintaining sodium and water balance
     - Five to eight percent have persistent glomerulonephritis, in much milder form, with abnormal urinary findings for 6 to 8 months
     - Less than 1% of cases develop rapidly progressive glomerulonephritis
     - One or two percent slowly progress to chronic glomerulonephritis
   - Adults
     - Sixty percent recover promptly
     - Three to five percent develop rapidly progressive glomerulonephritis
     - Thirty percent have persistent mild proteinuria, hematuria, or both, as well as hypertension

35. **What is the histologic substrate of rapidly progressive glomerulonephritis (RPGN), or crescentic glomerulonephritis?**
RPGN is associated with crescentic glomerulonephritis. Crescents found in more than 50% of glomeruli represent a sign of severe glomerular injury, which usually starts as focal and segmental necrotizing glomerulonephritis. This glomerular injury is associated with rupture of the GBM, which allows the entry of inflammatory cells and fibrinogen into the urinary space delimited by the Bowman capsule. Early crescents are composed of fibrin, inflammatory cells exudated into the urinary spaces, and proliferated epithelial cells of the Bowman capsule. The Bowman capsule may rupture, and the fibroblasts from the interstitium may invade the

glomerular urinary space and contribute to the transformation of early crescents into fibrotic older crescents. Thereafter fibroblasts predominate, and the cellular crescents will be replaced by collagen laid down by fibroblasts. Ultimately the collapsed remnants of the capillary loops and fibrotic crescents coalesce and the glomerulus undergoes hyalinization. See Fig. 15-4.

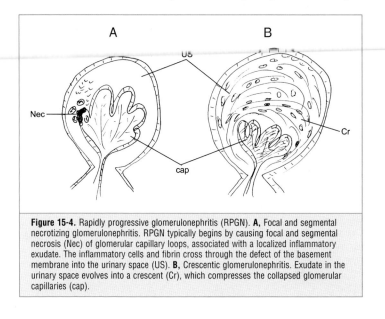

Figure 15-4. Rapidly progressive glomerulonephritis (RPGN). **A,** Focal and segmental necrotizing glomerulonephritis. RPGN typically begins by causing focal and segmental necrosis (Nec) of glomerular capillary loops, associated with a localized inflammatory exudate. The inflammatory cells and fibrin cross through the defect of the basement membrane into the urinary space (US). **B,** Crescentic glomerulonephritis. Exudate in the urinary space evolves into a crescent (Cr), which compresses the collapsed glomerular capillaries (cap).

36. **Discuss the causes of RPGN.**
    It is believed that RPGN is in most cases caused by immunologic mechanisms, although the exact pathogenesis of many cases remains unknown, and the glomeruli do not always contain immunoglobulins. RPGN is associated with 25% mortality and 40% progression to chronic end-stage kidney disease.
    RPGNs can be divided into three groups:
    - **Pauciimmune, antineutrophil cytoplasmic antibody-positive RPGN:** This group accounts for most cases of RPGN in adults. In adults older than 60 years, it accounts for 75% of cases. The glomeruli contain no immunoglobulin deposits or just a few minor aggregates of IgG or IgM and complement. This group of diseases includes pathologic and clinical entities such as:
      ○ Wegener granulomatosis
      ○ Microscopic polyarteritis nodosa
      ○ Churg–Strauss syndrome
    - **Immune complex–mediated glomerulonephritis:** This is the most common form of RPGN in childhood and in young adults younger than 20 years of age. The glomeruli show deposits of immune complexes. This group of diseases includes:
      ○ Postinfectious glomerulonephritis
      ○ Henoch–Schönlein purpura
      ○ SLE
      ○ IgA nephropathy
    - **Anti-GBM nephritis:** It is a rare form of RPGN, accounting for less than 10% of cases in all age groups. It is characterized by linear staining of GBM in immunofluorescence microscopic studies. It includes Goodpasture syndrome (antibodies to the globular part of collagen type IV and pulmonary hemorrhage).

37. **Which clinical symptoms and signs are found in both nephrotic and nephritic syndromes, and which are unique to each of these two syndromes?**
See Table 15-3 and Fig. 15-5.

TABLE 15-3. COMPARISON OF NEPHRITIC AND NEPHROTIC SYNDROMES

Sign/Symptom	Nephritic Syndrome	Nephrotic Syndrome
Proteinuria	++ to +++ +++	+++ (nephrotic range, >3.5 g/day)
Hypoalbuminemia	+	+++
Edema	++ to ++	++
Hematuria	++ and red blood cell casts	No
Oliguria	++++	No
Hyperlipidemia	No	+
Lipiduria	No	+
Hypertension	+	No

+, mild; ++, moderate; +++, severe.

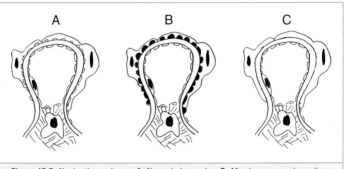

Figure 15-5. Nephrotic syndrome. **A,** Normal glomerulus. **B,** Membranous nephropathy. The glomerular basement membrane is covered with "lumpy-bumpy" subepithelial immune complex deposits. **C,** Minimal change ("nil") disease. The foot processes of the epithelial cell are fused. Otherwise, the glomerulus appears normal.

38. **Name the most common causes of nephrotic syndrome in children.**
In children younger than 15 years old, nephrotic syndrome is almost always caused by a primary kidney disease:
- Minimal change disease: 70%
- Focal segmental glomerulosclerosis: 10%
- Membranoproliferative glomerulonephritis: 10%
- Membranous glomerulonephritis: 5%
- Alport syndrome, IgA nephropathy, and all others: 5%

39. **What are the most common causes of primary nephrotic syndrome in adults?**
- Membranous nephropathy: 30%
- Minimal change disease: 10%
- Focal segmental glomerulonephritis: 35%
- Membranoproliferative glomerulonephritis type I or type II: 10%
- Membranous form of SLE: 5%
- IgA nephropathy and all other glomerular diseases: 15%

40. **What are the most common causes of secondary nephrotic syndrome in adults?**
Nephrotic syndrome may develop in the course of several systemic diseases. The most important systemic diseases that may be associated with nephrotic syndrome are:
- Diabetes mellitus (Because of the high prevalence of diabetes, it is overall the most common cause of nephrotic syndrome in adults.)
- SLE
- Amyloidosis
- Drug abuse nephropathy
- AIDS

41. **List the typical features of membranous nephropathy.**
- **Epidemiology:** Previously, this was the most common cause of primary nephrotic syndrome in adults.
- **Etiology:** Immune complexes deposition/formation in the glomeruli:
  ○ Primary idiopathic—cause unknown (most common)
  ○ Secondary—caused by prolonged antigenemia as in SLE, chronic viral hepatitis B and C, and in cancer patients who have circulating tumor antigens in blood
- **Pathogenesis:** Immune complex deposits on the subepithelial portion of the GBM, formed either in situ or through the filtering of immune complexes, and "get stuck" on the GBM.
- **Pathology:** There is diffuse thickening of GBM but no cellular proliferation in the glomeruli. Deposits seen on the subepithelial side of the GBM ("lumpy-bumpy") by electron microscopy and immunofluorescence.
- **Treatment:** It does not respond to corticosteroid treatment.
- **Prognosis and outcome:** The disease will progress to end-stage renal failure over a period of 10 to 15 years.

42. **List the typical features of minimal change disease.**
- It is also known as nil disease (from Latin *nihil,* "nothing") and in the clinical setting as lipoid nephrosis.
- It is the most common cause of nephrotic syndrome in children (90% of those younger than 5 years old and 50% of those younger than 10 years old, in comparison with 20% of adults).
- Etiology/pathogenesis is unknown. It is thought to be related to type IV hypersensitivity reaction or the effects of cytokines.
- **Pathology:** Microscopic and immunofluorescence findings are negative. The glomeruli appear normal.
- Electron microscopy shows reactive fusion of foot processes of epithelial cells.
- **Therapy:** It responds to corticosteroid treatment but may occasionally recur.

43. **What are the pathologic findings in focal segmental glomerulosclerosis?**
- It is the most common cause of nephrotic syndrome in adults.
- **Pathology:** There is sclerosis involving some parts of some glomeruli.
- FSG is classified etiologically as:
  ○ Primary (unknown cause)
  ○ Secondary, when part of a systemic disease or identifiable cause as in HIV infection, sickle cell anemia, intravenous drug abuse, or other forms of focal glomerulonephritis (e.g., IgA nephropathy)
- **Therapy:** It is unresponsive to steroid treatment.
- **Outcome:** The disease will usually progresses to end-stage kidney disease in 5 to 10 years.

44. **What is the most common form of HIV-associated nephropathy?**
Focal segmental glomerulosclerosis occurs in 5% to 10% of HIV-infected people. It presents as so-called collapsing glomerulopathy in which the glomeruli frequently undergo global sclerosis and renal failure develops at an accelerated rate.

45. **List the renal complications of HIV infection.**
Infection with HIV may be accompanied by complications related to superimposed opportunistic infections, intravenous drug abuse, or shock related to multiorgan failure in AIDS. The most common pathologic findings include:
- Focal segmental glomerular sclerosis
- Membranoproliferative glomerulonephritis
- Membranous nephropathy
- Tubulointerstitial nephritis
- Renal failure

46. **List key facts about IgA nephropathy (Berger disease).**
- The most common clinically recognized primary glomerular disease worldwide
- Focal and segmental glomerulopathy caused by the deposition of IgA in the mesangial areas
- Cause unknown; related to increased IgA in blood and the presence of polymeric IgA
- Affects children and young adults
- Clinically, has protean manifestations: Isolated hematuria and/or proteinuria, nephrotic syndrome, nephritic syndrome, chronic renal failure, and RPGN

47. **What are the most common clinical signs and symptoms of IgA nephropathy?**
- Gross hematuria following a respiratory infection
- Gastrointestinal infection or UTI in 55%
- Microscopic hematuria with or without proteinuria in 30%
  Hematuria is usually short-lived and lasts only a few days. It disappears spontaneously but recurs at unpredictable intervals. Renal function remains intact in most cases, but in 30% to 50% of cases, there is evidence of progressive loss of renal reserve and impending renal failure. See Fig.15-6.

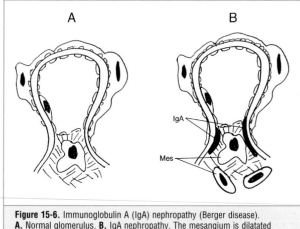

Figure 15-6. Immunoglobulin A (IgA) nephropathy (Berger disease). **A,** Normal glomerulus. **B,** IgA nephropathy. The mesangium is dilatated and contains deposits of IgA and an increased number of mesangial cells (Mes).

48. **What are the unfavorable prognostic signs in IgA nephropathy?**
- Onset in older adults (rather than in children and young adults)
- Heavy proteinuria

- Hypertension
- Extensive glomerulosclerosis (seen in renal biopsy)

49. **Which other disease besides IgA nephropathy is characterized by a deposition of IgA in the glomeruli?**
Henoch–Schönlein disease, a systemic disease of unknown etiology characterized by the deposition of IgA in the wall of small blood vessels, may affect the kidneys and presents with deposition of IgA in glomeruli.

50. **Define membranoproliferative glomerulonephritis (MPGN).**
MPGN is characterized by the formation of new membranes and proliferation of mesangial cells and exudation of inflammatory cells. New membrane formation can be recognized by light and electron microscopy as reduplication of GBM and widening of mesangial areas, which may impart a lobular appearance on the glomeruli.
Two types of primary MPGN are recognized:
- **MPGN-I:** This immune complex-mediated glomerulonephritis associated with deposition of immunoglobulins and complement in the subendothelial parts of the GBM.
- **MPGN-II:** Also known as "dense deposit disease," it is characterized by linear, dense deposits of C3 complement in the GBM (as seen using electron microscopy).
Clinically, primary MPGN most often affects children and young adults. It presents as nephrotic or nephritic syndrome and has a slowly progressive course. It does not respond to corticosteroid therapy and evolves into chronic end-stage renal disease in a period of 10–15 years.

51. **Explain the difference between primary and secondary MPGN-I.**
Primary MPGN-I is a disease of unknown etiology affecting children and young adults. Secondary MPGN-I occurs in the course of another systemic disease. It affects adults and can occur at any age. Morphologically, there are no differences between primary and secondary MPGN-I. Secondary MPGN-I can develop in the course of many chronic diseases characterized by chronic antigenemia, such as:
- SLE
- Cryoglobulinemia in the course of hepatitis virus C infection or malignant lymphoma
- HIV infection
- Bacterial endocarditis
- Schistosomiasis
- Neoplasms

52. **How often does SLE affect the kidneys?**
Signs of renal disease are found in 50% of patients at the time of diagnosis, and more than 80% of patients with SLE will develop some signs of renal disease at some time during the life span. The renal disease may be mild but is often a major feature of SLE and an important cause of mortality in these patients.

53. **Which parts of the kidney are affected in SLE?**
SLE is an immune complex–mediated systemic disease. Immune complexes are deposited in:
- **Glomeruli:** This is the most frequently affected part of the kidney. Because the immune complexes vary in size, solubility, and electric charge, they may be "trapped" on the subendothelial side, inside the GBM, or on the subepithelial side and the mesangium. Some immune complexes form intracapillary deposits (hyaline thrombi). Basement membranes lined with subendothelial immune complexes appear thickened and are called wire loops.
- **Blood vessels:** Immune complexes are usually deposited in arterioles.
- **Tubules and interstitial spaces:** Deposits are most often seen in the tubular basement membranes, but in severe disease, they may be found in the interstitial spaces as well.

54. **Why are kidney biopsies performed on patients with SLE?**
    - To establish the extent of renal involvement and determine the severity of disease
    - To classify the kidney disease (Classes I–VI)
    - To assess activity of glomerulonephritis
    - To determine the effects of treatment or progression of disease

55. **Why is it important to classify lupus nephritis?**
    Lupus nephritis is divided into six classes to aid in deciding how to treat it and for the sake of prognosis. Class I nephritis does not require treatment. Class IV requires aggressive immunosuppressive treatment, but even though it may respond, it still has the worst prognosis. Class V nephritis resembles idiopathic membranous nephropathy and does not respond to steroid treatment. See Table 15-4 and Fig. 15-7.

TABLE 15-4. CLASSIFICATION OF LUPUS NEPHRITIS		
Class	**Site of Immune Complex Deposition**	**Clinical Features**
Class I—No lesions	No deposits	No sign of renal disease
Class II—Mesangial GN	Mesangial	Mild hematuria/ proteinuria
Class III—Focal proliferative GN	Mesangial and subendothelial	Moderate GN
Class IV—Diffuse proliferative GN	Widespread	Severe GN
Class V—Membranous GN	Subepithelial	Nephrotic syndrome
Class VI—Chronic GN	Variable	Chronic GN

GN, Glomerulonephritis.

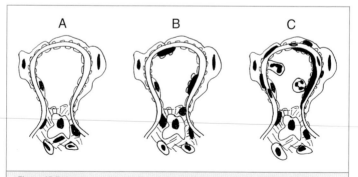

Figure 15-7. Lupus nephritis. **A,** Class II lesion. The glomerulus contains mesangial deposits of immune complexes and shows mesangial hypercellularity. **B,** Class III lesion. The glomerulus contains mesangial and subendothelial deposits of immune complexes and shows mesangial hypercellularity. **C,** Class IV lesion. The glomerulus shows mesangial, subendothelial, subepithelial, and intramembranous deposits of immune complexes and is hypercellular because of the proliferation of mesangial cells and leukocytes.

56. **How does diabetes mellitus damage glomeruli?**
Although the exact mechanism of glomerular injury caused by diabetes is not known, it seems that the injury is multifactorial and that several factors play a role:
- Hyperglycemia promotes nonenzymatic glycosylation of proteins in the GBM and mesangium.
- Metabolic disturbances affect the synthesis of main components of the GBM. This changes the ratio of collagen type IV to proteoglycans and glycoproteins such as laminin and fibronectin.
- Hemodynamic changes leading to glomerular hypertrophy and focal glomerular sclerosis occur.
- Infiltration of GBM with albumin and IgG (not immune mediated) plays a role in changing the permeability of the GBM.

57. **Define microalbuminuria.**
Microalbuminuria, defined as urinary albumin excretion of more than 300 mg/day, is an early sign of impending diabetic glomerulopathy that will be associated with nephrotic syndrome and progressive loss of glomerular functions. Progression of kidney disease can be slowed down by controlling hyperglycemia and hypertension.

58. **What are the pathologic features of diabetic glomerulopathy?**
Two forms of diabetic glomerulopathy are recognized:
- **Diffuse glomerulosclerosis:** It presents as widening of mesangial areas, increased number of mesangial cells, and thickening of GBM.
- **Nodular glomerulosclerosis (Kimmelstiel–Wilson disease):** This lesion, typical of diabetes, presents with characteristic round nodular masses segmentally in the peripheral mesangial portion of the glomeruli. The remaining glomerular loops show signs of diffuse glomerulosclerosis.

59. **Which renal diseases are caused by diabetes?**
- **Diabetic glomerulosclerosis:** It is associated with proteinuria, progressing to nephrotic syndrome or glomerular hyalinization and a loss of glomerular function and chronic renal failure.
- **Arteriolosclerosis:** Typically, the arterioles have thick hyalinized walls and narrow lumens. These changes are associated with hypertension.
- **Pyelonephritis:** High concentration of sugar in the interstitium promotes the growth of bacterial infections.
- **Papillary necrosis:** It results from diabetic microangiopathy and ischemia of the renal medulla.

60. **List key features of renal amyloidosis.**
Kidneys are often affected in both primary amyloidosis (e.g., deposition of AL amyloid in multiple myeloma) and secondary amyloidosis (e.g., deposition of AA amyloid in chronic suppurative conditions, such as purulent osteomyelitis or bronchiectasis).
- **Light microscopy:** It shows focal deposits of extracellular homogeneous eosinophilic material. Thickening of GBM may resemble diabetes or membranous nephropathy, and special stains must be used to make the correct diagnosis.
- **Special stain:** Congo red stains amyloid red, which becomes apple green birefringent on polarization.
- **Electron microscopy:** It shows typical 7- to 10-nm-thick fibrils with periodic beading. Amyloid deposits are found in:
  - Glomeruli (mesangial area and GBM)
  - Arterioles and arteries
  - Tubular basement membranes
- **Clinical findings:** Proteinuria is found in 100%, nephrotic syndrome in 75%, and hypertension in 50% of patients.
- **Outcome:** End-stage renal failure develops over 2 to 5 years. Kidneys infiltrated with amyloid remain large.

61. **Define chronic glomerulonephritis.**

Chronic glomerulonephritis is not a specific entity but an end stage of numerous acute or chronic glomerular diseases, such as acute poststreptoccocal glomerulonephritis, membranoproliferative glomerulonephritis, focal segmental glomerulosclerosis, or SLE nephritis.

DISEASES OF TUBULES AND INTERSTITIUM

62. **What are the causes of oliguria/anuria in ischemic or toxic acute tubular necrosis?**

Tubular epithelial cells are particularly sensitive to anoxia and toxins, which cause cell necrosis.

Debris resulting from the disintegration of cells fill the lumen and may block urine outflow and eventually increase intratubular pressure, thereby decreasing the GFR.

Fluid from the damaged tubules may leak into the interstitium. The outside pressure compressing the tubules contributes to their collapse.

Ischemic renal injury is also associated with intrarenal vasoconstriction that may cause reduced GFR and reduce the oxygen supply to the tubules even more. Ischemic injury of endothelial cells is associated with reduced release of nitric oxide (vasodilator) and increased secretion of endothelin (vasoconstrictor).

All these changes lead to reduced production of urine and cause oliguria.

63. **Name the three stages of acute tubular necrosis (ATN) following surgery.**
   - **Initiation stage:** The changes are related to reduced blood flow through the kidneys. During this phase, which typically lasts 24 to 36 hours, there is a decrease in urine output (400 to 600 mL/day) with a slight increase in BUN. The changes are reversible, and further progression can be prevented by proper maintenance of cardiac functions and hydration.
   - **Oliguric stage:** Urine volume is significantly reduced (40–400 mL/day), resulting in salt and water overload, rising BUN, hyperkalemia, and metabolic acidosis. Adverse effects of hyperkalemia may dominate.
   - **Polyuric stage:** Glomerular functions are reestablished, and the GFR returns to normal, but the regenerating tubules cannot concentrate the filtrate. Large quantities of dilute urine are formed. Polyuria is associated with a loss of sodium and potassium and may result in dehydration if not treated vigorously.

   In up to 50% of patients with ATN (especially following exposure to nephrotoxins), the oliguric stage never develops and renal injury immediately presents with polyuria.

KEY POINTS: DISEASES OF TUBULES AND INTERSTITIUM ✓

1. Tubular necrosis is the most common cause of oliguria or anuria after surgery, trauma, or circulatory collapse.

2. Pyelonephritis is a bacterial infection that is most often caused by an ascending route.

3. Urinary stones are found in 5% to 10% of Americans and are an important cause of kidney infection and urinary obstruction.

64. **How do drugs cause kidney injury?**
   - **Direct toxic injury:** This type of injury is predictable and dose dependent. Typically it occurs in cancer patients receiving cytotoxic drugs (e.g., cisplatinum).

- **Immunologic reaction:** Most often, it presents as acute tubulointerstitial nephritis (e.g., hypersensitivity to penicillin).
- **Papillary necrosis:** It is most often associated with an abuse of analgesics (e.g., phenacetin). These drugs inhibit prostaglandin synthesis and cause ischemia of the renal medulla.

65. **What is pyelonephritis?**
Pyelonephritis is a term used for bacterial infections of the kidney (i.e., infective tubulointerstitial nephritis). It can occur in an acute or a chronic form. This relatively common infection accounts for 20% of bacteremias in women and 2% or 3% of end-stage kidney disease patients in renal dialysis units.

66. **What are the most common causes of acute pyelonephritis?**
Eighty-five percent of cases of acute pyelonephritis are related to ascending infection with gram-negative bacteria, including *Escherichia coli* and *Proteus, Klebsiella, Enterobacter, Enterococcus,* and *Serratia* spp. Hematogenous infections with gram-positive pyogenic bacteria occur during bacteremia.
   A mnemonic for common gram-negative uropathogens is *KEEPS* (*Klebsiella, E. coli, Enterobacter, Pseudomonas aeruginosa,* and *Serratia*).

67. **What is the significance of the vesicoureteric reflux?**
The terminal portion of the ureters is embedded in the wall of the urinary bladder. The smooth muscle at the junction of the ureter and the urinary bladder acts as a valve, preventing the reflux of urine from the urinary bladder into the ureters. In normal individuals, the lumen of the ureter collapses when the bladder contracts during micturition. If the contraction of the smooth muscle occludes the ureter completely, a reflux can occur. Such a vesicoureteric reflux predisposes to pyelonephritis. It may be congenital or acquired:
- **Congenital vesicoureteric reflux:** This is found in 2% or 3% of preschool-age girls. It is not known why girls are more often affected than boys, but it probably relates to the male and female anatomies of that region.
- **Acquired vesicoureteric reflux:** Most often, this develops in men suffering from prolonged urinary obstruction (e.g., prostatic hyperplasia). Straining to overcome the effect of obstruction leads to increased intravesicular pressure and urinary bladder wall hyperplasia and hypertrophy. Bladder atony (e.g., paraplegia due to spinal cord injury) is also associated with reflux.

68. **What are the pathologic features of acute pyelonephritis?**
Acute pyelonephritis is a suppurative infection. Typical features include enlarged, swollen kidneys with small abscesses (yellow, pus-filled masses). It may be one-sided or bilateral. If the pus accumulates in the calices and pelves in obstructed urine, the kidney transforms into a "bag of pus" called pyonephros. Extension of suppuration through the renal capsule leads to the formation of perinephric abscess. Microscopically there is evidence of suppuration and destruction of tubules.

69. **List the most important conditions predisposing to acute pyelonephritis.**
- Urinary bladder obstruction (e.g., prostatic hypertrophy)
- Chronic cystitis
- Urinary stones
- Vesicoureteral reflux
- Pregnancy
- Preexisting renal lesions (e.g., gout nephropathy)
- Diabetes mellitus
- Instrumentation (catheterization is most common)
- Drug-induced tubular injury

70. **Describe the gross features of chronic pyelonephritis.**
    - Asymmetric involvement of kidneys: One kidney is usually more affected than the other.
    - Kidneys are small and irregularly shaped. The surface is scarred. This may be seen on x-ray.
    - At autopsy, renal parenchyma is firm (because of extensive fibrosis).
    - At autopsy when the kidneys are bisected, these scars are usually broad (U shaped) and involve the cortex and the medulla.
    - The pelvis contains irregular fibrous scars and is distorted (best seen using retrograde pyelography).

71. **What are the microscopic features of chronic pyelonephritis?**
    - There is infiltration of interstitial tissue with lymphocytes, plasma cells, and macrophages.
    - Fibrosis of interstitial spaces is noted.
    - There is loss of tubules, which are replaced by fibrosis and inflammatory cells.
    - Remaining tubules appear dilatated and atrophic and contain proteinaceous casts (called "thyroidization" because they resemble thyroid tissue).
    - Glomeruli cut off from the destroyed tubules undergo hyalinization, but many are still preserved.
    - Arteries show endarteritic narrowing of the lumen and fibrosis of media (reactive changes corresponding to involution of vasculature because there is a reduced demand for blood).

72. **What are the clinical features of chronic pyelonephritis?**
    - Gradual loss of renal function, especially in bilateral cases, when it may end in uremia
    - Hypertension
    - Flank pain and other signs of inflammation are vague
    - Urinary signs of bacterial infection are often missing

73. **Give the most common causes of papillary necrosis.**
    A mnemonic to remember is *diabetes*: diabetes, infection (pyelonephritis), analgesic abuse, blockade of urinary efflux (hydronephrosis), thrombosis-emboli, and sickle cell anemia.

74. **What is acute tubulointerstitial nephritis?**
    Acute tubulointerstitial nephritis is the accepted name for an immunologic kidney disease involving the tubules and adjacent interstitial spaces, most often related to drug hypersensitivity. Acute renal failure develops a few weeks to months after the onset of treatment. Pathologic examination reveals interstitial infiltrates of lymphocytes, eosinophils, macrophages, and tubular injury.

75. **How does multiple myeloma damage the kidneys?**
    Kidney injury is the most common cause of death in multiple myeloma. The kidney injury is multifactorial and is related to:
    - **Toxic effects of Bence Jones protein:** This protein is the light chain of immunoglobulin filtered through the glomeruli. It is toxic to tubular cells.
    - **Obstruction of tubules by casts:** Casts are formed from Bence Jones protein interacting with urinary glycoproteins.
    - **Amyloidosis:** AL amyloid formed from the light chains of immunoglobulin deposits in the glomeruli, blood vessels, and tubular basement membranes of tubules.
    - **Light chain nephropathy:** In some instances, the deposits of light chains do not become fibrillar and do not transform into AL amyloid. Nevertheless, these deposits damage the GBM and tubular basement membranes and cause renal failure.
    - **Hypercalcemia:** It leads to nephrocalcinosis and urinary stone formation.

76. **List the macroscopic and microscopic pathologic features of benign nephrosclerosis.**
    - Macroscopic features:
      - Kidneys are symmetrically reduced in size
      - The external surface of the kidney is finely granular, with scars that have a V shape, representing infarcts caused by the occlusion of medium-sized renal vessels. On cross-section, the cortex, is narrowed
    - Microscopic features:
      - Narrowed arterioles appear hyalinized, and arteries show fibrosis
      - Glomeruli are frequently sclerotic and obliterated
      - Tubules are atrophic, and there is tubular loss
      - Interstitial fibrosis replacing nephrons, associated with infiltrates of lymphocytes (no plasma cells)

77. **What are the pathologic features of malignant hypertension?**
    Malignant hypertension presents clinically with diastolic blood pressure over 130 mmHg, papilledema, retinopathy, and, in some patients, encephalopathy due to increased intracranial pressure. Microscopic findings include:
    - Hyperplastic arteriolopathy ("onion skin"–like smooth muscle cell hyperplasia)
    - Fibrinoid necrosis of arterioles and small arteries
    - Fibrinoid necrosis and microthrombi in segments of glomerular capillaries

78. **What is the most common cause of hemolytic uremic syndrome in children?**
    Intestinal infections with verocytotoxin-producing *E. coli* (0157:H7) cause 75% of cases of hemolytic uremic syndrome in children.

79. **What are the most common causes of renal infarcts?**
    Most renal infarcts result from thromboemboli or cholesterol emboli. These emboli typically originate from:
    - Mural thrombi in the left atrium in patients who have atrial fibrillation
    - Mural thrombi overlying the left ventricular myocardial infarction
    - Vegetations on mitral valve and aortic valve related to endocarditis
    - Aortic mural thrombi overlying atheromas
    - Cholesterol emboli from ruptured aortic atheromas

80. **Name the most common causes of diffuse cortical renal necrosis in pregnant women.**
    - Abruptio placentae
    - Amniotic fluid embolism
    - Disseminated intravascular coagulation
    - Hypotensive or septic shock

81. **What are the most common causes of obstructive uropathy?**
    - Congenital anomalies such as posterior urethral valves and urethral strictures, meatal stenosis, bladder neck obstruction, and ureteropelvic junction narrowing or obstruction
    - Urinary calculi
    - Benign prostatic hypertrophy
    - Tumors including carcinoma of the prostate, bladder tumors, contiguous malignant disease (retroperitoneal lymphoma), and carcinoma of the cervix or uterus
    - Uterus (pregnancy and uterine prolapse)
    - Neurogenic bladder (spinal cord damage)

82. **What are the pathologic changes caused in the kidney by urinary obstruction?**
    - Hydronephrosis, in which the pelvis and calices dilatate, and clear fluid accumulates in these spaces
    - Atrophy of the papillae, which appear blunted
    - Atrophy of the cortex and the entire kidney, typically seen in long-standing disease
    - Microscopically, accompanied by a loss of tubules and interstitial fibrosis

83. **How common are renal calculi in the United States?**
    Urolithiasis is a common clinical problem, affecting 5% to 10% of Americans. Men are affected more than women; peak onset of first symptoms is between 20 and 30 years of age. Stones are more common in the southeastern United States, the so-called stone belt.

84. **Name the four main types of renal calculi.**
    - **Calcium-containing stones:** 75% (composed of calcium phosphates or oxalates)
    - **Struvite stones:** 15% (composed of ammonium magnesium calcium phosphates)
    - **Uric acid stones:** 5%
    - **Cystine stones:** 1%

85. **What is the most common cause of renal calculi?**
    Urinary stones are often associated with increased urinary and serum concentration of substances found in the stones. Hypersaturation of urine with calcium is typically found in association with hypercalcemia, but some people have hypercalciuria without hypercalcemia. Hyperuricemia associated with increased excretion of uric acid in urine may lead to the formation of pure uric acid stones. However, hyperuricosuria may also promote the formation of calcium stones; the uric acid crystals formed under these conditions are considered to be the initial nidus for the crystalization of other salts. Cystine stones are found in children who have the inborn error of metabolism known as cystinosis.

86. **What is the chemical composition of urinary calculi caused by chronic urinary infection?**
    It is magnesium ammonium phosphate (struvite) stones. These stones arise in urine made alkaline (normal urine is acidic) by ammonia formed by urea-splitting bacteria, such as *Proteus* species and some species of *Staphylococcus*.

RENAL TUMORS

87. **Name three most important renal tumors.**
    - Renal cell carcinoma (RCC)—the most common renal tumor in adults
    - Wilms tumor—the most common tumor in infants and children
    - Transitional cell carcinoma of renal pelvis

88. **How common is renal cell carcinoma?**
    - It comprises 1% to 3% of all visceral cancers.
    - It represents 90% of all renal cancers.
    - There are 30,000 new cases diagnosed per year with 12,000 deaths per year in the United States.
    - The incidence is increasing for no clear reason.
    - The male-to-female ratio is 1.5:1.
    - Age of onset is 50 years and older.

89. **Discuss the evidence that some RCCs are familial and related to cancer genes.**
    - Most RCCs are sporadic and develop at random, but 5% are familial.
    - Loss of one allele of a tumor suppressor gene (called vHL) on chromosome 3 is found in 98% of sporadic RCCs. This gene is deleted in patients with von Hippel–Lindau disease, known to have a predisposition to RCC.
    - Approximately 40% of all patients with von Hippel–Lindau disease (characterized by retinal hemangiomas and cerebellar hemangioblastomas) develop RCC.
    - Autosomal dominant clear cell RCC occurs in some families.
    - Papillary type of RRC can be multifocal and hereditary.

KEY POINTS: RENAL TUMORS ✔

1. Renal cell carcinoma, the most common tumor of the kidney, presents in 50% of cases with hematuria.

2. Wilms tumors are malignant childhood tumors composed of renal blastema-like cells.

3. Transitional cell carcinomas of the renal pelvis are similar to those found in the ureters, urinary bladder, and posterior urethra.

90. **Describe the gross features of RCC.**
    - Size at the time of diagnosis varies from 2 to 20 cm or more (can be detected by computed tomography scan).
    - It is partially encapsulated, lobulated, growing by expansion and subsequently by infiltrating the surrounding renal parenchyma.
    - It is yellow on cross-section (tumor cells contain lipid and glycogen; histologically these cells appear clear).
    - It may show focal hemorrhage, necrosis, and prominent cystic degeneration.
    - Invasion of renal vein is a common mode of spread.
    - It may invade into perirenal fat, adrenal gland, and surrounding tissues.
    - Ther may be metastases to lungs (hematogenous) and local lymph nodes in the abdomen.

91. **List microscopic types of RCC.**
    - **Clear cell carcinoma (70%):** Clear cells may be arranged into tubules or solid nests.
    - **Papillary (15%):** It may be multifocal and familial.
    - **Chromophobe (5%):** It has excellent prognosis.
    Other morphologic subtypes are less common.

92. **What are the clinical signs and symptoms of RCC?**
    The classical triad comprising hematuria, flank pain, and an abdominal mass is found in only 10% of patients. The most frequent presenting manifestations are:
    - Hematuria: 60% (This is the most common finding, and it is most often microscopic and discovered by urinalysis.)
    - Pain: 45%
    - Flank mass: 20% (Only large tumors are palpable.)
    - Fever: 5%
    - Metastases as first sign of disease: 5%
    - Paraneoplastic syndromes: 5%

93. **What are the most common paraneoplastic syndromes in patients with RCC?**
RCC is a potential source of ectopic production of hormones and growth factors and may stimulate the production of amyloid. Paraneoplastic syndromes are so common that the tumor may present with a number of atypical symptoms. Hence it was nicknamed "internists' tumor." The most common paraneoplastic syndromes are:
- Erythrocytosis (related to erythropoietin)
- Hypercalcemia (due to parathyroid hormone or parathyroid-like polypeptide)
- Hypertension (due to renin secretion)
- Amyloidosis

94. **What is the 5-year survival rate of RCC?**
- Overall, the 5-year survival rate for RCC is approximately 45%.
- Tumors diagnosed early in the course of the disease (before metastases develop) have a good prognosis (>70% 5-year survival).
- Tumors invading the renal vein or the perinephric fat have a poor prognosis (15%–20% 5-year survival).
- There are many cases on record demonstrating that the metastases may regress after the primary tumor has been resected. The reasons for the regression of such metastases are not known.

95. **What is the most common renal tumor of infancy and childhood?**
Wilms tumor (also known as nephroblastoma) is the most common primary renal tumor of childhood.

96. **List the most important facts about Wilms tumor.**
- It accounts for 25% of all cancers in infancy and childhood.
- It is most often diagnosed between aged 2 and 5 years.
- It is rare after 10 years of age (98% <10 years).
- It is usually one sided but occasionally bilateral (5%–8%).
- Surgery combined with chemotherapy gives excellent results (95% cure).
- Children younger than 2 years have a better prognosis than older children.

97. **How many Wilms tumors are hereditary?**
- Only 5% of Wilms tumors are familial and thus obviously hereditary.
- An additional 5% of Wilms tumors may be related to genetic factors because these tumors occur in the context of developmental malformation syndromes:
  - WAGR syndrome (Wilms tumor, aniridia, genitourinary anomalies, and mental retardation)
  - Beckwith–Wiedemann syndrome (Wilms tumor, hemihypertrophy of the body, macroglossia, and visceromegaly)
- Familial and syndromic cases are bilateral in 20% of patients.
- Familial and syndromic cases may be associated with deletion of tumor suppressor genes (WT-1 or WT-2).
- Deletion of tumor suppressor gene WT-1 is also found in 10% of sporadic Wilms tumors.

98. **Describe the microscopic features of Wilms tumors.**
It is worth remembering that Wilms tumor is also known as nephroblastoma and is thus composed of cells found in the renal blastema (i.e., the fetal metanephros). Pathologists recognize three major components found in most tumors in varying proportions:
- **Blastema-like cells:** These "small blue cells" have a high nucleus:cytoplasm ratio and are classified as undifferentiated, or vaguely resembling fetal tissue.
- **Stromal cells:** These are spindle-shaped cells resembling fetal renal connective tissue. Stromal parts of the Wilms tumor may also contain heterotopic mesenchymal tissues (e.g., skeletal muscle cells or cartilage).

- **Epithelial cells:** These cells form tubules resembling those in the metanephros and the fetal kidney.

Some tumors contain more blastema-like cells, whereas others are more epithelial. Predominantly epithelial tumors have a better prognosis, but overall these tumors are also usually recognized in earlier stages (Stages I and II) than tumors composed of blastemal cells, which tend to be diagnosed in more advanced stages. The most important histologic finding predicting poor prognosis is anaplasia of tumor cells. Such cells show marked pleomorphism and have bizarre, large nuclei and abnormal mitoses. Anaplasia is found in tumors that are resistant to chemotherapy.

99. **List key facts about urothelial carcinomas of the renal pelvis.**
    - They are similar to transitional cell tumors of the urinary bladder.
    - They are most often papillary and exophytic but may also be invasive.
    - Transitional epithelial cells lining the papillae may detach and may be found in urine (important for diagnosis).
    - Even small tumors may cause hematuria, renal colic, or urinary obstruction and can be diagnosed in early stages of development.
    - Prognosis is good (up to 70% 5-year survival) because most tumors are exophytic papillary low-grade carcinomas. High-grade invasive tumors have poor prognosis (10% 5-year survival).

PATHOLOGY OF THE URINARY BLADDER

100. **How common are congenital anomalies of the urinary bladder?**
     Major anomalies are rare. Extrophy of the bladder resulting from the incomplete closure of the anterior wall of the bladder and the anterior abdominal wall results in a major defect that can be recognized at the time of birth.

101. **How common are infections of the urinary bladder?**
     Infectious diseases of the urinary bladder are very common. Such infections can present in the form of acute cystitis or chronic cystitis. In most instances, cystitis is caused by coliform bacteria, such as *E. coli* and *Proteus* sp.

102. **Is cystitis more common in women than in men?**
     Yes, because women have a shorter urethra than men and thus their urinary bladder is much more easily invaded by bacteria. Infection may be related to poor hygiene, intercourse, pregnancy, or genital infections. Chronic cystitis is a common disease in older men suffering from prostatic hyperplasia. Urinary stones are a common risk factor in both men and women.

KEY POINTS: PATHOLOGY OF THE URINARY BLADDER ✔

1. Cystitis, inflammation of the urinary bladder, is a common disease most often caused by coliform bacteria.

2. Transitional cell carcinomas are the most common tumors of the urinary bladder.

3. Prognosis of urinary bladder cancers depends on their histologic grade and clinical stage (i.e., depth of invasion and extent of spread).

103. **Is cystitis always caused by bacteria?**
No. Although gram-negative bacteria account for most cases of infectious cystitis, cystitis found in cancer patients or those with AIDS may be caused by viruses such as cytomegalovirus. In Egypt, cystitis is often caused by *Schistosoma haematobium*.

104. **Define interstitial cystitis.**
Interstitial cystitis is a chronic inflammation of the urinary bladder of unknown etiology. Typically it affects women and is clinically associated with severe pain that does not respond to conventional therapy. The diagnosis is based on clinical grounds and is confirmed by cystoscopy when the urologist may note "cracking" and fissuring of the urinary bladder mucosa distended by instillation of water during this diagnostic procedure. Some women develop chronic ulcers (Hunner ulcer). Histologic findings seen in urinary bladder biopsy are relatively nonspecific. Pathologists usually report that the bladder shows mild chronic inflammation and infiltration with mast cells.

105. **What is malakoplakia?**
Malakoplakia, literally "soft plaques," is a form of chronic cystitis characterized by the appearance of yellowish soft plaques covering the surface of the urinary bladder. Histologically, the lesions are composed of macrophages containing peculiar calcified cytoplasmic inclusions called Michaelis–Gutmann bodies. The exact pathogenesis of malakoplakia is not known. It is thought that malakoplakia is an unusual reaction to chronic *E. coli* infection. It may occur in other organs as well.

106. **Define iatrogenic cystitis.**
Iatrogenic cystitis (i.e., cystitis directly or indirectly related to medical treatment) is most often caused by:
- Instrumentation, such as catheterization or cystoscopy
- Radiation therapy (radiation cystitis)
- Chemotherapy (e.g., pseudomembranous cystitis found in patients treated with cyclophosphamide)
- Bacille Calmette–Guérin (BCG) treatment of bladder cancer (i.e., granulomatous inflammation following intravesical instillation of attenuated *Mycobacterium tuberculosis* strain of Calmette–Guérin).

107. **How common are tumors of the urinary bladder?**
Urinary bladder tumors are very common. Annually, there are 50,000 new cases diagnosed in the United States, and these tumors cause approximately 10,000 deaths per year (3% of all cancer-related deaths).

108. **Give the risk factors for urinary bladder cancer.**
- The most important risk factor is cigarette smoking.
- Industrial carcinogens, such as naphthylamine and benzidine, play a role among the workers in dye, rubber, plastic, and insulation industries.
- Schistosoma haematobium infection in Egypt is associated with an increased incidence of urinary bladder cancer.

109. **How are urinary bladder carcinomas classified histologically?**
Most urinary bladder carcinomas (>90%) are classified as urothelial or transitional cell carcinomas (TCCs). The remaining tumors are classified as squamous cell carcinomas or adenocarcinomas and occasionally as sarcomas. See Fig. 15-8.

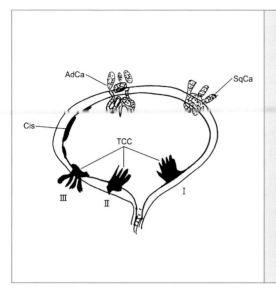

Figure 15-8. Urinary bladder cancer. Most urinary bladder cancers are classified as transitional cell carcinomas (TCCs). Histologically, there are three grades of TCCs: Stage I tumors are exophytic papillary lesions not invading the bladder wall. Stage II lesions are papillary lesions that also invade the muscle layer of the bladder wall. Stage III lesions are invasive tumors penetrating through the wall of the bladder and/or extending into adjacent tissues. Malignant tumors may also present as multifocal flat carcinomas in situ (Cis), adenocarcinomas (AdCa), and squamous cell carcinomas (SqCa).

110. **Describe how urinary bladder cancers appear on gross examination.**
    - **Papillary tumors:** Most small tumors are exophytic and project into the lumen of the bladder as wartlike papillary outgrowths. These tumors may be snared away during cystoscopy.
    - **Exophytic cauliflower-like tumors:** Larger tumors may be entirely exophytic, but some also have an invasive part.
    - **Flat lesions:** These are usually classified as carcinomas in situ.
    - **Ulcers:** Invasive tumors often present as ulcerations with indurated margins. These ulcerated tumors usually invade into the deeper layers of the urinary bladder wall and extend into the surrounding structures and pelvic organs.

111. **Why is it important to grade histologically TCCs of the urinary bladder?**
    The prognosis of TCCs depends on the grade and stage of the tumor. The grading is based on histologic examination. Well-differentiated transitional papillary tumors are Grade I. Papillary tumors composed of broad papillae and solid areas are Grade II. Solid, anaplastic tumors are Grade III. In general, the well-differentiated papillary exophytic tumors have a good prognosis, whereas poorly differentiated endophytic (invasive) tumors have a bad prognosis. The tumors that are predominantly papillary but also invade the bladder wall have an intermediate prognosis.

112. **Discuss how squamous cell carcinomas may arise in a transitional epithelium-lined organ such as the urinary bladder.**
    Squamous cell carcinomas originate in areas of squamous metaplasia that are typically found in chronic cystitis associated with urinary stones or parasitic infections. Thus it is not surprising that most urinary bladder carcinomas linked to chronic infection with *S. haematobium* are histologically classified as squamous cell carcinomas.

113. **What is the prognosis for TCCs of the urinary bladder?**
TCCs are treated surgically. The overall prognosis depends on the grade and stage of the tumor:
- Stage I: greater than 95% 10-year survival
- Stage II: 50% to 80% 5-year survival
- Stage III: 20% to 30% 5-year survival

114. **Do squamous cell carcinomas of the urinary bladder have a worse prognosis than TCCs?**
Yes. Overall, only 30% of all patients with squamous cell carcinoma survive more than 1 year after diagnosis.

WESTIES

1. http://www.ncbi.nlm.nih.gov/entrez/query.fcgi?db=PubMed
2. http://www-medlib.med.utah.edu/WebPath/webpath.html#MENU
3. http://www.uihealthcare.com/vh
4. http://www.mayoclinic.com/health/glomerulonephritis/DS00503
5. http://www.cancer.gov/cancertopics/types/kidney

BIBLIOGRAPHY

1. Chadban SJ, Atkins RC: Glomerulonephritis. Lancet 365:1797–1806, 2005.
2. Eddy AA, Symons JM: Nephrotic syndrome in childhood. Lancet 362:629–639, 2003.
3. Epstein JI, Amin MB, Reuter VR, et al: The World Health Organization/International Society of Urological Pathology consensus classification of urothelial (transitional cell) neoplasms of the urinary bladder. Am J Surg Pathol 22:1435–1448, 1998.
4. Hricik DE, Chung-Park M, Sedor JR: Glomerulonephritis. N Engl J Med 339:888–899, 1998.
5. Jennette JC, Falk RJ: Diagnosis and management of glomerular diseases. Med Clin North Am 81:653–676, 1997.
6. Kwoh C, Shannon MB, Miner JH, Shaw A: Pathogenesis of nonimmune glomerulopathies. Annu Rev Pathol 1:349–374, 2006.
7. Montironi R, Mikuz G, Algaba F, et al: Epithelial tumours of the adult kidney. Virchows Arch 434:281–290, 1999.
8. Schwartz MM, Lewis EJ: Rewriting the histological classification of lupus nephritis. J Nephrol 15(Suppl 6): S11–S19, 2002.
9. Vinen CS, Oliveira DB: Acute glomerulonephritis. Postgrad Med J 79:206–213, 2003.

CHAPTER 16

THE MALE GENITAL SYSTEM

Ivan Damjanov, MD, PhD

1. **What are the principal male genital organs?**
   - Testis
   - Epididymis
   - Vas deferens
   - Seminal vesicles
   - Prostate
   - Penis
   - Scrotum

2. **What are the most important diseases of the male genital system?**
   - Developmental disorders
   - Infections
   - Infertility
   - Tumors

KEY POINTS: DISEASES OF THE MALE GENITAL SYSTEM ✓

1. The most important diseases of the male genital system are infections and tumors.

2. Developmental disorders of the male genital system may have adverse effects on fertility or predispose to infections.

3. In young men, infections of the male genital system are mostly sexually transmitted, whereas in older men they are due to prostatic disease.

DEVELOPMENTAL DISORDERS

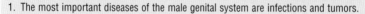

3. **What is the most common developmental abnormality involving the testis?**
   Cryptorchidism is the most common abnormality of the male genital tract. It is found in 3% of full-term infants but is much more common in prematurely born boys. It results from an incomplete descent of the testis into the scrotum. The testis may be "hidden" (as the term implies, *cryptos,* meaning "hidden" in Greek) in the abdominal cavity or inside the inguinal canal. Such testes can be repositioned into the scrotum surgically ("orchidopexy").

4. **What are the complications of cryptorchidism?**
   Cryptorchidism is associated with an increased incidence of:
   - **Infertility:** The testis retained in the abdominal cavity or the inguinal canal undergoes atrophy, and the seminal epithelium degenerates.
   - **Germ cell tumors:** The reasons for the increased incidence of germ cell tumors are not known.

5. **What is the difference between hypospadias and epispadias?**
The urethral meatus is normally located at the tip of the penis. The anomaly in which the opening of the urethra is found on the ventral surface of the penile shaft is called hypospadias. Opening of the penile urethra on the dorsal surface of the penis is called epispadias. Hypospadias is more common (1:1000 newborn males) than epispadias (1:30,000 newborn males). Hypospadias is a less severe anomaly, and it usually occurs in an isolated form. Epispadias often involves a longer segment of the penis and is often combined with extrophy of the urinary bladder. See Fig. 16-1.

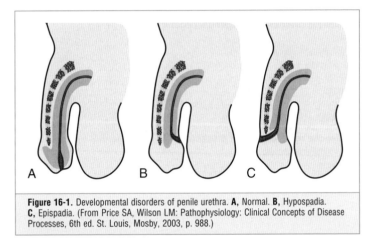

Figure 16-1. Developmental disorders of penile urethra. **A,** Normal. **B,** Hypospadia. **C,** Epispadia. (From Price SA, Wilson LM: Pathophysiology: Clinical Concepts of Disease Processes, 6th ed. St. Louis, Mosby, 2003, p. 988.)

6. **What is phimosis?**
Phimosis is an abnormality of the penis characterized by tight prepuce (foreskin) that cannot be retracted over the glans penis. Phimosis can be congenital or secondary to infections causing fibrosis of the foreskin. Circumcision is the treatment of choice.

7. **What is paraphimosis?**
Paraphimosis is a condition in which a tight prepuce is retracted over the glans but cannot be rolled back, thus strangulating the glans penis.

8. **What is inguinal scrotal hernia?**
Following the descent of the testis, the inguinal canal closes. If the canal remains open, abdominal contents can slide through the inguinal canal into the scrotum, resulting in a hernia. Hernia may be congenital or acquired because of a reopening of a previously closed inguinal canal.

9. **What is a hydrocele?**
A hydrocele is an accumulation of fluid in the scrotum, typically between the two layers of tunica vaginalis testis. This tunica is an extension of the mesothelium that envelops the testis during its descent.
  Normally the surfaces of tunica are kept wet with a few drops of fluid. Occasionally the amount of fluid will increase, often for no obvious cause. Similar hydrocele may develop because of infection of the testis and epididymis or due to a blockade of lymphatic drainage from the scrotum. Fluid also accumulates in the scrotum in generalized anasarca and also in the course of heart failure.

10. **What are the other scrotal disorders that may be confused with hydrocele?**
Hydrocele is diagnosed by palpating the scrotum and testes and by documenting fluid accumulation in the spaces limited by tunica vaginalis testis. This is best achieved by transluminating the scrotal contents with a flashlight placed behind the scrotum. Other conditions that may be mistaken for hydrocele are:
- **Epididymal cysts:** These cysts represent developmental recesses attached to the epididymis. If filled with sperm, they are called spermatocele.
- **Scrotal hernia:** Loops of the intestine may slide into the scrotum and present as a scrotal mass.
- **Varicocele:** This term is used for the varicous dilatation of the scrotal veins ("bag of worms" noticed on palpation).
- **Tumors:** In contrast to hydrocele, tumors do not transluminate.

INFECTIONS

11. **What is epididymoorchitis?**
Epididymoorchitis is an inflammation of the epididymis and testis. Infections reach the testis and epididymis hematogenously or by an ascending route from the urethra and ductus deferens. The most important pathogens include:
- Sexually transmitted pathogens, such as *Neisseria gonorrhoeae, Ureaplasma urealyticum,* and *Chlamydia trachomatis,* are typically found in young adults.
- Uropathogens, such as *Escherichia coli, Pseudomonas aeruginosa,* and *Klebsiella,* cause epididymoorchitis in the elderly suffering from prostatic hyperplasia and urinary tract infections.
- Viruses, such as the mumps virus, reach the scrotum testis through the hematogenous route and cause predominantly orchitis in children.

12. **What is balanitis?**
Balanitis is an inflammation of the glans penis. In men who are not circumcised, it is associated with an inflammation of the foreskin (balanoposthitis). Nonspecific bacterial balanitis is usually a consequence of poor hygiene.

13. **What are the common causes of ulceration on the glans penis?**
- **Genital herpes:** Herpes simplex virus 2 (HSV-2) infection presents with vesicles that ulcerate and heal by formation of crusts.
- **Syphilis:** Treponema pallidum infection may result in the formation of an ulceration (syphilitic chancre).
- **Chancroid:** Painful ulcer, associated with local swelling and enlargement of inguinal lymph nodes, is caused by Hemophilus ducreyi.

14. **How does gonorrhea present clinically?**
Infection with *N. gonorrhoeae* usually causes urethritis presenting with a purulent urethral discharge. If the discharge is examined under the microscope, *Neisseriae* may be seen as paired cocci (diplococci) in the cytoplasm of neutrophils in the smear.

15. **What is Peyronie disease?**
Peyronie disease is a fibromatosis of unknown etiology involving the fasciae of the penile shaft. Progressive fibrosis is associated with curvature of the penis and painful erection and intercourse.

NEOPLASMS AND RELATED CONDITIONS

16. **What is the most common neoplasm of the male genital tract?**
Prostatic carcinoma, a cancer of old age. In men younger than 40 years, testicular tumors are the most common genital cancer.

17. **List the most important facts about testicular tumors.**
    - They are uncommon tumors. Incidence is only 5 per 100,000 men.
    - They account for less than 1% of all malignant tumors in males.
    - Peak incidence in the 30- to 40-year-old age group. They are rare in prepubertal children and the elderly.
    - Most tumors (>90%) are of germ cell origin.
    - Most tumors (>90%) are malignant.
    - Serum tumor markers found in approximately 50% patients. These markers include alpha-fetoprotein (AFP) and human chorionic gonadotropin (hCG).
    - Platinum-based chemotherapy combined with surgery gives excellent results (>90% cure rate).

18. **What are the risk factors for testicular cancer?**
    - **Sex chromosome abnormalities:** Germ cell tumors occur at a rate of 25% in dysgenetic gonads, intersexes, hermaphrodites, and pseudohermaphrodites. Fortunately, these conditions are rare.
    - **Cryptorchidism:** This anomaly is associated with a 10-fold increase in the incidence of germ cell tumors. It is not known whether the tumors develop because the testis is in an abnormal location or whether the testis is retained because it is abnormal.

19. **Explain the histogenesis of testicular germ cell tumors.**
    Testicular germ cell tumors originate from intratubular germ cells, probably spermatogonia or primordial germ cells, that have undergone malignant transformation. Malignant transformation is accompanied by distinct morphologic changes that can be recognized histologically as carcinoma in situ or intratubular testicular germ cell neoplasia (ITTGCN). Malignant germ cells have enlarged, hyperchromatic nuclei and well-developed cytoplasm filled with glycogen. Such cells remain inside the tubules for variable periods of time and then give rise to invasive tumor cells that spread outside the seminiferous tubules.

KEY POINTS: NEOPLASMS AND RELATED CONDITIONS ✔

1. Testicular tumors are relatively rare but important because they affect men in their most productive years, between 30 and 40 years of age.

2. Testicular germ cell tumors account for 90% of all neoplasms of the testis, and they can be divided into two groups: seminomas and nonseminomatous germ cell tumors.

3. Prostate cancer, a neoplasm of older men, is the most common malignant tumor in males.

20. **How is ITTGCN diagnosed?**
    Intratubular preinvasive testicular germ cell tumors are usually diagnosed accidentally by testicular biopsy during the workup of infertility.

21. **How are testicular tumors classified clinically?**
    The histogenesis and pathologic classification of testicular tumors have been debated during the past 100 years, but no generally acceptable consensus has been reached. For practical purposes, it is thus most convenient to divide testicular germ cell tumors into two groups:
    - Seminomas (40%)
    - Nonseminomatous germ cell tumors (NSGCT) (40%)

Approximately 15% of tumors are composed of both seminomatous and nonseminomatous elements. Because the nonseminomatous elements are more malignant than the seminoma cells, clinically such mixed tumors are treated as if they were NSGCT. The remaining 5% of germ cell tumors comprise rare entities, such as yolk sac tumors of infants and young children, spermatocytic seminomas of the elderly, and rare benign teratomas.

22. **List key pathologic facts about seminomas.**
    - They are composed of a single cell type.
    - Tumor cells have clear cytoplasm, filled with glycogen.
    - Tumor cells are arranged into lobules surrounded by fibrous strand infiltrated with lymphocytes, macrophages, plasma cells, or giant cells. See Fig. 16-2.
    - On gross examination, the tumor appears lobulated and uniformly white or yellow on cross section.
    - Metastases are found first in paraaortic abdominal lymph nodes.

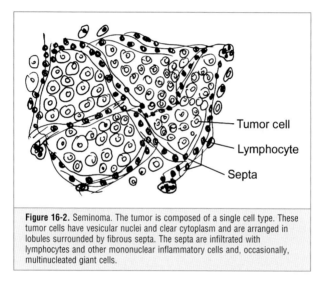

Figure 16-2. Seminoma. The tumor is composed of a single cell type. These tumor cells have vesicular nuclei and clear cytoplasm and are arranged in lobules surrounded by fibrous septa. The septa are infiltrated with lymphocytes and other mononuclear inflammatory cells and, occasionally, multinucleated giant cells.

23. **Describe the clinical course of the disease caused by seminomas.**
    - Most patients are 25 to 45 years of age.
    - Tumor presents as a scrotal mass.
    - Most tumors are diagnosed early while the tumor is limited to the testis; tumors with lymph node metastases are rare, and those with widespread metastases are uncommon today.
    - There are no serologic tumor markers for seminoma.
    - Treatment includes surgery, radiation therapy, and chemotherapy.
    - Cure rate is greater than 90%.

24. **List the key facts about the pathology of NSGCT.**
    - Histopathology highly variable.
    - Embryonal carcinoma (EC) cells are the stem cells of most NSGCT.
    - EC cells may proliferate as such, without differentiating into other cells, and such tumors are called embryonal carcinomas.
    - EC cells that differentiate into somatic tissues (e.g., neural tissue and cartilage) and extraembryonic tissues (e.g., yolk sac and trophoblastic cells) form heterogeneous tumors called teratocarcinomas.

- If the EC cells differentiate into trophoblastic cells that become the only malignant component of the tumor, the tumor is called choriocarcinoma.
- If the EC cells differentiate into yolk sac cells and the entire tumor is composed of these cells, the tumor is called yolk sac carcinoma.
- It the EC cells differentiate into somatic tissues, the tumor is called teratoma.

25. Describe the clinical course of the disease caused by NSGCT.
- Most patients are 20 to 45 years of age.
- The tumor presents as a scrotal mass.
- Metastases occur more often in NSGCT than in seminoma patients.
- Serologic tumor markers (AFP, hCG, or both) are found in more than 80% of patients.
- Treatment includes surgery combined with chemotherapy.
- Cure rate is approximately 90%.

26. What are mixed germ cell tumors?
This term is used for tumors composed of seminoma and NSGCT. Such tumors owe their malignancy primarily to the EC cells (i.e., the malignant stem cells of NSGCT) and are therefore clinically treated as NSGCT.

27. How common are pure embryonal carcinomas, choriocarcinomas, and yolk sac carcinomas in adult males?
All these tumors are rare. Most NSGCTs present as teratocarcinomas containing EC and other tissues that differentiate from these malignant stem cells. Pure embryonal carcinomas account for approximately 3% of all germ cell tumors. Pure testicular choriocarcinomas are extremely rare (1 case per 1000 testicular tumors). Pure yolk sac carcinomas are almost nonexistent in adult males.

28. Define yolk sac tumor.
Yolk sac tumor, also called endodermal sinus tumor, is a testicular tumor of early childhood. The following are key facts about this tumor:
- Most patients (99%) are younger than 4 years of age.
- Tumor is composed of cells resembling yolk sac. Remember that the yolk sac is an extraembryonic structure attached to the anterior abdominal wall of the early fetus. It involutes by the 16th week of pregnancy and is not found in adults. Thus yolk sac tumors are composed of extraembryonic tissues and, in a sense, resemble choriocarcinomas, another tumor composed of extraembryonic cells (i.e., placenta).
- Tumor cells arranged in several patterns, including glomeruloid structures known as Schiller–Duval bodies.
- AFP is found in the serum of all patients and is a good serologic marker.
- Cure rate is approximately 100%.

29. What are the sex cord cell tumors of the testis?
Sex cord cell tumors account for approximately 5% of all primary testicular tumors. This group of tumors includes:
- **Leydig cell tumor:** It is composed of solid masses of well-differentiated cells. These cells have round nuclei and well-developed eosinophilic cytoplasm. They resemble normal Leydig cells and may contain Reinke crystalloids.
- **Sertoli cell tumor:** Tumor cells form cords or tubules surrounded by a basement membrane.

30. **List the key facts about Leydig cell tumor.**
    - This tumor can develop at any age from infancy to old age.
    - Most tumors are benign, but some are malignant. Malignant Leydig cell tumors are low-grade malignancies and thus have a relatively favorable prognosis.
    - Histologic examination does not allow one to determine whether a tumor is benign or malignant.
    - Most tumors are hormonally active, but some are inactive.
    - Tumors may secrete androgens or estrogens
    - Excess androgen will cause premature puberty and macrogenitosomia in prepubertal boys, but it is usually unrelated to specific symptoms in adults.
    - Excess estrogen may cause gynecomastia in adult males.

31. **What are the most common testicular tumors in the elderly?**
    Primary germ cell or sex cord cell tumors are rare in the elderly. Most tumors in older men are metastases of lymphoma, prostatic carcinoma, or gastrointestinal cancer.

32. **List key facts about tumors of the penis.**
    - Penile cancer is rare in the United States but much more common in South America and underdeveloped countries of Asia and Africa.
    - Risk factors include poor hygiene and human papillomavirus (HPV) infection.
    - Almost all malignant tumors are classified as squamous cell carcinoma.
    - Most tumors present as ulcerations or mucosal indurated plaques.
    - Exophytic verrucous tumors (known as giant condyloma of Buschke and Lowenstein) are rare forms of low-grade squamous cell carcinoma.
    - Metastases occur in inguinal lymph nodes.
    - Five-year survival rate with modern therapy is 60%.

33. **Define Bowen disease and erythroplasia of Queyrat.**
    These names are used for the same disease. Traditionally, Bowen disease is the term used for the squamous carcinoma in situ on the shaft of the penis. Erythroplasia of Queyrat is a carcinoma in situ on the glans presenting in the form of red plaques. Invasive squamous cell carcinoma develops over time in 10% to 20% of these lesions.

34. **What is condyloma acuminatum?**
    Condyloma acuminatum or genital wart is a papilloma caused by HPV. Most often, they develop on the glans, but they may be found on the skin of the shaft of the penis. Papillomas are lined by hyperplastic squamous epithelium that shows koilocytosis, a typical feature of all HPV lesions. Condylomata acuminata are caused by HPV isotypes that do not cause cancer. Accordingly, these genital warts are not precancerous and do not progress to invasive carcinomas.

    Condylomata acuminata must be distinguished from condylomata lata, the flat papules of secondary syphilis. Condylomata lata may occur on genital organs but also in many other sites, especially palms and the plantar surface of the feet.

35. **What is the cause of nodular prostatic hyperplasia?**
    Nodular hyperplasia of the prostate, also known as benign prostatic hyperplasia (or, among surgeons, as benign prostatic hypertrophy [BPH]), is a common disease affecting many older men. The pathogenesis of this disease is not known, but it is thought that it occurs because of an altered normal ratio of testosterone to estrogen that develops in the elderly. It is thought that the cells of the central (periurethral) part of the prostate proliferate in response to a relative increase of estrogen or a reduction of testosterone in blood. It is not known why this hyperplasia:
    - Occurs predominantly in the central part of the prostate
    - Is more common in African American males than in Caucasians

- Shows geographic variation in various populations and is more common in the United States and Western Europe than in other areas of the world
- Is unrelated to cancer

36. **Describe the pathologic features of nodular prostatic hyperplasia.**
   - Gross appearance
     - Prostate enlarged, nodular, firm, and rubbery, weighing $2\times$ or more than normal
     - Periurethral (central) portion expanded by nodules that compress the peripheral part
     - Peripheral portion compressed into a "surgical capsule" (so called because the central nodular part can be shelled out of it during suprapubic prostatectomy)
     - Urethra is compressed and tortuous or deformed
     - Median bar may protrude into the urinary bladder and act like a "ball valve"
   - Microscopic appearance
     - Hyperplastic glands lined by columnar and cuboidal cells, often projecting into the lumen
     - Overall structure of the prostatic glands is preserved; all of them are composed of two layers: inner secretory epithelial cells and the outer basal cell layer
     - Stroma contains hyperplastic smooth muscle and fibroblastic cells
     See Fig. 16-3.

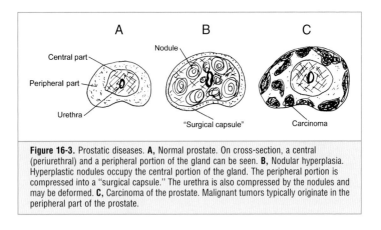

Figure 16-3. Prostatic diseases. **A,** Normal prostate. On cross-section, a central (periurethral) and a peripheral portion of the gland can be seen. **B,** Nodular hyperplasia. Hyperplastic nodules occupy the central portion of the gland. The peripheral portion is compressed into a "surgical capsule." The urethra is also compressed by the nodules and may be deformed. **C,** Carcinoma of the prostate. Malignant tumors typically originate in the peripheral part of the prostate.

37. **What are the pathologic changes caused by urinary obstruction caused by BPH?**
   - Tortuous and compressed urethra
   - Dilatated and hypertrophic urinary bladder (the wall shows intraluminal "trabeculation" due to smooth muscle cells hyperplasia and hypertrophy)
   - Cystitis
   - Calculi forming in the stagnant and infected urine
   - Prostatitis and epididymoorchitis due to extension of infections from the urinary bladder
   - Hydroureter and hydronephrosis (renal function may become compromised over time)

38. **What are the clinical features of benign prostatic hyperplasia?**
   - Symptoms pertain to the compression of the urethra and retention of urine
   - Dysuria (urge to urinate frequently, weak stream, halting, and incomplete emptying of the urinary bladder)
   - Urinary bladder infections
   - Urinary tract dysfunction due to obstructed urine flow

39. **How common is prostatic carcinoma?**
It is the most common tumor in males. Of cancer-related causes of death in males, it is second after lung cancer.

40. **List key facts about prostatic carcinoma.**
   - It is an old-age disease. Incidence increases proportionately with age.
   - The risks include racial and familial factors but are poorly defined.
   - Hormones play a role; carcinoma of the prostate never develops in men castrated before puberty.
   - Prostate-specific antigen (PSA) is used for screening and monitoring of tumors (test is sensitive but has low specificity).

41. **Describe the pathologic features of prostatic carcinoma.**
   - It shows multifocal induration, most often in the outer zones and posterior lobe (can be palpated on rectal examination).
   - Histologically, the tumors are adenocarcinomas with a desmoplastic stroma.
   - Tumor tends to invade nerves, seminal vesicles, and adjacent organs in the pelvis (urinary bladder and rectum).
   - Metastases to the local lymph nodes and bones are common.
   - Metastases are most often found in the vertebrae and sacrum.
   - Metastases often osteoblastic and associated with elevated serum alkaline phosphatase.

42. **What is the significance of Gleason classification?**
Gleason classification is used for grading prostatic carcinomas on a scale from 1 to 5. Low-grade tumors have a relatively good prognosis. High-grade tumors are invariably lethal.

43. **What is occult prostatic carcinoma?**
Prostatic carcinomas that are clinically inapparent and are found as microscopic lesions at autopsy or on random biopsy are called occult. Occult histologic carcinomas are found in approximately 30% of all 50-year-old men and up to 70% of those older than 80 years.

44. **What are the most useful techniques for diagnosing prostate carcinoma?**
   - **Biopsy:** It provides the definitive diagnosis and is easily performed.
   - **Ultrasound:** This technique is useful for localizing indurated "suspicious areas." Ultrasound-guided biopsy is more accurate than random biopsy.
   - **Computed tomography scanning:** This method is useful for assessing the extent of spread of prostate cancer and staging the disease.
   - **PSA:** This test is useful for screening populations at risk. However, elevated serum PSA may be encountered in association with BPH and prostatitis. Some undifferentiated prostatic carcinomas are associated with PSA in the normal range (<4 mg/mL).

45. **What is the prognosis of prostatic carcinoma?**
The prognosis depends on the stage and the grade of the tumor. Localized low-grade tumors are associated with good prognosis (95% 10-year survival rate). High-grade tumors extending to local tissues have a 50% 5-year survival rate. High-grade tumors that have metastasized to bones and distant sites have a poor prognosis (2- or 3-year survival).

46. **What is the treatment of prostatic carcinoma?**
Low-grade localized tumors, especially those discovered in older man aged over 70 years are best left alone; there is no definitive proof that early prostatectomy is useful in the treatment of such tumors. Some progress has been made in the radiation and chemical therapy of high-grade tumors, but the results are not encouraging.

47. **How are prostates resected?**
    Benign prostatic hyperplasia can be treated by transurethral resection (TUR), in common parlance compared with the "Roto-Rooter" approach to clogged house plumbing. Radical prostatectomy is used in the treatment of carcinomas.

48. **What are the consequences of prostatectomy?**
    The most common complications are incontinence and erectile dysfunction (impotence). Following radical prostatectomy for cancer, only 5% of patients retain normal sexual function, whereas 15% to 20% show some signs of urinary incontinence.

WESTES

1. http://www.cancer.gov/cancertopics/types/testicular/

2. http://www-medlib.med.utah.edu/WebPath/webpath.html#MENU

3. http://www.emedicine.com/med/topic3232.htm#section~future_and_controversies

4. http://www.emedicine.com/radio/topic574.htm

5. http://www.nlm.nih.gov/medlineplus/bladdercancer.html

BIBLIOGRAPHY

1. Bostwick DG, Qian J, Schlesinger C: Contemporary pathology of prostate cancer. Urol Clin North Am 30:181–207, 2003.
2. Burke HB, Bostwick DG, Meiers I, Montironi R: Prostate cancer outcome: epidemiology and biostatistics. Anal Quant Cytol Histol 27:211–217, 2005.
3. Cubilla AL, Velazques EF, Reuter VE, et al: Warty (condylomatous) squamous cell carcinoma of the penis. A report of 11 cases and proposed classification of "verruciform" penile tumors. Am J Surg Pathol 24:505–512, 2000.
4. Epstein JI. What's new in prostate cancer disease assessment in 2006? Curr Opin Urol 16:146–151, 2006.
5. Looijenga LH, Gillis AJ, Stoop HJ, et al: Chromosomes and expression in human testicular germ-cell tumors: insight into their cell of origin and pathogenesis. Ann N Y Acad Sci 1120:187–214, 2008.
6. Luzz GA, O'Brien TS: Acute epididymitis. BJU Int 87:747–755, 2001.
7. Montironi R, Mazzucchelli R, Scarpelli M, et al: Morphological diagnosis of urothelial neoplasms. J Clin Pathol 61:3–10, 2008.

CHAPTER 17

THE FEMALE GENITAL TRACT AND BREASTS

Ivan Damjanov, MD, PhD

1. **Name the principal parts of the female genital tract.**
   - Vulva
   - Vagina
   - Cervix
   - Uterus
   - Fallopian tubes
   - Ovaries

2. **What are the main diseases of the female genital system and breasts?**
   - Infections
   - Hormonally induced changes
   - Tumors

KEY POINTS: DISEASES OF THE FEMALE GENITAL TRACT ✔

1. The most important diseases of the female genital tract and breast are infections, hormonally related disorders, and tumors.

2. Female genital organs are affected by sexually transmitted disorders, which may ascend to the adnexa of the uterus and cause pelvic inflammatory disease (PID).

INFECTIONS

3. **How common are sexually transmitted diseases (STDs)?**
   They are very common. In the United States, there are approximately 5 million women infected with genital herpes simplex virus (HSV-2), 3 million infected with *Chlamydia trachomatis,* and 2 million genitally infected with human papillomavirus (HPV).

4. **What are the main signs and symptoms of STDs?**
   - Vaginal discharge
   - Vulvar lesions (e.g., vesicles and ulcers)
   - Pelvic pain or pelvic mass
   - Discomfort during intercourse (dyspareunia)

5. **Name the main viral pathogens causing infections of the lower female genital tract (vulva, vagina, and cervix).**
   - **HSV-2:** It causes vesicles, which coalesce and ulcerate. These vesicles appear 3 to 7 days after the infecting intercourse but in only approximately 30% of infected women. Ulcers may persist for 1 to 3 weeks but heal spontaneously without scarring. The virus migrates along the nerves to the lumbar ganglia, where it remains in a content form forever. The virus can be reactivated and descend to the vulva to produce recurrent vesicles.
   - **HPV:** The disease causes chronic infections, some of which heal spontaneously, whereas others ultimately lead to the formation of cancer. Giant vulvar wart is called condyloma acuminatum. HPV-related lesions of the vagina and the cervix are usually flat and are best recognized in Papanicolaou smear.

6. **What are the most common causes of vaginitis?**
   - ***Candida albicans:*** This fungus is found in the vagina of approximately 10% of women, who are usually unaware of the infection. Pregnancy, oral contraceptives, and diabetes promote fungal growth and cause the appearance of white patches on the mucosal surface and increased vaginal discharge with itching. Diagnosis is best made microscopically on wet mounts or Pap smear.
   - ***Trichomonas vaginalis:*** These flagellated protozoa are best diagnosed microscopically in freshly prepared wet mounts (i.e., smears of unfixed vaginal discharge, in which the protozoa keep moving). *T. vaginalis* is also visible on routine Pap smear.
   - ***Gardnerella vaginalis:*** This microbe grows in the vagina. The infection is best recognized on Pap smear by the appearance of "clue cells" (i.e., squamous cells covered with bacilli). Cytologic findings in various forms of vaginitis are illustrated in Fig. 17-1.

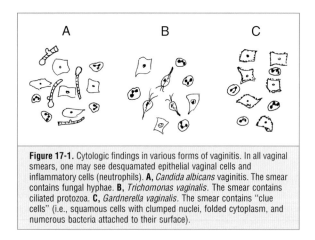

Figure 17-1. Cytologic findings in various forms of vaginitis. In all vaginal smears, one may see desquamated epithelial vaginal cells and inflammatory cells (neutrophils). **A,** *Candida albicans* vaginitis. The smear contains fungal hyphae. **B,** *Trichomonas vaginalis.* The smear contains ciliated protozoa. **C,** *Gardnerella vaginalis.* The smear contains "clue cells" (i.e., squamous cells with clumped nuclei, folded cytoplasm, and numerous bacteria attached to their surface).

7. **What is pelvic inflammatory disease (PID)?**
   In clinical practice, the term PID is used for extensive infections involving more than one part of the upper female genital tract. Infections of the fallopian tubes (salpingitis), which are almost invariably present, may be accompanied by endometritis or oophoritis and peritonitis. Pus tends to accumulate in the fallopian tubes (pyosalpinx), but it may penetrate into the pelvis, where it accumulates in the pockets formed by fibrous adhesions with other pelvic organs (e.g., tuboovarian abscess).

8. **Describe the most common causes of PID.**
   PID is most often a complication of sexually transmitted infections caused by *Neisseria gonorrhoeae* and *C. trachomatis*. Less often, PID is a complication of puerperal infections (i.e., polymicrobial ascending infection during delivery or abortion). In such cases, PID is caused by staphylococci, streptococci, or enteric bacteria, which usually invade the upper genital tract jointly from the infected uterus.

9. **List the clinical consequences of PID.**
   - Infertility due to occlusion of fallopian tubes
   - Chronic nonspecific infection, presenting with fever, malaise, and fatigue
   - Pelvic mass, which is tender and often associated with pain during urinary bladder distension, defecation, or intercourse (dyspareunia)
   - Peritonitis (peritoneal adhesions due to peritoneal spread of disease)
   - Septicemia (a rare systemic complication due to the entry of bacteria into blood)

VULVA AND VAGINA

10. **What are the most common diseases of the vulva?**
    The vulva is most often involved by infections, especially those that flourish in moist areas (e.g., candidiasis) or involve hair follicles (e.g., staphylococcal boils). Skin of the vulva may be involved with any other skin disease, such as psoriasis or eczema. Vitiligo (i.e., loss of pigmentation of unknown etiology) also may involve vulva.

11. **What is vulvar leukoplakia?**
    Leukoplakia, as implied by its name, is a whitish, plaquelike thickening of the mucosa noticed on naked-eye examination. This clinical term includes a number of pathologic entities:
    - Inflammatory dermatoses (e.g., psoriasis or eczema)
    - Lichen sclerosus, a disease of unknown etiology characterized by atrophy of the epidermis and sclerosing fibrosis of the underlying dermis
    - Squamous hyperplasia with hyperkeratosis and chronic dermal inflammation of unknown etiology
    - Neoplasms (e.g., vulvar intraepithelial neoplasia)

12. **What is a condyloma acuminatum?**
    Condyloma acuminatum is another name for genital warts, which are usually caused by HPV type 6 or 11.

KEY POINTS: VULVA AND VAGINA ✔

1. The vulva is commonly infected with human papillomavirus, which causes condylomata acuminata and may contribute to the pathogenesis of carcinoma.
2. Cancer of the vulva and vagina is most often classified as squamous cell carcinoma.

13. **What is koilocytosis?**
    Koilocytosis is a sign of HPV infection. The nuclei of infected squamous cells show irregular contours and appear crenated or "raisin-like." The nucleus is hyperchromatic, displaced laterally by clear cytoplasm. Hence the name, which in translation from Greek means "spoonlike cell." The virus particles can be seen in the nucleus on electron microscopy and are also demonstrable by immunohistochemistry.

14. **How common is carcinoma of the vulva?**

Carcinoma of the vulva is rare. Usually diagnosed in elderly women, it accounts for only 3% of all cancers of the female genital tract and is 8 times less common than cervical cancer.

15. **What is vulvar intraepithelial neoplasia (VIN)?**

VIN, also known as vulvar carcinoma in situ or Bowen disease, is a preinvasive squamous cell carcinoma. It is often multicentric, and like cervical or vaginal carcinoma, it is usually associated with HPV infection.

16. **Describe the histologic features of vulvar carcinoma.**

Most vulvar carcinomas are histologically classified as keratinizing or poorly differentiated (basaloid) squamous cell carcinomas. Other histologic forms, such as extramammary Paget disease or melanoma, are rare.

17. **How common is carcinoma of the vagina?**

Carcinoma of the vagina is rare, accounting for 1% of all female genital cancers.

18. **Discuss the histologic features of vaginal carcinoma.**

Most vaginal carcinomas diagnosed in adult women are of the squamous cell type. Clear cell adenocarcinomas are rare vaginal tumors, most of which were found in young women whose mothers took diethyl stilbestrol during pregnancy. Sarcoma botryoides is a rare vaginal tumor of girls younger than 5 years.

CERVIX

19. **What are the most common causes of cervicitis?**

Cervicitis occurs in several forms. Mucopurulent acute cervicitis is typically a feature of sexually transmitted infections and is most often caused by *Chlamydia* and *N. gonorrhoeae* invading the endocervix. These infections may persist and spread upward to cause endometritis or PID. Chronic persistent or recurrent infection of the squamous epithelium of the exocervix is typically caused by viruses—HPV and HSV-2. Mild, nonspecific chronic inflammation of the endocervix caused by vaginal saprophytic bacteria is found in many women but is of no clinical significance. In some women, it may lead to the formation of endocervical polyps, which cause "spotting."

20. **How common is cervical carcinoma?**

Invasive carcinoma of the cervix is the second most common malignant tumor of the female genital tract. Although only 13,000 new cases of invasive cervical carcinoma are diagnosed annually, approximately 1 million others are detected in the preinvasive stages by Pap smear and cured before they become invasive.

21. **Discuss the risk factors for cervical cancer.**

Infection with high-risk types of HPV (such as types 16, 18, 31, and 33) is the most important risk factor for cervical cancer. Other risk factors include becoming sexually active at an early age, having multiple sexual partners, and being multiparous. Cigarette smoking has an important cocarcinogenic role.

KEY POINTS: CERVIX ✔

1. Cervical carcinoma is related to human papillomavirus infection.

2. Cervical carcinoma and its precursors (cervical intraepithelial neoplasia) can be detected by vaginal exfoliative cytology (Pap smear).

22. **What is the most efficient way to diagnose cervical carcinoma?**
Tumor cells can be easily scraped from the cervix during routine gynecologic examination; thus Pap smears are the most efficient means for diagnosing preinvasive and invasive cervical carcinoma. Positive exfoliative cytology findings need to be confirmed by a biopsy, which is usually performed under colposcopic guidance. A colposcope, which serves as an intravaginal microscope, provides the gynecologist with a close-up magnified view of the cervix and allows him or her to take the tissue specimens from the pathologically altered portion of the cervix.

23. **Define cervical intraepithelial neoplasia (CIN).**
CIN represents a spectrum of neoplastic changes of the squamous epithelium of the cervix that have been recognized as precursors of invasive squamous cell carcinoma. CIN is graded on a scale from I to III, which can also be expressed descriptively as mild, moderate, or severe dysplasia, or carcinoma in situ. On Pap smear, these lesions are classified by cytologists as squamous intraepithelial lesions of low or high grade.

CIN I is usually caused by low-risk types of HPV. Koilocytic atypia is typically limited to the lower third of the squamous epithelium. If the atypia becomes more pronounced and extends toward the surface layers of the squamous epithelium, it is classified as moderate (CIN II). If the nuclear atypia can be found in all layers of the epithelium, which in such cases shows no signs of surface maturation, the cancer is classified as CIN III. Lesions classified as CIN II and CIN III are caused by high-risk types of HPV.

24. **Does CIN always progress to invasive carcinoma?**
Most CINs do not progress to invasive cancer. However, in each case, it is not possible to predict whether the lesion will progress to invasive cancer or regress. Therefore all CINs are treated as potential cancers. The chances that CIN will progress to invasive cancer depend on its grade. More than 85% of all CIN I cancers regress spontaneously, 10% progress to CIN III, and 2% or 3% progress to invasive cancer. Approximately 25% of all untreated cases of CIN III will progress to invasive carcinoma, usually within 10 years of diagnosis.

25. **How is CIN treated?**
The treatment of CIN depends on its grade and the extent of cervical involvement. Following initial biopsy, CIN I is followed up with regular Pap smears, colposcopic examinations, or both at regular time intervals. High-grade CIN must be removed surgically by conization (i.e., removal of the involved cone of tissue around the endocervical canal and the transformation zone by laser vaporization or cryosurgery). Women diagnosed with CIN are at risk of developing cancer of the cervix or carcinoma of the vulva and vagina and should be examined at regular time intervals for life.

26. **Describe the peak age incidence for CIN and invasive cervical carcinoma.**
The age of presentation of CIN I and CIN II peaks at 25 years. The incidence of CIN III reaches its peak between 35 and 40 years, and the peak for invasive cervical carcinoma is approximately 50 years. Assuming that a lesion arose as a CIN II at age 25 years, one can predict that an untreated lesion will progress to carcinoma in situ over 10 to 15 years and from carcinoma in situ to invasive cancer in the next 10 to 15 years.

27. **Has the peak age incidence for CIN and invasive cancer decreased during the past two decades?**
CIN is being diagnosed earlier. Epidemiologic data show that all forms of cervical neoplasia are being diagnosed in younger women compared with a few decades ago. In part, this is because sexual mores have changed and many women become sexually active at an earlier age.

It is also related to the widespread use of Pap smears in most developed countries. However, this does not explain the increased incidence of invasive cervical cancer in women younger than 35 years, which has been recorded worldwide.

28. How does invasive cervical carcinoma present on gross examination?
On gross examination, invasive cervical carcinoma may present in three forms:
- Ulceration
- Exophytic fungating mass
- Invasive lesion causing induration or deformities of the cervix ("barrel-shaped cervix")
  Microinvasive carcinoma is diagnosed unexpectedly in approximately 5% of cervical biopsies performed in patients thought to have CIN on colposcopic examination. Such microinvasive carcinomas do not have distinct macroscopic features, and the diagnosis is established only on finding nests of microscopic cancer cells superficially invading the endocervical stroma. Arbitrarily, it was decided to call carcinomas microinvasive if the invasion does not extend more than 5 mm from the nearest basement membrane delimiting the remaining preinvasive CIN.

29. What are the histopathologic features of invasive cervical carcinoma?
Approximately 85% of all cervical carcinomas are classified as squamous cell carcinomas. Adenocarcinomas originating from the endocervical glands account for approximately 10% of tumors. The remaining 5% of cancers comprise the less common variants, such as adenosquamous, neuroendocrine (oat cell), and undifferentiated carcinomas.

30. How does cervical carcinoma spread?
Cervical carcinoma tends to invade the vagina and parametria locally and also metastasize to the pelvic lymph nodes. Invasion of the rectum, urinary bladder, and distant metastases are found in later stages of cancer spread. Obstruction of the urinary outflow is a common cause of death.

31. What is the prognosis for survival of patients diagnosed with cervical cancer?
The prognosis of cervical cancer treated by hysterectomy with or without radiation depends primarily on the stage of the tumor at the time of diagnosis. The 5-year survival rate is as follows:
- **Stage I:** Limited to the cervix (80%–90%)
- **Stage II:** Involving the vagina, the upper third of the vagina, or the medial aspect of the parametria (75%)
- **Stage III:** Extending laterally to the pelvic wall or lower part of the vagina (35%)
- **Stage IV:** Extending beyond the true pelvis or with distant metastases (10–15%)

BODY OF THE UTERUS

32. Name the most important diseases of the body of the uterus.
- Hormonal disorders with dysfunctional endometrial bleeding or endometrial hyperplasia
- Tumors

33. What are the causes of dysfunctional uterine bleeding?
Dysfunctional uterine bleeding is defined as bleeding that does not have an organic cause and is presumptively related to some endocrine disturbance. The main causes are:

- **Failure of ovulation:** The normal menstrual cycle consists of a proliferative and a nonproliferative stage, separated by the midcyclic point of ovulation. At ovulation, the endometrium ceases to proliferate and enters a nonproliferative secretory phase. If ovulation does not occur, the endometrium will continue to proliferate until it outgrows its own blood supply. At that point, the surface portion of the endometrium becomes ischemic and starts dying off. This leads to bleeding, which typically occurs 2 or 3 weeks after the date of the "missed menstruation." Anovulatory bleeding occurs most often around puberty and menopause but may be caused by neuroendocrine disturbances (e.g., anxiety and anorexia nervosa), severe malnutrition, or debilitating diseases.
- **Luteal phase inadequacy:** If the corpus luteum does not secrete progesterone in adequate amounts, the level of progesterone may not be sufficient to transform fully the proliferative endometrium into a secretory endometrium. Such irregular maturation of the endometrium is usually associated with "spotting," premature onset of menstrual bleeding, or prolonged bleeding. Curetting of endometrium performed to determine the cause of bleeding often may also help reestablish the normal cycle. In many cases, irregular bleeding recurs; such women may have problems conceiving.

34. **What is endometrial hyperplasia?**
Endometrial hyperplasia, or excessive proliferation of endometrium, is thought to be caused by estrogenic stimulation, even though in most cases the cause of hyperestrinism cannot be identified. Identifiable causes include:
- Anovulatory hyperplasia in which estrogenic effect are not opposed by progesterone
- Exogenous estrogen in women on hormone replacement therapy
- Estrogen-producing ovarian tumors (e.g., theca or granulosa cell tumor)
- Polycystic ovary syndrome

KEY POINTS: BODY OF THE UTERUS ✔

1. Hormonal changes account for dysfunctional uterine bleeding, the most common form of vaginal bleeding in women.
2. Estrogen stimulation of the endometrium causes endometrial hyperplasia and plays an important role in the pathogenesis of endometrial carcinoma.
3. Endometrial carcinoma has an excellent prognosis if diagnosed early.
4. Leiomyomas of the uterus are the most common benign tumor of the female genital tract.

35. **Discuss how endometrial hyperplasia is diagnosed.**
Endometrial hyperplasia is diagnosed microscopically by the pathologist examining the tissue removed by endometrial biopsy or endometrial curettage. Histologically, there are three forms of endometrial hyperplasia, as shown in Fig. 17-2:
- **Simple hyperplasia:** The endometrium contains an increased number of dilatated glands.
- **Complex hyperplasia without atypia:** The glands appear crowded and are surrounded by relatively scant stroma. The glandular epithelium are lined by uniform cells, which show no nuclear atypia.
- **Complex hyperplasia with atypia:** The glands appear crowded and have an irregular shape, with stratification of cells that often protrude into the lumen. Nuclei of these glands show atypia, and sometimes it is not possible to distinguish them from well-differentiated adenocarcinoma. Some pathologists call it endometrial intraepithelial neoplasia.

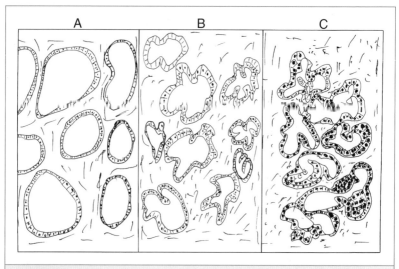

Figure 17-2. Endometrial hyperplasia. **A,** Simple hyperplasia. The endometrium contains an increased number of dilatated glands separated from each other by normal stroma ("Swiss-cheese pattern"). **B,** Complex hyperplasia without atypia. The endometrium contains an increased number of irregularly shaped glands surrounded by scant stroma. Glandular atypica is not accompanied by cytologic atypia. **C,** Complex hyperplasia with atypia. There is both histologic and cytologic atypia; the glands are irregular, and the cells forming the glands are hyperchromatic and vary in size and shape.

36. **What is the significance of endometrial hyperplasia?**
   Simple hyperplasia is a relatively innocuous lesion. Complex hyperplasia, however, can progress to cancer. Only 5% of complex hyperplasias without atypia ultimately progress to cancer. The rate of progression is much higher for complex hyperplasias with atypia; approximately 25% of all patients with these lesions will develop endometrial carcinoma.

37. **What are endometrial polyps?**
   Endometrial polyps are solitary fingerlike lesions found in the uterine cavity. Polyps are most likely benign tumors, but some authorities believe that they are nonneoplastic. They are covered by columnar epithelium similar to that covering the surface of the endometrium. Inside the polyp are cystic endometrial glands embedded in rather cellular and fibrotic stroma. Most polyps are diagnosed in perimenopausal women complaining of spotting or irregular bleeding. Polyps are easily removed by curettage.

38. **Name the most common tumors of the uterus.**
   The most common uterine tumor encountered in clinical practice is leiomyoma. The most common malignant tumor is adenocarcinoma of the endometrium.

39. **Are all endometrial tumors malignant?**
   Endometrial adenocarcinoma does not have a benign equivalent; if it did exist, it would be called endometrial adenoma. Hence, for practical purposes, all endometrial neoplasms should be considered malignant.

40. **How common are endometrial adenocarcinomas?**
   Endometrial adenocarcinoma is the most common invasive cancer of the female genital tract. There are approximately 35,000 new cases of endometrial cancer diagnosed annually in the United States. However, most of these cases are diagnosed in early stages when the cancer is curable; thus only 6000 women die every year of this cancer.

41. **Discuss the causes of endometrial cancer.**
Like endometrial hyperplasia, endometrial cancer is thought to be related to hyperestrinism. Endometrial hyperplasia is a common precursor and is the most important warning sign that an invasive carcinoma may develop. Other conditions associated with hyperestrinism, such as estrogen-producing ovarian lesions, are also associated with an increased incidence of endometrial cancer. Exogenous estrogens, especially if unopposed by progesterone, increase the risk of endometrial cancer 3 or 4 times.

42. **What are the epidemiologically identified risk factors for endometrial cancer?**
Risk factors associated epidemiologically with an increased incidence of endometrial cancer are:
- Obesity
- Diabetes
- Hypertension
- Infertility
- Early menarche, late menopause (i.e., a long reproductive life)
- Estrogen replacement therapy after menopause

43. **Is there a genetic predisposition to endometrial cancer?**
A genetic predisposition to endometrial cancer has been noted in women who have familial breast cancer. Lynch syndrome II is a hereditary condition with a high incidence of adenocarcinoma of the colon, endometrium, and breast.

44. **Describe the role of oncogenes and tumor suppressor genes in the pathogenesis of endometrial cancer.**
The role of these cancer genes has not been fully explored. Tumors that are not related to hyperestrinism, and those that have unusual histologic features may show overexpression of p53 and other cancer-related genes, but this is not proof that the oncogenes or tumor suppressor genes have a pathogenetic role in these lesions.

45. **How do endometrial carcinomas present on gross examination?**
- Exophytic, polypoid lesions protruding into the lumen
- Diffuse thickening of the endometrium
- Invasive infiltrative lesions extending into the myometrium
  See Fig. 17-3.

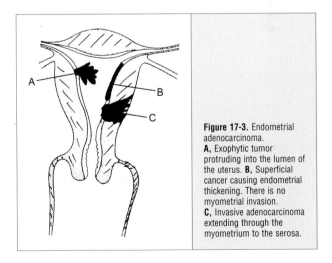

Figure 17-3. Endometrial adenocarcinoma. **A,** Exophytic tumor protruding into the lumen of the uterus. **B,** Superficial cancer causing endometrial thickening. There is no myometrial invasion. **C,** Invasive adenocarcinoma extending through the myometrium to the serosa.

46. **What are the typical microscopic features of endometrial carcinoma?**
Most endometrial carcinomas are composed of neoplastic glands that bear some resemblance to endometrial glands and therefore are called endometrioid adenocarcinomas. Some of these adenocarcinomas of the endometrium also show squamous differentiation. Less common forms of adenocarcinoma, such as papillary, serous, or clear cell adenocarcinoma, account for a minority of all cases.

47. **What is the prognosis for survival of patients diagnosed with endometrial carcinoma?**
The prognosis depends primarily on the stage of the tumor. The 5-year survival rate is as follows:
   - Stage I (tumor limited to neometrium or showing only superficial invasion of myometrium): 90%
   - Stage II (tumor involving the cervix or invading deeply into the myometrium): 50%
   - Stage III (tumor extending beyond the confines of the uterus but not outside the pelvis): 30%
   - Stage IV (tumor extending outside the pelvis and with distant metastases): 15%

48. **Where does endometrial cancer metastasize?**
Endometrial cancer metastases are found in lymph nodes of the pelvis, but some tumor cells may skip the pelvic nodes; these are then found in the periaortic nodes. Distant metastases in the lungs are found in approximately 40% of patients with advanced tumors. Histologic grade is also an important prognostic determinant. Uncommon histologic forms have a worse prognosis than typical endometrioid adenocarcinomas. Serous carcinomas are especially malignant tumors.

49. **What are leiomyomas?**
Leiomyomas are benign tumors of myometrium composed of smooth muscle cells. Because the smooth muscle cells in leiomyomas respond to estrogens like their nonneoplastic counterparts in the myometrium, it is self-apparent that most leiomyomas arise during the reproductive life of a woman. Leiomyomas are almost never found in prepubertal girls. After menopause, smooth muscle cells are lost, and these tumors therefore shrink in size and become fibrosed.

50. **How do leiomyomas present on gross examination?**
Leiomyomas have the appearance of well-circumscribed firm nodules. According to their location, they are classified as submucosal, intramural, or subserosal. On cross-sectioning, they have a whorled pattern, reflecting the fact that they are composed of bundles of smooth muscle cells. Leiomyomas are often multiple. See Fig. 17-4.

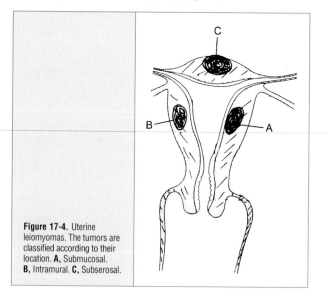

Figure 17-4. Uterine leiomyomas. The tumors are classified according to their location. **A,** Submucosal. **B,** Intramural. **C,** Subserosal.

51. **Which clinical symptoms are caused by leiomyomas?**
In most instances, leiomyomas are asymptomatic and are discovered by gynecologists during a routine pelvic examination. Because the tumors enlarge the uterus, they may cause a feeling of heaviness or compress the urinary bladder and rectum. Submucosal tumors may cause endometrial bleeding or interfere with the implantation of the fertilized ovum and thus cause infertility. Subserosal tumors, especially if pedunculated, may twist around their pedicles and become necrotic because of the torsion of their nutrient blood vessels. See Fig. 17-5.

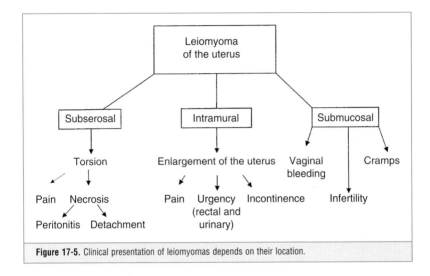

Figure 17-5. Clinical presentation of leiomyomas depends on their location.

52. **What is the risk of malignant transformation of leiomyomas?**
Malignant transformation of leiomyomas occurs extremely rarely, if ever. Leiomyosarcomas (i.e., malignant smooth muscle cell tumors of the uterus) are rare neoplasms, almost all of which originate de novo and are unrelated to the preexisting leiomyomas.

53. **Name the other tumors of the uterine body.**
Malignant transformation of endometrial stromal cells gives rise to tumors known as endometrial stromal sarcomas. Malignant tumors composed of neoplastic endometrial stroma and glands are called malignant mixed Müllerian tumors. These tumors are rare.

OVARIES

54. **Define ovarian cysts.**
Ovarian cysts are fluid-filled cavities lined by epithelium. In the ovary, most cysts develop from unruptured follicles and are therefore called follicular cysts. Other cysts represent cystic corpora lutea or inclusions of the surface epithelium. Ovarian cysts are usually small, solitary, and cause no clinical problems. Larger cysts need to be explored to ensure they are not neoplastic (i.e., cystadenomas and cystadenocarcinomas). See Fig. 17-6.

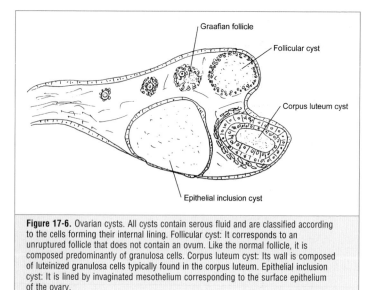

Figure 17-6. Ovarian cysts. All cysts contain serous fluid and are classified according to the cells forming their internal lining. Follicular cyst: It corresponds to an unruptured follicle that does not contain an ovum. Like the normal follicle, it is composed predominantly of granulosa cells. Corpus luteum cyst: Its wall is composed of luteinized granulosa cells typically found in the corpus luteum. Epithelial inclusion cyst: It is lined by invaginated mesothelium corresponding to the surface epithelium of the ovary.

55. **What is polycystic ovary syndrome?**
    Polycystic ovary syndrome, also known as Stein–Leventhal syndrome, is a hormonal disturbance of the hypothalamic-pituitary-ovarian-adrenal axis. Clinically it presents with menstrual irregularities, such as oligomenorrhea and amenorrhea; persistent anovulation in 40% of cases; obesity; and signs of virilization, such as hirsutism. Infertility is a major problem. The ovaries of these women contain numerous follicular cysts and show superficial fibrosis. Previously it was thought that the fibrosis of the superficial cortex was the cause of anovulation, but it is now known that the basic problem in such cases is hormonal.

KEY POINTS: OVARIES ✓

1. Ovarian enlargement can occur because of cysts or tumors.

2. Ovarian tumors can originate from the ovarian surface epithelium, germ cells, or sex cord cells.

3. Ovarian tumors are often malignant and tend to metastasize by peritoneal seeding.

56. **How common are ovarian tumors?**
    Ovarian tumors form the second most common group of tumors in the female genital tract. However, they have a mortality higher than that of any other female genital tract tumor. More women die of ovarian cancer than of all other female genital tract tumors combined, as shown in Table 17-1.

TABLE 17-1.	INCIDENCE OF GYNECOLOGIC CANCER IN THE UNITED STATES	
	New Cases	Deaths Due to Cancer
	(Number per Year)	(Number per Year)
Endometrium	35,000	6,000
Ovary	27,000	15,000
Cervix (invasive)	16,000	5,000
Vulva (invasive)	3,000	500
Vagina (invasive)	1,000	200

57. **How are ovarian tumors classified?**
Primary ovarian tumors can be classified histogenetically (i.e., according to their cell of origin) into three major groups:
- Tumors of surface epithelium
- Germ cell tumors
- Sex cord stromal tumors
See Fig. 17-7.

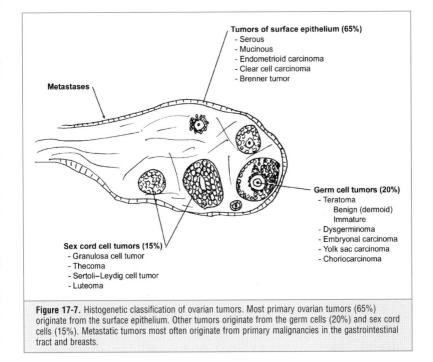

Figure 17-7. Histogenetic classification of ovarian tumors. Most primary ovarian tumors (65%) originate from the surface epithelium. Other tumors originate from the germ cells (20%) and sex cord cells (15%). Metastatic tumors most often originate from primary malignancies in the gastrointestinal tract and breasts.

58. **Are ovarian tumors more often benign or malignant?**
Benign tumors are more common. In women younger than 45 years, only 1 in 15 tumors is malignant. However, in women older than 50 years, 1 in 3 tumors is malignant.

59. **Describe the risk factors for ovarian tumors.**
The risk factors for ovarian tumors are not as well defined as those for other gynecologic cancers. Definite risk factors can be identified only in a minority of cases and include ovarian dysgenesis, familial cancer syndrome, and *BRCA1* and *BRCA2* gene mutations linked with an increased incidence of breast cancer. In most cases, ovarian cancer develops without any warning and cannot be linked with any environmental factors.

60. **Discuss whether oral contraceptives increase the incidence of ovarian cancer.**
Just the opposite is true. Widespread use of oral contraceptives has decreased the overall incidence of ovarian tumors.
    Most ovarian tumors originate from the surface epithelium, which is traumatized with each ovulation. During ovulation, the surface epithelium is disrupted to allow the expulsion of the oocytes. Because oral contraceptives prevent ovulation, it is thought that the reduced incidence of tumors is related to the reduced incidence of monthly trauma of the surface epithelium.
    In this context, it is worth noting that the egg-laying hen represents the best animal model of ovarian cancer. These hens, selected for their egg-laying capacity, succumb at a high rate to ovarian cancer. It is thought that the cancer of the ovary is directly related to the number of ovulation-related traumas of the surface epithelium. After ovulation, this epithelium proliferates to cover the defect, and during this proliferative event, it is probably exposed to carcinogens, which ultimately transform the surface epithelial cells into malignant cells.

61. **How are the surface epithelial tumors of the ovary classified?**
This group, which accounts for 70% of all ovarian tumors, comprises serous, mucinous, endometrioid, clear cell, and transitional (Brenner) tumors.
    To understand the histogenesis of these tumors, it is important to remember that the surface epithelial covering of the ovaries is composed of mesothelial cells. The same embryonic mesothelial cells have participated in the formation of the epithelium lining the inside of Müllerian ducts, which give rise to the fallopian tubes, uterus, endocervix, and the upper third of the vagina. Ovarian surface epithelium retains the capacity to differentiate like the invaginated portion of the embryonic mesothelium. Accordingly, during tumorigenesis, it can differentiate into serous epithelium similar to the tubal epithelium, endometrioid epithelium similar to the one in the uterus, and mucus-secreting endocervical epithelium and stratified squamous–transitional epithelium resembling that of the vagina or urinary bladder. This pluripotency of the ovarian surface epithelium accounts for the spectrum of histologic tumor types seen in this location.

62. **What are the most common ovarian surface epithelial tumors?**
The most common ovarian surface epithelial tumors are serous tumors. They are typically cystic and filled with clear serous fluid. Microscopically they may be benign (serous cystadenomas), borderline, or malignant (serous cystadenocarcinomas). Approximately 25% of benign and 50% of malignant serous tumors are bilateral.

63. **How can one distinguish benign serous tumors from serous cystadenocarcinomas?**
The definitive diagnosis of malignancy requires histologic examination of the tumor. Nevertheless, some macroscopic features can suggest the diagnosis of malignancy even during surgery or on gross pathologic examination. For example, malignant tumors tend to contain large solid areas with prominent foci of necrosis. The outgrowth of tumor cells through the capsule of the tumor is an ominous sign. The presence of tumor nodules on the peritoneum and ascites fluid that contains tumor cells are other signs of malignancy.

64. **Name the main features of ovarian mucinous tumors.**
Like serous tumors, mucinous ovarian tumors can be classified as benign, borderline, or malignant. They are also cystic. The cysts are lined with tall mucus-secreting cells and are therefore filled with viscous mucus.

65. **What is jelly-belly?**
Mucinous cystadenocarcinomas of the ovary metastasize by spreading and implanting all over the peritoneum of the abdominal cavity. These tumor implants continue to secrete mucus, which fills the abdominal cavity. This condition, called pseudomyxoma peritonei, is in popular terms known as "jelly-belly." Pseudomyxoma peritonei can result from the spread of other mucin-producing tumors as well and was described as a complication of mucinous tumors of the appendix, large intestine, stomach, and other parts of the digestive system.

66. **Do serous tumors of the ovary have a better or worse prognosis than mucinous tumors?**
Serous tumors are more often bilateral and malignant than mucinous tumors. Therefore mucinous tumors have a better prognosis.

67. **What are endometrioid carcinomas, and how do they differ from serous and mucinous tumors?**
Histologically endometrioid carcinomas resemble endometrioid adenocarcinomas.
    In contrast to serous and mucinous tumors, which are cystic, endometrioid adenocarcinomas are mostly solid. Serous and mucinous tumors are more often benign and also occur in a borderline form; endometrioid carcinomas are always malignant. Some authorities consider endometriosis as the benign precursor lesion of endometrioid carcinomas, but the transition cannot be convincingly demonstrated in most cases. Furthermore, endometriosis is common, affecting 10% to 15% of all women in one form or another, and endometrioid adenocarcinomas are rare.

68. **List the most important germ cell tumors of the ovary.**
    - Teratoma, the most common germ cell tumor
    - Dysgerminoma, ovarian equivalent of seminoma; malignant but radiosensitive and curable
    - Embryonal carcinoma, more malignant than dysgerminoma but still may respond to chemotherapy
    - Yolk-sac carcinoma (endodermal sinus tumor), malignant tumor that secretes alpha-fetoprotein
    - Choriocarcinoma, equivalent to gestational choriocarcinoma originating from the placenta in the uterus (This rare, highly malignant tumor secretes human chorionic gonadotropin [hCG].)

69. **What is a dermoid cyst?**
Dermoid cyst is another name for benign teratomas. These tumors tend to form cysts lined from inside with epidermis, which accounts for their popular name. Inside the cyst of these germ cell tumors, one may find sebaceous material, desquamated squames ("dandruff"), and hair. In the wall of these cystic tumors, one may find teeth, cartilage, or brain tissue, which proves that the tumor is a true teratoma (i.e., composed of derivatives of all three embryonic germ layers—ectoderm, mesoderm, and endoderm).

70. **What are immature teratomas?**
Teratomas that contain immature neural tissue may behave like malignant tumors and are therefore classified separately from benign teratomas. These tumors are more solid than benign teratomas (dermoid cysts).

71. **In which age group do ovarian germ cell tumors occur most often?**
In contrast to surface epithelial tumors, which occur more often in women older than age 35 years, germ cell tumors occur in younger women. Actually, teratomas are the most common ovarian tumor in women younger than age 25 years.

72. **How common are sex cord stromal tumors of the ovary?**
These tumors account for 10% of all ovarian tumors. They occur at any age and commonly secrete steroid hormones.

73. **List the most important sex cord stromal tumors.**
- **Fibroma:** This benign nonfunctioning tumor is composed of fibroblasts. It is the most common tumor in this group and may be associated with right-sided pleural effusion and ascites (Meigs syndrome). It is solid and white on cross-section and firm because of the abundance of collagen in its stroma.
- **Thecoma:** It is similar to fibroma. Thecoma is benign, solid, and firm, but on cross-section, it appears yellow. It is composed of spindle-shaped cells (theca cells) that contain fat and synthesize estrogens.
- **Granulosa cell tumor:** It is composed of granulosa cells that may secrete estrogens. This tumor is solid and yellow on cross-section and usually not as firm as fibromas and thecomas. Histologically it is composed of granulosa cells that may form Call–Exner bodies, such as the normal granulosa cells in ovarian follicles.
- **Sertoli–Leydig cell tumor (androblastoma):** This biphasic tumor contains cells resembling testicular Sertoli and Leydig cells. These tumors secrete androgens and cause virilization (deepening of the voice, facial and chest hirsutism, acne, clitoromegaly, amenorrhea, and infertility).
- **Hilar cell tumor:** Small tumor, yellow on cross-section. It is composed of Leydig cells and may secrete androgens.

74. **What is the prognosis of sex cord tumors?**
Most sex cord tumors are benign. Approximately 25% of all granulosa cell tumors are prone to recur or metastasize during the 10-year period after diagnosis and are considered low-grade malignant. Highly malignant tumors of this type are extremely rare. Sertoli–Leydig cell tumors also may be occasionally malignant.

75. **What are Krukenberg tumors?**
Krukenberg tumors are bilateral ovarian metastases of mucin-secreting gastrointestinal adenocarcinomas. Most often, these tumors are related to a gastric primary.

76. **List the serologic markers of ovarian tumors.**
- **Glycoprotein CA-125:** Marker of surface epithelial tumors but not specific enough for screening purposes
- **Estrogens:** Thecomas and granulosa cell tumors
- **Androgens:** Sertoli–Leydig and hilar cell tumors
- **Alpha-fetoprotein:** Yolk-sac carcinoma
- **Human chorionic gonadotropin:** Choriocarcinoma

DISEASES OF PREGNANCY

77. **How are infections transmitted transplacentally?**
- **Ascending infection:** Bacteria enter through the cervical canal and from the uterine cavity cross the fetal membrane.

- **Hematogenous infection:** Bacteria and other pathogens enter into the amniotic sac from the placental blood. This route of infection is favored by viruses (e.g., parvovirus and cytomegalovirus) and *Treponema pallidum*.

78. **Define ectopic pregnancy.**
Ectopic pregnancy is a consequence of abnormal implantation of the fertilized ovum outside of the uterus. Most commonly (95%), it occurs in the fallopian tubes, but it may also be found on the ovary, the pelvic peritoneum, and, rarely, the surface of the abdominal organs. Interstitial pregnancy resulting from the implantation of the ovum in the intrauterine portion of the fallopian tubes is also considered to be ectopic.

79. **How is ectopic pregnancy diagnosed?**
Ectopic pregnancy, which occurs in 1% of all pregnancies, should be suspected in any woman who believes that she is pregnant and has a positive pregnancy test but complains of pelvic pain or discomfort. The fallopian tube distended by the developing embryo and placenta may rupture, and a massive hematoperitoneum may develop if the condition is not recognized. If diagnosed in time, the pregnancy can be removed from the distended fallopian tube laparoscopically. If this is not feasible, the fallopian tube must be resected together with the embryo and the placenta.

KEY POINTS: DISEASES OF PREGNANCY ✔

1. Most pathologic changes of pregnancy are related to placentation.

2. Examples include ectopic implantation, abnormal placentation (e.g., placenta accreta), abnormal formation of chorionic villi (as in hydatidiform mole), and gestational trophoblastic neoplasia (choriocarcinoma).

80. **Discuss gestational trophoblastic disease.**
This term comprises three pathologic entities: benign hydatidiform mole, a locally invasive mole, and an overly malignant choriocarcinoma.

81. **What is hydatidiform mole?**
Hydatidiform mole is a developmental abnormality of the placenta that occurs in pregnancies resulting from faulty fertilization. In rare cases (1:2000 pregnancies), only the placenta develops. It consists of numerous vesicles and occurs in two forms:
- **Complete hydatidiform mole—46,XX karyotype:** However, both sets of 23 chromosomes are derived from the father. This process, called androgenesis, is accompanied by a loss of maternal chromosome and the reduplication of the male chromosome set contributed by the sperm.
- **Partial mole—triploidy (69,XXY):** In this condition, the abnormal placenta is attached to a partially formed fetus. Partial moles result from diandry (i.e., fertilization by two sperms), leading to an extra set of chromosomes (3 × 23 = 69).
See Fig. 17-8.

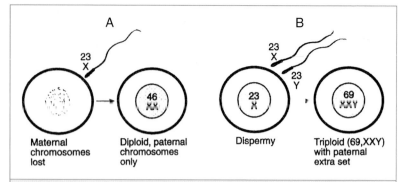

Figure 17-8. Histogenesis of hydatidiform moles. **A,** Complete hydatidiform mole results from androgenesis, a process in which all the chromosomes are of paternal origin. Typically the nucleus of the ovum is lost, and all the chromosomes found in the zygote (fertilized ovum) are derived from the sperm. The zygote is diploid (46,XX). Because a single sperm contributes only 23 chromosomes, the full complement of 46 chromosomes is achieved by reduplication of that haploid set. **B,** Partial mole. The ovum is fertilized by two sperms, a process called dispermy. The zygote is triploid (69,XXY or 69,XYY).

82. **What is the clinical significance of hydatidiform mole?**
Today most molar pregnancies are diagnosed by ultrasound in the early stages of pregnancy and can be completely evacuated by curettage. Nonetheless, approximately 10% of complete moles become locally invasive, and 2% or 3% give rise to choriocarcinomas. Partial moles generally do not predispose to choriocarcinoma.

83. **What is choriocarcinoma?**
Choriocarcinoma is a rare but highly invasive malignant tumor composed of malignant mononuclear cytotrophoblastic and multinucleated syncytiotrophoblastic cells. It develops in 1 in 30,000 pregnancies. Very young and older women (younger than 20 and older than 40 years) are most often affected. Approximately 50% of choriocarcinomas arise from preexisting complete hydatidiform moles, 25% originate from residual chorionic villi after an abortion, and 25% arise after a normal pregnancy.

84. **Does gestational choriocarcinoma differ from germ cell–derived choriocarcinomas?**
Choriocarcinoma arising from the placenta carries paternal genes that are foreign to the host. In contrast, choriocarcinoma arising from the host's own germ cells has the same genes as the host. This accounts for the fact that the gestational choriocarcinomas are readily curable with chemotherapy, which probably also stimulates the host's immune system in the defense against the choriocarcinoma cells. On the other hand, germ cell choriocarcinomas are incurable.

85. **What is preeclampsia?**
Preeclampsia is a disease of pregnancy presenting proteinuria, hypertension, and edema. Typically these symptoms occur in the third trimester. Primiparous women older than 35 years are at highest risk. If untreated, preeclampsia may progress to eclampsia, which has the same clinical findings but also presents with seizures.

86. **Describe the pathogenesis of preeclampsia.**
The exact pathogenesis of preeclampsia is not known. Most evidence suggests that the crucial changes occur in the uteroplacental bed and the spiral arteries, which do not seem to be able

to provide enough blood to the placenta. Spiral arteries are not invaded by trophoblast and retain their musculoelastic wall. These arteries therefore do not dilatate but retain their thick muscle layer. Furthermore, these blood vessels show signs of acute atherosis in which foamy macrophages accumulate in the intima narrowing the lumen of the vessel. Some blood vessels show fibrinoid necrosis. All these vascular changes cause placental ischemia and a release of placenta-derived cytokines, which damage the endothelial cells in the maternal organism. Proteinuria, edema, and hypertension result from glomerular injury, which is the most prominent pathologic finding in the majority of affected women. Disseminated intravascular coagulation develops, and if the microthrombi occlude, cerebral blood vessel seizures ensue.

87. **List the causes of spontaneous abortion.**
    - **Fetal factors:** These include chromosomal abnormalities, major developmental abnormalities, infections, or metabolic disorders that cause fetal demise.
    - **Maternal factors:** These are usually less obvious and include postulated endocrine dysfunction or insufficiency of the cervix.
    - **Placental factors:** These include infections and poorly defined conditions known as placental insufficiency.

88. **What is placenta accreta?**
    Placenta accreta results from an abnormal attachment of the placenta to the underlying uterus. The reason for the abnormal implantation seems to be related to the inability of the affected uterus to form a decidual layer, which normally provides a buffer zone between the chorionic villi and myometrium. The placental villi invade without any resistance into the muscular layer of the uterus. According to the extent of invasion of the uterine wall, abnormal placentas can be classified as:
    - **Placenta accreta:** The chorionic villi reach the myometrium but do not invade into it.
    - **Placenta increta:** The chorionic villi invade beyond the endometrium into the myometrium.
    - **Placenta percreta:** The chorionic villi penetrate through the entire myometrium and may reach the serosal surface.
    See Fig. 17-9.

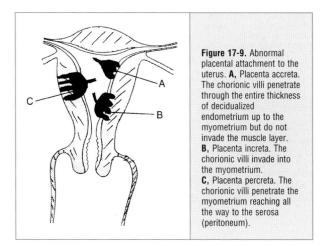

Figure 17-9. Abnormal placental attachment to the uterus. **A,** Placenta accreta. The chorionic villi penetrate through the entire thickness of decidualized endometrium up to the myometrium but do not invade the muscle layer. **B,** Placenta increta. The chorionic villi invade into the myometrium. **C,** Placenta percreta. The chorionic villi penetrate the myometrium reaching all the way to the serosa (peritoneum).

89. **What are the major causes of bleeding from the pregnant uterus?**
    - **Premature separation of the placenta:** This may cause a retroplacental hematoma or bleeding through the cervical orifice. A major form of separation is known as abruptio placentae.
    - **Placenta accreta:** Bleeding in the third trimester is the most common presenting sign of this condition.
    - **Placenta previa:** Abnormally implanted placenta covering the internal os of the end of the cervical canal may present with repeated bouts of bleeding during the entire pregnancy.
    - **Imminent or incipient abortion:** Termination of pregnancy can be related to a variety of fetal or maternal causes.
    - **Gestational trophoblastic disease:** These neoplastic proliferations of placental cells often present with bleeding.

BREAST

90. **Discuss the most important mass lesions of the breast biopsied or excised by surgeons.**
    Pathology reports indicate that the most common microscopic finding in breast biopsies is fibrocystic change (40%). Traumatic fat necrosis, duct ectasia, chronic mastitis, and similar nonneoplastic changes represent 15% of cases. Benign tumors are found in 5% and malignant tumors in 10% of biopsies. In 30% of cases, there are no microscopic abnormalities. These statistical data reflect current widespread use of mammography and the awareness of breast carcinoma among women in the United States. See Fig. 17-10.

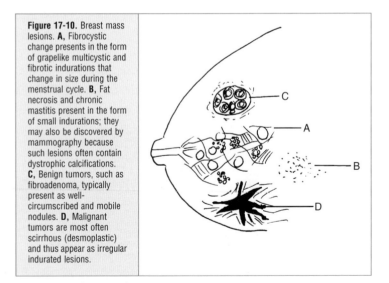

Figure 17-10. Breast mass lesions. **A,** Fibrocystic change presents in the form of grapelike multicystic and fibrotic indurations that change in size during the menstrual cycle. **B,** Fat necrosis and chronic mastitis present in the form of small indurations; they may also be discovered by mammography because such lesions often contain dystrophic calcifications. **C,** Benign tumors, such as fibroadenoma, typically present as well-circumscribed and mobile nodules. **D,** Malignant tumors are most often scirrhous (desmoplastic) and thus appear as irregular indurated lesions.

91. **What is fibrocystic change of the breast?**
    Fibrocystic change (also known as nonproliferative breast changes) includes a spectrum of macroscopic and microscopic changes in the female breasts resulting from an exaggerated and coordinated response of mammary ducts and stroma to cyclic hormonal stimulation that occurs in the normal menstrual cycle. It includes three main histologic changes:
    - **Fibrosis:** The dense interlobular fibrous tissue expands into the lobules, replacing the loose intralobular connective tissue.
    - **Cystic dilatation of ducts:** Strands of fibrous tissue constrict the ducts segmentally so that the normal secretions cannot pass out. This leads to distal dilatation of these terminal ducts.
    - **Adenosis:** This term denotes changes resulting from the proliferation of terminal duct cells, which are usually grouped around the centrally located dilatated ducts.

92. **What are the features of proliferative breast disease without atypia?**
    This name is applied to a group of lesions resulting from proliferation of ducts and stroma. It includes the following pathologic changes:
    - Florid epithelial hyperplasia
    - Sclerosing adenosis
    - Papillomas and papillomatosis
    - Fibroadenomatous hyperplasia

    These changes rarely form discrete masses and are usually diagnosed by biopsy of mammographically identified suspicious areas in the breast. Women with these lesions have a slightly increased risk for cancer (1.5–2 times).

KEY POINTS: BREAST ✔

1. Fibrocystic change is the most common cause of palpable masses in the breast.

2. In young women, benign fibroadenomas account for most neoplasms.

3. Breast cancer is the most common malignant tumor in females.

4. Breast cancer occurs in several histologic forms, but more than two thirds of carcinomas are of the invasive ductal type.

93. **What is the most common benign breast tumor?**
    The most common benign breast tumor is fibroadenoma. It is composed of elongated ducts surrounded by loose fibrous stroma. These tumors are well circumscribed from the normal breast and typically present as easily movable spherical masses in the breasts of young women in the 20- to 35-year- age group.

94. **What is phyllodes tumor?**
    Phyllodes tumors are closely related to fibroadenomas. Their name is derived from the Greek term for "leaf": on cross-sectioning, they appear leaflike, like an open book. Like fibroadenomas, they are composed of an epithelial and a stromal neoplastic component. The stroma shows increased cellularity and, in a minority of cases, even anaplasia. Most phyllodes tumors are benign. Malignant phyllodes tumors are locally invasive and may recur after incomplete excision. Metastasizing malignant phyllodes tumors are rare.

95. **What are intraductal papillomas?**
Intraductal papillomas are benign tumors of the major lactiferous ducts. Because of their intraductal growth pattern and a papillary structure, these tumors are easily torn away, which leads to bleeding from the nipple. Small duct papillomas are part of the proliferative breast diseases without atypia.

96. **How common is breast cancer?**
Breast cancer is the most common malignant tumor and the second most common cause of cancer-related mortality in women in the United States.

97. **List the main risk factors for breast cancer.**
The incidence of breast cancer is clearly associated with aging. Other established risk factors are as follows:
- Family history (mother and sisters): 2–9 times higher risk than population at large
- Menstrual history (early menarche–late menopause): 2 times higher risk
- Pregnancy (early pregnancy and lactation are protective): 3 times higher risk
- Proliferative breast disease and hyperplasia: 2 times higher risk
- Atypical hyperplasia: 4 times higher risk
- Carcinoma in situ: 8 times higher risk

98. **In which part of the breast are most carcinomas located?**
Most of the normal glandular tissue of the breast is located in the upper outer quadrant; thus more than 50% of all cancers originate in that location. The central area is the site of origin of 20% of tumors, and the other three quadrants are the site of origin of the remaining 30% of cancers. See Fig. 17-11.

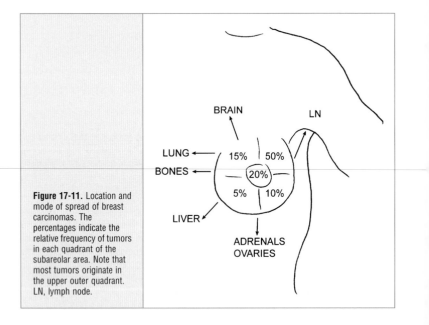

Figure 17-11. Location and mode of spread of breast carcinomas. The percentages indicate the relative frequency of tumors in each quadrant of the subareolar area. Note that most tumors originate in the upper outer quadrant. LN, lymph node.

99. **Discuss how breast cancers are classified.**

Breast cancers are classified according to their site of origin into ductal (90%) and lobular (9%) carcinomas. Fewer than 1% of tumors are sarcomas, lymphomas, and other rare entities. According to their growth pattern, carcinomas are divided into two major groups:
- Noninvasive carcinomas
- Invasive carcinoma

100. **What is intraductal carcinoma?**

Intraductal carcinoma, or ductal carcinoma in situ (DCIS), is the preinvasive form of breast carcinoma. In most instances, it is clinically inapparent and is discovered incidentally during histologic examination of breast tissue identified as abnormal by mammography. It is the most common form of newly diagnosed breast carcinoma.

101. **Do all intraductal carcinomas evolve into invasive breast carcinoma if left untreated?**

The answer to this question cannot be given because a controlled study would be difficult to perform. The available data show that the progression to invasive cancer depends on the histologic type of DCIS. The most ominous are the DCIS that show central necrosis (comedo-type necrosis, so named because the necrotic material can be expressed by late pressure, as in skin "blackheads," or comedos). These high-grade DCIS lesions progress to invasive carcinoma in approximately 40% of cases, and the progression of lower-grade lesions is probably in the range of 20%.

102. **Define lobular carcinoma in situ (LCIS).**

LCIS is the preinvasive form of lobular carcinoma. It is considerably less common than DCIS. In approximately 30% of cases, it will progress to invasive carcinoma. These lesions are often bilateral. LCIS should be treated as a sign of increased risk for invasive cancers, some of which develop on the biopsied breast, whereas others arise on the other side.

103. **How are invasive breast carcinomas classified?**

Approximately two of three invasive breast carcinomas are classified as "invasive ductal carcinoma, not otherwise specified." The remaining cancers are classified as follows:
- Lobular carcinomas
- Tubular carcinomas
- Medullary carcinomas
- Rare forms of cancer
- Colloid mucinous carcinomas

104. **Why are invasive ductal carcinomas of the breast also called scirrhous carcinomas?**

Invasive ductal breast carcinomas evoke a dense fibroblastic response in the host tissue, which imparts these tumors with a rock-hard consistency. Such desmoplastic tumors are called scirrhous carcinomas (from the Greek word *scirrhous,* meaning "hard").

105. **Explain why scirrhous breast carcinomas appear whitish and gritty on sectioning in the pathology laboratory.**

The dense collagen is white—remember the white appearance of aponeuroses enveloping the meat in inexpensive steak. In addition, there may be deposits of calcium that appear chalky white—chalk is mostly calcium phosphate.

106. **Why does breast cancer cause retraction of the nipple and skin ("peau d'orange")?**

The desmoplastic reaction caused by an infiltrating ductal carcinoma resembles an irregular scar, which deforms and causes retraction of the nipple. The connective tissue that fills the papillary dermis between the hair follicles gives the skin an indurated appearance, accentuating the normal follicular indentations, which appear like dimples on the surface of an orange.

107. **Which histologic or anatomic compartment of the breast is most often invaded by infiltrating duct carcinoma?**
Infiltrating duct carcinoma typically does not respect anatomic borders and invades the normal breast at random. Invasion of the fat tissue often can be seen on gross examination as stellate white tissue extending into the yellow fat tissue. Invasion of blood vessels, lymphatics, and perineural spaces can be seen on microscopic examination.

108. **Discuss Paget disease of the breast.**
Paget disease of the breast is a term used for infiltrating ductal carcinomas involving the epidermis of the nipple and the areola. It can be recognized clinically as a reddened, moist, or scaly skin lesion resembling eczema. Histologically, the epidermis appears infiltrated with large mucopolysaccharide-filled tumor cells, which are most prominent in the basal portion of the epidermis. Tumor cells may form small groups and extend to the surface, causing ulceration, often with superimposed infection. The prognosis of Paget disease of the breast depends on the extent of the underlying infiltrating ductal carcinoma.

109. **Which histologic forms of invasive breast carcinoma have a more favorable prognosis than the "garden variety" infiltrating ductal carcinoma?**
Three histologic subtypes of breast cancer that carry a better prognosis are:
- Medullary carcinoma
- Colloid or mucinous carcinoma
- Tubular carcinoma
    Unfortunately, these tumors with favorable prognosis account for only 2% or 3% of all breast cancers.

110. **What is medullary carcinoma?**
By remembering that medulla of the bone marrow and medulla oblongata of the brain are soft, one will also understand why these soft, often bulky tumors are called medullary carcinomas of the breast.
    In contrast to rock-hard scirrhous carcinomas that have an abundant connective tissue stroma, medullary carcinomas contain almost no connective tissue and are therefore soft. They are composed of sheets of tumor cells infiltrated with lymphocytes. These lymphocytes represent an immune response that contributes to the more favorable prognosis assigned to medullary carcinoma.

111. **Define colloid carcinoma.**
Colloid or mucinous carcinomas are rare tumors composed of mucin-producing cells floating in loose mucinous extracellular material that they have excreted into the interstitial spaces of the breast. The tumor is soft, jellylike, and usually described as "gelatinous." It occurs in older women and has a better prognosis than infiltrating ductal carcinoma.

112. **What is infiltrating lobular carcinoma?**
As implied in the name, lobular carcinomas originate in the lobules. They are composed of small, uniform cells with round nuclei invading the perilobular connective tissue in a single-file pattern. Invasive tumor cells often form concentric layers around the lobules and terminal ducts filled with lobular carcinoma in situ imparting the tissue with a targetoid ("bull's-eye") appearance.

113. **Does lobular carcinoma have a better prognosis than infiltrating ductal carcinoma?**

Compared stage by stage, lobular carcinomas have the same prognosis as infiltrating ductal carcinomas. However, it is important to remember that 20% of all lobular carcinomas are bilateral. Therefore any suspicious lesion in the contralateral breast should be biopsied, and a follow-up of the apparently healthy breast is mandatory.

114. **Describe how breast carcinomas metastasize.**

Breast cancers spread locally through the lymphatics and distally through the blood circulation. Axillary lymph nodes are usually the first to be involved. Tumors located in the inner quadrants metastasize into the lymph nodes along internal mammary arteries. The most common sites for distant metastases are lungs, liver, bones, and, for unknown reasons, adrenals. The brain may be involved in terminal cases.

115. **Name the most important prognostic factors of breast cancer.**

The most important prognostic factor is the stage of the tumor. Obviously, the best prognosis is assigned to noninvasive intraductal carcinomas. The prognosis of histologic typing of breast carcinoma is also important. Unfortunately, the tumors that have a good prognosis (medullary, colloid, and tubular) are rare. Other prognostic factors currently being investigated but already used in many medical centers on a routine basis are:

- **Estrogen receptors and progesterone receptors:** Tumors expressing these receptors tend to respond better to chemotherapy, which may be supplemented with an estrogen receptor blocker such as tamoxifen.
- **Chromosomal aneuploidy and proliferation index:** These parameters, usually determined by flow cytometry or the fluorescence in situ hybridization technique, provide data on the aggressiveness of the tumor.
- **Overexpression of oncogenes and loss of tumor suppressor genes:** HER2/neu protein, an equivalent of growth factor receptor, is an oncogene that plays a role in the pathogenesis of breast cancer, and its overexpression is associated with poor prognosis.

116. **How does the staging determine the 5-year survival rate of women with breast carcinomas?**

- Stage I (localized tumor, <2 cm in diameter): 87%
- Stage II (2- to 5-cm tumor and local lymph node metastases): 75%
- Stage III (tumor >5 cm with lymph nodes involvement on the same side, skin involvement or chest wall fixation): 46%
- Stage IV (tumor of any size with distant metastases): 13%

117. **Should a woman who has no evidence of breast cancer recurrence for 10 years be considered cured of her disease?**

Generally, she is not likely to have more recurrences. Nevertheless, late recurrences have been noted, even after more than 10 years.

118. **How common is cancer of the male breast?**

- Male breast cancer is 100 times less common than breast cancer in women.
- Histologically it has the same features as the more common cancer of the female breast, but it tends to invade more rapidly. At the time of diagnosis, 50% of tumors have already metastasized.

119. **Describe the difference between mastectomy and lumpectomy.**

Mastectomy, which the surgeon can perform as a simple mastectomy or radical mastectomy, involves removal of the entire breast and, in the radical form, the lymph nodes as well. Lumpectomy (also referred to as breast-conserving surgery) involves only excision of the tumor from the breast. It may be accompanied by axillary lymph node removal.

WEBSITES 🌐

1. http://www.ncbi.nlm.nih.gov/entrez/query.fcgi?db=PubMed

2. http://www-medlib.med.utah.edu/WebPath/webpath.html#MENU

3. http://www.uihealthcare.com/vh

4. http://mammary.nih.gov

5. http://www.mayoclinic.com/health/ovarian-cancer/DS00293

BIBLIOGRAPHY

1. Fackenthal JD, Olopade OI: Breast cancer risk associated with BRCA1 and BRCA2 in diverse populations. Nat Rev Cancer 7:937–948, 2007.

2. Feeley KM, Wells M: Hormone replacement therapy and the endometrium. J Clin Pathol 54:435–440, 2001.

3. Folsom AR, Anderson JP, Ross JA: Estrogen replacement therapy and ovarian cancer. Epidemiology 15:100–104, 2004.

4. Moulder S, Hortobagyi GN: Advances in the treatment of breast cancer. Clin Pharmacol Ther 83:26–36, 2008.

5. Payne SJ, Bowen RL, Jones JL, Wells CA: Predictive markers in breast cancer—the present. Histopathology 52:82–90, 2008.

6. Reinhardt MJ: Gynecologic tumors. Recent Results Cancer Res 170:141–150, 2008.

7. Rubin SC: Cervical cancer: successes and failures. CA Cancer J Clin 51:89–91, 2001.

8. Sawaya GF, Brown AD, Washington AE, Garber AM: Current approaches to cervical cancer screening. N Engl J Med 344:1603–1607, 2001.

9. Silverstein MJ: Ductal carcinoma in situ of the breast. Annu Rev Med 51:17–32, 2000.

10. Tavassoli FA: Ductal intraepithelial neoplasia of the breast. Virchows Arch 438:221–227, 2001.

CHAPTER 18

THE ENDOCRINE SYSTEM

Ivan Damjanov, MD, PhD

1. **Which organs belong to the endocrine system?**

   The endocrine system consists of cells that secrete hormones and includes:

   - Parts of the central nervous system, such as the hypothalamus
   - Organs composed predominantly of endocrine cells, such as the pituitary gland, the thyroid gland, the parathyroid glands, and the adrenals
   - Organs that have a major endocrine component, such as the testis, ovary, and endocrine pancreas (islets of Langerhans)
   - Dispersed endocrine system of the respiratory and gastrointestinal mucosa

2. **What are hormones?**

   Hormones are biologically active substances secreted by one cell that stimulate other cells. Traditionally this term was reserved for endocrine substances (i.e., secreted into the blood and carried by circulation to their distant target organs). This concept was broadened and today includes a variety of substances that exert:

   - Paracrine stimulation (i.e., act on adjacent cells in the tissue of their origin)
   - Autocrine stimulation (i.e., act on the cell that has produced the substance)
   - Neurocrine stimulation (i.e., substances produced by neurons that act on nonneuronal cells)
     See Fig. 18-1.

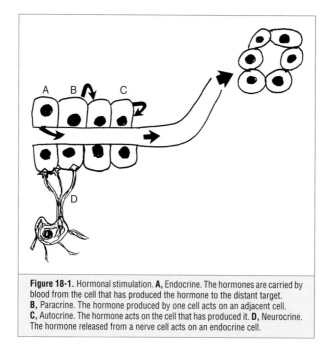

Figure 18-1. Hormonal stimulation. **A,** Endocrine. The hormones are carried by blood from the cell that has produced the hormone to the distant target. **B,** Paracrine. The hormone produced by one cell acts on an adjacent cell. **C,** Autocrine. The hormone acts on the cell that has produced it. **D,** Neurocrine. The hormone released from a nerve cell acts on an endocrine cell.

3. **What are the main types of hormones?**

   Biochemically, hormones can be classified as:
   - Peptides, such as insulin, prolactin, or parahormone
   - Amines, such as epinephrine, histamine, or serotonin
   - Steroids, such as cortisol, estrogens, or androgens

4. **What are the differences between peptide and amine hormones versus steroid hormones?**

   In general, peptide and amine hormones are stored inside the cells of their origin in the form of dense neuroendocrine granules that can be seen by electron microscopy. These hormones act on receptors on the plasma membrane of target cells, which in turn activate a signaling system in the cytoplasm. The impulse is transmitted from the plasma membrane to the DNA by secondary messengers. In contrast to these hormones, steroids are not stored in granules but are synthesized on external stimulation by trophic hormones (e.g., adrenocorticotropic hormone [ACTH] stimulates the synthesis of glucocorticoids). Steroid hormones have receptors in the nucleus of their target cells, and their action on the nuclear DNA does not require activation of a cytoplasmic messenger system. See Fig. 18-2.

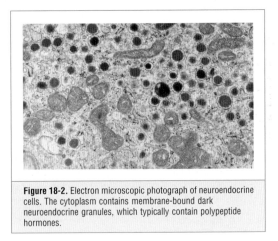

Figure 18-2. Electron microscopic photograph of neuroendocrine cells. The cytoplasm contains membrane-bound dark neuroendocrine granules, which typically contain polypeptide hormones.

5. **How do endocrine disorders present clinically?**

   Endocrine disorders present clinically as:
   - Hypofunction (i.e., reduced production of specific hormones)
   - Hyperfunction (i.e., increased production of specific hormones)
   - Mass lesions (i.e., enlargement of the endocrine organ due to an underlying neoplasia or hyperplasia)

6. **Is the enlargement of endocrine glands always associated with their hyperfunction?**

   The enlargement of endocrine glands may be accompanied by overproduction of hormones, no obvious hormonal changes, or reduced hormonal output. For example, thyroid enlargement in Graves disease is associated with hyperthyroidism. Nodular goiter is most often euthyroid. Anaplastic carcinoma may completely destroy the normal thyroid and cause hypothyroidism.

PITUITARY

7. Where is the normal pituitary located?
The pituitary is located in the sella turcica, a concavity of the sphenoid bone that forms a part of the base of the skull. Enlargement of the pituitary can cause an expansion of the sella turcica that can be seen by x-ray.

8. To which other organ is the pituitary anatomically linked?
The pituitary is attached to the brain by a stalk, composed of blood vessels of the pituitary portal system and axonal extensions of hypothalamic nerves. Transection of the pituitary stalk causes hypopituitarism. It will hinder the influx of blood that contains the hypothalamic-releasing factors (i.e., neuropeptides that normally stimulate the cells in the anterior lobe of the pituitary). The transection of axons that serve as conduits for the transport of oxytocin and antidiuretic hormone (ADH) from the hypothalamus into the posterior lobe of the pituitary will prevent the entry of these hormones into the blood and thus cause diabetes insipidus.

9. Why does enlargement of the pituitary impair vision?
Enlargement of the pituitary will cause compression of the optic chiasm, which is overlying the membranous covering of the sella turcica. Compression of the central portion of the chiasm leads to a loss of lateral visual fields of both eyes, known as bilateral hemianopsia.

10. What are the main cell types of the pituitary?
The anterior pituitary consists of four functional cell types that can be identified immunohistochemically using the antibodies to specific pituitary hormones. These cells are:
- Somatotrophs, producing growth hormone
- Lactotrophs, producing prolactin
- Corticotrophs, producing ACTH
- Thyrotrophs, producing thyroid-stimulating hormone (TSH)
- Gonadotrophs, producing follicle-stimulating hormone (FSH) and luteinizing hormone (LH)
Cells that do not react with antibodies to any of the previously mentioned hormones are called null cells and represent either undifferentiated stem cells or exhausted and nonfunctioning cells. Some nonfunctioning cells have prominent eosinophilic cytoplasm and contain numerous mitochondria. These cells are called oncocytes. The posterior lobe of the pituitary is composed of axonal processes of hypothalamic neurons and does not contain hormone-producing cells.

KEY POINTS: PITUITARY ✓

1. Adenomas are the most common pathologic lesion of the pituitary.
2. Pituitary adenomas may be hormonally inactive or produce excess prolactin, growth hormone adrenocorticotropic hormone, thyrotropin, or gonadotropins.
3. Loss of anterior pituitary leads to panhypopituitarism, and the loss of posterior pituitary leads to deficiency of antidiuretic hormone ADH and diabetes insipidus.

11. Are the pituitary tumors composed of the same cells as the normal pituitary?
Most pituitary tumors are monoclonal and are composed of a single cell type corresponding to one of the six cell types found in the normal anterior lobe of the pituitary. Axons of the posterior pituitary do not form tumors.

12. **What is the most common tumor of the pituitary?**
    Most pituitary tumors (>95%) are benign and classified as adenomas. Most adenomas are composed of a single cell type and secrete only one hormone. Prolactinomas, which account for approximately 30% of all pituitary tumors, are the most common pituitary neoplasm.

13. **Are all pituitary tumors hormonally active?**
    Approximately 80% of all pituitary tumors are hormonally active. In the remaining 20% of cases, the pituitary tumors are composed of hormonally inactive cells, which may compress the normal gland and cause hypopituitarism. Small clinically undiagnosed pituitary tumors may be found accidentally in 20% of routine adult autopsies.

14. **What is the most common cause of hyperpituitarism?**
    Pituitary adenomas are the most common cause of pituitary hyperfunction syndromes. Carcinomas and hyperplasias account for no more than 5% or 6% of all cases.

15. **What are the most common signs and symptoms caused by the local mass effect of pituitary tumors?**
    - Increased intracranial pressure (headache, nausea, and vomiting)
    - Radiographic changes in the sella turcica
    - Bitemporal hemianopsia due to the compression of the optic chiasm
    - Hypopituitarism or diabetes insipidus

16. **What are the main clinical features of hyperprolactinemia?**
    In women of reproductive age, hyperprolactinemia causes amenorrhea and galactorrhea. In men, the symptoms are more subtle and may include loss of libido and infertility.

17. **Why is hyperprolactinemia usually treated with bromocriptine?**
    In normal circumstances, pituitary lactotrophs are inhibited by dopamine and therefore do not secrete prolactin. Many cases of hyperprolactinemia are related to a loss of this dopaminergic inhibition. Bromocriptine, a dopamine agonist, will inhibit prolactin secretion and cause regression of lactotroph hyperplasia and even microscopic prolactinomas. Larger tumors that do not respond must be removed surgically, usually by a transethmoidal approach.

18. **What are the clinical manifestations of growth hormone-secreting tumors?**
    In growing children and adolescents, growth hormone–secreting adenomas cause gigantism, whereas in adults, these tumors cause acromegaly.

19. **What are the features of acromegaly?**
    The most prominent findings are the marked enlargement of hands and feet, nose, and jaws ("acra," i.e., protruding terminal parts). These externally visible changes are accompanied by internal organomegaly and metabolic disorders (diabetes, hypertension, etc.). The most common findings are illustrated in Fig. 18-3.

20. **What is Cushing disease?**
    Cushing disease is hypercortisolism caused by an ACTH-secreting tumor. Because the ACTH molecule contains a fragment that has a melanocyte-stimulating function, the disease is associated with hyperpigmentation of the skin.

21. **How do gonadotroph adenomas present clinically?**
    These tumors do not produce distinct clinical syndromes and are usually diagnosed only after they have attained a size that will cause a mass effect. Menstrual abnormalities, infertility, and various nonspecific hormonal changes are found in some patients.

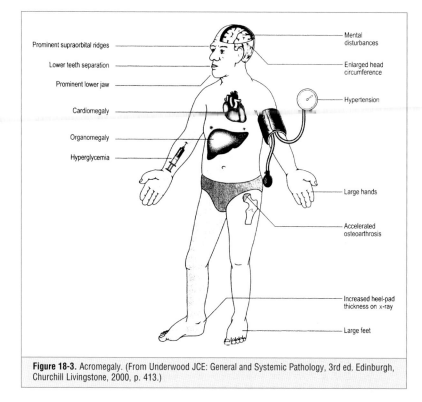

Figure 18-3. Acromegaly. (From Underwood JCE: General and Systemic Pathology, 3rd ed. Edinburgh, Churchill Livingstone, 2000, p. 413.)

22. **What are null cell adenomas?**
Null cell adenomas are hormonally inactive tumors recognized by their mass effect. Large tumors may cause hypopituitarism.

23. **What is the anatomic substrate of hypopituitarism?**
Clinical signs of hypopituitarism appear after a loss of 75% or more of the anterior pituitary.

24. **What are the most common causes of hypopituitarism?**
   - Tumors, especially nonfunctioning adenomas and primary or metastatic carcinomas
   - Stalk lesion due to surgery, trauma, or neoplasms of the brain
   It is worth remembering that pituitary insufficiency may be caused by several pathologic processes that all begin with the letter "i":
   - Invasion of the pituitary, pituitary stalk, or the hypothalamic nuclei by tumors
   - Injury (e.g., head trauma with basal fractures or brain surgery)
   - Infarction (e.g., postpartum pituitary necrosis known as Sheehan syndrome)
   - Irradiation (for brain tumors or base of the skull and ear, nose, and throat tumors)
   - Immune diseases (e.g., sarcoidosis and autoimmune hypophysitis)
   - Infection (e.g., basal meningitis and tuberculosis)
   - Inborn errors of metabolism (mostly childhood diseases; in adults the most common is iron deposition in hemochromatosis)
   - Idiopathic (after all other causes have been excluded)

25. **What is Sheehan syndrome?**

    Sheehan syndrome is also known as postpartum pituitary necrosis. Previously it was the most common form of ischemic necrosis of the pituitary, but it is rare today. It develops due to massive blood loss at the time of delivery, causing hypoperfusion of the pituitary that has undergone physiologic hyperplasia during pregnancy. Symptoms include hypothyroidism, adrenal insufficiency, and amenorrhea.

26. **What is the empty sella syndrome?**

    This term is applied to a variety of conditions in which the sella turcica appears "empty." In primary empty sella syndrome, which rarely presents with hypopituitarism, the pituitary atrophy is related to a compression by the cerebrospinal fluid and arachnoidea that invaginate into the sella through a defect in the diaphragm. Secondary empty sella is a consequence of surgical intervention or radiation therapy.

27. **What is diabetes insipidus?**

    Diabetes insipidus is a syndrome characterized by polyuria, polydipsia, and renal loss of water due to a deficiency of ADH. It may be caused by injury of the hypothalamus, pituitary stalk, or posterior pituitary.

28. **What is the syndrome of inappropriate ADH secretion?**

    This syndrome, characterized by excessive renal retention of water and dilutional hyponatremia, is caused by hyperproduction of ADH. The most common causes of ADH overproduction are small cell lung cancer, chronic lung disease, and hypothalamic lesions.

29. **What is craniopharyngioma?**

    Craniopharyngiomas are tumors originating from remnants of the Rathke pouch, the embryonic anlage of the anterior pituitary. These tumors occur in children and young adults, and they are located in the suprasellar space, causing lesions of the hypothalamus and the pituitary stalk.

THYROID

30. **How does the thyroid develop?**

    The thyroid develops during early embryonic life from the outpouching of the pharyngeal epithelium at the base of the tongue. This epithelium proliferates and forms the thyroglossal duct, which extends caudally, finally forming the thyroid on the anterior side of the neck. The thyroglossal duct involutes normally during fetal life, but if this involution is not complete its remnants give rise to thyroglossal duct cysts.

31. **What are the basic functional units of the thyroid?**

    Thyroid cells are arranged into functional units called follicles. Follicles are lined by cuboidal epithelium surrounding the centrally located colloid, composed of thyroglobulin.

32. **How is thyroxine formed?**

    Thyroxine (tetraiodothyronine or T4) is formed from thyroglobulin by follicular cells. Follicular cells stimulated by TSH pinocytose thyroglobulin and transform it into T4 and, to a lesser extent, triiodothyronine (T3). T4 and T3 are released into the blood, where they circulate predominantly bound to thyroid-binding globulin (TBG) but also in a free form.

KEY POINTS: THYROID ✓

1. The most common cause of thyroid enlargement is goiter caused by thyroid follicular hyperplasia.

2. Graves disease is the most common cause of hyperthyroidism, and Hashimoto thyroiditis the most common cause of hypothyroidism.

3. Follicular adenomas are the most common benign thyroid tumors, whereas papillary carcinomas are the most common malignant tumors.

33. **What are goitrogens?**
Goitrogens are substances such as propylthiourea that interfere with the synthesis of T4 and T3. In an effort to compensate for the reduced production of T4 and T3, thyroid follicles enlarge and become lined by hyperplastic epithelium. Inefficient synthesis of T3/T4 leads to an accumulation of colloid in follicles. These dilatated follicles cause enlargement of the thyroid known as goiter or struma.

34. **Which thyroid cells produce calcitonin?**
Calcitonin is a hormone that stimulates the uptake of serum calcium into the bones. It is produced by parafollicular or C cells of the thyroid.

35. **What is the most common cause of hyperthyroidism?**
Graves disease, an autoimmune disease associated with diffuse enlargement of the thyroid, accounts for 85% of the cases of hyperthyroidism.

36. **Can multinodular goiter cause hyperthyroidism?**
Yes. Some goiters contain hyperfunctioning thyroid cells, which form nodules detectable by radioactive iodine scanning ("hot nodules"). Solitary hyperfunctioning nodules in an otherwise normal thyroid represent benign tumors (adenomas) that account for a small percentage of hyperthyroidisms.

37. **What are the clinical features of hyperthyroidism?**
Symptoms of hyperthyroidism are caused by hypermetabolism and excessive stimulation of the sympathetic system. Increased metabolic rate is accompanied by hyperactivity and subsequent fatigue, heat intolerance, and weight loss. The most important signs and symptoms related to major organ systems are:
- **Cardiovascular system:** Tachycardia, increased cardiac output, increased incidence of atrial fibrillation, and palpitations
- **Nervous system:** Nervousness, anxiety, hyperkinesia, and tremor
- **Skeletal muscles:** Muscle weakness and wasting
- **Gastrointestinal system:** Increased appetite, intestinal hypermotility, and diarrhea
- **Skin:** Excessive sweating
- **Bones:** Osteoporosis

38. **Is exophthalmos found in all forms of hyperthyroidism?**
No. Exophthalmos is found only in patients with Graves disease. It is associated with lymphocytic infiltrates in the retroorbital tissues. External eye muscles are particularly affected and appear swollen. This enlargement of the retroorbital tissue and orbital muscles leads to proptosis (anterior displacement of the eyeball). The weakness of eye muscles results in functional disturbances such as diplopia and inability to read. During physical examination, these patients show conjunctival congestion and palpebral symptoms ("lid lag" and "lid retraction").

39. **Which laboratory tests are most useful for diagnosing hyperthyroidism?**
    The most useful tests are based on the measurements of TSH, T4, and T3 (total and free form). Increased serum TBG (in pregnancy) or decreased TBG (in cirrhosis) may influence the concentration of T3/T4 in blood. Radioactive iodine uptake is followed by a thyroid scan to determine whether the entire thyroid is hyperfunctioning or whether the disease is caused by a hyperfunctioning nodule.

40. **What are the possible causes of hypothyroidism?**
    Hypothyroidism may be related to three sets of causes:
    - Structural defect (lack of thyroid cells)
    - Functional defect in the synthesis of T4 and T3
    - Extrathyroid disease (hypothalamic or pituitary lesion)
      For an extended list of possible causes of hypothyroidism, use the mnemonic *add iodine*:
      Autoimmune diseases (Hashimoto disease, Riedel thyroiditis)
      Developmental (agenesis of the thyroid)
      Dietary (goitrogens in food such as turnips, rutabaga, and cassava)
      Iodine deficiency (in endemic areas)
      Oncologic diseases (destruction of thyroid by cancer)
      Drugs (propylthiouracyl, methimazole, and lithium)
      Iatrogenic interventions (surgical thyroidectomy, radiation therapy)
      Nonthyroidal defects (e.g., TBG deficiency)
      Endocrine diseases (pituitary insufficiency and hypothalamic defects)

41. **What is the most common cause of hypothyroidism?**
    Hashimoto (autoimmune) thyroiditis is the most common cause of hypothyroidism in the United States, as well as in other developed countries that use iodized salt. In some underdeveloped mountainous regions of Asia (Himalayas) or South America (Andes), iodine deficiency is a significant cause of goiter, which may be accompanied by hypothyroidism.

42. **What is the cause of cretinism?**
    Cretinism is a term used for hypothyroidism of infancy and early childhood. Previously, it was endemic in iodine-deficient areas. Today it is rare in the United States and is most often caused by congenital agenesis of the thyroid or inborn errors of iodine metabolism and thyroid hormone synthesis.

43. **What are the clinical features of cretinism?**
    Hypothyroidism of infancy and early childhood retards the somatic growth and affects the development of the central nervous system. These children have short stature and are mentally retarded. Their faces have coarse features and a protruding tongue.

44. **What is myxedema?**
    Myxedema is a term used to denote edema of the skin and internal organs due to the accumulation of hygroscopic glycosaminoglycans that typically occurs in hypothyroidism of adulthood. By inference, the term myxedema has become a synonym for hypothyroidism.

45. **What are the features of hypothyroidism?**
    The lack of thyroid hormones slows the metabolism and most body functions. The clinical picture is dominated by bradycardia and reduced cardiac output, constipation, and decreased sweating. Coarse facial features due to edema of the dermis are typical.

46. **What is the most common cause of thyroiditis?**
    Thyroiditis, an inflammation of the thyroid, most often has an autoimmune pathogenesis. Simple chronic lymphocytic thyroiditis is usually subclinical and is diagnosed histologically as an incidental finding at autopsy. Like all other thyroid diseases, it occurs more often in females than

males. The most common form of thyroiditis associated with clinical symptoms is Hashimoto disease. Infectious thyroiditis is rare.

47. **What is Hashimoto thyroiditis?**
Hashimoto thyroiditis is an autoimmune disease causing progressive loss of thyroid tissue, which is replaced by lymphoid cells. Both T and B cells play a pathogenic role in the destruction of thyroid follicles. The disease is often associated with other autoimmune diseases and is 10 to 20 times more common in women than in men. A familial and HLA (human leukocyte antigen) related clustering of cases suggests a genetic predisposition.

48. **Which antibodies are found in Hashimoto thyroiditis?**
Almost all patients with Hashimoto thyroiditis have antibodies to thyroglobulin and thyroid peroxidase (an enzyme located in the microvilli on the apical, or inner, cell membrane of thyroid follicular cells). However, these antibodies are nonspecific signs of thyroid injury and occur in other thyroid disorders as well. Antibodies to the TSH receptor, like those in Graves disease, are also found. However, in Hashimoto disease anti-TSH antibodies do not stimulate thyroid cells but rather have a blocking effect, which accounts for the hypothyroidism in most cases.

49. **What is the pathogenesis of Hashimoto thyroiditis?**
The cause and the pathogenesis of Hashimoto thyroiditis are not known. It is an autoimmune disease in which the loss of suppressor T-cell activity leads to overproduction of antibodies to thyroid antigens and an unregulated function of T cytotoxic cells, which destroy the thyroid follicles and cause hypothyroidism. Antithyroglobulin antibodies are found in serum and are useful for the diagnosis of this disease.

50. **What is the appearance of the thyroid in Hashimoto disease?**
The thyroid is diffusely enlarged in most cases. Histologically the parenchyma is infiltrated with lymphocytes and plasma cells replacing thyroid follicles. Lymphocytes may form germinal centers reminiscent of those normally found in lymph nodes. The remaining thyroid follicles vary in size and shape and are typically lined by cuboidal cells that have eosinophilic granular cytoplasm. These cells, known as oncocytes or Hürthle cells, contain numerous mitochondria in their cytoplasm but are inefficient producers of thyroxine.

51. **What malignancy develops most often in Hashimoto thyroiditis?**
Like many other autoimmune disorders, Hashimoto thyroiditis is associated with an increased incidence of B-cell lymphoma, which usually presents as a low-grade lymphoma limited to the thyroid. Papillary carcinoma, a low-grade epithelial malignant tumor of the thyroid, also occurs more often in thyroids affected by Hashimoto disease.

52. **What is subacute thyroiditis?**
Subacute thyroiditis, also known as granulomatous or de Quervain thyroiditis, is a disease of unknown etiology. In many instances, the symptoms appear following an upper respiratory tract infection, suggesting that the thyroid disease also has a viral etiology. Histologically, the thyroid contains numerous giant cell-rich granulomas developing around ruptured thyroid follicles. Subacute thyroiditis has a sudden or somewhat insidious onset. Symptoms appear suddenly and include pain in the neck, fever, and slight enlargement of the thyroid, which is sensitive to palpation. The disease has a self-limited course with a recovery in 4 to 6 weeks. The release of thyroglobulin from destroyed follicles may cause transient hyperthyroidism.

53. **What is lymphocytic thyroiditis?**
Lymphocytic thyroiditis, also known as painless or subacute lymphocytic thyroiditis, is a common pathologic finding of questionable significance. This diagnosis is made in 10% of thyroids examined at autopsy. Some patients have clinical signs and symptoms of transient, self-limited hyperthyroidism that last a few weeks. In most instances, however, the pathologic

diagnosis of lymphocytic thyroiditis made at autopsy or in thyroids resected for some other reason cannot be related to specific thyroid function.

54. **What is Graves disease?**
Graves disease is an autoimmune disease presenting with hyperthyroidism and exophthalmos and, less commonly, localized pretibial dermal swelling (myxedema).

55. **How common is Graves disease?**
Graves disease is common, affecting probably 1% or 2% of all women in the United States. It is 7 times more common in women than in men. It shows familial clustering, high concordance in monozygotic twins, and an association with some HLA haplotypes and other autoimmune diseases, suggestive of a genetic predisposition.

56. **What is the pathogenesis of Graves disease?**
Although it is well known that Graves disease is mediated by antibodies to the TSH receptor on thyroid follicular cells, the reasons for the appearance of these antibodies are not known. The overproduction of antibodies is most likely secondary to the loss of regulatory T-cell functions and the suppression of autoantibody production. Antibodies binding to the TSH receptor activate adenylate cyclase and thus stimulate the overproduction of thyroid hormones and thyroid cell hypertrophy and hyperplasia. Exophthalmos is also immune mediated. Both the thyroid and the retroorbital ocular muscle are infiltrated with B lymphocytes. The mechanism of exophthalmos is not known.

57. **What are the morphologic features of Graves disease?**
The thyroid is diffusely enlarged, hyperemic, and soft. Histologically, the gland consists of tall columnar hyperplastic thyroid cells lining the follicles and forming micropapillary projections or solid cords. The colloid is pale and shows peripheral scalloping due to rapid uptake of thyroglobulin by the hyperfunctioning thyroid cells. The stroma contains infiltrates of lymphocytes, which occasionally form aggregates.

58. **What are the signs and symptoms of Graves disease?**
Hyperthyroidism causes hypermetabolism and symptoms such as fever, tachycardia, and increased intestinal motility. The basal metabolism rate is increased. Typical laboratory findings include elevated serum T4 and T3 and low TSH accompanied by increased radioactive iodine uptake diffusely into the entire thyroid.

59. **What is goiter?**
Goiter is enlargement of the thyroid. It may be diffuse or multinodular. Enlargement of the thyroid is usually related to a defect in the synthesis of thyroid hormones, evoking a compensatory hyperplasia of thyroid cells. The inefficient synthesis of thyroid hormones results in accumulation of colloid inside the follicles (colloid goiter). Irregular proliferation of thyroid cells coupled with degenerative changes that evoke hemorrhage, fibrosis, and calcification will cause transformation of simple colloid goiters into nodular goiter.

60. **What is the difference between sporadic and endemic goiter?**
Sporadic goiter, the most common form of thyroid enlargement in the United States, is a disease that usually affects young women. Although it may be related to the ingestion of goitrogens, such as Brussels sprouts, cabbage, or cauliflower, in most instances the cause remains undetermined. Thyroid enlargement represents a "cosmetic defect" but is not accompanied by hypo- or hyperthyroidism. Endemic goiter is a term used to denote thyroid enlargement found in more than 10% of the population. It is always related to iodine deficiency, and it occurs typically in mountainous areas of underdeveloped countries. The symptoms of the disease are related to the mass effect of the enlarged thyroid gland.

61. **What is the morphology of nodular goiter?**
The thyroid is enlarged and consists of multiple nodules composed of follicles that vary in size and shape. Some follicles are dilatated and lined by flattened atrophic epithelium, whereas others are lined by normal or even hyperplastic epithelium. The interfollicular stroma is fibrotic, and many nodules have a fibrous capsule resembling the capsule of a benign tumor. Secondary degenerative changes are common and include hyalinization, calcification of the stroma, cystic degeneration of parenchyma, hemorrhage, and necrosis leading to cystic cavities filled with fluid.

62. **Do multinodular goiters cause hyperthyroidism?**
Most patients with multinodular goiters are euthyroid. The enlarged thyroid may contain a solitary or multiple hyperfunctioning "hot" nodules. Toxic multinodular goiter associated with exophthalmos and pretibial myxedema, called Plummer syndrome, is clinically similar to Graves disease. Multinodular goiter is rarely associated with hypothyroidism.

63. **What are thyroid adenomas?**
Most thyroid adenomas present as well-encapsulated nodules, measuring, on average, 3 to 10 cm in diameter. These benign tumors represent clonal proliferation of follicular cells resembling adult or embryonic or fetal thyroid cells. Several histologic variants have been identified. Histologic subclassification of adenomas is of no clinical significance. Well-differentiated follicular carcinomas may be composed of cells that are indistinguishable from those in adenomas, and in such cases the diagnosis of malignancy is established by demonstrating penetration of tumor cells through the capsule or invasion of blood vessels.

64. **Do all thyroid adenomas take up radioactive iodine?**
Most adenomas do not take up radioactive iodine and present as cold nodules on thyroid radionucleotide scans. Radioactive iodine scans cannot distinguish benign nonfunctioning adenomas from thyroid carcinomas, which also present as cold nodules. Approximately 10% of solitary cold nodules are carcinomas. Approximately 5% of thyroid adenomas present as hot nodules. Hot nodules are almost never malignant.

65. **How common are thyroid carcinomas?**
Thyroid carcinomas are rare and account for only 1.5% of all malignant tumors of internal organs. It is worth remembering that:
- Most tumors (80%) are low-grade papillary carcinomas.
- Most tumors arise in middle-aged adults.
- Women are more often affected than men, except for the rare tumors of children and the elderly, which show no sex predilection.

66. **What are the risk factors for thyroid cancer?**
Risk factors for thyroid cancer include:
- Ionizing radiation
- Autoimmune thyroid diseases
- Iodine deficiency
- Genetic factors
The incidence of thyroid cancer is increased in people who were exposed to ionizing radiation during childhood. Increased incidence has been noticed in men and women treated by x-rays for acne during puberty and those who survived the atomic blast in Japan during World War II or the Chernobyl nuclear plant accident in Ukraine in 1986.
Hashimoto thyroiditis is associated with an increased incidence of thyroid epithelial tumors and lymphomas. Endemic goiter in iodine-deficient areas of the world is associated with an increased incidence of follicular carcinoma. Medullary carcinoma shows familial clustering, and in some cases it is one of the tumors of the syndrome of multiple endocrine neoplasia (MEN-2). Such tumors show rearrangement of chromosome 10 containing the RET protooncogene.

The RET oncogene is mutated in approximately 95% of patients with MEN-2. The RET oncogene also plays a role in the pathogenesis of some papillary carcinomas.

67. **List the most important histologic forms of thyroid cancer.**
    - Papillary carcinoma (70%)
    - Follicular carcinoma (15%)
    - Medullary carcinoma (5%)
    - Undifferentiated (anaplastic) carcinoma (2%–3%)

    Histologic features of these tumors are illustrated in Fig. 18-4.

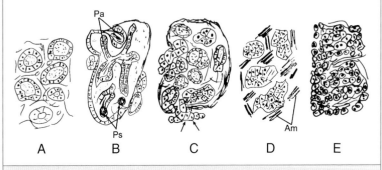

Figure 18-4. Thyroid tumors. This drawing illustrates the salient features of main thyroid cancers. **A,** Normal thyroid consists of follicles filled with colloid. **B,** Papillary carcinoma consists of papillae (Pa) that have a central connective tissue core lined by cuboidal cells. Tumor cells have clear nuclei with finely dispersed chromatin. There are scattered calcifications ("psammoma bodies" [Ps]). **C,** Follicular carcinoma is composed of irregular follicles. Tumor cells also form solid cords or nests. The lesion is encapsulated, but the tumor cells invade beyond the capsule into the adjacent tissue. **D,** Medullary carcinoma consists of solid nests of tumor cells and extracellular amyloid in the stroma (Am). **E,** Anaplastic undifferentiated carcinoma consists of solid masses of anaplastic cells showing marked pleomorphism. Many cells are very large and binucleated.

68. **List key facts about papillary carcinoma of the thyroid.**
    - It is the most common malignant tumor of the thyroid.
    - It affects women more often than men.
    - It may occur in early adulthood and throughout adult life (20–60 years of age).
    - It has a good prognosis in most instances (10-year survival >90%), but some tumors in older patients have a less favorable prognosis.

69. **Describe the morphology of papillary carcinoma of the thyroid.**
    Most tumors present as small nodules without sharp margins, but larger tumors may not have a distinct capsule. Microscopically the tumor is composed of cuboidal cells lining the fibrovascular papillae. Foci of calcification (psammoma bodies) are common. Tumor cell nuclei contain cytoplasmic inclusions or appear "empty" and are described as "Orphan Annie eyes." These nuclear features are important for making the fine needle aspiration biopsy diagnosis of papillary carcinoma and in tumors that do not form obvious papillae (follicular variant of papillary carcinoma).

70. **How do papillary carcinomas metastasize?**
    Papillary carcinomas have a tendency to invade lymphatics and metastasize early to ipsilateral lymph nodes on the neck. This local spread does not worsen the prognosis, which is usually excellent (98% 10-year survival rate). Less favorable variants and tumors that invade

the blood vessels are occasionally found. Papillary carcinoma of the elderly has a less favorable prognosis.

71. **What is follicular carcinoma of the thyroid?**
Follicular carcinoma accounts for approximately 15% of thyroid malignancies and is the second most common thyroid cancer. Typically tumors begin as encapsulated lesions that break through the capsule and invade the normal thyroid or adjacent tissues. On gross examination such encapsulated tumors are indistinguishable from benign adenomas. Other tumors begin as indistinct foci of atypical cells invading the normal thyroid. Histologically tumors are composed of cuboidal cells forming follicles filled with colloid or solid nests and strands of less differentiated cells.

72. **How do follicular adenomas differ from follicular carcinomas?**
The well-differentiated follicular carcinomas may be indistinguishable from adenomas, and the only evidence that a tumor is malignant is the extension of tumor cells beyond the capsule, invasion of lymphatics and blood vessels, or, even more convincing, distant metastases. Less differentiated tumors show cellular anaplasia and more obvious signs of invasive growth, as well as distant hematogenous metastases.

73. **What are the clinical features of follicular carcinoma?**
Follicular carcinomas usually present as slowly enlarging, painless nodules. As a rule, these tumors appear as cold nodules on scintigrams, but some concentrate radioactive iodine. Surgical treatment is curative in more than 80% of cases, and no additional treatment is necessary. Approximately 20% recur locally, and up to 15% may have distant hematogenous metastases. Radioactive iodine may be used for radiotherapy of tumors that take up iodine. The overall prognosis is excellent, and the 10-year survival rate is higher than 90%. The prognosis depends on the size of the tumor, the extent of spread, and the degree of differentiation of the tumor cells.

74. **What is medullary carcinoma?**
Medullary carcinoma is a rare malignant tumor accounting for 5% of all thyroid tumors. It is composed of parafollicular C cells secreting calcitonin. Calcitonin may serve as the precursor for amyloid that is deposited in the stroma of these tumors. Most medullary carcinomas occur sporadically, but in 20% of cases, they are familial and associated with MEN-2A or MEN-2B. The 5-year survival rate for sporadic tumors is 50%, but familial tumors have a better prognosis, in part because they are discovered earlier with screening of family members at risk.

75. **What is anaplastic carcinoma of the thyroid?**
Anaplastic carcinoma is a rare, but highly lethal, tumor that occurs in the elderly. All patients die, usually within 2 years of diagnosis. Histologically, the tumors are composed of undifferentiated cells that may be pleomorphic, small, or spindle shaped. These tumors invade local neck structures and metastasize to distant sites.

PARATHYROID

76. **How many parathyroid glands does a healthy person have?**
Most people have four parathyroid glands, but 10% of normal people have only two or three parathyroids. These small organs, measuring 3 or 4 mm in diameter, are located on the posterior surface of the thyroid, but in some cases they may descend during fetal development into the mediastinum, and some become embedded in the thymus. Knowledge of these anatomic facts is important for surgeons, who must identify all parathyroids before removing the one that is abnormal.

77. **How is the secretion of parathyroid hormone controlled?**
Parathyroid hormone secretion is controlled by the concentration of free calcium in blood. Low blood calcium stimulates the release of parathyroid hormone, which will restore the low calcium to its normal level. This is accomplished by:
- Stimulating the release of calcium from the bones
- Increased calcium absorption in the intestine
- Increased reabsorption of calcium in the renal tubules
- Increased conversion of vitamin D into its active 1,25-dihydroxy form
- Increased urinary phosphate excretion

78. **Besides the overproduction of parathyroid hormone (PTH), what are the other major causes of hypercalcemia?**
The most important causes of hypercalcemia are:
- Parathyroid hormone excess
- Parathyroid hormone-related protein excess
- Tumors

79. **What is PTH-related protein?**
Parathyroid hormone–related protein (PTHrP) is a polypeptide normally produced by squamous epithelial cells of the skin. It binds to receptors for PTH and thus has the same effects on calcium homeostasis as PTH. PTHrP is the cause of hypercalcemia in people with squamous cell carcinomas, most often originating from bronchi. Malignant tumors metastatic to the bones cause hypercalcemia by directly destroying bone or indirectly by activating osteoclasts through the action of tumor necrosis factor-a and interleukin-1.

KEY POINTS: PARATHYROID

1. Hyperparathyroidism is much more common than hypoparathyroidism.
2. Parathyroid adenomas are the most common cause of hyperparathyroidism, which is typically associated with hypercalcemia and a variety of clinical symptoms involving the neuromuscular, skeletal, renal, and cardiovascular system.
3. Hypoparathyroidism is most often caused by accidental removal of parathyroids during surgery.

80. **What is the most common cause of hyperparathyroidism?**
Hyperparathyroidism is most often caused by a parathyroid adenoma, which accounts for 80% of cases. Primary parathyroid hyperplasia accounts for 15% and parathyroid carcinoma for 5% of cases. Most adenomas (95%) are sporadic, but some (5%) occur in the context of MEN-1. Approximately 10% to 20% of sporadic adenomas are associated with a mutation of parathyroid adenoma 1 protooncogene, located on chromosome 11 next to the PTH regulatory gene.

81. **How are parathyroid adenomas distinguished morphologically from parathyroid hyperplasia or parathyroid carcinoma?**
Parathyroid adenomas present as nodular enlargement of one parathyroid gland, whereas the size of the other three glands remains normal. Occasionally a rim of compressed normal parathyroid may be seen at one pole of the adenoma or carcinoma. In contrast, parathyroid hyperplasia leads to an enlargement of all four parathyroid glands. Parathyroid carcinomas may be indistinguishable from parathyroid adenomas, and the only definitive sign that a tumor is malignant is the presence of metastases. Histologic examination of parathyroids is of limited value: both the adenomas and carcinomas and the hyperplastic parathyroids are composed of relatively uniform "water-clear" or oxyphil cells. These cells "squeeze out" the fat cells normally found in the parathyroid glands.

82. **Which pathologic changes are caused by hyperparathyroidism?**
Hyperparathyroidism causes changes in several organs:
- Bone erosion and restructuring (Osteoclasts stimulated by PTH cause resorption of bone trabeculae. At the same time, there is increased osteoblastic activity and new bone formation. Fragile bones fracture easily, causing bleeding, fibrosis, and osteoclastic resorption of bone (osteitis fibrosa cystica). In severe cases, osteoclasts and fibroblasts form tumorlike lesions resembling giant cell tumors of bone, known as brown tumor of hyperparathyroids.)
- Renal calcification and stone formation
- Metastatic calcifications in various sites

83. **What are the signs and symptoms of hyperparathyroidism?**
The laboratory findings are diagnostic and include increased serum ionized calcium, low phosphorus, and high parathyroid hormone. Clinical symptoms are, in part, due to the pathologic changes in the bones and kidneys as well as functional changes in the gastrointestinal tract (constipation, nausea, peptic ulcer, and pancreatitis) and neuromuscular disorders (muscle weakness, depression, lethargy, and even seizures). These manifestations of hyperparathyroidism are known as "painful bones, renal stones, abdominal groans, and mental moans." See Fig. 18-5.

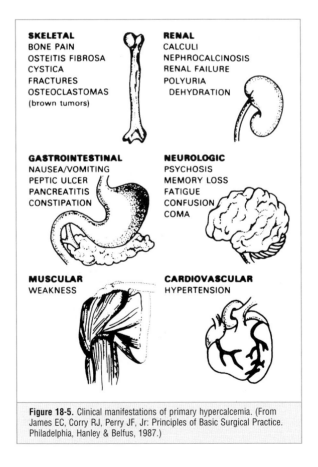

Figure 18-5. Clinical manifestations of primary hypercalcemia. (From James EC, Corry RJ, Perry JF, Jr: Principles of Basic Surgical Practice. Philadelphia, Hanley & Belfus, 1987.)

84. **What is the most common cause of secondary hyperparathyroidism?**
It is chronic renal failure. End-stage kidney disease impairs the excretion of phosphate, causing hyperphosphatemia, which depresses the serum calcium. Low levels of serum calcium trigger a release of PTH and parathyroid hyperplasia, which develops over time. An excess of PTH will cause bone lesions (renal osteodystrophy) similar to, but usually less severe than, those found in primary hyperparathyroidism. Laboratory findings include high PTH, high calcium, and high phosphate levels.

85. **What is tertiary hyperparathyroidism?**
Secondary hyperparathyroidism of chronic renal failure usually recedes following renal transplantation or efficient renal dialysis. If the stimulated parathyroids remain active even after the metabolic consequences of renal disease have been corrected, a parathyroidectomy may be the only way to correct this tertiary hyperparathyroidism.

86. **What are the most common causes of hypoparathyroidism?**
Hypoparathyroidism is a rare disorder that is most often caused by accidental parathyroidectomy during neck surgery for thyroid or other cancer. Some patients treated surgically for primary hyperparathyroidism develop hypoparathyroidism.
   Congenital parathyroid aplasia in DiGeorge syndrome, mutations of the calcium-sensing receptor (PCAR1), and destruction of parathyroids in pluriglandular autoimmune and familial endocrine insufficiency syndrome are rare causes of hypoparathyroidism.

87. **What are the clinical features of hypoparathyroidism?**
Diagnostic laboratory findings include low serum calcium, high phosphate, and low PTH concentration. Hypocalcemia leads to increased neuromuscular irritability and hyperreflexia, which can be demonstrated by eliciting the Chvostek or Trousseau signs. Mental and neurologic symptoms predominate and include depression, paranoia, and signs of intracranial hypertension. Cataracts develop due to calcifications of the lenses. Cardiac conduction defects are common.

88. **How is hypoparathyroidism treated?**
All forms of hypoparathyroidism respond well to supplementation of diet with calcium and vitamin D.

ADRENAL GLANDS

89. **What are the three zones of the adrenal cortex?**
The adrenal cortex consists of zona glomerulosa, the source of aldosterone; zona fasciculata, accounting for 75% of the total cortex and the source of glucocorticoids; and zona reticularis, a narrow juxtamedullary rim of cells, the source of sex steroids.

90. **What are the three principal endocrine syndromes caused by hyperfunction of adrenal cortex?**
The principal adrenocortical hyperfunction syndromes are:
- Hypercortisolism (Cushing syndrome)
- Hyperaldosteronism (Conn syndrome)
- Adrenogenital syndrome

91. **What is the most common cause of Cushing syndrome?**
Exogenous steroids used in the treatment of autoimmune disease (e.g., rheumatoid arthritis) and renal diseases (e.g., nephrotic syndrome) are the most common cause of hypercortisolism. Less common causes include:
- Pituitary tumors secreting ACTH (Cushing disease)
- Paraneoplastic syndromes due to ACTH-secreting tumors (e.g., lung cancer)
- Adrenal cortical lesions (adenoma, carcinoma, or nodular hyperplasia)

A mnemonic to remember the causes of Cushing syndrome is *ACTH:*

Adrenal disease (adenoma, carcinoma, and hyperplasia)

Cushing's disease (pituitary tumor secreting ACTH)

Tumor secreting ACTH (most often small cell carcinoma of the lung)

Hormonal therapy (with corticosteroids)

92. **What are the laboratory findings in Cushing syndrome?**

Cushing syndrome caused by adrenal lesions is characterized by increased serum concentration of corticol and low ACTH. In Cushing disease caused by pituitary tumors, both cortisol and ACTH blood levels are elevated. ACTH secretion from the pituitary or from a lung tumor is unresponsive to inhibition with dexamethasone. Excess cortisol is associated with an increased excretion of 17-hydroxycorticosteroids in urine. Hypercortisolism is associated with a loss of normal diurnal cyclic secretion of cortisol.

93. **What are the pathologic findings in the adrenal glands of patients showing signs of hypercortisolism?**

The morphologic changes in the adrenal depend on the cause of hypercortisolism. Exogenous corticosteroids cause adrenal cortical atrophy. Diffuse bilateral hyperplasia is typical of pituitary and ectopic ACTH stimulation and is also found in two thirds of primary adrenal hypercortisolism. Adenomas and carcinomas are yellow neoplasms expanding and replacing the normal adrenal. The benign tumors have similar histologic features as the malignant ones. Carcinomas are usually larger, show invasive growth, and tend to metastasize.

KEY POINTS: ADRENAL GLANDS ✔

1. Adrenal diseases result from hyperfunction of the entire adrenal gland or its specific parts: zona glomerulosa, fasciculata, and reticularis of the cortex and adrenal medulla.

2. Adrenal cortical hyperfunction or hypofunction can be a consequence of pituitary disease or endogenous adrenal disorders.

3. Adrenal tumors usually produce hormones and are associated with distinct clinical syndromes.

4. Adrenal cortical insufficiency is caused most often by autoimmune destruction of the adrenal glands.

94. **What are the clinical features of Cushing syndrome?**

The excess of corticosteroids causes complex metabolic abnormalities, including diabetes, redistribution of fat (moon face, buffalo hump, etc.), atrophy of the skin and bones, neuropsychiatric disturbances, and menstrual irregularities.

The symptoms and signs of Cushing disease can be remembered with the mnemonic *buffalo hump:*

Buffalo hump

Unusual behavior (depression, personality changes, and fatigability)

Facial features (moon face, hirsutism in women)

Fat accumulation (obesity)

ACTH (and cortisol) in blood ↑; ACTH and dexamethasone test abnormalities

Loss of muscle mass (thin legs and arms; protruding abdomen due to weak abdominal muscles)

Overextended skin (striae with easy bruisability due to weak vessels)

Hypertension
Urinary cortisol ↑ and 17-hydroxycorticosteroids ↑
Menstrual irregularities
Porosity of bones (osteoporosis)
See Fig. 18-6.

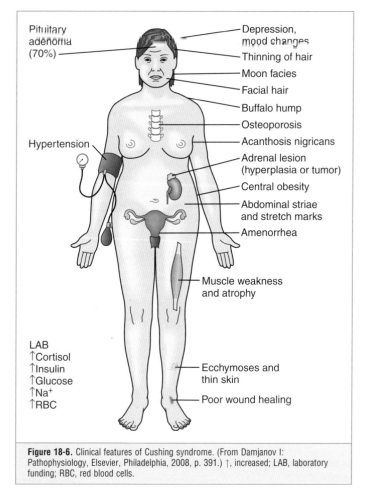

Figure 18-6. Clinical features of Cushing syndrome. (From Damjanov I: Pathophysiology, Elsevier, Philadelphia, 2008, p. 391.) ↑, increased; LAB, laboratory funding; RBC, red blood cells.

95. **What are the causes of hyperaldosteronism?**
Hyperaldosteronism may be classified as primary or secondary. Primary hyperaldosteronism is caused by tumors originating from the zona glomerulosa of the adrenal cortex. Secondary hyperaldosteronism is a consequence of the stimulation of the adrenal cortex by the renin–angiotensin system. The most common conditions associated with secondary hyperaldosteronism are:

- Congestive heart failure
- Atherosclerosis of the aorta and arteriolonephrosclerosis causing hypoperfusion of the kidneys
- Chronic renal disease
- Pregnancy
- Cirrhosis of the liver due to hypoalbuminemia and reduced effective plasma volume

96. **Describe the clinical findings in primary hyperaldosteronism**

Primary hyperaldosteronism caused by adrenal cortical adenomas (80%) or primary adrenal cortical hyperplasia (15%) is also known as Conn syndrome. The following are clinical features:
- More common in women than in men (2:1)
- Hypertension
- Weakness, paresthesias, and even tetany
- Hypokalemia with hypernatremia and metabolic alkalosis
- Polyuria—urine has low fixed specific gravity and does not respond to vasopressin
- Renin values in serum typically low

97. **Define adrenogenital syndrome.**

Adrenogenital syndrome results from abnormal production of adrenal androgens. Typically it is associated with either androgen excess or deficiency. It may be congenital, which is typically related to a genetic deficiency of an enzyme in the steroid metabolic pathway, or acquired, typically associated with adrenal tumors.

98. **What are the symptoms of adrenogenital syndrome?**

The symptoms depend on the type of abnormality and whether it occurs in females or males, in infants or adults.

Congenital adrenal hyperplasia in female neonates is usually associated with virilization of external genitalia including clitoral hypertrophy, fusion of the labia, and general signs of pseudohermaphroditism. In postpubertal females, virilization is usually caused by tumors, and it includes menstrual abnormalities, hirsutism, deepening of the voice, and baldness.

99. **What is the most common form of congenital adrenal hyperplasia?**

The most common form of congenital adrenal cortical hyperplasia is caused by 21-hydroxylase deficiency. This genetic defect, inherited as an autosomal recessive trait, occurs at a rate of 1:12,000 births and accounts for more than 90% of all cases of congenital adrenal hyperplasia. The deficiency of 21-hydroxylase leads to an increased production of progesterone, 17-OH-progesterone, and dehydroepiandrosterone (DHEA), as well as a reduced formation of cortisol and aldosterone. DHEA leads to virilization of female genitalia of these newborns, and the lack of aldosterone leads to loss of sodium and retention of potassium. The treatment includes administration of glucocorticoids and, if necessary, aldosterone. Severe virilization may require surgical reconstruction of external genitalia.

100. **What are the causes of primary adrenal insufficiency in adults?**

Adrenal insufficiency can be classified as primary or secondary. Primary insufficiency is a consequence of the destruction of adrenal glands. Secondary insufficiency results from a deficiency of ACTH and is a consequence of hypopituitarism.

The most important causes of primary adrenal insufficiency in adults are:
- Autoimmune adrenalitis (the disease of President John F. Kennedy; 70%)
- Infections
  - Human immunodeficiency virus
  - Tuberculosis (rare in Western countries)
  - Histoplasmosis and other disseminated fungi
- Hemorrhage (Waterhouse–Friderichsen syndrome in meningococcemia)
- Metastatic tumors (e.g., breast carcinoma and bronchial carcinoma)
- Amyloidosis
- Sarcoidosis

101. **What is the most common cause of acute adrenal insufficiency?**
The most common cause of acute adrenal insufficiency is sudden withdrawal of steroids from patients treated with steroids for rheumatic or other chronic diseases. Waterhouse–Friderichsen syndrome with bilateral adrenal hemorrhage or trauma in patients who have subclinical adrenal insufficiency may also provoke acute adrenal crisis.

Adrenal crisis is clinically characterized by complete vascular collapse, renal shutdown, and severe pain in the abdomen, back, and legs.

102. **What are the symptoms of Addison disease?**
Addison disease, or chronic adrenal cortical insufficiency, is a rare disease (incidence of 4:100,000). However, it is a medical emergency that needs to be treated as soon as possible after diagnosis. The symptoms and signs of Addison disease are mostly related to dehydration and loss of sodium. They include:
- Weakness and fatigue
- Dehydration (observe the skin, oral mucosa, and eyes) and fever
- Hypotension and tachycardia
- Nausea, vomiting, diarrhea, and abdominal cramping
- Hyperpigmentation of skin (due to increased ACTH secretion)

103. **What are the laboratory findings in Addison disease?**
The deficiency of steroid hormones results in a disturbance of mineral and water maintenance, abnormal metabolism of glucose, and alterations of pH. The main findings include:
- Hyponatremia (<130 mEq/L)
- Hyperkalemia (>5 mEq/L)
- Na:K ratio of $<20:1$
- Hypoglycemia (<50 mg/dL)
- Metabolic acidosis with low bicarbonate (<28 mEq/L)
- Azotemia
- ACTH increased in primary and low in secondary Addison disease
- Cortisol low in blood and ketosteroids low in urine

104. **What is the difference between adrenocortical adenomas and carcinomas?**
See Table 18-1.

TABLE 18-1. MAJOR DIFFERENCES BETWEEN ADENOMA AND CARCINOMA		
	Adenoma	Carcinoma
Size	Small (1–3 cm), may be multiple	Large (>10 cm)
Shape	Nodule, well circumscribed	Irregular mass, invasive
Color	Yellow or brown, uniform	Variegated (yellow, white, brown, or red)
Hormonally active	Yes or no	Yes or no

105. **What is the function of the adrenal medulla?**
The adrenal medulla is composed of cells that secrete epinephrine and norepinephrine. Epinephrine is the main catecholamine produced by the adrenal medulla, in contrast to sympathetic ganglia, which produce predominantly norepinephrine.

Adrenal medulla is part of the sympathetic system and is important for the regulation of blood pressure. Catecholamines released from the adrenal medulla also have metabolic effects. The following are the most important effects of catecholamines:
- They increase blood pressure, skeletal muscle blood flow, skeletal contractility, heart rate, blood glucose, lipolysis
- They decrease visceral blood flow, gastrointestinal contractility, urinary output

106. **List the most important tumors of the adrenal medulla.**
- Pheochromocytoma
- Neuroblastoma (in children)
- Ganglioneuroma

107. **What are pheochromocytomas?**
Pheochromocytomas are tumors of the adrenal medulla. Most tumors occur in adults but may also be found in children. Because most pheochromocytomas secrete catecholamines, these tumors are usually associated with arterial hypertension. Hypertension is typically paroxysmal (i.e., presents with sudden onset of blood pressure elevation) and is resistant to standard antihypertensive therapy. Typically it is associated with increased excretion of urinary metanephrine and vanillylmandelic acid.

108. **What is the rule of five 90% for pheochromocytomas?**
- 90% of tumors originate from the adrenal, 10% from extraadrenal paraganglia.
- 90% of tumors are functional and cause hypertension, 10% are nonfunctional.
- 90% are benign, 10% are malignant.
- 90% are unilateral and solitary, 10% are bilateral or multiple.
- 90% are sporadic, 10% occur in multiple endocrine adenomatosis type 2A and 2B.

109. **What are adrenal neuroblastomas?**
- Neuroblastomas are malignant tumors composed of primitive nerve cell precursors derived from the neural crest.
- Most neuroblastomas (>80%) are diagnosed in children younger than age 5 years.
- Most tumors are found in the adrenals.
- Histologically identical tumors can originate from paraganglia in the abdomen, thorax, and cerebral tissue.
- Hematogenous metastases occur early and frequently involve the skeleton, liver, and other organs.
- Most tumors respond well to chemotherapy, but the prognosis depends on the stage (i.e., extent of metastasis): Stage I and II tumors have a 5-year survival of more than 90%, whereas Stage III and IV tumors have a survival of less than 30%.

110. **What is the difference between neuroblastoma, ganglioneuroblastoma, and ganglioneurocytoma?**
Neuroblastomas are composed of undifferentiated neuroblasts, which focally may show some signs of abortive differentiation into neural cells. If this differentiation proceeds and the tumor contains both undifferentiated neuroblasts and ganglion cells, it is called ganglioneuroblastoma. Such tumors are still malignant because the undifferentiated neuroblasts can metastasize and kill the host. If the tumor consists of fully differentiated ganglion cells and mature nerves, it is called a ganglioneurocytoma. Such tumors do not contain malignant neuroblasts and are benign.

111. **What are multiple endocrine neoplasia syndromes?**
This term comprises three familial syndromes inherited as autosomal dominant traits: MEN-1, MEN-2A, and MEN-2B.

MEN-1 is related to a deletion of a tumor suppressor gene on chromosome 11. It presents with:

- Parathyroid hyperplasia or adenoma (95%)
- Islet cell neoplasia or hyperplasia (80%)—most often gastrinoma causing Zollinger–Ellison syndrome (peptic ulcers)
- Pituitary adenoma (60%)
  Other tumors, such as adrenocortical adenomas and thyroid adenomas, occur less often.
  MEN 2A is related to mutation of the RET tyrosine kinase domain. It presents with:
- Medullary carcinoma of the thyroid (99%)
- Pheochromocytoma (50%)
- Parathyroid adenoma or hyperplasia (20%)
  MEN-2B is related to mutation of RET tyrosine kinase, which is, however, different from that found in MEN-2A. It presents with the same findings as MEN-2A, but patients also have numerous mucocutaneous neuromas (e.g., on the tongue, eyelids, and intestines).

WEBSITES

1. http://www.ncbi.nlm.nih.gov/entrez/query.fcgi?db=PubMed

2. http://www-medlib.med.utah.edu/WebPath/webpath.html#MENU

3. http://www.thyroidmanager.org/

4. http://www.mic.ki.se/Diseases/C19.html

5. http://www.endocrineweb.com/

BIBLIOGRAPHY

1. Boscaro M, Barzon L, Fallo F, Sonino N: Cushing syndrome. Lancet 357:783–791, 2001.
2. Dayan CM: Interpretation of thyroid function tests. Lancet 357:619–624, 2001.
3. Findling JW, Raff H: Cushing's syndrome: important issues in diagnosis and management. J Clin Endocrinol Metab 91:3746–3753, 2006.
4. Grinspoon SK, Biller BM: Laboratory assessment of adrenal insufficiency. J Clin Endocrinol Metab 79:923–931, 1994.
5. Klein I, Ojamaa K: Thyroid hormone and the cardiovascular system. N Engl J Med 344:501–509, 2001.
6. Krempl GA, Medina JE: Current issues in hyperparathyroidism. Otolaryngol Clin North Am 36:207–215, 2003.
7. Nygaard B: Hyperthyroidism. Am Fam Physician 76:1014–1016, 2007.
8. Sosa JA, Udelsman R: New directions in the treatment of patients with primary hyperparathyroidism. Curr Probl Surg 40:812–849, 2003.
9. Weetman AP: Graves' disease. N Engl J Med 343:1236–1248, 2000.

CHAPTER 19

THE SKIN

Ivan Damjanov, MD, PhD

1. **What are the three main layers of the skin?**
   - Epidermis, composed of four or five layers of squamous epithelium
   - Dermis, composed of connective tissue (Its upper part extending between the rete ridges of the epidermis is called papillary dermis, whereas the lower part is called reticular dermis. In some portions of the body, the dermis also contains hair follicles and sweat and sebaceous glands. Dermis contains blood vessels and nerves.)
   - Subcutis, composed of fat tissue and connective tissue arranged to provide support to the upper layers of the skin and link them to the underlying muscles and bones

2. **What are the most important features of skin lesions?**
   Dermatology is a visual discipline, and it relies on accurate macroscopic and microscopic description of skin lesions. Thus it is important to pay attention to the basic characteristics of each lesion, including its:
   - Size
   - Color
   - Location and distribution
   - Consistency
   - Shape
   - Surface characteristics

3. **How are skin lesions classified?**
   In clinical practice, it is customary to classify skin lesions as primary or secondary. Primary skin lesions include macules, papules, patches, plaques, nodules, cysts, wheals, vesicles, bullae, and pustules. Secondary skin lesions are related to the progression of the disease but may also be caused by scratching, trauma, or treatment. This group of lesions includes crusts, erosions, ulcers, fissures, excoriations, scars, and scales (Figs. 19-1 and 19-2).

4. **What is the difference between a macule and a papule?**
   Macules are flat lesions presenting as a change in the color of skin, whereas papules are slightly elevated. For example, a freckle (ephelis) is a macule, whereas a congenital mole (intradermal nevus) is a papule. Some childhood exanthemas, such as measles, present in the form of a widespread maculopapular rash—that is, red macules, which are flat, and papules, which are slightly raised. Very large macules are called plaques.

5. **What is the difference between a papule and a nodule?**
   Papules are small, slightly elevated solid skin lesions measuring less than 0.5 cm. In practice, this means they can be covered with the flat end of a pencil. Nodules are deeper seated and larger, measuring more than 0.5 cm in diameter. Most skin tumors present as nodules, but obviously some can be diagnosed early in their development while they are still smaller than 0.5 cm. (*Continued on p. 390*)

Primary Skin Lesions

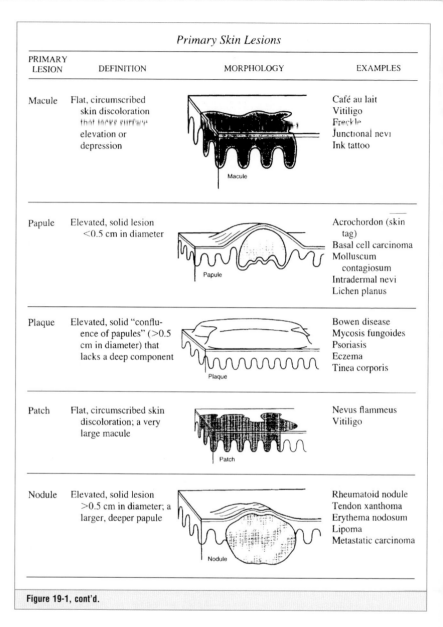

PRIMARY LESION	DEFINITION	MORPHOLOGY	EXAMPLES
Macule	Flat, circumscribed skin discoloration that lacks surface elevation or depression	Macule	Café au lait Vitiligo Freckle Junctional nevi Ink tattoo
Papule	Elevated, solid lesion <0.5 cm in diameter	Papule	Acrochordon (skin tag) Basal cell carcinoma Molluscum contagiosum Intradermal nevi Lichen planus
Plaque	Elevated, solid "confluence of papules" (>0.5 cm in diameter) that lacks a deep component	Plaque	Bowen disease Mycosis fungoides Psoriasis Eczema Tinea corporis
Patch	Flat, circumscribed skin discoloration; a very large macule	Patch	Nevus flammeus Vitiligo
Nodule	Elevated, solid lesion >0.5 cm in diameter; a larger, deeper papule	Nodule	Rheumatoid nodule Tendon xanthoma Erythema nodosum Lipoma Metastatic carcinoma

Figure 19-1, cont'd.

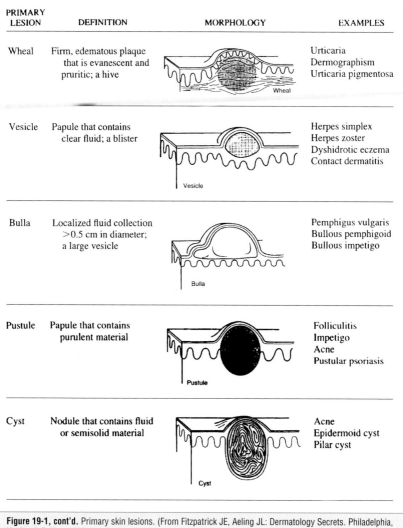

PRIMARY LESION	DEFINITION	MORPHOLOGY	EXAMPLES
Wheal	Firm, edematous plaque that is evanescent and pruritic; a hive	Wheal	Urticaria Dermographism Urticaria pigmentosa
Vesicle	Papule that contains clear fluid; a blister	Vesicle	Herpes simplex Herpes zoster Dyshidrotic eczema Contact dermatitis
Bulla	Localized fluid collection >0.5 cm in diameter; a large vesicle	Bulla	Pemphigus vulgaris Bullous pemphigoid Bullous impetigo
Pustule	Papule that contains purulent material	Pustule	Folliculitis Impetigo Acne Pustular psoriasis
Cyst	Nodule that contains fluid or semisolid material	Cyst	Acne Epidermoid cyst Pilar cyst

Figure 19-1, cont'd. Primary skin lesions. (From Fitzpatrick JE, Aeling JL: Dermatology Secrets. Philadelphia, Hanley & Belfus, 1996, pp. 9–10.)

Secondary Skin Lesions

SECONDARY LESION	DEFINITION	MORPHOLOGY
Crust	A collection of cellular debris, dried serum, and blood; a scab. Antecedent primary lesion is usually a vesicle, bulla, or pustule	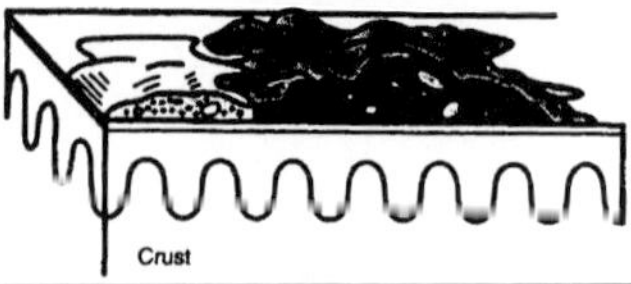 Crust
Erosion	A partial focal loss of epidermis; heals without scarring	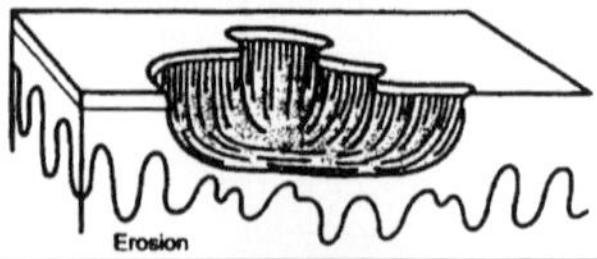 Erosion
Ulcer	A full-thickness, focal loss of epidermis and dermis; heals with scarring	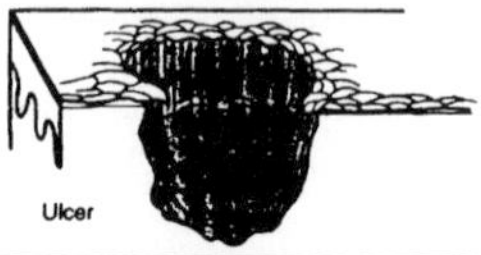 Ulcer
Fissure	Vertical loss of epidermis and dermis with sharply defined walls; crack in skin	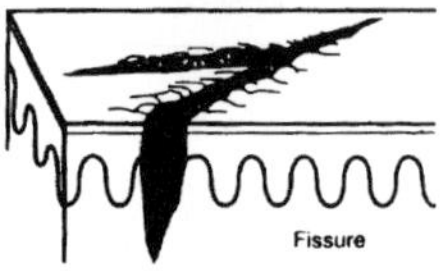 Fissure
Excoriation	Linear erosion induced by scratching	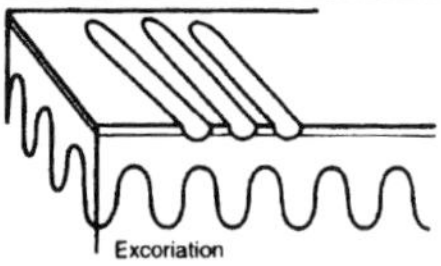 Excoriation
Scar	A collection of new connective tissue; may be hypertrophic or atrophic. Scar implies dermoepidermal damage	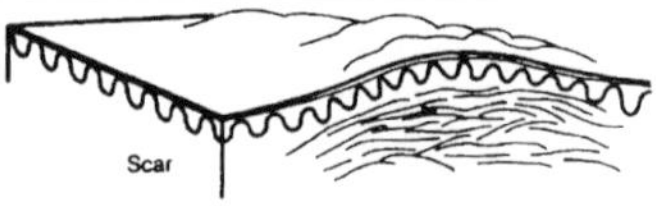 Scar
Scale	Thick stratum corneum that results from hyperproliferation or increased cohesion of keratinocytes	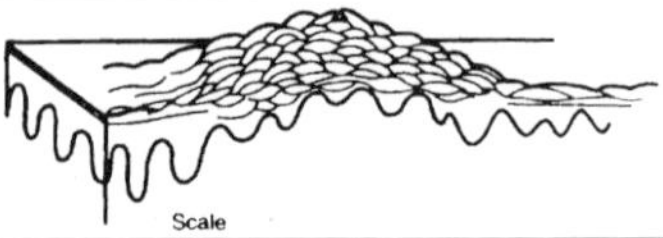 Scale

Figure 19-2. Secondary skin lesions. (From Fitzpatrick JE, Aeling JL: Dermatology Secrets. Philadelphia, Hanley & Belfus, 1996, pp. 10–11.)

6. **What is the difference between a plaque and a papule?**

   Like papules, plaques are slightly elevated skin lesions, but they measure more than 0.5 cm in diameter. Plaques often arise by a confluence of multiple papules. In contrast to nodules, plaques appear relatively flat and do not have a deeper dermal component. Plaques are typical of eczema, a common skin lesion that may have many mechanisms.

7. **What is the difference between a wheal, a papule, a plaque, and a nodule?**
   Wheals are solitary or grouped, raised, soft skin lesions. Wheals are larger than papules and more elevated than a plaque. In contrast to nodules, which are firm and develop over a longer period of time, wheals are soft, edematous, and of recent onset. Wheals are often pruritic, red or pale, and often tend to disappear without any consequences. Wheals are typically caused by allergies. Dermal edema due to a release of histamine from mast cells is the underlying cause of wheals in dermographism.

8. **What is the difference between a vesicle and a bulla?**
   Vesicles are slightly raised skin lesions filled with fluid. Grouped vesicles are typical of herpes simplex infection. Larger vesicles measuring more than 0.5 cm are called bullae. In common parlance, bullae are called blisters.

9. **What is the difference between a vesicle and a pustule?**
   Vesicles are filled with serous fluid, whereas pustules contain pus. Upon infection, vesicles transform into pustules.

10. **What is the difference between a cyst and a bulla?**
    Cysts are cavities lined by an epithelial layer. Cysts develop from invaginations of surface epithelium or obstruction of excretory ducts of skin appendages. They may contain fluid and thus have some common features with bullae. However, bullae do not have a defined epithelial lining and typically develop fast, whereas cysts develop over a prolonged period of time. Epidermal inclusion cysts filled with desquamated epithelium and keratin may resemble nodules.

11. **What is a crust?**
    Crust, also known as a scab, is the material typically found on the surface of scratches or wounds. It consists of coagulated plasma, cell debris, and extravasated blood cells.

12. **What is the difference between erosion and an ulcer?**
    Erosions are superficial defects of the epidermis above the epidermodermal basement membrane. Ulcers are deeper defects involving both the epidermis and the dermis. Erosions heal without scarring, whereas the healing of ulcers involves granulation tissue and scar formation. Linear erosions caused by scratching are called excoriations.

CLASSIFICATION OF SKIN DISEASES

13. **How are skin diseases classified etiologically?**
    Skin diseases can be classified according to their causation into several categories:
    - Congenital (e.g., congenital ichthyosis and congenital nevus)
    - Diseases caused by chemical or physical irritants (e.g., burns, frostbite, ulcers caused by exposure to caustic materials, and dust-induced eczema)
    - Infectious diseases (e.g., viral exanthemas of childhood, such as rubella or varicella, and impetigo caused by pus-forming cocci)
    - Immunologic diseases (e.g., poison ivy and atopic dermatitis)
    - Idiopathic diseases (e.g., psoriasis and epidermolysis bullosa; many chronic skin diseases are poorly understood and fall into this category. Some of these diseases have a hereditary component and have a tendency to occur in families.)
    - Neoplastic diseases (e.g., squamous cell carcinoma and malignant melanoma)

14. **How are skin diseases classified according to their duration?**
    Like all other diseases, skin disease can be classified as acute or chronic. Acute diseases may heal, recur, or progress to chronic diseases. Chronic diseases can be preceded by an acute

stage, but many of them begin insidiously without a distinct acute phase, lasting without an obvious end. The best example of such a chronic disease, psoriasis, is a common chronic disease that has no obvious beginning and rarely, if ever, any end.

15. **How are skin diseases classified according to their distribution?**
Skin diseases may be localized and limited to an area of the body, or they may involve the entire body. For example, bacterial folliculitis may be limited to the face, whereas viral exanthemas, such as measles, involve the entire body. Many systemic diseases, such as systemic lupus erythematosus (SLE), have skin manifestations and at the same time involve many internal organs.

KEY POINTS: SKIN LESIONS ✔

1. Various macroscopic and histologic skin lesions must be correlated with clinical data or biopsied for microscopic examination in order to formulate the correct diagnosis.

2. Many viruses, bacteria, fungi, and parasites affect the skin, causing lesions of the epidermis, dermis, or subcutis.

3. Immunologic diseases of the skin include reactions to foreign antigens (as in poison ivy) or autoantigens (as in systemic lupus erythematosus).

4. There are many skin diseases of unknown etiology, but the most common is psoriasis, which affects 1% or 2% of the total population.

5. Skin lesions are found in the course of many metabolic, hormonal, immunologic, circulatory, and neoplastic diseases.

16. **How are skin diseases classified microscopically?**
Pathologists can classify most skin diseases into several categories, which then must be correlated with clinical data to arrive at the final clinical–pathologic diagnosis. General categories of skin diseases recognized in skin biopsies are too broad. For example, chronic dermatitis may be caused by immune mechanisms, infections, or irritation. It is thus common to classify skin diseases according to the way they involve the skin. These categories include:
- Diseases of the epidermis (e.g., psoriasis, ichthyosis, and pemphigus vulgaris)
- Diseases of the dermal–epidermal interface (e.g., epidermolysis bullosa, bullous pemphigoid, erythema multiforme, and lupus erythematosus)
- Diseases of the superficial and deep vascular bed (e.g., urticaria, cutaneous vasculitis, and contact dermatitis)
- Disorders of the dermal connective tissue (e.g., systemic sclerosis)
- Inflammatory disorders of the panniculus adiposus (e.g., erythema nodosum, erythema induratum, and arthropod infestations)
- Skin neoplasms

17. **What is eczema?**
The clinical term eczema (from the Greek word meaning to "boil over") is probably the best example of the vagueness of some dermatologic terms. In acute stages, it presents in the form of erythematous, oozing, or crusted papules, which then become crusted in the chronic stages. Eczema is a reaction pattern and may be a manifestation of:
- Atopic dermatitis
- Allergic dermatitis
- Irritant dermatitis

- Drug reaction
- Photosensitivity reaction
- Idiopathic diseases (e.g., seborrheic keratosis)

INFECTIOUS DISEASES

18. **What are the main infectious skin pathogens?**
    - Viruses, such as herpes simplex virus or human papillomavirus
    - Bacteria, such as *Staphylococcus aureus* and *Streptococcus*
    - Fungi, such as Dermatophytes (e.g., *Trichophyton* sp.)
    - Parasites, such as *Sarcoptes scabiei*

19. **Which skin diseases are caused by herpes viruses?**
    Herpes viruses (HSVs; Fig. 19-3) cause several skin diseases:
    - HSV-1 is the cause of herpetic vesicles on the lips (herpes labialis), also known as cold sores. Histologically, the vesicles contain fluid and detached epithelial cells containing intranuclear viral inclusions.
    - HSV-2 is the cause of genital vesicles (herpes genitalis).
    - Varicella-zoster virus is the cause of chickenpox in children. Reactivation of the same virus causes shingles (herpes zoster) in adults.
    - HSV-8 is the cause of Kaposi sarcoma in AIDS patients.

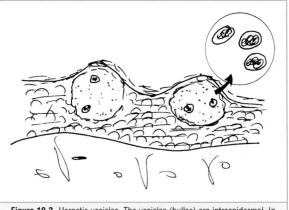

Figure 19-3. Herpetic vesicles. The vesicles (bullae) are intraepidermal. In addition to fluid, these vesicles contain enlarged keratinocytes, which are typically multinucleated and have "ground-glass" nuclei filled with viral particles *(inset)*. Viral particles can be seen only by electron microscopy, but they can also be demonstrated by immunohistochemistry with antibodies to herpes virus.

20. **Which skin diseases are caused by human papillomaviruses?**
    Human papillomaviruses are DNA viruses that are classified into more than 70 subgroups. Some of these viruses have a predilection for certain anatomic sites, causing clinically identifiable skin lesions known as verrucae or warts (Fig. 19-4).

- **Verruca vulgaris (common wart):** These rough-surfaced, hyperkeratotic papules usually appear on hands. May be solitary or multiple. Histologically, the warts show papillomatosis (formation of papillae that have a central vascular connective tissue core and are covered with thick epithelium), acanthosis (i.e., thickening of the epithelium), granular layer thickening, and hyperkeratosis.
- **Verruca plana (flat wart):** These small (2–5 mm), flat-topped, multiple hyperpigmented multiple papules appear on the face and hands of children.
- **Verruca plantaria (plantar wart):** It is a thick hyperkeratotic, often painful lesion on the soles.
- **Condyloma acuminatum (anogenital wart):** These moist, cauliflower-like exuberant growths appear on the penis or vulva.

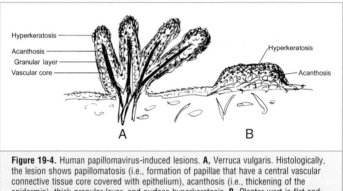

Figure 19-4. Human papillomavirus-induced lesions. **A,** Verruca vulgaris. Histologically, the lesion shows papillomatosis (i.e., formation of papillae that have a central vascular connective tissue core covered with epithelium), acanthosis (i.e., thickening of the epidermis), thick granular layer, and surface hyperkeratosis. **B,** Plantar wart is flat and shows hyperkeratosis and acanthosis.

21. **Do warts ever become malignant?**
    Although warts contain HPV virions, there is no evidence that the subtypes of HPV causing skin warts are carcinogenic. Hence common warts do not transform into carcinoma.

22. **What is impetigo?**
    Impetigo is a superficial skin infection caused by gram-positive bacteria. *Staphylococcus aureus* is the most common cause. Most often, the disease presents in the form of superficial pustules on the faces of small children. Histologically, the pus accumulates in the upper part of the epidermis. The pustules rupture easily and heal without scarring.

23. **What is folliculitis?**
    Folliculitis is a bacterial infection of the hair follicles characterized by an accumulation of pus around the hair shaft. Infection is most often caused by *S. aureus* and involves hairy areas of the skin, such as the buttocks and thighs, bearded part of the face, and the scalp. Suppuration extending into the perifollicular soft tissue may lead to formation of abscesses, which are known as furuncles or boils. Confluent boils form indurated masses that are dark bluish black and are thus known as carbuncles (name derived from a cognate for carbon). See Fig. 19-5.

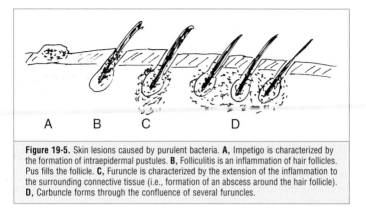

Figure 19-5. Skin lesions caused by purulent bacteria. **A,** Impetigo is characterized by the formation of intraepidermal pustules. **B,** Folliculitis is an inflammation of hair follicles. Pus fills the follicle. **C,** Furuncle is characterized by the extension of the inflammation to the surrounding connective tissue (i.e., formation of an abscess around the hair follicle). **D,** Carbuncle forms through the confluence of several furuncles.

24. **What is acne?**
    Acne vulgaris is a disorder of the pilosebaceous units of the skin. The disease is multifactorial and involves:
    - Overproduction of sebum by the sebaceous glands attached to the hair follicle (Androgenic hormones stimulate the production of sebum, and accordingly the disease is more prominent in men than in women.)
    - Obstruction of the pilosebaceous canal by keratin plugs
    - Distention of the pilosebaceous canal by sebum and keratin
    - Proliferation of anaerobic bacteria such as Propionibacterium acnes
    - Secondary infection by pus-forming bacteria, which leads to folliculitis and abscess formation

25. **What is cellulitis?**
    Cellulitis is diffusely spreading suppurative infection of the dermis and soft tissues. Most often, it is caused by *Streptococcus pyogenes.* This beta-hemolytic group A streptococcus secretes lytic enzymes (streptokinase, DNAse, and hyaluronidase), which facilitate the spreading of the infection through the tissues.

26. **What is erysipelas?**
    Erysipelas is a superficial cellulitis with prominent involvement of lymphatics, usually caused by group A beta-hemolytic *Streptococcus pyogenes.* Most often, it occurs on the face, arms, and legs. Redness and swelling of the affected area are accompanied by regional lymphadenitis and systemic symptoms, such as high fever and chills.

27. **What is hydradenitis suppurativa?**
    Hydradenitis suppurativa is an infection of apocrine glands in the axilla and the anogenital region, most often caused by *Staphylococcus aureus.*

28. **What are dermatophytes?**
    Dermatophytes are fungi that live in the keratinized surface layer of the skin. The most common human pathogens belong to the *Trichophyton, Microsporum,* and *Epidermophyton* species.
    Dermatophytes produce tinea, commonly known as ringworm. Tinea cruris is known as jock itch, and tinea pedis is known as athlete's foot. Tinea capitis, a fungal infection of the scalp most often found in children, may cause loss of hair (alopecia). Onychophytosis is nail infection caused by fungi of the *Trichophyton* species.

29. **What are deep fungal infections?**
Infections of the deeper portions of the skin may occur because of the entry of invasive fungi through damaged skin or hematogenously during a fungemia. Such infections are caused by *Blastomyces, Coccidioides, Histoplasma, Cryptococcus,* and other fungi that affect internal organs.

30. **What is a mycetoma?**
Mycetomas are chronic suppurative infections of the subcutis and soft tissues of feet, arms, or back characterized by marked swelling and formation of pus draining sinus tracts. Despite their name, which implies that these lesions are a manifestation of mycotic infections, only a minority of mycetomas are caused by fungi. The most common causes of mycetomas are filamentous bacteria such as *Nocardia* and *Actinomyces*.

31. **What is scabies?**
Scabies is caused by a mite, *Sarcoptes scabiei*. The female mite burrows into the stratum corneum, depositing eggs, which hatch within a few days, causing irritation and itching. These parasites live only on humans and are transmitted from one person to another during direct contact and only rarely by fomites.

32. **What is pediculosis?**
Pediculosis, an infestation with lice, may involve the scalp, hairy parts of the body, or the genital area. The head louse is most often found in school-age children. These lice and their eggs can be easily found attached to the hair. The body louse typically affects poor people living in overcrowded tenements and those who rarely clean their clothes. These lice live in the clothes and do not attach to the skin except for short periods during feeding. The pubic louse, also know as crabs, is typically transmitted during sexual contact. It can be easily found on the shaft of pubic hair, but it may attach to the hair of the axillary area, eyelashes, and even scalp and body hair.

IMMUNOLOGIC SKIN DISEASES

33. **What is the difference between allergic and autoimmune diseases of the skin?**
Allergic skin diseases represent a response to exogeneous allergens. On the other hand, autoimmune diseases, such as SLE, are based on an abnormal immune response to endogenous antigens, or antigens that have not been fully identified. Endogenous antigens eliciting autoimmune diseases include denatured proteins or nucleic acids, so-called hidden antigens that are normally sequestered from the body's immune system. Such antigens are capable of inducing an autoimmune reaction when released into the circulation (e.g., thyroglobulin sequestered in thyroid follicles or the spermatozoa, located in the seminiferous tubules).

34. **Which hypersensitivity reactions affect the skin?**
Four hypersensitivity reactions are generally recognized, and all can affect the skin.
   ■ Type I hypersensitivity reaction, or atopic reaction, is based on the reaction of antigens with the immunoglobulin (Ig) E bound to the surface of mast cells in the skin. Degranulation of mast cells leads to the formation of wheals (hives), which result from the increased permeability of blood vessels induced by histamine. Bee stings, allergic reactions to drugs, and atopic dermatitis of childhood are other examples of type I hypersensitivity.
   ■ Type II hypersensitivity reaction, or cytotoxic cell reaction, is mediated by antibodies that attach to antigens on the surface of epidermal cells (as in pemphigus vulgaris) or the epidermal–dermal basement membrane (as in bullous pemphigoid). Type II hypersensitivity reaction leads to the formation of bullae.
   ■ Type III hypersensitivity reaction is based on the deposition of preformed circulating antigen–antibody complexes along the epidermal–dermal basement membrane (as in SLE) or in the vessel wall (as in hypersensitivity vasculitis).

- Type IV hypersensitivity reaction is based on the reaction of T lymphocytes and is typically induced by foreign antigens, as in contact dermatitis (e.g., poison ivy). It may be accompanied by the formation of granulomas, as in hypersensitivity to *Mycobacterium tuberculosis* or *Mycobacterium leprae*. Sarcoidosis is a type IV hypersensitivity reaction to unknown antigens.

35. **What is pemphigus vulgaris?**
    Pemphigus vulgaris (from the Greek word *pemphix,* "bubble") is a chronic disease characterized by the formation of blisters over large surfaces of skin and oral mucosa. It is mediated by cytotoxic autoantibodies that bind to the surface of epidermal cells, causing acantholysis and intraepidermal fluid accumulation. The autoantigen has been identified as a component of desmosomes, called desmoglein III.
    Pemphigus vulgaris most often affects middle-aged people but can occur at any age. In approximately 60% of cases, it begins with oral lesions. The skin bullae rupture, and the entire surface may become denuded. Corticosteroids provide relief, but if no treatment is given, the disease may be lethal.

36. **What is bullous pemphigoid?**
    Bullous pemphigoid (Fig. 19-6) is a blistering autoimmune disease resembling pemphigus vulgaris. In contrast to pemphigus, it rarely affects oral mucosa. Bullous pemphigoid is mediated by antibodies to glycoproteins in the lamina lucida of the epidermal–dermal basement membrane. Deposition of antibodies along the epidermal–dermal basement membrane leads to the formation of bullae. Typically such vesicles and bullae are subepidermal (i.e., between the basement membrane and the basal layer of the epidermis that was lifted off the basement membrane).

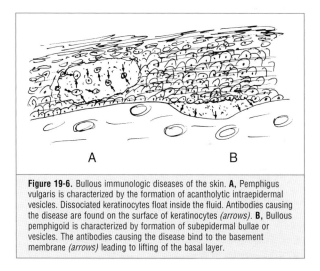

Figure 19-6. Bullous immunologic diseases of the skin. **A,** Pemphigus vulgaris is characterized by the formation of acantholytic intraepidermal vesicles. Dissociated keratinocytes float inside the fluid. Antibodies causing the disease are found on the surface of keratinocytes *(arrows)*. **B,** Bullous pemphigoid is characterized by formation of subepidermal bullae or vesicles. The antibodies causing the disease bind to the basement membrane *(arrows)* leading to lifting of the basal layer.

37. **How can pemphigus vulgaris be distinguished from bullous pemphigoid?**
    In contrast to pemphigus vulgaris, which may be fatal if not treated with corticosteroid, bullous pemphigoid is a relatively benign disease. Skin biopsy is useful to distinguish these diseases one from another.
    In pemphigus vulgaris, the bullae are intraepidermal, whereas in bullous pemphigoid the bullae are subepidermal because the fluid accumulates between the damaged epidermal–dermal basement membrane and the basal layer of the epidermis. By immunofluorescence microscopy, one can see deposits of IgG along the cell membrane of epidermal cells in pemphigus

vulgaris. In bullous pemphigoid, the deposits of IgG are linear along the epidermal–dermal basement membrane.

In pemphigus vulgaris, the layers of the unblistered skin can be separated from each other by applying gentle pressure. By putting a finger on the patient's skin and rubbing it, one can feel that the surface layers are moving over the basal layer and ultimately a bulla will form. This Nikolsky sign cannot be elicited in bullous pemphigoid.

38. **What is the difference between bullous pemphigoid and epidermolysis bullosa?**
In contrast to bullous pemphigoid, an autoimmune disease of middle-aged people, epidermolysis bullosa is a term denoting a number of congenital blistering diseases. In epidermolysis bullosa, the bullae develop because of a congenital defect involving a component of the epidermal–dermal basement membrane or the basal layer keratinocytes. Bullae may start appearing in early life and even during intrauterine life.

39. **What is dermatitis herpetiformis?**
Dermatitis herpetiformis is a chronic autoimmune skin disease characterized by recurrent eruptions of itchy vesicles surrounded by erythematous patches. The disease is mediated by deposits of IgA along the epidermal–dermal junction, especially at the tips of dermal papillae. Subepidermal vesicles form and are accompanied by infiltrates of neutrophils in their wall. Most patients also have celiac sprue. Both the intestinal and the skin disease respond favorably to a gluten-free diet.

40. **What is lichen planus?**
Lichen planus is a skin disease thought to be mediated by T lymphocytes. It typically presents in the form of violaceous papules on the inner side of the wrist, small papules or blisters on the soles and palms, or as white lacy eruptions on mucosal surfaces (e.g., oral or genital mucosa). Scratching or minor trauma can cause additional lesions. Histologically, the skin or the mucosae contain bandlike infiltrates along the epidermal–dermal junction, destroying the basal layer of the epithelium. Such lesions heal spontaneously or with steroid treatment. Depigmentation or hyperpigmentation is seen at the site of healed lesions.

41. **What are the skin lesions of SLE?**
Lupus erythematosus is a systemic disease characterized by the deposition of immune complexes along the dermal–epidermal junction and lymphocytic infiltrates around the blood vessels and the skin appendages. Skin lesions are found in 85% of all patients with this disease. These lesions may present as a fairly characteristic rash on sun-exposed surfaces (e.g., typical "butterfly rash" on the nose and cheeks) or in the form of nonspecific skin lesions. The lesions may appear acutely or may be chronic (e.g., chronic discoid lupus). See Fig. 19-7.

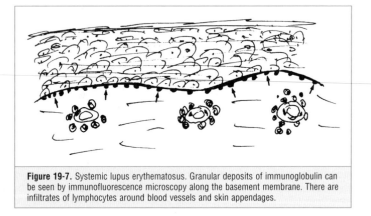

Figure 19-7. Systemic lupus erythematosus. Granular deposits of immunoglobulin can be seen by immunofluorescence microscopy along the basement membrane. There are infiltrates of lymphocytes around blood vessels and skin appendages.

42. **What is the lupus band test?**

    Lupus band test is a term used to describe the typical immunofluorescence microscopy findings in the skin of patients who have lupus erythematosus. The test includes a skin biopsy. The sample is immediately frozen and sectioned with a cryostat, and the frozen sections are stained with fluoresceinated antibodies to IgG. In patients affected with lupus, these antibodies bind to the IgG deposited in a granular manner along the epidermal–dermal junction. Microscopically, these deposits appear in the form of a finely granular band, which accounts for the name of the test.

IDIOPATHIC SKIN DISEASES

43. **What is psoriasis vulgaris?**

    Psoriasis, as its official Latin name (*vulgaris*) implies, is a common skin disease affecting 1% or 2% of the total population. The cause of the disease is not known, but it runs in families and obviously has a hereditary basis. Its pathogenesis is not known, but it appears that the basic defect lies in the hyperproliferation of epidermis and abnormal keratinization. It has a chronic course characterized by exacerbations and remissions. In approximately 10% of cases, it is accompanied by destructive joint disease.

44. **What are the pathologic features of psoriasis?**

    The skin lesions appear in the form of scaly, silvery plaques, most often on the extensor surfaces of extremities (i.e., over the elbows and knees). Trauma apparently plays a role because lesions tend also to appear at the site of wounds and obviously traumatized skin (Koebner phenomenon). Skin of the face and the scalp may also be involved. Histologically, psoriatic lesions show thickening of the epidermis with club-form elongation of rete ridges. The surface of the epidermis is covered with parakeratosis, which accounts for the silvery scales seen on gross examination. Aggregates of neutrophils in the stratum corneum (Munro microabscesses), and subcorneal pustules of Kogoj are typically found. Between the elongated rete ridges, there are dermal papillae that contain prominent capillary loops extending almost to the surface. By scratching the surface epidermis, one can easily expose the capillary loops and thus induce punctate bleeding. This clinical test is known as Auspitz sign. See Fig. 19-8.

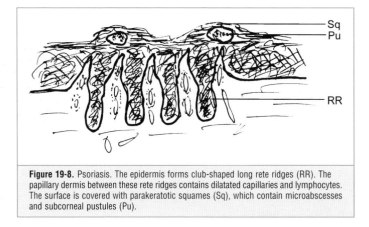

Figure 19-8. Psoriasis. The epidermis forms club-shaped long rete ridges (RR). The papillary dermis between these rete ridges contains dilatated capillaries and lymphocytes. The surface is covered with parakeratotic squames (Sq), which contain microabscesses and subcorneal pustules (Pu).

45. **What is erythema multiforme?**

    Erythema mutiforme is a relatively common disease of unknown etiology considered to be a form of hypersensitivity or hyperreaction to a variety of agents. In some cases, it is related to a well-defined autoimmune disease, such as SLE, and in some instances it is a paraneoplastic manifestation of internal malignancy. It may be related to various infections, and in some instances it is a reaction to drugs.

    As implied in its name, its presentation varies and may include a spectrum of skin lesions— maculea, papulee, bliotere, and co forth. Target lesions that have a red center surrounded by a pale halo are typical but not always present. The epidermis of such lesions may show necrosis of the basal layer, which leads to the formation of bullae. A severe generalized form of erythema multiforme, characterized by peeling of skin all over the body, is called Stevens–Johnson syndrome. It is associated with high mortality.

46. **What is erythema nodosum?**

    Erythema nodosum is a common skin disease of unknown etiology. It may be associated with some other diseases, or the skin lesions may appear without any obvious cause. It appears clinically as tender red nodules, most often on the anterior shin. The disease has a self-limited course, and the lesions regress after approximately 1 month. Histologically, it is a panniculitis, with infiltrates of lymphocytes and macrophages in the connective tissue septa of the subcutaneous fat tissue. Vasculitis of subcutaneous small blood vessels is also evident.

47. **What is pityriasis rosea?**

    Pityriasis rosea is a common, acute, self-limited skin disease of unknown etiology that affects young people. It starts with the appearance of a red patch surrounded by a rim ("collarette") of scales. These scales correspond histologically to parakeratosis. The "herald patch" is followed a few days or weeks later by a crop of smaller scaly lesions on the trunk and proximal extremities. The center of these lesions becomes red, and the scales remain only at the periphery. Similar "pityriasiform" skin eruptions occur in other skin diseases, but these are less common than pityriasis rosea.

48. **What is seborrheic dermatitis?**

    Seborrheic dermatitis is a skin disease of unknown etiology. In infants, it presents in the form of patches and dry scales on the scalp as cradle cap or as reddened skin in the groin as diaper rash. In adults, the scalp shows excessive formation of dandruff and is greasy and inflamed. The face and the chest also show scaly lesions.

NEOPLASMS

49. **How common are skin tumors?**

    Skin tumors are common. First, skin is a very large organ. Second, skin is exposed to numerous exogenous influences, some of which (e.g., ultraviolet light) are carcinogenic. Finally, because of their superficial location, skin tumors are much more easily noticed than tumors of internal organs. Skin tumors are usually not included in official statistics dealing with tumors of internal organs.

50. **How are skin tumors classified?**

    As in other organs, skin tumors can be benign or malignant. These growths can arise from cells in the epidermis or dermis and subcutis. Accordingly, it is best to classify primary skin tumors histogenetically, taking into account their cell of origin. Major groups of skin neoplasms are:
    - Tumors of keratinocytes (e.g., squamous cell carcinoma) and their precursors in the basal layer of skin (e.g., basal cell carcinoma)
    - Tumors of melanocytes (e.g., malignant melanoma)

- Tumors of Merkel cells (Merkel cell carcinoma)
- Tumors of Langerhans cells (Langerhans cell histiocytosis)
- Tumors of skin appendages (e.g., sebaceous gland adenocarcinoma)
- Tumors of connective tissue cells (e.g., hemangioma)
- Tumors of hematopoietic and lymphoid cells (e.g., lymphoma of the skin)

Most important among these various tumors are those of keratinocytes and melanocytes. It should be noted that the skin may be involved by metastatic tumors. Lymphomas of the skin may arise in the skin, but more often they are a sign of dissemination of a malignancy that originated in the lymph nodes or the bone marrow.

51. **What are the most important neoplasms arising from keratinocytes and their precursors in the basal layer of the skin?**
This group of lesions includes:
- Benign tumors: seborrheic keratosis
- Premalignant lesions: actinic keratosis
- Invasive malignant tumors—basal cell carcinoma and squamous cell carcinoma

52. **What is seborrheic keratosis?**
Seborrheic keratosis (Fig. 19-9) is a term used for benign epithelial growths that occur in older people. These benign tumors appear on the extremities, trunk, or face in form of slightly elevated flat papules. Typically they are covered with scales, may be brownish and appear "greasy." Microscopically, they are composed of upward-proliferating mature epithelial cells, often surrounding invaginations or round spaces filled with keratin ("horn cysts"). Because of their exophytic growth, these tumors appear "stuck on" normal skin and can be scraped off easily with a sharp instrument.

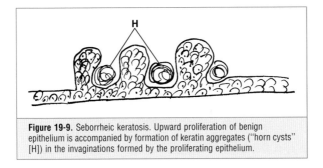

Figure 19-9. Seborrheic keratosis. Upward proliferation of benign epithelium is accompanied by formation of keratin aggregates ("horn cysts" [H]) in the invaginations formed by the proliferating epithelium.

KEY POINTS: NEOPLASMS ✓

1. Seborrheic keratosis is the most common benign epidermal tumor, whereas basal cell carcinoma is the most common malignant tumor.

2. Basal cell carcinomas differ from squamous cell carcinomas in that the former do not metastasize, whereas the latter will metastasize if not removed on time.

3. Pigmented lesions of the skin include benign lesions (e.g., freckles and moles), which are common, and malignant tumors (malignant melanomas), which are relatively rare.

53. **What is the significance of seborrheic keratosis?**
Seborrheic keratosis is one of the most common skin lesions removed by dermatologists. Because of its relatively rapid growth, it may be mistaken for a malignancy. Pigmented lesions may be mistaken for melanoma. It is important to assure the patient that the lesions have nothing to do with skin cancer and are not premalignant, even though in some cases similar papules may recur. In rare instances, the appearance of multiple papules of seborrheic keratosis may be a sign of internal malignancy.

54. **What is basal cell carcinoma?**
  - It is the most common malignant tumor of the skin.
  - It is a locally invasive tumor and almost never metastasizes.
  - Typically it is located on the sun-exposed areas of the skin and thus pathogenetically related to ultraviolet light exposure.
  - It is most commonly found on the face.
  - Tumors appear in the form of waxy papules or small nodules covered with pearly squames and a central crater.
  - Tumor cells invade the dermis and form nests rimmed by palisaded basal cells. These cells resemble those in the basal layer of the skin (Fig. 19-10).
  - Excision of the tumor with wide margins is usually curative, but untreated tumors can invade into deeper parts of the skin and even erode bones or metastasize.

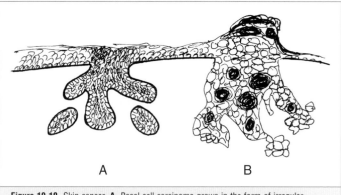

Figure 19-10. Skin cancer. **A,** Basal cell carcinoma grows in the form of irregular extensions and nests composed of basal cells. The nests are enclosed by a basement membrane rimmed by palisaded basal cells. **B,** Squamous cell carcinoma grows in the form of irregularly shaped tongues invading the dermis. Tumor cells vary in size and shape and form round keratin pearls.

55. **What is squamous cell carcinoma?**
  - It is a locally invasive malignant tumor that can metastasize (1%–2%).
  - It occurs on sun-exposed skin and is more common in fair-skinned people than in those who have more pigment.
  - It is most often found on the face, preferentially involving the lower lip.
  - Pathogenesis of this tumor is linked to exposure to ultraviolet light.
  - Other possible pathogenetic influences are less common but should be mentioned. Squamous cell carcinomas may occur in burn scars, chronic skin ulcers, at the site of

draining sinuses (e.g., overlying chronic osteomyelitis), following x-radiation/treatment, and following prolonged exposure to arsenic (vineyard workers).

■ Often preceded by preinvasive intraepithelial malignancies known as actinic keratosis (solar keratosis) or carcinoma in situ.

■ Histologically the tumors are composed of malignant epithelial cells that tend to keratinize and form "keratin pearls" (*see* Fig. 19-10).

■ Squamous cell skin carcinomas are microscopically indistinguishable from squamous cell carcinomas in other sites, such as those originating in the cervix, vulva, penis, mouth, esophagus, or bronchi.

56. **What is actinic keratosis?**
Actinic keratosis is a form of intraepidermal malignancy typically found on sun-exposed areas of the skin. It presents in the form of patches that have a rough surface and appear hyperkeratotic. Histologically the lesion contains atypical hyperchromatic neoplastic cells, which are limited to the lower half of the epidermis. The surface of the lesions is covered with parakeratosis. Actinic keratosis may progress to carcinoma in situ and invasive squamous cell carcinoma. It may be multifocal and is often found in the skin adjacent to invasive squamous cell carcinoma.

57. **Is carcinoma in situ always found on sun-exposed skin?**
Like actinic keratosis, carcinoma in situ is found most often on the sun-exposed skin of the face, arms, or chest. However, it may occur on sun-protected areas and on the mucosal surfaces as well. Carcinoma in situ of the skin and anogenital area is also known as Bowen disease. It presents in the form of erythematous patches. Histologically, the malignant cells permeate the entire epidermis but do not invade the basement membrane.

58. **What are the most important pigmented skin lesions?**
Benign pigmented skin lesions are common. They include:

■ Freckle (ephelis) is a pigmented macule composed of normal melanocytes, which overreact to sunlight by producing melanin at a rapid rate. The number of melanocytes is not increased (Fig. 19-11).

■ Lentigo is a pigmented lesion containing an increased number of melanocytes with a hyperpigmentation of adjacent keratinocytes. In contrast to ephelis, lentigo does not darken

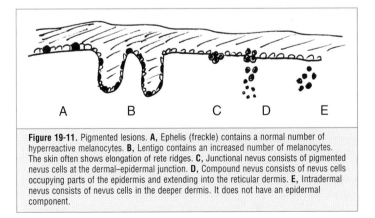

Figure 19-11. Pigmented lesions. **A,** Ephelis (freckle) contains a normal number of hyperreactive melanocytes. **B,** Lentigo contains an increased number of melanocytes. The skin often shows elongation of rete ridges. **C,** Junctional nevus consists of pigmented nevus cells at the dermal–epidermal junction. **D,** Compound nevus consists of nevus cells occupying parts of the epidermis and extending into the reticular dermis. **E,** Intradermal nevus consists of nevus cells in the deeper dermis. It does not have an epidermal component.

upon exposure to sunlight. Histologically the involved skin shows elongation of rete ridges, thus bringing the pigmented cells closer one to another.

- Solar lentigo (also known as liver spots or senile lentigo) are pigmented lesions on the face or the dorsum of the hand of elderly people. Histologically these lesions are identical to regular lentigos.
- Melanocytic nevus (also known as mole) is a hamartoma composed of melanocytes. Nevi may be congenital or acquired. Congenital nevi are found in approximately 1% of all newborns. Acquired nevi appear later, usually at puberty, and involute spontaneously in old age.
- Malignant melanomas are malignant tumors composed of melanocytes.

59. **How are melanocytic nevi classified histologically?**
Nevi are classified according to the location of melanocytes (nevus cells) into three groups:
- **Junctional nevus:** In this lesion, the nevus cells are located at the interface between the epidermis and dermis (*see* Fig. 19-11).
- **Compound nevus:** In this lesion, the nevus cells are at the interface between the epidermis and dermis and also in the reticular dermis.
- **Intradermal nevus:** In this lesion, the nevus cells are located in the deeper dermis, and there is no junctional activity.

60. **What are blue nevi?**
Blue nevi are composed of heavily pigmented dendritic melanocytes located in the reticular dermis. Because the light reflected from these deeply seated pigmented cells must pass through a thicker layer than that of superficially located melanocytes, the lesions appear bluish gray rather than black. With a few rare exceptions, blue nevi are almost always benign.

61. **What are dysplastic nevi?**
Dysplastic nevi are pigmented lesions that clinically and histopathologically differ from regular nevi and thus appear atypical. This term is poorly defined and often misused, and a National Institutes of Health consensus conference recommended that the term dysplastic be abandoned and replaced by atypical nevus. Nevertheless, some facts deserve to be mentioned.
- An increased incidence of melanoma in atypical nevi has been documented, but the exact risk remains disputed. The estimates range from 1% to 40%.
- Familial atypical mole-melanoma syndrome, a rare hereditary condition, is a proof that some melanomas have a genetic basis. Among the members of these families there is an increased incidence of atypical nevi and an increased incidence of melanomas has been recorded.
- Histologic criteria for diagnosing atypical nevi have not been universally accepted. Accordingly, the recorded incidence of atypical nevi varies from 2% to 8% among pigmented lesions removed from adults and examined microscopically.
- Atypical nevi may give rise to melanoma in situ or invasive melanoma. This transition can be recognized with certainty only by microscopic examination of biopsied lesions. Accordingly, any suspicious mole, especially those larger than 6 mm in diameter, must be removed and examined microscopically.
- Clinical features suggesting an atypical nevus are their size (>6 mm), irregular borders, and variegated color (shades of brown, tan, and light red). A "fried egg" appearance (dark center surrounded by less pigmented rim that has indistinct margins) is often cited as typical for these atypical nevi.

62. **What is a malignant melanoma?**
Malignant melanoma (MM) is a malignant tumor of melanocytes. Most often, these tumors originate in the skin, but they may also arise in the eyes. Occasionally these tumors originate in internal organs, probably from displaced melanocytes. Melanocytes derived from the neural

crest do not have epithelial features; therefore these tumors are not classified as carcinomas. Classifying them as sarcomas (because these tumor cells contain vimentin in their cytoskeleton, like other sarcomas) or neuroepithelial malignancies (because they originate from the neural crest) would also not be appropriate. Hence malignant melanomas are in a category by themselves.

63. **How common are malignant melanomas?**
Excluding other forms of skin cancer, MM accounts for 2% of all malignant neoplasms in humans and is responsible for 1% of all cancer deaths. Approximately 25,000 new cases of MM are diagnosed annually in the United States, and approximately 6,000 deaths per year are attributed to MM. The following are other important facts:
- The incidence of MM is increasing at a rapid rate all over the world.
- It is estimated that 1 in 100 infants born in 2008 will develop a melanoma during their lifetime.
- Exposure to the sun or artificial UV light plays an important pathogenetic role.
- Pale-skinned people (especially those who always burn and never tan) are at highest risk.

64. **How are MMs classified?**
There are four histopathologic forms of melanoma:
- Lentigo maligna
- Superficial spreading
- Nodular
- Acral lentiginous

65. **Which is the most common form of MM?**
Superficial spreading melanomas account for 75% of all MMs diagnosed in the United States. Nodular melanomas (15%), lentigo maligna (5%), and acral lentiginous melanoma (2%–3%) are less common.

66. **On which part of the body do melanomas occur most often?**
- MM can occur in any location.
- In men, melanomas are found most often on the trunk, and in women most often on the extremities.
- Lentigo maligna tends to develop on sun-exposed skin of the face and the head and neck region.
- Acral lentiginous melanomas occur on palms and soles and the nail bed.

67. **What is the peak age for the occurrence of MMs?**
MMs are most often diagnosed in the 40- to 60-year age group, with the peak incidence at 50 years of age. However, MMs can occur in young people as well, and it is currently the most commonly diagnosed cancer in women aged 25 to 29 years. Lentigo maligna melanoma tends to occur in older people, and its peak incidence is at 70 years of age.

68. **Can malignant melanomas develop in dark-skinned people of African or Indian origin?**
Acral lentiginous melanoma is the most common form of malignant melanoma in dark-skinned people. Other forms of melanoma can also occur but are rare.

69. **How do melanomas arise?**
- Fifty percent of all melanomas arise in acquired melanocytic nevi.
- Forty percent develop from melanocytes in normal skin.
- MMs rarely develop from small congenital nevi. Large congenital nevi give rise to MMs in approximately 6% of cases.

- Atypical nevi have the highest risk for developing into melanomas, but these pigmented lesions are less common than regular melanocytic nevi.

70. **How are melanomas recognized clinically?**
Definitive diagnosis of melanoma requires microscopic confirmation, and two thirds of all lesions suspected to be MMs turn out not to be malignant. Nevertheless, a high degree of suspicion is required for early diagnosis of lesions that are still completely curable. To this end, clinicians use the mnemonic ABCD of malignant melanoma, which stands for

- **A**symmetry: All irregularly shaped asymmetrical lesions should be removed and sent for pathologic examination.
- **B**orders and bleeding: All pigmented lesions that have irregular borders or bleed spontaneously or upon minor trauma should be treated as potentially malignant.
- **C**olor: Irregularly pigmented moles or those that change color should be removed.
- **D**iameter: All acquired pigmented lesions that cannot be covered with the blunt end of the pencil (>6 mm) should be excised.

71. **How do MMs grow?**
The initial lesion, malignant melanoma in situ, may spread through the epidermis or become invasive and spread into the dermis. Intraepidermal radial growth is typical of superficial spreading MM and lentigo maligna, whereas vertical growth is typical of nodular melanoma. Untreated radial phase lesions will, over time, enter a vertical growth phase.

72. **How are malignant melanomas staged histologically?**
MMs are staged histologically according to the system developed by Clark (Fig. 19-12):

- Level I—melanoma in situ; tumor cells confined to the epidermis
- Level II—tumor cells cross the basement membrane but do not fill the papillary dermis
- Level III—tumor cells fill the papillary dermis but do not extend beyond an imaginary line drawn over the tips of the rete ridges
- Level IV—tumor cells extend into the reticular dermis
- Level V—tumor cells extend into the subcutis

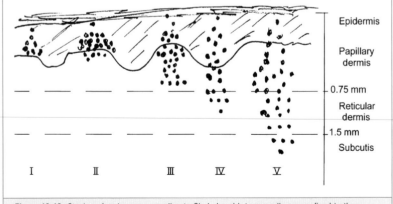

Figure 19-12. Staging of melanoma according to Clark. Level I: tumor cells are confined to the epidermis. Level II: cells extend into papillary dermis but do not fill it. Level III: cells fill the papillary dermis but do not extend into the reticular dermis (i.e., beyond the tip of rete ridges). Level IV: cells extend into the reticular dermis. Level V: tumor cells extend into the subcutis.

Five-year survival for patients with surgically resected Level I lesions is 100%, for Level II lesions is 90%, for Level III lesions is 70%, for Level IV lesions is 40%, and for Level V lesions is 25%.

The Breslow system of staging is similar but is easier to reproduce because it is based on measuring the thickness of the tumor. According to the Breslow system, MMs that have not invaded beyond 0.75 mm have a cure rate close to 100%. The 5-year survival rate for patients with tumors that measure 0.75 to 1.5 mm is 90% to 95%; that of patients with tumors 1.5 to 4.0 mm is 60% to 75%, and that of patients with tumors thicker than 4 mm is less than 50%.

73. **How are malignant melanomas staged?**
The American Joint Commission on Cancer (AJCC) staging is based on the TNM (Tumor, Node, Metastases) system, in which Stage I has a 95% 5-year survival rate, Stage II 80%, Stage III 50%, and Stage IV 20%. Histologic staging (i.e., the depth of tumor invasion into the skin) is important for Stage I and II tumors. After lymph node metastases are identified, and the tumor is Stage III, the histologic staging of the skin lesion is not important. Stage IV MM is reached when the tumor metastasizes to the viscera.

74. **What is Merkel cell carcinoma?**
Merkel cell carcinoma, also known as primary neuroendocrine carcinoma of the skin, is a rare but highly malignant tumor. Approximately 50% of tumors arise on the head and neck area of elderly people, but it may occur in younger people and at other sites of the body. In approximately 70% of cases, the tumor has already metastasized at the time of diagnosis. The 5-year survival rate is 40% to 60%.

75. **What is Langerhans cell histiocytosis?**
Langerhans cell histiocytosis (also known as histiocytosis X) may present with dermal involvement during the dissemination of the disease. Dermal infiltrates are composed of cells that have the immunohistochemical and ultrastructural features of epidermal Langerhans cells. A primary form of the disease occurs in children younger than 2 years of age and is known as Letterer–Siwe disease.

76. **What is mycosis fungoides?**
Mycosis fungoides is a malignant T-cell lymphoma involving the skin. Tumor cells have the phenotype of CD4+ T helper cells.

77. **What is the most common connective tissue tumor of the skin?**
Hemangiomas and dermatofibromas are probably the most common benign skin tumors. Some hemangiomas are congenital and may be classified as hamartomas.

DERMAL MANIFESTATIONS OF INTERNAL DISEASES

78. **What causes acanthosis nigricans?**
Acanthosis nigricans, which presents with hyperpigmentation of the intertriginous areas (axilla and groin) and the neck, is a paraneoplastic condition most often associated with adenocarcinoma of the stomach.

79. **What causes hyperpigmentation of the skin?**
Hyperpigmentation can be a consequence of hyperestrinism and is common in pregnancy or in women taking estrogenic hormones and contraceptive pills. Addison's disease, associated with compensatory hypersecretion of adrenocorticotropic hormone (which has a melanocyte-stimulating effect), and hemochromatosis also cause hyperpigmentation.

80. **What causes hypopigmentation?**
Localized depigmentation, known as vitiligo, is a disease of unknown etiology and pathogenesis. In some instances, it is associated with systemic autoimmune diseases or diabetes mellitus.

81. **Which internal diseases are often associated with pruritus?**
    Pruritus or itching is a common symptom in jaundiced patients and thus may be encountered in those suffering from obstructive jaundice, primary biliary cirrhosis or drug-induced jaundice. Uremia caused by end-stage kidney disease is also accompanied by profound itching. Diabetes mellitus is typically associated with anogenital pruritus, probably associated with infections related to glucosuria.

82. **Which internal diseases are associated with pyoderma gangrenosum?**
    Pyoderma gangrenosum presents as a pustule that spreads laterally, undergoing central ulceration. The inflammation also involves the adjacent soft tissues, and the entire area appears indurated. Pyoderma gangrenosum is a common complication of ulcerative colitis but may occur in Crohn disease, leukemia, rheumatoid arthritis, and other diseases.

83. **Which internal diseases cause hirsutism?**
    Increased hair growth on the face or chest of women is a symptom of androgen excess encountered with some tumors, such as Sertoli–Leydig cell tumors of the ovary or adrenal cortical tumors. It also occurs in polycystic ovary syndrome.

84. **Which internal diseases are accompanied by increased hair loss?**
    Hair loss (alopecia) may occur in many chronic debilitating diseases or endocrine disorders (e.g., hypothyroidism). Cytotoxic drugs typically cause hair loss.

WEBSITES 🌐

1. http://tray.dermatology.uiowa.edu/DPT/Path-Index.htm

2. http://dermatlas.med.jhmi.edu/derm/

3. http://www.ncbi.nlm.nih.gov/entrez/query.fcgi?db=PubMed

4. http://www-medlib.med.utah.edu/WebPath/webpath.html#MENU

5. http://telemedicine.org/stamford.htm

BIBLIOGRAPHY

1. Anhalt GJ, Diaz LA: Research advances in pemphigus. JAMA 285:652–654, 2001.
2. Byers HR, Bhawan J: Pathologic parameter in the diagnosis and prognosis of primary cutaneous melanoma. Hematol Oncol Clin North Am 26:717–736, 1998.
3. Edman RL, Klaus SN: Is routine screening for melanoma a benign practice? JAMA 284:883–886, 2000.
4. Kwong L, Chin L, Wagner SN: Growth factors and oncogenes as targets in melanoma: lost in translation? Adv Dermatol 23:99–129, 2007.
5. Paus R, Cotsarelis G: The biology of hair follicles. N Engl J Med 341:491–497, 1999.
6. Reinhardt MJ: Cutaneous melanoma. Recent Results Cancer Res 170:151–157, 2008.
7. Rossi R, Mori M, Lotti T: Actinic keratosis. Int J Dermatol 46:895–904, 2007.
8. Rudikoff D, Lebwohl M: Atopic dermatitis. Lancet 351:1715–1720, 1998.
9. Stollery N. Disorders of keratinisation. Practitioner 251:60–65, 2007.
10. Yancey KB, Egan CA: Pemphigoid: clinical, histologic, immunopathologic, and therapeutic considerations. JAMA 284:350–356, 2000.

CHAPTER 20

BONES AND JOINTS

Ivan Damjanov, MD, PhD

1. **What are the main anatomic portions of tubular long bones?**
   The midportion of a tubular long bone is called the diaphysis. The articular portion of these bones is called epiphysis. The part of the bone between the epiphysis and the diaphysis is called the metaphysis. In growing bones of children and adolescents, the midportion of the metaphysis contains the physis or the cartilaginous growth plate. The calcifying growth plates, easily recognizable on x-ray, are called secondary ossification centers, in contrast to primary ossification centers, a term used for the subperiosteal cortical bone formation. See Fig. 20-1.

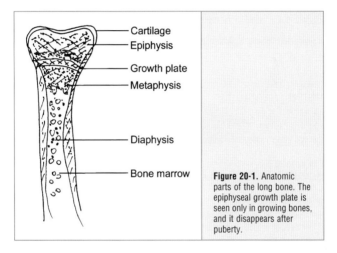

Cartilage
Epiphysis
Growth plate
Metaphysis
Diaphysis
Bone marrow

Figure 20-1. Anatomic parts of the long bone. The epiphyseal growth plate is seen only in growing bones, and it disappears after puberty.

2. **Name the main bone-forming cells in the bone.**
   - **Osteocytes:** These mature resting cells are involved in the maintenance of the basic functional and anatomic units of the bone, called osteons. Osteocytes also participate in the maintenance of the blood concentration of calcium and phosphates.
   - **Osteoblasts:** These bone-forming cells synthesize osteoid and participate in its calcification. Osteoblasts can be stimulated by parathyroid hormone, vitamin D, and estrogens.
   - **Osteoclasts:** These bone-resorbing cells are closely related to macrophages. Thus they are derived from the same bone marrow precursors responding to granulocyte-macrophage colony-stimulating factor (GM-CSF) and macrophage colony-stimulating factor. In contrast to mononuclear macrophages, osteoclasts are multinucleated.

   In addition to these cells, which are related to the formation, maintenance, and resorption of the bone matrix, bones contain other cells that can be found in anatomic sites, such as fibroblasts and blood vessels. The joint surface of the mature bone and the growth plate of the growing long bones contain cartilage cells. The bone marrow contains hematopoietic and fat cells.

3. **What is the difference between lamellar and woven bone?**
Newly formed bone, composed of haphazardly arranged strands of collagen, appears like woven cloth when examined microscopically under polarized light. Gradually, it transforms into lamellar bone, composed of parallel arrays of mineralized osteoid. Woven bone is formed in growing children, whereas lamellar bone, which is stronger and more resistant to stress, is a typical component of adult bones.

4. **What are the most important bone diseases?**
   - Developmental disorders
   - Metabolic disorders
   - Fractures
   - Infectious diseases
   - Tumors

KEY POINTS: DISEASES OF BONES AND JOINTS ✔

1. Bones are affected by numerous developmental, metabolic, infectious, and neoplastic diseases and are also prone to mechanical trauma.

2. Genetic disorders may result in the formation of short, deformed, or structurally abnormal bones.

3. Joints are affected mostly by inflammatory and degenerative diseases.

DEVELOPMENTAL ABNORMALITIES

5. **What is adactyly?**
A congenital abnormality characterized by an absence of fingers.

6. **What is amelia?**
A congenital abnormality characterized by an absence of upper or lower extremities or both.

7. **Define arachnodactyly.**
Arachnodactyly (literally, "spiderlike fingers") is a feature of Marfan syndrome. It can be found in other disorders involving genes that encode extracellular matrix proteins, such as Ehlers–Danlos syndrome. However, many legendary violinists, such as Paganini, and pianists, such as Rubinstein, had long fingers but were otherwise normal. Hence, long fingers are not necessarily stigmata of a congenital disorder.

8. **What is syndactyly?**
A congenital abnormality characterized by fusion of the fingers or the toes. It results from defective apoptosis of interdigital cells in the fetal limb buds.

9. **Explain the pathogenesis of achondroplasia.**
An autosomal dominant form of congenital dwarfism caused by abnormal formation of the epiphysial growth plate of long tubular bones. The defect lies in the gene encoding the fibroblast growth factor receptor-3 (FGF-3), which plays a critical role in the growth of cartilage. In normal circumstances, FGF-3 inhibits the proliferation of cartilage cells, but this inhibition does not take place in people with a mutated receptor. These people have broad epiphysial growth plates composed of constantly proliferating cartilage cells that are not replaced by osteoblasts. Accordingly, tubular bones do not grow longitudinally. The affected person has short limbs, a normal trunk, and a relatively large head. Approximately 80% of all achondroplastic dwarfs have normal parents, and their disease is caused by a new mutation.

10. **What is osteogenesis imperfecta (OI)?**
    Also known as "brittle bone disease," OI is not a single disease. It occurs in four forms, all of which are related to the mutation of the genes encoding the chains of type I collagen. The defects in the synthesis of collagen type I cause osteopenia and make bones weak and fragile.

11. **How does OI present?**
    Severe forms of OI, such as OI type II, may present with multiple fractures during fetal life and are usually fatal. Milder forms of OI may present with stunted growth and increased fragility of bones, predisposing affected people to fractures even after minimal injury.

12. **What are the typical extraskeletal manifestations of osteogenesis imperfecta?**
    All tissues containing collagen type I, which is actually present in various amounts in most organs, may be affected. However, these defects remain mostly inapparent. Visible abnormalities include blue sclerae and dental defects. Hearing defects are common because of abnormalities in the middle and inner ear.

13. **List the causes of dwarfism.**
    - Defects in bone formation, such as achondroplasia and osteogenesis imperfecta, and various mucopolysaccharidoses
    - Pituitary abnormalities associated with growth hormone secretion
    - Deficiency of growth hormone receptor (Laron-type dwarfism)
    - Deficiency of thyroid hormones (cretinism)

14. **What is osteopetrosis?**
    Osteopetrosis, or marble bone disease, is a genetic disorder characterized by abnormal thickening of bones. It is related to some undefined defect in the function of osteoclasts, which do not resorb the bone. The bones grow but are not remodeled and ultimately obliterate the marrow spaces. Such bones are fragile and easily broken. Anemia caused by the compression of the hematopoietic bone marrow by sclerotic bone is common.

METABOLIC DISORDERS

15. **Define osteopenia.**
    Osteopenia (literally, "lack of bone") is a radiologic term used to denote a decreased amount of bone visible on x-ray. It can be congenital or acquired and includes many pathologic entities, such as osteogenesis imperfecta, osteoporosis, and osteomalacia.

16. **What is osteoporosis?**
    Osteoporosis (literally, "increased porosity of bones") is a form of osteopenia characterized by decreased bone mass. It may be localized (e.g., in a limb immobilized by a cast after fracture) or generalized, as typically seen in postmenopausal women.

KEY POINTS: METABOLIC DISORDERS ✓

1. Osteoporosis is the most common form of bone loss (osteopenia).

2. Osteomalacia is related to vitamin D deficiency.

3. Several hormones affect the bones, but the parathyroid hormone has the most pronounced effects on bone formation, maintenance, and resorption.

17. **Discuss the difference between primary and secondary osteoporosis.**

Primary osteoporosis, an age-related, accelerated bone loss, occurs without obvious or well-defined reasons. Secondary osteoporosis is related to various metabolic, endocrine, or nutritional disorders. Typical examples of secondary osteoporosis are:

- Endocrine deficiencies, such as hypogonadism, anorexia nervosa, and ovarian failure
- Endocrine hyperfunction, such as in hypercortisolism, hyperthyroidism, and hyperparathyroidism
- Gastrointestinal diseases resulting in malabsorption
- Bone marrow malignancies, such as multiple myeloma, lymphoma, and metastatic carcinoma
- Drugs, such as corticosteroids, heparin, chemotherapeutic agents, cyclosporine, and anticonvulsants
- Alcohol abuse

18. **What are the risk factors for developing osteoporosis?**

- **Age:** Osteoporosis is an age-related disease, and its incidence increases with advanced years.
- **Genetic factors:** Osteoporosis runs in families and is considered to be a multifactorial disease. People who have thin bones and a small skeleton are more likely to develop osteoporosis than those who have a large frame (peak bone mass).
- **Sex:** Women are more susceptible to osteoporosis than men.
- **Hormones:** Deficiency of estrogen in the postmenopausal period accelerates osteoporosis. Estrogen replacement therapy may retard the development of osteoporosis.
- **Nutritional status:** Calcium and vitamin D are essential for the maintenance of the skeleton, and a deficiency of these nutrients promotes osteoporosis.
- **Physical activity:** Reduced physical activity promotes osteoporosis.
- **Environmental factors:** Cigarette smoking and alcohol abuse promote osteoporosis.

19. **Is primary osteoporosis a single entity?**

Primary osteoporosis is not a single pathologic entity. Two distinct types of primary osteoporosis are recognized:

- Type 1 primary osteoporosis typically occurs in postmenopausal women. It is caused by increased activity of osteoclasts, related to decreased levels of estrogen in the circulation. Lack of estrogen is associated with an increased release of cytokines, such as interleukin (IL)-1 and IL-6, which stimulate osteoclasts.
- Type 2 primary osteoporosis, known as senile osteoporosis, affects both men and women. The pathogenesis of loss is not understood. Bone loss in this form of bone atrophy is not related to an increased osteoclastic activity, and the cause of bone loss is obscure.

20. **Which bones are affected most by osteoporosis?**

Type 1 (postmenopausal) osteoporosis primarily affects bones that have a large cancellous compartment, such as vertebral bodies. Compression fractures of vertebral bodies are thus common in this condition.

Type 2 (senile) osteoporosis leads to thinning of the cortical portion of long bones, which become fragile. Stress fractures of weight-carrying bones, especially the femur, are common in this form of osteoporosis.

21. **How is osteoporosis diagnosed clinically?**

In most instances, osteoporosis is asymptomatic, and the diagnosis of this disease is usually made accidentally during a workup for another disease or following bone fracture. Radiologists can recognize osteopenia after the bone loss exceeds more than 30% to 40% of the total bone mass. Osteopenia does not necessarily mean that the bone loss is due to osteoporosis; osteomalacia can also produce the same radiologic changes. Accordingly, to document osteoporosis one must use additional methods developed to measure bone density. Such techniques (e.g., single-energy photon absorptiometry) are rarely used except in research studies in highly specialized centers.

22. **Does osteoporosis cause biochemical abnormalities that can be detected in the clinical laboratory?**

    The typical laboratory tests used for assessing bone diseases give normal results in osteoporosis. Accordingly, one can expect that serum levels of calcium, phosphate, parathyroid hormone, and alkaline phosphatase will be within normal limits.

23. **Can osteoporosis be diagnosed histologically by bone biopsy?**

    Bone biopsy is diagnostic in advanced osteoporosis. In such cases, the bone spicules are thinner than normal because of an even loss of mineral and nonmineral (osteoid) components of the bone. Unfortunately, given the great variation in the appearance of normal bone spicules, mild osteoporosis cannot be detected so easily.

24. **What is osteomalacia?**

    Osteomalacia (literally, "softening of bones") is a metabolic disorder characterized by inadequate mineralization of osteoid. Osteomalacia of growing children is called rickets.

25. **What is the cause of osteomalacia?**

    The most common cause of osteomalacia is vitamin D deficiency due to inadequate nutrition or inadequate sun exposure, which is necessary for endogenous production of vitamin D in the skin. Other causes include:

    - Abnormal vitamin D metabolism (e.g., deficiency of vitamin D receptors or deficiency of 1-hydroxylase, an enzyme that transforms the 25(OH)2 vitamin D in the kidneys into the active form 1,25(OH)2 of vitamin D)
    - Phosphate deficiency states encountered in some inborn errors of metabolism, such as renal Fanconi syndrome (renal wastage of phosphate, amino acids, and glucose)
    - Paraneoplastic tumor-associated phosphaturia
    - Defective mineralization of osteoid due to genetic deficiency of alkaline phosphatase (congenital hypophosphatasia)

26. **Discuss the histologic features of osteomalacia.**

    In osteomalacia, the bone trabeculae are of normal thickness, but they are incompletely calcified. The central core of these bone spicules is normally calcified, but their peripheral portion is composed of uncalcified osteoid. These seams of uncalcified osteoid are lined by numerous osteoblasts.

27. **What are the typical clinical laboratory findings in osteomalacia?**

    Vitamin D deficiency is associated initially with low blood levels of calcium and phosphate and a normal level of parathyroid hormone (PTH). PTH elevation that occurs subsequently may raise the blood levels of phosphate. Increased activity of osteoblasts is associated with an elevation of blood alkaline phosphatase.

28. **What are the clinical features of osteomalacia?**

    Clinical symptoms of osteomalacia are nonspecific and usually include vague deep skeletal pain, gradual deformity of weight-carrying bones (e.g., deformity of femur and tibia), and a predisposition to fractures. X-rays show osteopenia and radiolucent bands (pseudofractures or Looser's zones). Vertebral bodies are typically biconcave because of the central compression of softened vertebrae by intervertebral disks. In contrast to osteoporosis, which is irreversible, the changes of osteomalacia can be reversed by supplementing the diet with adequate amounts of vitamin D and by normalizing the metabolism of calcium.

29. **How does hyperparathyroidism affect the bones?**

    Hyperparathyroidism is associated with increased bone resorption and replacement of bone trabeculae with fibrous tissue. Histologically, the affected bones contain increased numbers of osteoclasts. These multinucleated cells are most prominent inside the lacunae (i.e., invaginations of the bone trabeculae undergoing resorption). The weakened trabeculae fracture and cause bleeding. The fibrous tissue replacing the bone will therefore contain not only fibroblasts but also hemosiderin-laden macrophages.

30. **Are the bone lesions of hyperparathyroidism localized or diffuse?**
    Although the parathyroid hormone affects the entire skeleton, some bones react more prominently than others. The skeletal changes are thus diffuse, but locally they may present in the form of tumoral swelling and cystic bone destruction. Three pathologic lesions are typically recognized:
    - **Osteitis fibrosa:** Fibrous tissue replacing bone trabeculae in numerous bones or the entire skeleton.
    - **Osteitis fibrosa cystica (von Recklinghausen disease):** Cystic lesions caused by extensive resorption of cortical bone and subsequent cystic expansion of the bone defect.
    - **Brown tumor of hyperparathyroidism:** Expansile, tumorlike proliferations of osteoclasts, resembling neoplastic giant cell tumors of bones. Because of early diagnosis and better treatment of hyperparathyroidism, brown tumors are rare today.

31. **Where are the changes caused by hyperparathyroidism best recognized?**
    Hyperparathyroidism leads to the resorption of cortical bone, which is more affected than the cancellous bone. The most typical changes are seen in the middle phalanges of the index and middle fingers.

32. **What is renal osteodystrophy?**
    The term renal osteodystrophy is used to describe a set of changes seen in the bones of patients suffering from chronic renal insufficiency. It is not a unique pathologic entity, and the diagnosis is usually made only by correlating the clinical, x-ray, laboratory, and pathologic findings.

33. **What are the pathologic features of renal osteodystrophy?**
    In most instances, the bone changes are a combination of those seen in osteomalacia and hyperparathyroidism. In a dynamic renal osteodystrophy, there is also osteoporosis. Some cases show marked osteosclerosis alternating with osteoporosis, a pattern described by British radiologists as "rugger (rugby) jersey spine."

34. **Why do patients on chronic renal dialysis have bone disease?**
    Patients on chronic renal dialysis show deposition of aluminum and iron in the bones. Aluminum, derived from dialysis solutions, inhibits mineralization of osteoid and contributes to osteomalacia. Deposits of amyloid derived from b2 microglobulin are also found in such patients.

35. **What is Paget disease of bone?**
    Paget disease of bone (also known as osteitis deformans) is a disease of unknown etiology, characterized by abnormal remodeling and thickening of bones. Viral particles have been found in the bone cells on electron microscopy, but the significance of this finding is unknown.

36. **How common is Paget disease?**
    Approximately 1% of all Caucasian men older than 50 years have some signs of Paget disease; however, the condition is rare in other races. The importance of Paget disease lies in the fact that it is one of the predisposing factors for bone sarcoma in adults.

37. **Explain the evolution of bone changes in Paget disease.**
    Paget disease has three phases:
    - Osteolytic phase, characterized by increased osteoclastic activity
    - Mixed osteoclastic and osteoblastic phase
    - Osteosclerotic or burnt-out phase

Only the histologic features of the third phase are pathognomonic. In this phase, the bone shows a typical mosaiclike pattern of thick osteons, composed of woven bone that appears like a jigsaw puzzle.

38. **What are the clinical features of Paget disease?**
Paget disease is usually asymptomatic and is incidentally discovered as thickening of bones during routine radiologic examinations or following unexplained elevation of alkaline phosphatase in the blood. The disease may be monostotic or polyostotic. Thickened bone may cause enlargement of the head (e.g., hats do not fit anymore), deafness or visual disturbances (because of the compression of cranial nerves), or sciatica (due to compression of lumbar nerve roots). Although the bones are thick, they are brittle and prone to fractures (chalkstick fractures). Bow leg deformities are common. Most of the laboratory findings (including serum calcium, phosphate, and parathyroid hormone) are within normal limits, but the blood alkaline phosphatase levels are elevated. The urine may contain increased amounts of calcium in the osteolytic phase of the disease.

Osteogenic sarcomas develop at an increased rate in patients suffering from Paget disease. In the polyostotic form of Paget disease, these tumors may be multifocal.

39. **Describe how clinical laboratory data help in the diagnosis of metabolic bone diseases.**
The clinical laboratory has an invaluable role in the study of bone diseases that present radiologically as osteopenia or osteopenia combined with osteosclerosis. The complete workup of the patient will typically require information on the serum calcium, phosphate, and alkaline phosphatase, which then can be supplemented with more expensive tests, such as measurement of PTH and vitamin D in blood. Typical findings are listed in Table 20-1.

TABLE 20-1. LABORATORY FINDINGS IN METABOLIC BONE DISEASES

	Calcium	Phosphate	Alkaline Phosphatase	PTH	Vitamin D
Osteoporosis	N	N	N	N	N
Osteomalacia	Low	High or low	High	N	Low/N
Hyperparathyroidism	High	Low	N or high	High	N
Renal osteodystrophy	N or low	High	High	High	N

N, Normal; *PTH*, parathyroid hormone.

FRACTURES

40. **Are all fractures caused by trauma?**
Most, but not all, fractures are caused by obvious trauma incurred through a fall or extraneous force. Fractures related to repeated minor or inapparent trauma (e.g., prolonged march and sports injuries) are called stress fractures. Fractures that occur in pathologically altered bones, during normal activity and seemingly unrelated to trauma, are called pathologic fractures.

41. **List three examples of pathologic fractures.**
- Fracture of the femur invaded by tumor
- Fracture of leg bones in Paget disease
- Compression fracture of vertebrae in osteoporosis

42. **What is the difference between complete and incomplete fractures?**
Complete fractures result in bone fragments that are separated from each other. Comminuted fracture is a complete fracture in which the bone is broken into numerous fragments. Displaced fracture denotes that the fractured bone parts have moved out of alignment. In incomplete fractures, the continuity of bones is not disrupted. These are also called greenstick fractures. Spiral fracture of the long bones is another form of incomplete fracture.

43. **What is the difference between closed and open fractures?**
   - **Closed (simple) fracture:** The overlying soft tissue and skin are intact.
   - **Open (compound) fracture:** The gaping fracture site communicates with the outside world and is typically infected.

44. **What is callus?**
Callus is the Latin name for the hardening of the skin, such as on feet constantly traumatized by tight shoes. The same term is used in bone pathology for the hardening of the connective tissue that fills the gap between two bone fragments at the site of fracture.

45. **How do bone fractures heal?**
The healing of bone fractures is a continuous process that can be divided into three stages:
   - **Provisional callus (procallus):** It forms during the first week after fracture and is composed of granulation tissue, newly formed cartilage, and osteoid. It is typically fusiform, filling the defect caused by fracture, but also bulging over the edges of the fractured bone fragments.
   - **Fibrocartilaginous callus:** Formed during the second week from the procallus, it consists of more abundant collagenous matrix, cartilage, and osteoid that is in the process of calcification.
   - **Fibroosseous callus:** It is composed of haphazardly arranged bone spicules surrounded by connective tissue. Over time, the bone spicules are reformed and realigned to correspond to preexisting bone lost by fracture.

46. **What is osteonecrosis?**
Osteonecrosis is a clinical term used for localized death of bone due to infarcts. Thus, this lesion is also called avascular necrosis: To emphasize that these lesions are not caused by infection, they are also called aseptic necrosis.
   Foci of osteonecrosis can be found in many locations and may be solitary or multiple. Depending on their anatomic location, they can be classified as:
   - **Medullary:** It involves the bone marrow and internal cancellous bone of long and short bones.
   - **Cortical:** It involves the subchondral or subperiosteal cortex of long bones.

47. **What are the main causes of osteonecrosis?**
Although it is assumed that osteonecrosis results from ischemia, its true cause is not evident in most cases, and in such instances the disease is considered to be idiopathic. For example, it is not known why chronic alcoholics often develop osteonecrosis of the head of the femur. Idiopathic osteonecrosis necessitates approximately 50,000 femoral head replacements annually in the United States.
   Idiopathic osteonecroses in children and adolescents often have clinical eponyms. For example, osteonecrosis of the head of the femur, typically found in 3- to 10-year-old boys, is known as Legg–Calvé–Perthes disease. Osteonecrosis of the epiphysial tubercle of the tibia is known as Osgood–Schlatter disease.

48. **What are the most important identifiable causes of osteonecrosis?**
   - Trauma
   - Corticosteroids
   - Radiation therapy
   - Systemic diseases, such as sickle cell anemia, systemic lupus erythematosus, polycythemia, and gout
   - Emboli (e.g., thromboemboli or air emboli in caisson disease)

49. **What is the clinical presentation of osteonecrosis?**
    Clinical symptoms depend on the location of the infarct. Subchondral and subperiosteal foci of osteonecrosis cause pain and may lead to fracture of the affected bone. The subperiosteal necrotic bone is replaced by newly formed bone spicules, a process called creeping substitution. Subchondral bone heals slowly, and the cartilage overlying the necrotic bone may detach and float away into the joint space. These changes predispose to degenerative joint disease. Medullary infarcts are usually silent and discovered only accidentally during x-ray studies performed for some other reason.

OSTEOMYELITIS

50. **What is osteomyelitis?**
    Osteomyelitis is inflammation of bones, most often caused by bacteria. It evolves because of:
    - Direct implantation of bacteria into the bone by trauma, penetrating wounds, or surgery
    - Hematogenous spread from some other site of infection and during sepsis (Drug addicts are prone to hematogenous osteomyelitis. Aseptic [avascular] foci of osteonecrosis may become infected, most often in children suffering from sickle cell anemia.)
    - Local extension from infected joints or adjacent soft tissues (the least common form of infection)
    - Spread of dental infection (Infections of the mandible or maxilla, usually in the form of a periodontal abscess, are a common form of osteomyelitis.)

51. **List the most common causes of osteomyelitis.**
    - *Staphylococcus aureus* is overall the most common cause of osteomyelitis. It is the most common cause of hematogenous osteomyelitis in children and adolescents and in postsurgical bone infections.
    - Mixed infection is typically found after trauma and penetrating bone wounds.
    - *Salmonella* infection is common in sickle cell anemia patients.
    - *Mycobacterium tuberculosis* infection may complicate pulmonary tuberculosis, but it is rare in the United States.

KEY POINTS: FRACTURES AND INFLAMMATION ✔

1. Most fractures are caused by trauma or stress, but some also occur because of endogenous pathologic changes in the bones (pathologic fractures).

2. Osteonecrosis may have many causes, but most often it is a consequence of ischemic infarction (also known as aseptic necrosis).

3. Inflammation of bones is most often caused by bacteria that reach the bones hematogenously or by direct implantation during trauma.

52. **Which bones are most often affected by osteomyelitis?**
    Any bone may become infected. If one excludes the dental infection of jaws and posttraumatic infections, the most commonly infected bones are the long bones of the extremities and the vertebrae.

53. **What is the pathogenesis of acute osteomyelitis?**
    Typical hematogenous infection starts most often in the metaphyseal portion of growing long bones. The bacteria enter the bone through the nutrient arteries and reach the highly vascularized growth plate, where they exit into the interstitial spaces. The infection site attracts neutrophils, and the entire area becomes edematous. Because of space limitation and the rigid structure of the bone, the exudates inside the bone cavity will compress the capillaries and

prevent the inflow of blood. This will cause ischemic necrosis of the infected bone and will facilitate the formation of an intraosseous abscess. The pus may spread through the Haversian canals or penetrate underneath the periosteum, which will further compromise the blood supply of the infected bone. A large abscess may develop, and the pus may spread into the adjacent soft tissue. Draining sinuses may form on the surface of the skin or into the articular cavity.

54. **What is the pathogenesis of chronic osteomyelitis?**
Chronic osteomyelitis results from incompletely healed or persistent suppurative acute infection. Lytic enzymes released from the inflammatory cells cut channels through the bone, leading to the formation of bone fragments that ultimately detach from the main bone mass. Such a piece of dead bone, called sequestrum, may float inside the abscess cavity. The wall of the abscess cavity is composed of newly formed bone, which is called involucrum. Sinus tracts draining the pus from the abscess to the surface of the body are called cloacae. Chronic bone abscess fully enclosed by sclerotic bone is called Brodie abscess.

55. **Name the most important complications of chronic osteomyelitis.**
   - **Deformities of bones:** For example, tuberculous spondylitis (osteomyelitis involving the vertebral column, also known as Pott disease) may result in a hunchback deformity.
   - **Pathologic fractures:** Damaged bones tend to fracture upon minimal impact.
   - **Systemic effects:** These include fever, fatigue, leukocytosis, and elevated erythrocyte sedimentation rate.
   - **Amyloidosis:** Like any other chronic suppuration, chronic osteomyelitis can stimulate the production of serum amyloid-associated protein (SAAP), which is then deposited in the kidneys, liver, blood vessels, and other sites typical of secondary amyloidosis.
   - **Squamous cell carcinoma:** The skin at the edges of the sinus tracts draining the pus from the infected bone may, over time, undergo malignant transformation.

BONE TUMORS

56. **How are bone tumors classified?**
As in any other organ, tumors are classified according to their biologic behavior as benign or malignant. Benign tumors are more common than malignant ones. Many benign tumors are small and asymptomatic (e.g., osteochondroma) and are not even recognized clinically. Malignant tumors can be primary or metastatic. Metastases to the bones are more common than primary malignant tumors. According to their cell of origin and histologic features, primary bone tumors can be classified as being composed of:
   - Bone-forming cells (e.g., osteoma, osteoblastoma, and osteosarcoma)
   - Cartilage-forming cells (e.g., chordoma and chondrosarcoma)
   - Osteoclastic cells (e.g., giant cell tumor)
   - Fibroblastic cells (e.g., fibrosarcoma and malignant fibrous histiocytoma)
   - Undifferentiated cells (e.g., Ewing sarcoma)
   - Hematopoietic and lymphoid cells (e.g., multiple myeloma, leukemia, and lymphoma)

57. **How are bone tumors diagnosed?**
Most bone tumors are diagnosed on the basis of local symptoms that they produce, such as pain due to compression of nerves or swelling of the extremities. Further workup of the patient is performed by a diagnostic team, which includes an orthopedic surgeon, a radiologist, and a pathologist. Accordingly, all bone tumors are diagnosed only by correlating the following:
   - Clinical data, such as age, sex of the patient, family history, previous diseases, and location of the tumor
   - X-ray findings, indicating whether the tumor is most likely benign or malignant
   - Histopathologic data, essential for diagnosing the tumor as benign or malignant and for further classifying the tumor as bone-forming, cartilaginous, or other

58. Name the most important data for the diagnosis of bone tumors.
- **Age:** Most bone tumors show an age-dependent occurrence. For example, osteosarcomas and Ewing sarcomas are tumors of childhood and adolescence, whereas chondrosarcoma usually occurs after 40 years of age.
- **Anatomic site:** For example, osteosarcomas occur predominantly in the long bones of the extremities, whereas chondrosarcomas tend to involve the axial skeleton of the body (i.e., the bones of the pelvis, shoulder, and vertebrae).
- **Part of the bone involved by the tumor:** For example, osteosarcomas tend to occur in the metaphysis of long bones, whereas Ewing sarcoma involves the diaphysis. See Fig. 20-2.

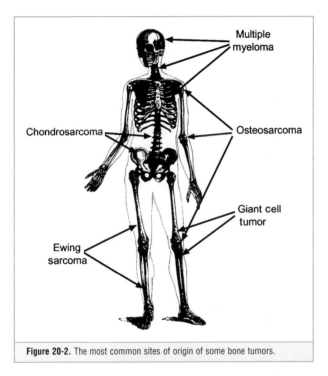

Figure 20-2. The most common sites of origin of some bone tumors.

KEY POINTS: BONE TUMORS

1. Osteosarcoma, the most common bone tumor in children and young people, typically originates from the metaphysis of long bones.

2. Chondrosarcoma, the most common malignant bone tumor of adults, occurs mostly in the axial skeleton.

3. Ewing's sarcoma, a tumor of undifferentiated medullary cells, typically develops in the diaphysis of long bones of young people.

59. **Which tumors occur most often in the epiphysis of long bones?**
Epiphysis of long bones is the most common site of origin of giant cell tumors of bone.

60. **Which tumors occur most often in the metaphysis of long bones?**
Osteosarcoma is the most common malignant tumor of the metaphysis of long bones. Nonossifying fibroma is the most common benign tumor in this location. Other bone-forming and cartilaginous benign tumors can also occur but are less common.

61. **Name the types of tumors that occur most often in the diaphysis of long bones.**
Ewing sarcoma is the most common tumor of the diaphysis of long bones in children. Malignant diaphyseal tumors in adults are most often metastases from some other primary site.

62. **Which tumors occur most often in the short bones of the hands and feet?**
Enchondromas are the most common bone tumors in these locations. Typically they are diagnosed in 20- to 50-year-old men, who are more often affected than women. Enchondromas can easily be removed surgically, but some recur. Multiple enchondromas may occur in some familial syndromes, such as Ollier disease (enchondromatosis, typically one sided) or Mafucci syndrome (associated with multiple hemangiomas). Multiple enchondromas are at risk of becoming malignant, in contrast to solitary enchondromas of small bones, which undergo malignant transformation only exceptionally.

63. **What is the most common benign tumor of bones?**
Osteochondroma, a small outgrowth of bone capped with cartilage, is the most common benign tumor. Because many of these tumors remain clinically undetected, their exact incidence is not known.

   Also known as exostosis, this benign tumor usually presents as mushroom-shaped outgrowths on the lateral sides of the metaphysis of long bones. Most often, they are located around the knee joints of young adults. Although they start growing in childhood, it is only in late adolescence that they reach a size at which they become clinically apparent. Such lesions present as slow-growing "bumps" that may become painful because of nerve compression or fracture.

64. **Define osteomas.**
Osteomas are solitary benign bone tumors of the head bones. Most of them are actually developmental abnormalities rather than tumors. These tumors grow slowly and rarely produce symptoms. Histologically, they are indistinguishable from normal bone. Osteomas are associated with colonic polyps in familial Gardner syndrome.

65. **What kind of lesions are nonossifying fibromas?**
Nonossifying fibromas are benign fibroblastic tumors originating in the subperiosteal cortex of the metaphysis of long bones, typically the distal femur and proximal tibia. These tumors originate in cortical fibrous defects, which are developmental defects found by x ray in at least 30% to 40% of children. Most ossifying fibromas are diagnosed radiologically in adolescents or young adults and can be cured by curettage.

66. **Name the main risk factors for osteosarcoma.**
Most osteosarcomas develop in people who have no known predisposing conditions. In a minority of cases (referred to as secondary osteosarcomas), there are identifiable risk factors, such as:
- **Retinoblastoma (Rb-1) gene mutation or deletion:** Osteosarcomas develop at an increased rate in adolescents who had retinoblastoma as infants or young children.
- **Radiation therapy or exposure to radioactive isotopes:** The best known example is the epidemic of osteosarcomas that occurred in the early 20th century in women who

painted the dials of watches with radioactive phosphorus. These women licked the brushes used for painting the dials, and the radioactive phosphorus from the paint accumulated in the jaw bones, causing osteosarcomas over time.

- **Paget disease:** Most osteosarcomas of old age develop in patients who have Paget disease. The reasons for this association are not known.

67. **List the most important facts about osteosarcomas.**
    - The most common primary bone tumor
    - Peak incidence in second decade of life
    - Occurs preferentially in the metaphysis of long bones of the extremities
    - Approximately 60% of cases found around the knee joint
    - Invades locally and metastasizes hematogenously to the lungs
    - Very malignant (Without therapy there is high mortality; combined chemotherapy with surgery is curative in 80% of childhood and adolescent tumors; old-age osteosarcomas have a less favorable response to therapy. See Fig. 20-3.)

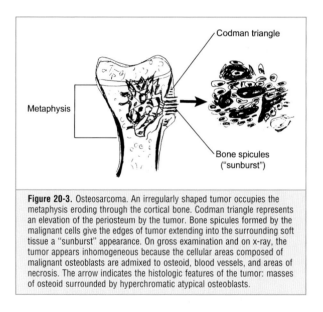

Figure 20-3. Osteosarcoma. An irregularly shaped tumor occupies the metaphysis eroding through the cortical bone. Codman triangle represents an elevation of the periosteum by the tumor. Bone spicules formed by the malignant cells give the edges of tumor extending into the surrounding soft tissue a "sunburst" appearance. On gross examination and on x-ray, the tumor appears inhomogeneous because the cellular areas composed of malignant osteoblasts are admixed to osteoid, blood vessels, and areas of necrosis. The arrow indicates the histologic features of the tumor: masses of osteoid surrounded by hyperchromatic atypical osteoblasts.

68. **Name the salient pathologic features of osteosarcoma.**
    - Tumor originates inside the metaphysis, expanding the bone. It infiltrates the cortex and the medullary cavity but usually does not cross the epiphysial cartilage plate and does not extend into the joint cavity.
    - The tumor may lift up the periosteum, producing the so-called Codman triangle, which is visible on x-ray.
    - The tumor forms bone spicules that are visible on x-ray ("sunburst appearance") and give the tumor a gritty texture on sectioning.
    - Microscopically, the tumor is composed of neoplastic osteoblasts, which form osteoid or calcified bone spicules.
    - Other mesenchymal elements may be present, such as fibroblasts, chondroblasts, and numerous blood vessels.

- Several microscopic subtypes are recognized, such as classical osteosarcoma, chondroblastic, fibroblastic, telangiectatic, and others, but histologic subtyping is of no clinical significance.

69. **List the most important facts about chondrosarcoma.**
    - It is the second most common primary malignant bone tumor.
    - Its peak incidence in the 40- to 60-year-old age group.
    - It involves the axial skeleton—pelvis, vertebra, shoulder, and proximal parts of the femur and radius.
    - Most tumors develop de novo, but some occur in preexisting enchondromas and may be familial.
    - Chondrosarcomas are slower-growing tumors than osteosarcomas. Untreated tumors generally have a better prognosis than osteosarcomas. Chondrosarcomas do not respond well to chemotherapy.
    - Prognosis depends on the resectability of the tumor, its histologic grade, and the presence or absence of hematogenous metastases.
    - Five-year survival is as follows: Grade I tumors, up to 90%; Grade III tumors, 40%. See Fig. 20-4.

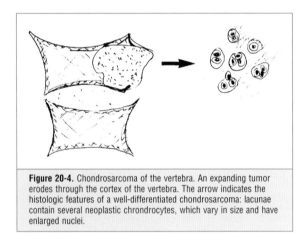

Figure 20-4. Chondrosarcoma of the vertebra. An expanding tumor erodes through the cortex of the vertebra. The arrow indicates the histologic features of a well-differentiated chondrosarcoma: lacunae contain several neoplastic chrondrocytes, which vary in size and have enlarged nuclei.

70. **What are the salient pathologic features of chondrosarcoma?**
    - Cartilage-forming tumors develop in the medullary cavity, expanding and eroding the cortical bone.
    - On gross examination, cartilage appears white, glistening, and gritty.
    - Microscopically, it is composed of cells lying inside the lacunae surrounded by cartilaginous matrix.
    - Tumors are histologically graded (I–III), depending on the degree of differentiation. Grade I tumors resemble normal cartilage, whereas Grade III tumors are anaplastic.

71. **What is Ewing sarcoma?**
    Ewing sarcoma is a tumor composed of undifferentiated primitive cells of uncertain histogenesis. It is thought to develop from primitive mesenchymal cells in the bone marrow of long bones, but it can also occur in extraskeletal sites. It is thought to be related to the primitive neuroectodermal tumors of soft tissues, which show the same chromosomal abnormalities as the Ewing tumor.

72. **List the most important facts about Ewing sarcoma.**
    - It is the second most common tumor of bones in children and adolescents (after osteosarcoma).
    - Its peak incidence in the 5- to 20-year-old age group.
    - It is most often located in the diaphysis of long bones of extremities, but it may involve ribs and pelvic bones as well.
    - It may metastasize early to other bones and thus appear multifocal.
    - Metastases to the lungs, liver, brain, and other organs are common.
    - In the past, prognosis was dismal, but with chemotherapy 75% of children survive 5 years.

73. **What are the salient pathologic features of Ewing sarcoma?**
    - Tumor originates in the medullary portion of the diaphysis of long bones. Tumor cells penetrate into the cortical bone, raising the periosteum. The periosteum forms new bone in a typical concentric manner, giving the bone an "onion-skin" appearance on x-ray.
    - Histologically the tumor is composed of solid sheets of small blue cells (i.e., cells that have a nucleus surrounded by scant cytoplasm and therefore appear blue in routine histologic sections).
    - Tumor cells contain glycogen in their cytoplasm, like many other embryonic primitive cells. Therefore, tumor cells stain with PAS stain.
    - Diagnostic chromosomal translocation (11;22) (q24;q12) is found in essentially all tumors and is an important diagnostic finding. See Fig. 20-5.

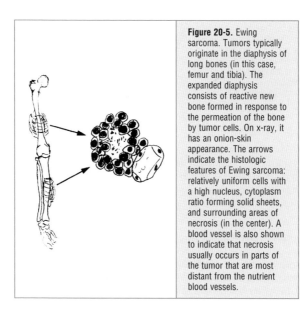

Figure 20-5. Ewing sarcoma. Tumors typically originate in the diaphysis of long bones (in this case, femur and tibia). The expanded diaphysis consists of reactive new bone formed in response to the permeation of the bone by tumor cells. On x-ray, it has an onion-skin appearance. The arrows indicate the histologic features of Ewing sarcoma: relatively uniform cells with a high nucleus, cytoplasm ratio forming solid sheets, and surrounding areas of necrosis (in the center). A blood vessel is also shown to indicate that necrosis usually occurs in parts of the tumor that are most distant from the nutrient blood vessels.

74. **Which other "small blue tumors" should be considered in the differential diagnosis of Ewing sarcoma?**
Other small blue cell tumors that may involve the bones of children and adolescents are neuroblastoma, malignant lymphomas, rhabdomyosarcoma, and osteosarcoma. These tumors usually can be distinguished from Ewing sarcoma by means of immunohistochemistry. Chromosomal studies may also be useful because Ewing sarcoma has diagnostic chromosomal features.

75. **Define giant cell tumor of bones.**
Giant cell tumor of bones (Fig. 20-6) is a benign tumor composed of spindle-shaped mononuclear cells resembling fibroblasts and multinucleated giant cells resembling osteoclasts. The salient features of these tumors are as follows:
- They account for 20% of all bone tumors.
- Peak incidence is in the 20- to 40-year-old age group.
- Located in the epiphysis of long bones, mostly around the knee joint.
- Radiologically, the tumor appears as a benign expansile mass.
- Most tumors are benign but tend to recur if incompletely removed by curettage. Occasionally, sarcomatous transformation may occur.

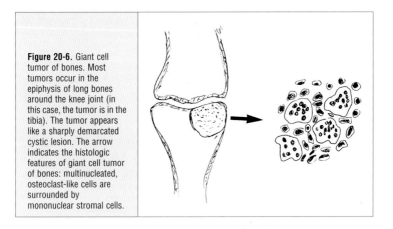

Figure 20-6. Giant cell tumor of bones. Most tumors occur in the epiphysis of long bones around the knee joint (in this case, the tumor is in the tibia). The tumor appears like a sharply demarcated cystic lesion. The arrow indicates the histologic features of giant cell tumor of bones: multinucleated, osteoclast-like cells are surrounded by mononuclear stromal cells.

76. **Which tumors metastasize most frequently to the bones?**
The most common malignant tumors metastasizing to the bones of adults are carcinomas of the prostate, breast, lung, kidney, gastrointestinal tract, and thyroid. Neuroblastoma of Infancy and childhood commonly metastasizes to the bones.

77. **Which primary bone malignancy presents radiologically with multiple punched-out lesions in adults?**
Multiple myeloma typically presents with multiple lytic lesions. The lesions are most prominent in the skull bone, ribs, and vertebrae (i.e., bones that contain hematopoietic bone marrow). Malignant tumors, such as breast or prostate cancer, spread to bones and may cause multiple lytic lesions. Multiple lytic lesions of bones in children may be a feature of neuroblastoma or Ewing sarcoma.

JOINT DISEASES

78. **Name the most important joint diseases.**
Almost all joint diseases (arthropathies) are associated with some inflammation and are therefore called arthritis. Arthritides are pathogenetically classified as:
   - Infectious (e.g., arthritis of Lyme disease and gonococcal arthritis)
   - Autoimmune (e.g., rheumatic arthritis)
   - Degenerative (e.g., osteoarthritis)
   - Metabolic (e.g., gout)
   Malignant tumors of joints are rare and of limited clinical significance. Apparently, these constantly moving parts of the body are not the best place for tumor cells to grow.

79. **Define osteoarthritis.**
Osteoarthritis, also called degenerative joint disease (DJD), is a chronic disease characterized by progressive degeneration, destruction, and loss of articular cartilage.
   It occurs in two forms:
   - **Primary DJD:** Occurs mostly in the elderly without an obvious cause
   - **Secondary DJD:** Affects joints damaged by another disease (e.g., mucopolysaccharidosis), congenital malformation (e.g., congenital subluxation of the hip), or trauma

80. **What are the most important facts about osteoarthritis?**
   - Very common disease
   - Age related (80% of all 80-year-old men and women have some signs of DJD)
   - More common in women than in men
   - Cause unknown in most cases
   - Progressive and often crippling

KEY POINTS: JOINT DISEASES ✓

1. Osteoarthritis, also known as degenerative joint disease, is a multifactorial disease affecting mostly older people.

2. Rheumatoid arthritis, a common systemic autoimmune disease of women, causes chronic inflammation and deformities of joints.

3. Gout is a common cause of metabolic arthropathy, most often presenting with painful swelling of the metatarsophalangeal joint of the great toe.

81. **What is the pathogenesis of osteoarthritis?**
The pathogenesis of osteoarthritis is not known. Hypothetical factors that may play a role include:
   - **Wear and tear of articular cartilage:** This hypothesis explains the high prevalence of DJD in the elderly, but unfortunately, DJD also occurs in younger people. Hence age-related wear and tear is not the only cause.
   - **Mechanical injury:** Weight-carrying joints are more often affected than other joints, and the disease is more prominent in people who abuse their joints. However, small joints of fingers are also affected, which shows that other factors must play a pathogenetic role.
   - **Metabolic injury of chondrocytes:** Research data point to abnormalities in the synthesis of proteoglycans and collagen type II and an increased release of lytic enzymes that may

damage or weaken the extracellular matrix of the joint cartilage. No definitive proof is available to support any of the proposed hypotheses.

82. **Name the joints most often affected by osteoarthritis.**
    - Large joints of lower extremities—knee and hip
    - Vertebral joints—lower cervical and lumbar joints
    - Distal and proximal interphalangeal joints (Note: Osteophytes in distal interphalangeal DJD cause Heberden nodes.)
    - First carpometacarpal joint
    - First tarsometatarsal joints

83. **What are the pathologic features of osteoarthritis?**
    The changes seen in the joints affected by osteoarthritis include (Fig. 20-7):
    - **Degenerative changes in the articular cartilage:** These changes include fraying, splitting, and cracking of the cartilage. Fragmented cartilage forms so-called joint mice, which may float freely in the articular cavity.
    - **Ulceration of the cartilage:** Loss of cartilage exposes the underlying bone to undue pressure and rubbing with the joint surface on the opposing side.
    - **Subchondral sclerosis:** The constant pressure on the bone denuded of cartilage leads to sclerosis. This process is called eburnation because the thickened bone resembles ivory.
    - **Subchondral cysts:** Degenerative changes in the stressed bone often become cystic.
    - **Osteophytes:** These spurs form from reactive new bone, project on the lateral sides of the joint, and mechanically irritate the adjacent soft tissues.

    These pathologic changes can be recognized on x-ray and are important for the radiologic diagnosis of osteoarthritis.

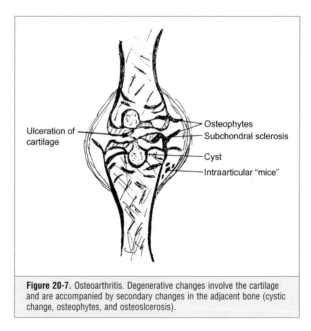

Ulceration of cartilage

Osteophytes
Subchondral sclerosis
Cyst
Intraarticular "mice"

Figure 20-7. Osteoarthritis. Degenerative changes involve the cartilage and are accompanied by secondary changes in the adjacent bone (cystic change, osteophytes, and osteosclerosis).

84. **List the most common clinical features of osteoarthritis.**
    - Pain, dull and deep seated; it can be aggravated by movement
    - Stiffness of joints, most prominent in the morning or after resting
    - Crepitus, a sound elicited by the opposing joint surfaces; found in advanced cases only
    - Swelling and effusion, which may not be prominent
    - Heberden nodes involving the finger joints

85. **What is rheumatoid arthritis?**
    Rheumatoid arthritis (RA) is a chronic systemic disease of unknown etiology causing inflammation of diarthrodial joints. In addition to arthritis, it may present with a number of extraarticular disorders. It affects 1% or 2% of the total adult population and is more common among women than men by a ratio of 3:1.

86. **Explain the pathogenesis of RA.**
    The pathogenesis of RA is not known. Available data indicate that it is immune mediated and that it develops in people with a genetic predisposition.

87. **Does RA have a genetic basis?**
    - RA has a tendency to occur in families, but a distinct pattern of inheritance has not been identified.
    - Monozygotic twins show a 30% concordance for RA.
    - More than 70% of patients have a specific pentapeptide sequence motif in the human leukocyte antigen (HLA)-II region (HLA-DRB1 gene), suggesting a genetic predisposition.

88. **Is RA associated with any disorders of humoral or cellular immunity?**
    There is evidence for both abnormal humoral and cell-mediated immunity:
    - Many patients with RA have autoreactive antibodies. These antibodies [usually IgM], which react with the Fc component of the IgG, can be detected in the blood as rheumatoid factor in approximately 75% of patients with RA.
    - Approximately 25% of patients have antinuclear antibodies (ANAs).
    - Synovial tissue of inflamed joint is infiltrated with plasma cells that secrete antibodies into the synovial fluid.
    - Synovial tissue contains activated oligoclonal T-helper lymphocytes and secretes cytokines. Cytokines such as tumor necrosis factor and IL-1 stimulate the proliferation of synovial lining cells and promote resorption of cartilage.
    - Macrophages in the inflamed joint tissue collaborate with the T lymphocytes. Macrophages also secrete cytokines. Lytic enzymes released from macrophages destroy cartilage and promote inflammation.

89. **Is rheumatoid factor diagnostic of RA?**
    No. Rheumatoid factor is found in only 75% of patients with RA. Furthermore, it may be present in the serum of patients who do not have RA. Rheumatoid factor has been associated with systemic lupus erythematosus, Sjögren syndrome, and various infectious diseases, such as infectious mononucleosis, viral hepatitis, and malaria tuberculosis.

90. **Name the joints most often affected by RA.**
    RA may affect any joint. Joints are usually affected symmetrically and appear swollen, tender, and warm. Small hand joints, especially proximal interphalangeal and metacarpophalangeal joints, are often involved. Foot joints, especially the metatarsophalangeal joint, wrists, elbows, and ankles are also often involved.

91. **What are the pathologic features of RA?**
    RA is associated with intraarticular inflammation characterized by the formation of copious granulation tissue interposing itself between the joint surfaces. This granulation tissue is called pannus (meaning "cloak" in Latin). All the other pathologic findings are secondary to this inflammation.

For the sake of completeness, the following is a list of typical pathologic findings in a joint affected by RA:

- **Chronic inflammation of the synovium:** The synovial folds are hyperplastic and infiltrated with B and T lymphocytes, macrophages, and plasma cells. Numerous newly formed blood vessels are present. Lymphocytes may aggregate into lymphoid follicles (Allison–Ghormley bodies).
- **Exudation of cells, fluid, and fibrin into the articular cavity:** Fibrin may aggregate into small bodies ("rice bodies"). Inflammatory cells are mostly neutrophils, but in prolonged inflammation, lymphocytes account for 50% of all cells.
- **Erosion of cartilage:** The inflammatory cells and cytokines or enzymes released from them destroy the cartilage and expose the underlying bone. Because of the loss of the cartilage, the joint space appears narrower on x-ray.
- **Periarticular osteoporosis:** Interleukins, prostaglandins, and other products of inflammatory cells stimulate osteoclasts and promote bone loss. Distinct periarticular osteoporosis can be recognized on x-ray.
- **Ankylosis:** The pannus interposed between the two articular surfaces erodes the bone. At the same time, the granulation tissue "matures" and becomes more fibrotic. After some time, the pannus may transform into a collagenous scar that limits the mobility of the joint. Bony ankylosis is found in some cases.
- **Deformities of joints:** Because of contraction of the scarred joint capsule, long-lasting RA leads to typical joint deformities. These are clinically known as "opera-glass deformity" (because of ulnar deviation of the fingers).

See Fig. 20-8.

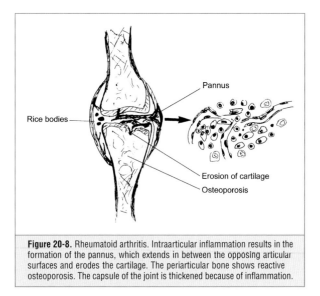

Figure 20-8. Rheumatoid arthritis. Intraarticular inflammation results in the formation of the pannus, which extends in between the opposing articular surfaces and erodes the cartilage. The periarticular bone shows reactive osteoporosis. The capsule of the joint is thickened because of inflammation.

92. **What are the extraarticular lesions of RA?**

Extraarticular manifestations of RA include:

- Subcutaneous rheumatoid nodules
- Lymphadenopathy and splenomegaly
- Anemia

- Dry mouth and dry eyes (secondary Sjögren syndrome)
- Pneumonitis with interstitial fibrosis and nodules
- Pericarditis
- Uveitis and scleritis

93. **Explain what rheumatoid nodules are.**
Rheumatoid nodules develop in 30% patients with RA. These nodules are located most often on the extensor side of the forearm. Histologically, in the center of the nodules is fibrinoid necrosis of collagen surrounded by palisading macrophages and lymphocytes. Rheumatoid nodules are not diagnostic of RA and may be found in other diseases, such as granuloma annulare.

94. **How is RA diagnosed clinically?**
The American Rheumatism Association has formulated criteria for diagnosing RA. See Table 20-2.

TABLE 20-2. REVISED CRITERIA FOR CLASSIFICATION OF RHEUMATOID ARTHRITIS (1987)
Any four of the following findings must be present
Symptoms lasting at least 6 months
Morning stiffness for more than 1 hour
Arthritis involving three or more joints
Arthritis of hand joints
Symmetric arthritis
Rheumatoid nodules
Rheumatoid factor in serum
Radiographic changes typical of rheumatoid arthritis
Modified from Arnett FC, et al: The American Rheumatism Association 1987 revised criteria for classification of rheumatoid arthritis. Arth Rheum 31:315–324, 1988.

95. **List the differences between RA and osteoarthritis.**
See Table 20-3.

TABLE 20-3. MAJOR DIFFERENCES BETWEEN RHEUMATOID ARTHRITIS AND OSTEOARTHRITIS		
	Rheumatoid Arthritis	**Osteoarthritis**
Pathogenesis	Inflammatory (possibly immune)	Degenerative (possibly wear and tear)
Age, peak (years)	30–40	60–80
Sex	Female:male = 3:1	Male = female
Joint involvement	Symmetric	Asymmetric
Preferential sites	Small joints of hand (pannus)	Weight-bearing joints (degeneration of cartilage)

(Continued)

TABLE 20-3. MAJOR DIFFERENCES BETWEEN RHEUMATOID ARTHRITIS AND OSTEOARTHRITIS (CONTINUED)		
	Rheumatoid Arthritis	**Osteoarthritis**
Pathology		
Joint	Ankylosis	Osteoporosis
Bone	Osteosclerosis	Ostoophytoc
Extraarticular	Rheumatoid nodules	No
Internal organs	Yes	No
Systemic findings	Yes	No

96. **What is juvenile RA ?**

Juvenile RA (JRA) is used for a variant of RA that begins before the age of 16 years. In most instances, it is seronegative (i.e., there is no rheumatoid factor [RF]). Complete remission can be induced in up to 75% of patients. It may present in three forms:
- JRA with systemic onset (also known as Still disease) is found in 20% of patients. This disease typically begins with fever, rash, generalized lymphadenopathy and splenomegaly, leukocytosis, and thrombocytosis.
- JRA with pauciarticular onset, found in 40% of cases, typically affects girls. It is ANA positive and often associated with iridocyclitis.
- JRA with polyarticular onset, found in 40% of cases, resembles adult RA. RF is positive in a minority of these patients, but they have a worse prognosis than others.

97. **What is spondyloarthropathy?**

Spondyloarthropathy is a term used for diseases that involve the joints of the vertebral column. Previously, these diseases were considered to be variants of RA, but now it is known that they are unique entities. This group includes ankylosing spondylitis, Reiter syndrome, psoriatic arthritis, and arthritis associated with inflammatory bowel diseases. In addition to the fact that all of these diseases involve the vertebral joints and the sacrum, they have some common features:
- Seronegativity (no RF or ANAs)
- Association with some class I major histocompatibility antigens (e.g., HLA-27)
- Early onset (i.e., affecting younger people)
- Asymmetry in involvement of diarthrodial joints

98. **What is ankylosing spondylitis?**
- Seronegative arthropathy preferentially involving the vertebral column and the sacrum.
- It affects mostly men (male-to-female ratio, 3:1); symptoms begin appearing in the 20- to 40-year-old age group.
- More than 90% of all patients have HLA-B27.
- Destruction of joints leads to fusion of vertebrae ("bamboo spine" on x-ray).
- Limited chest expansion (because of the costovertebral joint involvement) and back pain relieved by activity are early signs. A typical bent-over posture develops over time.
- Peripheral joint involvement is asymmetrical.
- Systemic symptoms found in 30% of patients include ocular, neurologic, cardiovascular, and pulmonary findings.

99. **What is Reiter syndrome?**
This syndrome includes a clinical triad:
- Seronegative arthritis
- Urethritis
- Conjunctivitis

The disease usually develops in HLA-B27-positive people (60%–90%) after an acute infection. Such infections are classified as sexually transmitted or dysenteric. Reiter syndrome preceded by a sexually transmitted disease usually occurs in 20- to 40-year-old men and is thought to be a complication of *Chlamydia trachomatis* infection. Enteric infections that precede Reiter syndrome may be caused by a variety of bacteria.

100. **What are the common forms of infectious arthritis?**
Infectious arthritis may evolve because of the extension of infections from adjacent structures (bone and soft tissues) or hematogenous spread. The latter route of infection is much more common. The most important examples are:
- Arthritis of Lyme disease: Infection with *Borrelia burgdorferi,* transmitted by ticks such as *Ixodes dammini,* typically presents in the first stage with skin lesions. In the second stage, there may be involvement of the heart and central nervous system, and amigratory arthritis may develop. In approximately 10% of patients, chronic arthritis develops, typically involving the knee joints. Histologically, the synovium of these inflamed joints shows perivascular infiltrates of lymphocytes and plasma cells, as in syphilis. Silver stain may be used to demonstrate the spirochetes in the tissue.
- Gonococcal arthritis follows genital infections.
- Suppurative arthritis caused by staphylococci or mixed bacteria may be encountered in immunosuppressed drug addicts prone to septicemia.

101. **What is pigmented villonodular synovitis?**
Villous outgrowth of intraarticular synovial fronds is considered by some to be a reactive change and a benign neoplasm by others. These exuberant fronds filling the joint cavity consist of proliferating synovial lining cells, fibroblasts, angioblasts, and hemosiderin-laden macrophages, which impart a brownish color to the lesion.
The knee joint is involved in 80% of cases.

102. **What is gout?**
Gout is a metabolic disease characterized by hyperuricemia (>7 mg/dL) and deposition of urate crystals in various sites, most often joints, subcutaneous soft tissues, and kidneys.

103. **What is the difference between primary and secondary gout?**
Primary gout is idiopathic (i.e., unrelated to a known cause or disease). It accounts for 90% of all cases of gout. Hyperuricemia results most often from an impaired urinary excretion of urates and less often because of overproduction.
Secondary gout is a complication of other diseases or their treatment. Hyperuricemia can occur because of:
- Overproduction of uric acid from nucleic acids: This typically occurs following chemotherapy, when massive tumor-cell killing is associated with a release of DNA and RNA, which are catabolized to uric acid. Conditions characterized by cellular hyperproliferation such as psoriasis also predispose to gout.
- Underexcretion of uric acid in the kidneys, as seen in patients who have end-stage kidney disease: Renal toxicity of lead accounts for saturnine gout, which is also related to underexcretion of uric acid.

104. **What is the pathogenesis of joint disease in gout?**
Deposition of urate crystals in the joints may cause an acute or chronic inflammation of the affected joint. The disease may be monoarticular or polyarticular. Acute attacks of gout arthropathy begin with the deposition of insoluble uric acid crystals in tissues. These crystals activate complement, which generates chemotactic fragments, attracting neutrophils into the area.
   Chronic gout arthropathy results from massive aggregates of uric acids, which form nodular masses protruding into the joint and eroding the joint surfaces of the bones (chronic tophaceous gout).

105. **Name the joints most often affected in gout.**
The metatarsophalangeal joint of the great toe is the most often involved joint, accounting for the term podagra ("foot-trap"), by which gout was once known. Ankle, knee, wrist, and elbow are also often involved.

106. **What are the histopathologic features of a tophus?**
Tophus consists of aggregates of uric acid crystals, which typically elicit a foreign body reaction with numerous multinucleated giant cells and mononuclear histiocytes surrounding the crystals. In properly fixed tissue (i.e., in 100% alcohol because uric acids are eluted from tissues by water-containing fixative, such as formalin), the uric acid crystals appear birefringent under polarized light.

107. **Do tophi occur only in the joints?**
No. Tophi occur most often in the subperiosteal parts of the bones, but they may occur in many other tissues as well. Clinically, the bone lesions must reach a size of 5 mm to be recognized on x-ray. The subcutaneous nodules are usually found overlying the joints or on the ear lobe. Large multiple tophi are sometimes seen deforming the fingers and the metacarpophalangeal joints.

108. **List the most important clinical facts about gout.**
   - It is a common disease inherited as a multifactorial trait. 20% patients have a family history of gout.
   - Males are affected preferentially (male-to-female ratio, 9:1).
   - Its onset is in the 20- to 40-year-old age group.
   - Monoarthritis is more common than polyarthritis.
   - Attacks tend to recur at unpredictable times. The intervals between the attacks (called intercritical intervals) are often long but tend to become shorter as the disease progresses.
   - Renal calculi represent the most important extrarticular complication (found in 10% of cases).
   - End-stage renal disease was a common cause of death in the past, but with modern treatment it has become less common.

109. **What are the risk factors for gout?**
Hyperuricemia is found in approximately 15% of all adults, but only 10% of these develop attacks of gout. The disease is obviously multifactorial and has a hereditary basis, but some preventable and treatable factors may influence its occurrence and precipitate the attacks. These risk factors include the following:
   - Obesity and hyperlipidemia in general
   - Hypertension
   - Alcoholism
   - Drugs, such as diuretics (e.g., thiazides), cyclosporine, ethambutol, and so on.

110. **Describe pseudogout.**

Pseudogout, also known as chondrocalcinosis, is a common joint disease caused by deposition of calcium pyrophosphate dihydrate (CPPD) crystals. Most often, it is asymptomatic, but it may simulate gout and osteoarthritis.

X-ray signs of pseudogout may be seen in 5% of 70 year olds and in more than 50% of those older than 90 years of age. However, only a minority of these people will develop signs of arthritis, which may resemble gout or osteoarthritis.

Diagnosis is made by finding linear calcifications in the articular cartilage and by identifying CPPD crystals in the joint fluid. These crystals are rod shaped or rhomboid and are birefringent under polarizing light.

111. **Which other systemic diseases may affect joints?**

Joints are commonly involved in most autoimmune diseases, also known as connective tissue diseases, including the following:

- Systemic lupus erythematosus
- Polyarteritis nodosa
- Systemic sclerosis (scleroderma)
  A variety of other diseases can affect joints, such as:
- Sickle cell anemia
- Hemophilia (hemarthrosis)
- Acromegaly
- Hemochromatosis

WEBSITES

1. http://www.ncbi.nlm.nih.gov/entrez/query.fcgi?db=PubMed

2. http://www-medlib.med.utah.edu/WebPath/webpath.html#MENU

3. http://courses.washington.edu/bonephys/

4. http://www.nlm.nih.gov/medlineplus/osteoporosis.html

5. http://bonetumor.org/

BIBLIOGRAPHY

1. Akerstrom G, Hellman P: Primary hyperparathyroidism. Curr Opin Oncol 16:17, 2004.

2. Creamer P, Hochberg MC: Osteoarthritis. Lancet 350:503–509, 1997.

3. Dorfman HD, Czerniak B: Bone cancers. Cancer 75:203–210, 1995.

4. Kennedy JG, Frelinghuysen P, Hoang BH: Ewing sarcoma: current concepts in diagnosis and treatment. Curr Opin Pediatr 15:53–57, 2003.

5. Lane NE: Clinical practice. Osteoarthritis of the hip. N Engl J Med 357:1413–1421. 2007.

6. Learmonth ID, Young C, Rorabeck C: The operation of the century: total hip replacement. Lancet 370: 1508–1519, 2007.

7. Painter SE, Kleerekoper M, Camacho PM: Secondary osteoporosis: a review of the recent evidence. Endocr Pract 12:436–445, 2006.

8. Tak PP, Bresnihan B: The pathogenesis and prevention of joint damage in rheumatoid arthritis. Arth Rheum 43:2619–2633, 2000.

9. Watts NB: Focus on primary care: Postmenopausal osteoporosis. Obstet Gynecol Surv 55(Suppl 3):S49–S55, 2000.

10. Yaw KM: Pediatric bone tumors. Semin Surg Oncol 16:173–183, 1999.

CHAPTER 21

SKELETAL MUSCLES

Ivan Damjanov, MD, PhD

1. **Describe the basic structure of skeletal muscles.**

   The basic histologic component of all skeletal muscles is the skeletal muscle cells, also known as muscle fibers or myofibers. Myofibers are grouped into larger units called muscle fascicles, which are enveloped together by connective tissue (called epimysium) into anatomically recognized muscles. Epimysium extends internally between fascicles, forming septa that are called perimysium. Perimysium extends into still thinner strands, called endomysium, enveloping individual myofibers (muscle cells). The connective tissue skeleton attaches the muscles to the tendons and bones. It supports the muscles and contains the blood vessels and nerves.

2. **What is a neuromuscular motor unit?**

   A motor unit comprises the lower motor neuron located in the anterior horn of the spinal cord and the muscle fibers that it innervates. The size of each motor unit varies. In lower extremities, individual axons form numerous branches that innervate several hundred muscle fibers, whereas in the eye muscles, most motor units are composed of only 20 muscle cells.

3. **Explain how muscle fibers are classified.**

   Muscle fibers are classified as type I or type II, depending on their biochemical and functional properties. Type I fibers are also known as red or slow-twitch fibers, whereas type II fibers are known as white or fast-twitch fibers.

   In some animals, such as chickens, white and red fibers are grouped into individual skeletal muscles. White muscles of the breast are responsible for the fast movement of wings. The slow-twitch, red muscle fibers, used for prolonged (sustained) action, are found in the leg muscles. In human muscles, type I and type II muscles are not segregated into distinct anatomic muscles and are usually found intermixed in a checkerboard manner.

   Whether a muscle fiber will be of one or another type depends on the innervation the cells receive. Reinnervation can thus change one muscle fiber type into another.

4. **How can one recognize these two types of muscle fibers?**

   In routine hematoxylin and eosin (H&E)-stained microscopic sections, type I and type II muscle fibers cannot be distinguished from one another. However, these fibers can be identified by enzyme histochemical stains that differentiate type I and type II fibers. Type I fibers have numerous mitochondria and stain strongly with mitochondrial stains, whereas type II fibers contain fewer mitochondria and thus appear paler in these sections.

5. **How common are muscle diseases?**

   Cumulatively, skeletal muscles represent the largest organ in the body. Muscles are often traumatized or involved in various metabolic, autoimmune, and infectious diseases. In most cases, the underlying pathology of these secondary muscle diseases is not studied in greater detail and remains unknown. For example, there are no "hard data" about fibromyalgia, even though this disease is diagnosed daily by most family practitioners. Most people who have muscle aches during a bout of flu probably have a form of viral myositis, but few physicians will go to the trouble of proving it. These common diseases are not studied by pathologists, and because so little is known about them, medical students and residents can be assured that the pathology of these everyday diseases will not show up on medical school or board examinations.

6. **List the typical symptoms and signs of muscle diseases.**
   - Weakness or paralysis
   - Atrophy (i.e., muscle wasting)
   - Hypertrophy or pseudohypertrophy (typically caused by infiltration of muscles by fat cells)
   - Irregular contractions, spasms, or fasciculations (defined as irregular contractions of muscle fibers belonging to the same motor unit)
   - Pain and tenderness to palpation

7. **Explain how muscle diseases are classified etiologically.**
   Muscle diseases are classified according to their causation as:
   - Neurogenic (denervation atrophy; e.g., due to nerve transection)
   - Genetic (e.g., muscular dystrophies)
   - Metabolic (e.g., endocrine myopathies, as in hypothyroidism and Addison disease)
   - Toxic (e.g., heavy metals, drugs, and alcohol)
   - Immunologic (e.g., dermatomyositis or polymyositis, and myasthenia gravis)
   - Infectious (e.g., viral myopathy and muscle abscess)
   - Traumatic (e.g., rhabdomyolysis following crush injury)
   Another way to remember the causes of muscle diseases is the mnemonic *genetic*:
   Genetic
   Endocrine
   Neurogenic
   Ethanol (alcoholic)
   Toxic
   Inflammatory (immune and infectious)
   Crush injury (trauma)

8. **Is muscle biopsy the definitive approach to diagnosing muscle diseases?**
   Unfortunately not. Muscles have a limited capacity to respond to injury, and the changes seen in muscle biopsy specimens are often nonspecific. Accordingly, muscle biopsy findings can be meaningfully interpreted only in the context of other clinical and laboratory data.
   Muscle diseases are associated with three morphologic patterns, and the changes seen in the biopsied muscle often do not provide definitive answers about the causes of the disease. These three patterns are:
   - **Myopathic pattern:** The muscle fibers show signs of injury or necrosis usually associated with an inflammatory response and repair in the form of fibrosis and limited attempts at regeneration. These findings indicate that the primary site of injury is the muscle.
   - **Neuropathic pattern:** The muscle fibers show signs of atrophy caused by denervation. The muscle changes are obviously secondary to a nerve injury or diseases of the nervous system.
   - **Normal muscle histology:** The most important disease in which signs of muscle weakness are not associated with any microscopically visible changes in the muscle biopsy is myasthenia gravis. Some of the muscle diseases presenting on normal light microscopic findings will show ultrastructural changes visible by electron microscopy (e.g., mitochondrial myopathy).

9. **Name the clinical differences between primary myopathies and neurogenic muscle disease.**
   The differences between primary myopathies and neurogenic muscle diseases are not always obvious. Some of the most important clinical signs and symptoms favoring one or another of these diseases are given in Table 21-1.

TABLE 21-1. DIFFERENCES BETWEEN PRIMARY MYOPATHIES AND NEUROGENIC MUSCLE ATROPHY

	Muscle Disease	
Signs/Symptoms	Myopathy	Neurogenic Muscle Atrophy
Muscles involved	Proximal extremity	Distal extremity
Bilateral	Usually	Yes and no
Muscle appearance	Tender or painful	Not sensitive
	Swollen or normal	Atrophic
Cramps/fasciculations	No	May be present
		No loss of sensation ("glove and stocking" pattern)
Onset	Gradual	Often sudden
Systemic disease	Common	Usually not present
Electromyography	Yes	Yes
Creatine phosphokinase	Elevated	Normal
Antinuclear antibody	Often elevated	No

NEUROGENIC MUSCLE ATROPHY

10. **What could cause neurogenic muscle atrophy?**
    Denervation of muscle fibers could result from many injuries of the upper (cortical) or lower (spinal) motor neuron or their axons. Salient examples are given in Table 21-2.

TABLE 21-2. CAUSES OF NEUROGENIC MUSCLE ATROPHY

Location of Injury	Example
Upper (cortical) motor neuron	Apoplexy
Axon of the upper motor neuron	Spinal cord
Lower (spinal) motor neuron	Poliomyelitis, amyotrophic lateral sclerosis*
Axon of the lower motor neuron	Nerve transection, peripheral neuropathy
Axonal branches	Diabetes

*It can involve both the lower and the upper motor neurons.

11. **Define peripheral neuropathy.**
    The term peripheral neuropathy is used to describe a number of diseases of peripheral nerves that present with a loss of motor or sensory functions and are accordingly classified as

primary motor, primary sensory, or sensorimotor neuropathies. According to the involvement of nerves, clinicians distinguish three forms:

- **Polyneuropathy:** It is characterized by random involvement of numerous nerves, as typically seen in Guillain–Barré syndrome and other systemic diseases (e.g., diabetes).
- **Mononeuropathy:** It presents with single nerve involvement, as in carpal tunnel syndrome, in which the ulnar or radial nerves are compressed by the connective tissue in the carpal tunnel.
- **Mononeuritis multiplex:** It presents with involvement of several major nerves unrelated to each other, as in polyarteritis nodosa or leprosy.

12. **What are the causes of peripheral neuropathy?**
   In the United States, the most common cause of peripheral polyneuropathy is diabetes mellitus. Diabetes is a microangiopathy, so the lesions are caused in part by ischemia and in part by the metabolic changes that affect axons and myelin sheaths. Alcohol (ethanol) is another common cause of neuropathy. Nerve biopsy is often used to determine the cause of neuropathy and to prescribe treatment.

   To remember that diabetes is the most common cause of peripheral neuropathy and to make other possible causes of this ailment easier to remember, use the mnemonic *diabetic*:
   Diabetes
   Immune disorders (Guillain–Barré syndrome, polyarteritis nodosa, and amyloidosis)
   Alcohol
   B vitamin deficiencies (e.g., beri-beri [B1] and pellagra [B6 niacin])
   External pressure (e.g., carpal tunnel, Paget disease, osteophytes, and tumor)
   Therapeutic (toxins such as lead and hydrocarbon solvents [from glue sniffing]; drugs [such as nitrofurantoin, cisplatinum, and isoniazid])
   Infections (e.g., leprosy, diphtheria, and acquired immune deficiency disease)
   Congenital (e.g., Charcot–Marie–Tooth disease, Dejerine–Sottas disease, Refsum disease, etc.)

13. **Discuss the two typical microscopic patterns of neurogenic muscle atrophy.**
   - **Fascicular atrophy:** Loss of motor neurons in the cortex or spinal cord leads to atrophy of entire fascicles of skeletal muscle. Most commonly, this type of atrophy is seen in children and adolescents affected by spinal muscular atrophy, an autosomal recessive disease caused by mutations of a gene on chromosome 5. In adults, it may be caused by cortical or spinal cord lesions resulting from cardiovascular accident or traffic injuries. Amyotrophic lateral sclerosis and poliomyelitis cause similar changes.
   - **Single muscle fiber atrophy:** Atrophic muscle fibers, which appear angulated and compressed by surrounding normal muscle fibers, are distributed at random. They may be either type I or type II fibers. Atrophy of this type develops due to a loss of single axonal branches and is most often a complication of diabetes.
   These two types of muscle fiber atrophy are illustrated in Fig. 21-1.

14. **Is neurogenic muscle atrophy irreversible?**
   No. Regeneration of transected peripheral nerves can occur, and today it is common medical practice to surgically reconnect the proximal and distal parts of severed nerves. The distal part of the axon will initially degenerate (Wallerian degeneration), but the sprouting axonal branches from the proximal part will replace the damaged axons and reestablish contact with the muscle fibers. Such muscle will resume full function and over time will become as strong as the original muscle prior to the injury.

15. **Describe the histologic appearance of the reinnervated muscle.**
   The reinnervated muscle appears indistinguishable from normal muscle in routine H&E histologic sections. However, in freshly frozen tissue sectioned with a cryostat and stained with

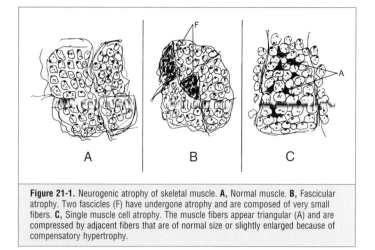

Figure 21-1. Neurogenic atrophy of skeletal muscle. **A,** Normal muscle. **B,** Fascicular atrophy. Two fascicles (F) have undergone atrophy and are composed of very small fibers. **C,** Single muscle cell atrophy. The muscle fibers appear triangular (A) and are compressed by adjacent fibers that are of normal size or slightly enlarged because of compensatory hypertrophy.

an enzymatic method for demonstrating oxidative enzymes, one will notice that the type I and type II muscle fibers are no longer distributed in a typical checkerboard pattern. Segregation or type-specific grouping of type I and type II muscle fibers is typical of reinnervated muscles. See Fig. 21-2.

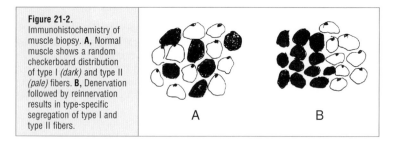

Figure 21-2. Immunohistochemistry of muscle biopsy. **A,** Normal muscle shows a random checkerboard distribution of type I *(dark)* and type II *(pale)* fibers. **B,** Denervation followed by reinnervation results in type-specific segregation of type I and type II fibers.

MUSCULAR DYSTROPHIES AND CONGENITAL MYOPATHIES

16. **What are muscular dystrophies?**
    Muscular dystrophies are a heterogeneous group of primary muscle diseases historically grouped together because they:
    - Have a genetic basis and occur in families
    - Show preferential involvement of certain muscle groups, as shown in Fig. 21-3
    - Have a consistent clinical presentation, such as age of onset and progression of muscle weakness

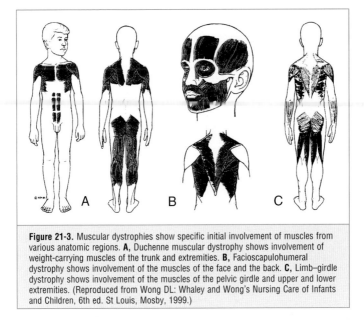

Figure 21-3. Muscular dystrophies show specific initial involvement of muscles from various anatomic regions. **A,** Duchenne muscular dystrophy shows involvement of weight-carrying muscles of the trunk and extremities. **B,** Facioscapulohumeral dystrophy shows involvement of the muscles of the face and the back. **C,** Limb–girdle dystrophy shows involvement of the muscles of the pelvic girdle and upper and lower extremities. (Reproduced from Wong DL: Whaley and Wong's Nursing Care of Infants and Children, 6th ed. St Louis, Mosby, 1999.)

17. **Name the most important forms of muscular dystrophy.**
    See Table 21-3.

TABLE 21-3. MUSCULAR DYSTROPHIES

Disease (Dystrophy)	Inheritance	Age of Onset (Years)	Distribution (Involved Muscles)
Duchenne type	XR	3–5	Generalized
Becker	XR	10–20	Generalized
Facioscapulohumeral	AD	10–30	Face, neck, shoulders
Oculopharyngeal	AD	30–40	Extraocular and pharyngeal
Limb–girdle	AR > AD	Variable	Limbs and trunk
Myotonic	AD	10–15	Face and extremities

AD, Autosomal dominant; *AR,* autosomal recessive; *XR,* X-linked recessive.

18. **What is the cause of Duchenne muscular dystrophy (DMD)?**
    DMD is an X-linked recessive disease caused by a mutation of the gene encoding dystrophin. The dystrophin gene is located on the X chromosome. In most instances, the gene mutation involves a deletion, but frameshift mutations and point mutations also occur.

19. **Describe the function of dystrophin.**
    Dystrophin is a cytoplasmic protein normally found in the skeletal muscle, heart muscle, and nerve cells. In muscle, it is located in the subsarcolemmal portion of the cytoplasm linking the contractile filaments to the cell membrane. It is involved in maintaining the cell structure of the myocytes and enabling them to contract. Muscle cells lacking dystrophin degenerate and die.

20. **What are the histopathologic features of DMD?**
    The muscle fibers lose their normal shape and disintegrate. The fragmented myofibrils are taken up by macrophages or replaced by fibrous tissue. There are also scattered reserve cells that try to replace the dead myofibrils. The remaining muscle fibers undergo hypertrophy. See Fig. 21-4.

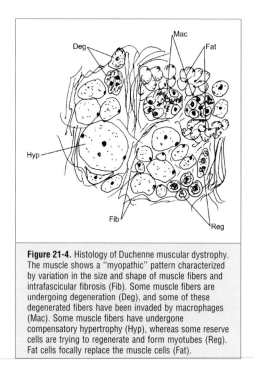

Figure 21-4. Histology of Duchenne muscular dystrophy. The muscle shows a "myopathic" pattern characterized by variation in the size and shape of muscle fibers and intrafascicular fibrosis (Fib). Some muscle fibers are undergoing degeneration (Deg), and some of these degenerated fibers have been invaded by macrophages (Mac). Some muscle fibers have undergone compensatory hypertrophy (Hyp), whereas some reserve cells are trying to regenerate and form myotubes (Reg). Fat cells focally replace the muscle cells (Fat).

21. **What is pseudohypertrophy?**
    Lost skeletal muscle cells are typically replaced in DMD by fibroblasts and adipocytes (fat cells). Copious fat cells may increase the size of such muscles, which may appear hypertrophic. Because this muscle enlargement is not true muscular hypertrophy, such muscles are soft on palpation and weak. Pseudohypertrophy most prominently involves calf muscles. See Fig. 21-5.

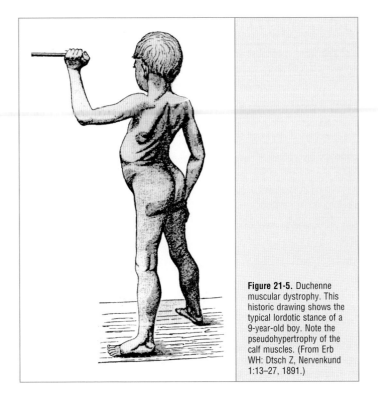

Figure 21-5. Duchenne muscular dystrophy. This historic drawing shows the typical lordotic stance of a 9-year-old boy. Note the pseudohypertrophy of the calf muscles. (From Erb WH: Dtsch Z, Nervenkund 1:13–27, 1891.)

22. **List the most important facts about DMD.**
   - X-linked recessive; hence, it affects only boys.
   - It begins in early childhood as weakness of pelvic and leg muscles (the child cannot get up from a sitting position and will use hands to "crawl up the body"). See Fig. 21-6.
   - It is rapidly progressive and invariably fatal.
   - Affected boys are wheelchair bound by school age, bed bound by puberty, and dead by 20 years of age.
   - Heart disease (cardiomyopathy) and slow mental development accompany the muscle disease.

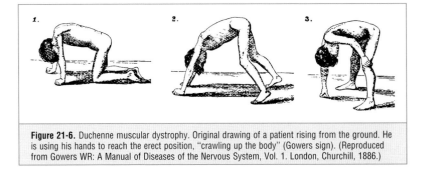

Figure 21-6. Duchenne muscular dystrophy. Original drawing of a patient rising from the ground. He is using his hands to reach the erect position, "crawling up the body" (Gowers sign). (Reproduced from Gowers WR: A Manual of Diseases of the Nervous System, Vol. 1. London, Churchill, 1886.)

KEY POINTS: DISEASES OF SKELETAL MUSCLES ✓

1. Loss of innervation may cause single muscle fiber atrophy or, if more pronounced, fascicular muscle atrophy.

2. Neurogenic atrophy is potentially reversible, as seen in reinnervation after surgical repair of transected nerves.

3. Muscular dystrophy and congenital myopathies are genetic diseases that may present with muscle weakness in childhood or later in adult life.

4. Inflammatory myopathies are usually immunologically mediated but may also be of viral, bacterial, and parasitic origin.

5. Myasthenia gravis results from the immunologic blockade of neural impulse transmission at the neuromuscular junction.

6. Tumors of the skeletal muscles are clinically grouped together with other soft tissue tumors.

23. **How is DMD diagnosed?**
    - Typical clinical presentation is in preschool-age boys.
    - Family history is positive in 70% of cases (30% are new mutations).
    - Creatine kinase (CK) is elevated in blood.
    - Muscle biopsy shows typical myopathic changes.
    - No dystrophin is seen in muscle biopsy tissue (by immunohistochemistry in slides or by Western blot on electrophoresed tissue extracts).

24. **Do carrier mothers of patients with DMD have any symptoms?**
    No, they are asymptomatic. However, 70% have elevated CK in blood, suggesting a subclinical (mild) muscle disease. The carrier gene can be detected in these women by means of molecular biology.

25. **Discuss the difference between DMD and Becker muscular dystrophy.**
    Becker dystrophy is a milder form of DMD, usually starting around puberty and not becoming lethal until late adulthood. Most patients live 40 to 50 years.
    Like DMD, Becker dystrophy is related to a mutation of the dystrophin gene. The mutation is milder, allowing the synthesis of dystrophin, which is of abnormal molecular weight. Dystrophin can be demonstrated immunohistochemically in some muscle fibers, but it is missing from most others.

26. **List the important autosomal muscular dystrophies.**
    This group of hereditary muscle diseases is too large to be memorized. It includes more than 200 genetic entities, most of which have been identified with the advent of molecular biology. Clinically, these rare diseases have been classified according to the distribution of involved muscles and named accordingly (e.g., facioscapulohumeral or limb–girdle dystrophies).
    Some of these dystrophies are inherited as autosomal dominant traits (e.g., facioscapulohumeral or oculopharyngeal muscular dystrophies); some are inherited as autosomal recessive (e.g., congenital muscular dystrophy due to laminin mutation). The largest and most heterogeneous group is made up of the limb–girdle dystrophies, which can be inherited as either autosomal dominant or autosomal recessive traits.

27. **What are sarcoglycans and dystroglycans?**
Sarcoglycans and dystroglycans are transmembrane proteins found in the plasma membrane of skeletal muscle cells. They form complexes linking the dystrophin with the pericellular matrix proteins (e.g., laminin). Mutations of genes encoding these proteins cause various dystrophies of the limb-girdle type.

28. **Define myotonic dystrophy.**
Myotonic dystrophy is an autosomal dominant disease caused by the mutation of myotonin protein kinase. The gene contains a triple nucleotide repeat, which is amplified in affected people and even more so in their offspring. The disease causes weakness and atrophy of muscles but involves other organs as well. Like other triple nucleotide repeat-related diseases, the severity of symptoms increases with every generation, and the symptoms appear earlier in life.

29. **Is the muscle biopsy useful in the diagnosis of myotonic dystrophy?**
Pathologically, the disease may present with myopathic changes, which are nonspecific or otherwise indistinguishable from those in other dystrophies. However, often the histologic changes are more characteristic and include an increased number of centrally located nuclei and ring fibers. Enzyme histochemistry may show selective atrophy of type I fibers.

30. **What are the clinical features of myotonic dystrophy?**
The disease usually begins in late childhood or adolescence with symptoms of abnormal gait or hand weakness. In adult patients, typical findings include the following:
- Atrophy and weakness of hand and foot muscles
- Facial muscle loss ("hatchet-man facial expression")
- Cataracts of early onset
- Frontal baldness
- Testicular atrophy
- Cardiomyopathy
- Glucose intolerance

31. **What are ion channel myopathies?**
This group of autosomal dominant muscle diseases (also known as "channelopathies") is related to mutations of genes that code the plasma membrane proteins, forming the channels for the transmembrane passage of sodium, potassium, calcium, and chloride ions. Clinically, these diseases present with periodic hypotonic paralysis or myotonia (inability to relax muscle after contraction).

32. **What are congenital myopathies?**
This group includes several muscle diseases, such as central core disease and nemaline myopathy, which are inherited as autosomal dominant or recessive traits. The underlying gene defect has been identified in many of these diseases. These diseases share certain common features, such as:
- Onset in infancy and childhood
- Generalized hypotonia and muscle weakness ("floppy child syndrome")
- Nonprogressive or slowly progressive course

33. **Name the inborn errors of metabolism that cause myopathies.**
Many inborn errors of metabolism cause myopathies, especially those involving the intermediary metabolism of lipids (e.g., carnitine palmitoyltransferase deficiency) and carbohydrates (e.g., deficiency of muscle phosphorylase in glycogenosis type V [McArdle disease]).

34. **What are mitochondrial myopathies?**
Mitochondrial myopathies are rare diseases involving the genes that code the respiratory enzymes located in the mitochondria. The abnormally large mitochondria can be seen on electron microscopy in the muscle biopsy. Mutations may involve the nuclear genes or

mitochondrial genes. Because the mitochondria are contributed at the time of fertilization by the maternal gamete (oocyte), mitochondrial myopathies encoded by mitochondrial genes are maternally transmitted. Myopathy is usually associated with other symptoms, usually pointing to central nervous system abnormalities. The best-known diseases in this group are:

- Myoclonic epilepsy with ragged red fibers
- Mitochondrial encephalopathy with lactic acidosis and strokelike episodes
- Leber hereditary optic neuropathy

INFLAMMATORY MYOPATHIES

35. **What is the most common cause of clinically important inflammatory myopathies?**
Most inflammatory myopathies encountered in clinical practice have an autoimmune pathogenesis. These diseases involve more than one group of muscles and are therefore called polymyositis. Polymyositis may present in several forms:
- Isolated muscle disease
- Part of an autoimmune systemic disease, such as systemic lupus erythematosus or Sjögren disease
- Part of dermatomyositis

36. **List the salient clinicopathologic features of polymyositis.**
- Gradual onset of proximal muscle weakness of arms and legs (e.g., while lifting objects or walking up stairs)
- Muscle pain, tenderness, and fleeting arthralgia
- Dysphagia, cough, and dyspnea
- Laboratory findings: CK elevated (5- to 30-fold), positive antinuclear antibodies test, anti-Jo-1 antibody (positive in 70% cases)
- Electromyogram shows "myopathic changes"
- Muscle biopsy shows interstitial infiltrates of lymphocytes (mostly CD8 T-cytotoxic lymphocytes), plasma cells, macrophages, and muscle cell necrosis
  See Fig. 21-7.

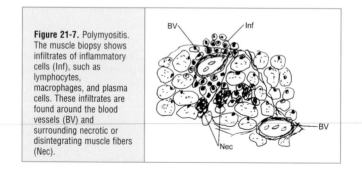

Figure 21-7. Polymyositis. The muscle biopsy shows infiltrates of inflammatory cells (Inf), such as lymphocytes, macrophages, and plasma cells. These infiltrates are found around the blood vessels (BV) and surrounding necrotic or disintegrating muscle fibers (Nec).

37. **What is dermatomyositis?**
Dermatomyositis is an autoimmune disease resembling polymyositis; however, it also includes skin changes that appear on the face, chest, and extremities. It occurs in two age groups:
- **Adolescents:** In this group, girls predominate. Periorbital "heliotropic" rash is a common feature.

- **Older age group:** In this group, men and women are affected to the same extent. The disease is associated with underlying malignancies in approximately 15% of cases.

38. **Discuss the differences between dermatomyositis and polymyositis.**
Polymyositis is a cell-mediated muscle disease mediated by CD8+ T-cytotoxic lymphocytes, whereas dermatomyositis seems to be an antibody-mediated disease. Immunohistochemical studies of muscle show deposits of immunoglobulin (Ig) G, IgM, and complement in the walls of small blood vessels in the muscle and perivascular infiltrates of plasma cells and B lymphocytes and mostly CD4+ helper T lymphocytes. Because of the vascular changes, there is ischemic atrophy of muscle fibers grouped at the periphery of the fascicles. This perifascicular atrophy, combined with the deposition of immunoglobulins in the vessel walls, is diagnostic of dermatomyositis, even if the muscle shows scant infiltrates of inflammatory cells.

39. **What are the most important infectious forms of myositis?**
    - **Viral myositis:** It is typically a fleeting, self-limited disease that occurs in the course of many systemic viral diseases, such as flu or childhood exanthemas. Coxsackie B virus infection (Bornholm disease) is known to be associated with muscle pain and may be complicated with myocarditis.
    - **Bacterial myositis:** It presents as a localized infection in the form of purulent infections and abscesses. It occurs in muscles in the vicinity of infected wounds or infected injection sites (e.g., in drug addicts). Tetanus and gas gangrene are serious complications of wound infection with *Clostridia* organisms.
    - **Parasitic myositis:** Trichinosis, the most common parasitic myositis results from the infestation of skeletal muscles with *Trichinella spiralis* following ingestion of inadequately prepared pork.

DISEASES OF THE NEUROMUSCULAR JUNCTION

40. **What are the diseases that may affect the transmission of impulses from the nerve to the muscle at the neuromuscular junction?**
    - **Myasthenia gravis:** In this disease the antibodies to the acetylcholine (Ach) receptor block the binding of Ach released from the nerve to the receptors on the surface of the muscle membrane.
    - **Lambert–Eaton syndrome:** This disease is caused by antibodies to calcium channels in the nerve ending. These antibodies block the flow of calcium and thus inhibit the transmission of nerve impulses.
    - **Botulism:** The neurotoxin from *Clostridium botulinum* blocks the release of Ach from the nerve endings and may cause widespread paralysis and death.
    - **Tick paralysis:** Certain ticks produce a toxin that inhibits the release of Ach, which may cause paralysis of muscles.

41. **List the key features of myasthenia gravis.**
    - It is autoimmune disease caused by antibodies to Ach receptors at the neuromuscular plate.
    - It affects 3 in 100,000 people. There are two age peaks: 20 to 30 years (women) and 50 to 60 years (men).
    - Thymic hyperplasia (65%) and thymoma (15%) are found among younger patients.
    - Microscopically muscle appears normal.
    - Muscle weakness is generalized but usually fluctuating and becoming more pronounced toward the end of the day.
    - Weakness most prominently affects extraocular eyes (ptosis and diplopia).
    - Electromyography shows progressively weaker contraction of muscles on repeated stimulation.

- The Tensilon (edrophonium) test provides immediate improvement because this drug inhibits acetylcholinesterase.
- Antibodies to acetylcholine receptor present in the serum of 80% of patients. See Fig. 21-8.

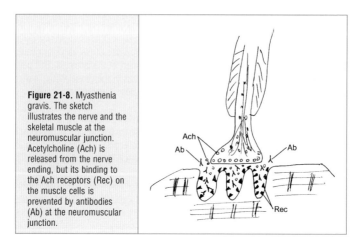

Figure 21-8. Myasthenia gravis. The sketch illustrates the nerve and the skeletal muscle at the neuromuscular junction. Acetylcholine (Ach) is released from the nerve ending, but its binding to the Ach receptors (Rec) on the muscle cells is prevented by antibodies (Ab) at the neuromuscular junction.

NEOPLASMS

42. **What are the most common tumors of the skeletal muscle?**
Benign tumors of the muscle typically originate from fibroblasts and blood vessels. These small nodules, such as hemangioma, benign fibrous histiocytoma, and lipoma, are usually inconsequential. Malignant tumors are rare and include those that are typically classified as soft tissue sarcomas:

- **Rhabdomyosarcoma:** This is a striated muscle fiber tumor that is most often found in children. It is highly malignant but responds well to chemotherapy.
- **Malignant fibrous histiocytoma:** This is tumor of fibroblast and histiocyte-like cells. It is the most common sarcoma of soft tissues in adults.
- **Liposarcoma:** This is a tumor of fat cells and is found mostly in adults. Several subtypes including low-grade and high-grade tumors.
- **Synovial sarcoma:** This is a tumor composed of undifferentiated mesenchymal cells (has no connection to synovium). It is typically a tumor of young adults, highly malignant, and resistant to therapy.
- **Leiomyosarcoma:** A tumor of smooth muscle cells, most often originating from muscle cells in arteries. Microscopically it is similar to uterine or gastrointestinal smooth muscle cell tumors.

WESTES

1. http://www.ncbi.nlm.nih.gov/entrez/query.fcgi?db=PubMed

2. http://www-medlib.med.utah.edu/WebPath/webpath.html#MENU

3. http://www.neuro.wustl.edu/neuromuscular/index.html

BIBLIOGRAPHY

1. Alexanderson H, Lundberg IE: Inflammatory muscle disease: clinical presentation and assessment of patients. Curr Rheumatol Rep 9:273–279, 2007.

2. Anderson JR: Recommendations for the biopsy procedure and assessment of skeletal muscle biopsies. Virchows Arch 431:227–233, 1997.

3. Cohn RU, Campbell KP: Molecular basis of muscular dystrophies, Muscle Nerve 23:1456 1471, 2000.

4. Dalakas MC, Hohlfeld R: Polymyositis and dermatomyositis. Lancet 362:971–982, 2003.

5. Deconinck N, Dan B: Pathophysiology of Duchenne muscular dystrophy: current hypotheses. Pediatr Neurol 36:1–7, 2007.

6. Griffin TA, Reed AM: Pathogenesis of myositis in children. Curr Opin Rheumatol 19:487–91, 2007.

7. Irani S, Lang B: Autoantibody-mediated disorders of the central nervous system. Autoimmunity 41:55–65, 2008.

8. Lisi MT, Cohn RD: Congenital muscular dystrophies: new aspects of an expanding group of disorders. Biochim Biophys Acta 1772:159–172, 2007.

9. Mendell JR, Boué DR, Martin PT: The congenital muscular dystrophies: recent advances and molecular insights. Pediatr Dev Pathol 9:427–443, 2006.

CHAPTER 22

THE CENTRAL NERVOUS SYSTEM

Péter Molnár, MD, DSc

1. **What are the most important diseases of the central nervous system (CNS)?**
   - Developmental disorders
   - Physical injury of the brain and spinal cord
   - Vascular disorders
   - Infections
   - Autoimmune diseases
   - Neurodegenerative diseases
   - Nutritional, metabolic and toxic brain diseases
   - Neoplasms

REACTION OF THE CENTRAL NERVOUS SYSTEM TO INJURY

2. **List the most important pathologic reactions of neurons.**
   - **Acute injury:** This is most commonly caused by hypoxia/ischemia but also under the influence of toxic or infectious agents that can kill neurons. Affected neurons have pyknotic nuclei and an acidophilic cytoplasm, which stains intensely red with eosin ("red is dead") in standard hematoxylin and eosin (H&E) slides.
   - **Axonal reaction:** It occurs following transection or other severe injury of the axon and is characterized by histologic and ultrastructural changes in the cytoplasms of the neuron (perikaryon). Following axonal injury, the perikaryon swells. Ultrastructurally, the ribosomes of rough endoplasmic reticulum (RER) are lost. This degranulation of the RER, which in the neurons is called Nissl substance, is visible by light microscopy as a loss of basophilia and is called chromatolysis.
   - **Formation of neuronal inclusions:** Neuronal inclusions can be intracytoplasmic or intranuclear. Typical examples include lipofuscin (i.e., the cytoplasmic brown "wear and tear" pigment of aging) and viral inclusions (cytoplasmic inclusions, e.g., the Negri bodies in rabies; nuclear inclusions such as those seen in herpes encephalitis and known as Cowdry type A bodies; or nuclear and cytoplasmic inclusions such as in cytomegalovirus infection).
   - **Aggregation of abnormal proteins:** Cytoplasmic bodies are found in neurons in several neurodegenerative diseases, such as the formation of neurofibrillary tangles in Alzheimer disease or the formation of cytoplasmic Lewy bodies made out of α-synuclein in Parkinson disease.
   - **Neuronophagia:** Phagocytosis of damaged neurons by microglial and inflammatory cells is a common reaction to CNS injury in various infectious or toxic diseases.

3. **What is the most common cellular reaction to CNS injury?**
   Gliosis is the most common reaction of the CNS to injury. It presents in the form of hypertrophy and hyperplasia of fibrillary astrocytes, some of which acquire abundant cytoplasm and transform into so called gemistocytes. Cytoplasmic extensions of these astrocytes form a dense meshwork of "glial fibrils," which results in the formation of the so-called glial scar. Glial scars differ from scars in other organs in that they are devoid of collagen.

KEY POINTS: REACTION OF THE CENTRAL NERVOUS SYSTEM TO INJURY ✓

1. Neurons are the most vulnerable cells of the central nervous system.

2. The response to injury of the central nervous system includes glial cell reactions and circulatory changes and edema.

---

4. **How do microglial cells respond to CNS injury?**
   Microglia cells are bone-marrow-derived macrophages that accumulate at the site of CNS injury, forming glial nodules. Activated microglial cells show nuclear elongation resulting in rod cells. Microglia cells take part in phagocytosis of dying neurons, a process known as neuronophagia.

5. **What are the common forms of cerebral edema?**
   Three forms of cerebral edema are recognized: vasogenic, cytotoxic, and interstitial.
   - **Vasogenic edema:** It is characterized by the accumulation of fluid in between the neurons and glial cells and most prominently in the Virchow–Robin spaces around the blood vessels. It develops as a consequence of blood–brain barrier dysfunction. Fluid escapes from the vascular space into the interstitial space of the parenchyma across the cytoplasm of vascular endothelial cells or between these cells through the disrupted tight junctions. It may be localized (e.g., around a tumor or an abscess) or generalized (e.g., in encephalitis or following head trauma).
   - **Cytotoxic edema:** In this form of edema, the fluid accumulates inside the cells. It is most frequently caused by ischemia, hypoxia, or both, which lead to hydropic swelling of neurons and glial cells.
   - **Interstitial edema:** It is the result of increased intracerebral influx of CSF through the ependymal lining. Fluid from the ventricles enters into the periventricular white matter, typically under conditions associated with an increased intraventricular CSF pressure. This form of edema is typically a complication of hydrocephalus.

6. **Describe the gross appearance of the brain with generalized vasogenic edema.**
   Typical features seen at autopsy include:
   - Gyri are flattened and broad.
   - Sulci are narrowed and slitlike.
   - Lateral ventricles are compressed.
   - On sectioning of the unfixed brain at autopsy, the brain is heavier than normal and soft, and the fluid seeps from the cut surfaces.
   - Signs of cerebral or cerebellar herniation are evident.

7. **Describe various forms of intracranial cerebral or cerebellar herniations.**
   Herniations (Fig. 22-1) occur as a result of increased intracranial volume. Most often, they accompany space-occupying lesions, such as tumors, hematomas, or abscesses, but they may also be caused by trauma. The displacement of parts of the brain is morphologically most evident at three herniation sites:
   - **Cingulate herniation (subfalcine herniation):** It results from a unilateral hemispheric mass lesion (e.g., abscess, hematoma, and tumor) that expands the volume of one hemisphere, dislocates the midline structures (midline shift), and forces the ipsilateral cingulate gyrus to be compressed ("herniate") underneath the falx cerebri. Focal necrosis and hemorrhage may develop in the herniated tissue together with distant reduction of blood flow (i.e., compression of the anterior cerebral artery).

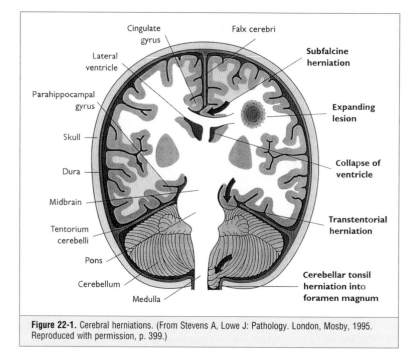

Figure 22-1. Cerebral herniations. (From Stevens A, Lowe J: Pathology. London, Mosby, 1995. Reproduced with permission, p. 399.)

- **Transtentorial herniation (uncinate herniation):** It is caused by the expansion of one or both supratentorial tissue compartments (cerebral hemispheres). The uncus gyri hippocampi is displaced on one or both sides and is herniated underneath the free edge of the rigid cerebellar tentorium. Simultaneously, the ipsilateral third cranial nerve is compressed between the tentorium and the expanding temporal lobe, as indicated by the dilatation of the ipsilateral pupil plus abnormal eye movements on the same side.
- **Tonsillar herniation:** It may develop unilaterally or bilaterally and is a life-threatening condition because the herniated cerebellar tonsils that are forced into the foramen magnum compress the vital respiratory and cardiac centers within the medulla oblongata. Compression of vital centers may cause cardiac or respiratory paralysis (or both).

DEVELOPMENTAL DISORDERS

8. **Define dysraphic malformations and list the most common forms of this malformation.**
   Dysraphic malformations result from a failure of the dorsal closure of the fetal neural tube. Two main forms of dysraphism are recognized: cranial and spinal. Both occur in several subtypes.
   - **Cranial dysraphism:** It is associated with incomplete formation of the skull and occurs most often as anencephaly or encephalocele. This severe cerebral malformation is usually incompatible with life.
   - **Spinal dysraphism:** This group of developmental disorders includes spina bifida occulta, meningocele, meningomyelocele, and rachischisis, all of which are characterized by variably severe defective closure (most commonly) of the lumbosacral segment of the neural tube, vertebral arches, and, in the most severe cases, the skin. Severe forms of spinal dysraphism are not compatible with life. Spina bifida occulta, however, is not life threatening and is typically accompanied only by neurologic defects affecting the lower extremities.

9. **List the most frequent causes of congenital CNS malformations.**
   The cause of most congenital CNS malformations is unknown. The following are among the known causes:
   - Fetal intrauterine infections such as those causing the TORCH complex, which includes toxoplasmosis, rubella, cytomegalovirus (CMV), herpes virus, and others such as syphilis, listeriosis, leptospirosis, and viral infection with varicella-zoster virus, Epstein–Barr and so on, etc.; human immunodeficiency virus 1 (HIV-1) infection during fetal life may also cause CNS lesions.
   - Chromosomal abnormalities (trisomy 13–15 and 18)
   - Fetal alcohol syndrome
   - Dilantin (phenytoin) and other antiepileptic drugs

PHYSICAL INJURY

10. **What are the main forms of spinal cord or brain injury caused by physical forces?**
    Skull fractures are often accompanied by parenchymal injuries, which include:
    - **Contusions ("bruising"):** This type of injury results from rapid deceleration or acceleration of the skull and the brain. Typically it involves a coup lesion at the site of the impact of force or a contrecoup contusion, diametrically opposite to it.
    - **Lacerations (tearing of tissue):** It is a severe form of brain injury typically seen in vehicular accidents. It is associated with bleeding and high mortality.
    - **Diffuse axonal injury:** It is usually found in the parasagittal or deep centroaxial white matter. Such injury results from the action of shearing forces in laminar planes within the brain and is frequently accompanied by focal hemorrhages.
    - **Tearing of cerebral blood vessels:** This traumatic vascular injury is accompanied by bleeding.
    - **Penetrating wounds:** These are most often caused by bullets.

KEY POINTS: PHYSICAL INJURY ✔

1. Physical injury may directly damage the brain and the spinal cord, or it may cause hemorrhages, which cause secondary brain lesions.

2. Hemorrhages into various compartments of the intracranial space produce distinct clinical syndromes, but all of them may be lethal.

11. **Describe the most common spinal cord injuries.**
    Concussions, contusions, lacerations, and penetrating injuries are similar to those elsewhere within the CNS. Unique to the spinal cord are the hyperextension and hyperflexion injuries.
    - **Hyperextension injury:** It typically occurs in the cervical spine and is caused by sudden posterior displacement of the head that causes rupture of the anterior spinal ligament. The so-called posterior angulation of the cervical vertebrae is accompanied by contusion of the posterior segment of the cervical spinal cord.
    - **Hyperflexion injury:** It also affects the cervical spine and results from trauma that leads to a compression of one of the cervical vertebrae. Such a "teardrop" fracture of the vertebral body is usually caused by an impact force that rapidly drives the head down and forward. This is accompanied by anterior angulation and consecutive anterior contusion of the cervical spinal cord.

12. **What are the most important forms of intracranial bleeding?**
   Cranial–cerebral trauma often results in hemorrhage into one of the intracranial compartments. The most important forms of intracranial hemorrhage or hematoma are:
   - Epidural hematoma
   - Subdural hematoma
   - Subarachnoid hematoma
   - Intracerebral (parenchymal) hemorrhage
   - intraventricular hemorrhage, also known as hematocephalus internus

13. **What is epidural hematoma ?**
   Epidural hemorrhage results from bone fractures at the base of the skull that tear the middle meningeal artery. Arterial bleeding leads to the formation of a hematoma in the virtual space between the inner aspect of the cranial bones and the dura mater. Hematoma that forms under arterial pressure grows progressively, and without proper surgical intervention, it is invariably fatal within several hours after injury.

14. **What is subdural hematoma?**
   Subdural hemorrhage stems from traumatically severed "bridging veins" that connect superficial cerebral veins and the dural venous sinuses. This venous bleeding may stop on its own as soon as the pressure outside the veins exceeds the pressure inside the vascular lumen. However, as the blood clots and the external pressure on the bridging veins decreases, bleeding may resume even after minor cranial trauma. Subdural hematomas are typically found following repeated traumatic head injuries, as in:
   - Chronic alcoholics who tend to often stumble and fall
   - Elderly people, especially those who are hospitalized or stay in nursing homes and often fall out of bed
   - Boxers
   Subdural hematomas may present with neurologic symptoms, but many remain undetected during life and are discovered only at autopsy.

VASCULAR DISORDERS

15. **List the most common aneurysms found in the CNS.**
   An aneurysm is a circumscribed, segmental dilatation of an artery. The most important forms of intracranial aneurysms are:
   - **Berry aneurysms:** These small saccular aneurysms are typically found in and around the circle of Willis at the base of the brain. They develop at the site of arterial branching corresponding to the congenital weakest part of the vessels. The rupture of these aneurysms leads to a usually fatal subarachnoid and/or intraparenchymal/intraventricular hemorrhage.
   - **Atherosclerotic aneurysms:** These aneurysms may involve the extraparenchymal or intracranial arteries. Most often, they are asymptomatic and rarely rupture.
   - **Hypertensive microaneurysms:** Long-standing hypertension leads to deposition of lipid–hyaline substances within the wall of small branches of penetrating arteries and arterioles. These deposits weaken the vessel wall and cause microscopic Charcot–Bouchard aneurysms.

KEY POINTS: VASCULAR DISORDERS ✓

1. Stroke can be caused by intracerebral hemorrhage or infarction.

2. Ischemia of the brain may cause only transient functional changes or a variety of lesions, such as watershed infarct and laminar necrosis.

16. **What are cerebral arteriovenous malformations?**
    Arteriovenous malformations (AVMs) result from defective formation of capillaries in a normal part of the brain. The arterial blood thus enters directly into the veins, usually by way of arteriovenous anastomoses that form at the defective site. Typical AVMs consist of tortuous arteries and veins that form cortical–subcortical networks of "wormlike" arteriovenous shunts embedded in hemosiderin–laden glial tissue. AVMs have a high blood flow, often pulsate, and may be a source of mixed parenchymal/subarachnoidal bleeding and seizures.

17. **List the most important causes of nontraumatic intracerebral hemorrhage (i.e., hemorrhagic strokes).**
    - **Hypertension:** Chronic, severe (usually uncontrolled), systemic hypertension is the most common cause of hemorrhagic stroke. Hypertension accelerates arteriosclerosis of the larger arteries and also causes lipohyalinosis of the smaller branches promoting the development of rupture-prone Charcot–Bouchard aneurysms. Hypertensive hemorrhages occur most often within the basal ganglia and less commonly in the cerebellum or the medulla oblongata.
    - **Coagulation abnormalities:** Most often, this kind of hemorrhage occurs in terminal stages of leukemia and severe thrombocytopenia.
    - **Rupture of berry aneurysms:** Because the blood exits the ruptured arteries under pressure, it may penetrate into the cerebral parenchyma and even into the ventricles. Thus the blood may be found not only in the subarachnoid space but also inside the brain (mixed bleeding: subarachnoidal plus parenchymal/intraventricular).

18. **What are the most common sites of hypertensive cerebral hemorrhages?**
    - Basal ganglia and thalamus (65%)
    - Pons (15%)
    - Cerebellum (10%)

19. **What are the pathologic consequences of global cerebral ischemia?**
    Generalized reduction of available oxygen that affects the whole CNS may cause:
    - **Transient ischemic attacks (TIAs):** These lack morphologic sequelae.
    - **Focal neuronal death:** Typically it first affects the most vulnerable neurons (e.g., hippocampus and Purkinje cells).
    - **Watershed infarcts:** Typically these occur in hypotensive condition (e.g., cardiogenic shock or massive bleeding) and affect the border zones between the supply area of two major arteries (e.g., area supplied by anterior and middle cerebral artery).
    - **Laminar necrosis:** This form of necrosis typically affects the deep layers of the cerebral cortex—that is, the area that receives the blood from the blood vessels entering the cortex from the surface of the brain ("short penetrators").

20. **What are the most important causes of occlusion of cerebral arteries?**
    - **Thrombi:** Most thrombi form over ruptured atheromas. They account for 80% cerebral infarcts.
    - **Thromboemboli:** Most of these stem from the heart chambers or valves and the large arteries.

INFECTIONS

21. **What are the most common routes of entry of infectious agents into the intracranial space?**
    - **Vascular spread:** Most infectious agents reach the brain and the meninges through the arterial bloodstream. Venous blood may serve as a carrier of infectious agents from the infected periocular and perinasal tissues.

- **Direct extension from adjacent structures:** Such infection may spread from the infected middle ear or sinuses. Herpes virus residing in the trigeminal ganglion of latently infected people can also spread into the brain.
- **Ascending neural route:** Some viruses, such as rabies, ascend into the brain along the axons of peripheral nerves.
- **Penetrating wounds:** Bacteria can be inoculated directly into the brain by bullets and sharp objects, such as a knife, or by direct entry through an open or surgical wound

22. **What are the most important infectious diseases of the CNS ?**
    - **Meningitis:** Infection may be limited to the subarachnoid space (leptomeningitis) or may spread into the brain (meningoencephalitis). Such infection may be classified as acute or chronic. According to the appearance of the cerebrospinal fluid one can classify meningitis as purulent (bacterial) or serous (viral).
    - **Encephalitis:** Inflammation of the brain is most often caused by viruses. It may be diffuse (i.e., involve the entire brain) or localized to a part of the brain. It may be combined with meningitis (meningoencephalitis).
    - **Brain abscess:** This purulent localized infection of the brain is typically caused by bacteria. Abscesses may be solitary or multiple (usually in sepsis).

23. **List the most common causes of acute bacterial meningitis.**
    The infection can be caused by a variety of microorganisms. *Streptococcus pneumoniae* has become the most common cause because immunization has eliminated many other causes such as *Hemophilus influenzae.* In neonates it is most commonly caused by *Escherichia coli* and group B streptococci. Among children and young adults, an important cause is *Neisseria meningitidis* (meningococcus), which may cause miniepidemics among army recruits or in student camps. Gram-negative bacteria (*E. coli, Klebsiella,* and *Enterobacter*) cause meningitis in immunosuppressed people following brain trauma or brain surgery.

24. **Describe the gross and microscopic findings in acute bacterial meningitis.**
    - The brain is edematous and congested.
    - The subarachnoid space is filled with a purulent exudate. The pus is most obvious in the sulci of the convexity and the subarachnoid cisterns at the base of the brain.
    - Microscopically the exudate in the subarachnoidal space consists predominantly of live and dead neutrophils.

25. **List the most important causes of chronic meningitis.**
    Acute meningitis caused by bacteria resistant to treatment may become chronic, but even in this circumstance, the exudate remains purulent. This prolonged purulent meningitis must be distinguished clinically and for treatment purposes from chronic meningitis caused by pathogens that typically cause chronic diseases. Such chronic meningitis typically has an insidious onset and may last weeks or months. Chronic meningitis may be a feature of:
    - Tuberculosis (prevalent in developing countries but rare in the United States)
    - Fungal diseases, especially in immunosuppressed people suffering from acquired immune deficiency syndrome (AIDS)
    - Lyme disease caused by *Borrelia burgdorferi*
    - Syphilis caused by *Treponema pallidum* (CNS infection is a feature of tertiary syphilis.)

26. **Describe the pathologic findings in chronic meningitis.**
    The pathologic findings in various forms of chronic meningitis vary depending on the causative pathogen. The infection is usually more circumscribed than in acute meningitis and may be localized to parts of the brain. For example, tuberculous meningitis typically involves the basal

cisterns and the lateral sulci that contain gelatinous whitish gray material. Histologically, these lesions contain caseating granulomas. In secondary and tertiary syphilis, the meninges show focal irregular thickening. These changes are most prominent around the spinal cord but may be seen over the convexity of the brain or over the cerebellum. Histologically, thickened meninges contain infiltrates of lymphocytes and plasma cells, typically arranged around the meningeal blood vessels. Tertiary syphilis may also present in the form of a granulomatous inflammation (gumma of syphilis).

27. **List the most important causes of viral meningitis.**
Viral meningitis (also known as aseptic meningitis) may occur as part of a systemic viral disease (e.g., varicella, mumps, and measles), or it may be limited to the CNS. The latter may be sporadic (e.g., herpes virus infection) or epidemic (e.g., arboviruses transmitted by arthropods such as eastern or western equine encephalitis), and is often associated with encephalitis (i.e, meningoencephalitis).

28. **What is tabes dorsalis?**
Tabes dorsalis (Fig. 22-2) is a manifestation of tertiary syphilis involving the lumbar spinal cord. Syphilitic meningitis leads to fibrosis, compressing the posterior nerve roots. In normal circumstances, these afferent nerves, originating from the spinal ganglia, form the posterior columns in the spinal cord, and transmit proprioceptive and sensory impulses. Wallerian degeneration that results from the injury of axons entering the spinal cord results in posterior columns. Clinically, these patients experience loss of vibration and proprioception, which affects their gait. Joint degeneration resulting in deformities (Charcot joints) is commonly found.

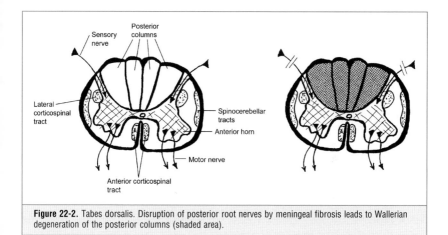

Figure 22-2. Tabes dorsalis. Disruption of posterior root nerves by meningeal fibrosis leads to Wallerian degeneration of the posterior columns (shaded area).

29. **What are the typical clinical features of acute and chronic meningitis?**
- Headache, usually of sudden onset and quite severe; often localized to the forehead
- Fever (high, over 40°C in acute bacterial, but less prominent in aseptic meningitis)
- Prodrome often seen in viral diseases, but bacterial infection may have a sudden onset
- Nausea and vomiting
- Stiff neck

- Mental confusion, somnolence, photophobia, seizures, and neurologic symptoms
- Kernig sign (hip flexion induces knee pain)
- Brudzinski sign (upon flexion of the neck, there is spontaneous similar movement of the hips and knees)
- Increased cerebrospinal fluid (CSF) pressure with changes in the biochemical composition of CSF
  See Table 22-1.

TABLE 22-1. CEREBROSPINAL FLUID IN VARIOUS FORMS OF MENINGITIS

	Cells	Protein	Glucose
	(0–10 mm^3)	(Normal <40 mg/dL)	(Normal 40–60 mg/dL)
Bacterial	Neutrophils	↑	↓
Tuberculous	Lymphocytes	↑	↓
Viral	Lymphocytes*	↑	Normal

*In acute viral encephalitis, neutrophils may be present during the first 24 to 48 hours. However, in viral meningitis, the exudation is considerably less prominent than in bacterial infection (>1000 cells/μL). Exudate in bacterial infection is typically purulent, and the cerebrospinal fluid appears cloudy or even yellow.

30. **List the complications of meningitis.**
    - Hydrocephalus resulting from obstruction of CSF due to scarring of meninges
    - Neurologic defects due to destruction of underlying brain
    - Epilepsy due to focal damage of the brain or scarring of meninges
    - Abscess formation in the brain or subdural spaces (especially in children)
    - Spinal or cranial nerve compression or constriction as in tabes dorsalis

31. **List key facts about the pathogenesis and pathology of cerebral abscesses.**
    - Localized suppuration of the brain is caused by pyogenic bacteria (*Streptococcus pneumoniae* or *Staphylococcus aureus*) presenting clinically as a destructive, space-occupying lesion.
    - It may be solitary (developing from local foci of infection) or multiple (in sepsis and septic embolism from endocarditis). It is also a complication of suppurative meningitis.
    - Solitary abscesses may evolve from suppurative infection of nasal sinuses (frontal lobe), the middle ear, and mastoid bone (temporal lobe or cerebellum).
    - Solitary hematogenous abscess is usually a consequence of septic embolization from infected endocardial valves. Emboli cause a cerebral infarct, which then becomes infected and transforms into an abscess.

32. **List key facts about the clinical presentation of cerebral abscess.**
    - General signs and symptoms of infection and increased intracranial pressure (e.g., somnolence and papilledema). Progressive intracranial hypertension may cause hemiplegia, seizures, and even coma.
    - CSF finding is nonspecific and nondiagnostic in the majority of cases (10% bacterial culture positive).
    - Computed tomography (CT) shows typical ring-enhancing lesions.
    - Without surgery and chemotherapy, it is fatal in most cases.

KEY POINTS: INFECTIONS AND IMMUNOLOGIC DISEASES ✔

1. Infections of the central nervous system (CNS) may present as meningitis, encephalitis, or brain abscesses.

2. The most common causes of CNS infections are viruses and bacteria, but patients with acquired immune deficiency syndrome may also have parasitic and fungal infections.

3. Infections cause distinct changes in the cerebrospinal fluid that can be analyzed in the sample obtained by spinal tap.

4. Creutzfeld–Jakob disease is a spongiform encephalopathy caused by prions.

5. Multiple sclerosis is an immunologic disease characterized by multifocal demyelinization of the CNS.

33. **List key facts about viral encephalitis.**
    - It is often associated with meningitis (meningoencephalitis).
    - Most infections are hematogenous.
    - It may be diffuse or preferentially localized to specific areas (e.g., poliomyelitis affects the anterior horns of the spinal cord, and herpes simplex virus affects the temporal lobe).
    - Some infections occur in previously healthy people (e.g., epidemic arthropod-borne encephalitis, rabies, and poliomyelitis), but many are found more often or exclusively in immunosuppressed people (e.g., CMV encephalitis).
    - Virus may remain in latent form (e.g., herpes simplex virus in trigeminal nerve) and become reactivated by events that change the interaction between the host and the virus.

34. **What are the microscopic findings in viral infection?**
    - Perivascular infiltrates of lymphocytes (perivascular cuffing)
    - Neural injury followed by phagocytosis of damaged and killed cells by microglia cells and macrophages (neuronophagia and microglial nodules)
    - Intraneural inclusions are seen in some diseases but not in others
    - Edema and widening of the perivascular spaces
    - Concomitant meningitis (meningoencephalitis)
      See Fig. 22-3.

35. **List viral infections associated with cellular inclusions visible by light microscopy.**
    - There is CMV enlargement of cells, which contain typical bluish "owl-eyed" intranuclear inclusions. The cytoplasm also contains virions and appears bluish.
    - Herpes simplex virus is associated with "smudgy" or more distinct Cowdry type A nuclear inclusions that are surrounded by an empty delimiting space. Herpetic inclusions are found in neurons, glia cells, and endothelial cells.
    - Rabies infection is accompanied by the formation of cytoplasmic inclusions (Negri bodies) in neurons.
    - Measles virus causing subacute sclerosing panencephalitis forms intranuclear inclusions in neurons. The inclusions have a clear halo around them.
    - JC papova virus–induced progressive multifocal leukoencephalopathy presents with "ground-glass" intranuclear inclusions in oligodendroglia cells.

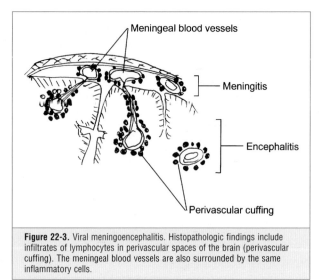

Figure 22-3. Viral meningoencephalitis. Histopathologic findings include infiltrates of lymphocytes in perivascular spaces of the brain (perivascular cuffing). The meningeal blood vessels are also surrounded by the same inflammatory cells.

36. **What are the typical features of arthropod-borne viral encephalitides?**
   - The virus resides in animal hosts (e.g., horses).
   - The virus is carried by arthropods (e.g., mosquitos or ticks).
   - The disease is often epidemic.
   - Diffuse encephalitis presents pathologically with perivascular lymphocytic infiltrates and widespread foci of necrosis involving the white and gray matter.
   - Necrotizing vasculitis and neuronophagia are often prominent.

37. **List the salient features of CMV encephalitis.**
   - It is the most important opportunistic viral CNS infection in immunocompromised people.
   - It may also occur as part of TORCH syndrome in neonates.
   - Pathology shows hemorrhagic, necrotizing encephalitis.
   - There is no preferential location; it may involve any part of the brain, the ependymal lining of ventricles (ependymitis), and choroid plexus.
   - On microscopy, CMV-infected cells appear enlarged and contain viral inclusions in their cytoplasm and nucleus. These inclusions are found in neurons, glia cells, and endothelial cells, as well as ependymal cells and cells of the choroid plexus.
   - Calcification of old lesions is a common feature, especially in neonates.

38. **List key facts about poliomyelitis.**
   - It is extremely rare in the United States, the disease has been fully controlled by preventive immunization at an early age.
   - Enterovirus infection by the fecal–oral route begins as a gastroenteritis.
   - The virus spreads hematogenously to the spinal cord, causing meningoencephalitis.
   - The motor neurons of the anterior horn are preferentially infected by virus and destroyed after a short phase of aseptic meningoencephalitis.
   - Severe flaccid paralysis of variable severity ensues.
   - Unless there is severe bulbar paralysis, most patients will have only limited consequences (motor defects).
   - Severe cases are lethal. Death may be caused by involvement of respiratory muscles.

39. **Describe the pathology of rabies.**
   - Rabies virus is caused by an enveloped, single-stranded RNA virus (rhabdovirus).
   - The virus is transmitted by the bite (infected saliva) of carnivore wild animals (e.g., foxes, bats, and dogs).
   - The virus reaches the CNS by centripetal axoplasmic flow, and it reaches the viscera (salivary glands) by intraaxonal centrifugal propagation.
   - Lymphocytic perivasculitis is seen around small vessels within the brain stem, basal ganglia, or hypothalamus.
   - Negri bodies are found most prominently in the hippocampus, Purkinje cells, and the brain stem.
   - Infection is accompanied by almost no glial inflammatory reaction in the brain.
   - Clinically, there is generalized encephalopathy, presenting with irritability, seizures, contracture of the pharyngeal muscles (hydrophobia—inability to swallow water), and, terminally, delirium.
   - Preventive immunization and serial vaccination of infected people are effective. After the virus reaches the brain, death is inevitable.

40. **How does HIV-1 infection affect the CNS?**
   - Subacute encephalitis causing the AIDS dementia complex (dementia, apathy, depression, ataxia, bowel and bladder incontinence, and seizures).
   - Vacuolar myelopathy (extensive vacuolation of the posterior/lateral columns, similar to subacute combined degeneration) is probably caused by impaired vitamin B_{12} metabolism; it causes ataxia and spastic paraparesis.
   - It leads to AIDS-related peripheral neuropathy—acute and chronic demyelinating polyneuropathy and various other neuropathies due to segmental demyelination, axonal degeneration, and infiltration of neural structures by mononuclear inflammatory cells.
   - Opportunistic infections occur, most commonly caused by *Toxoplasma gondii, Cryptococcus neoformans, Candida albicans,* and *Aspergillus fumigatus.*

41. **What are the typical pathologic findings in HIV encephalopathy?**
   - Mild cerebral atrophy with moderately widened sulci and dilatated ventricles
   - Typical but not diagnostic histologic findings include widely scattered microglial nodules with multinucleated giant cells in the subcortical white matter, diencephalon, and brain stem with focal necroses and gliosis; swollen endothelial cells and perivascular foamy macrophages; and axonal swelling and gliosis occurring multifocally in the white matter

42. **What is progressive multifocal leukoencephalopathy (PML)?**
   PML is a JC virus infection (no relationship to Jakob–Creutzfeldt disease). The virus infects oligodendroglia cells, characterized by nuclear inclusions and relentlessly progressive demyelination of variable-sized areas within the brain stem, cerebrum, and cerebellum. The affected foci are rich in foamy macrophages, and there is an axonal reduction. Reactive, often bizarre, irregular, giant astrocytes with hyperchromatic, often multiple nuclei that may raise the suspicion of tumor in stereotactic brain biopsies are characteristic components of foci of destruction.

43. **What are the most important features of cryptococcal infection?**
   - *Cryptococcus neoformans* is excreted by pigeon feces from which infection occurs via inhalation.
   - Most often it is an opportunistic infection in immunodeficient people suffering from AIDS, lymphoma, and leukemia, or it occurs during cytotoxic and steroid treatment.
   - It occurs as a chronic meningitis/meningoencephalitis with meningeal fibrosis leading to hydrocephalus. The subarachnoid exudate has a gelatinous consistency.
   - Diagnosis is made by identifying cryptococci in the CSF. These fungi have a proteoglycan capsule and can be demonstrated in India ink preparations.

- Extension of infection to the brain leads to formation of cystic lesions showing minimal inflammatory reaction.
- Untreated infections are fatal.

44. List key facts about CNS toxoplasmosis.
- *Toxoplasma gondii* infection of the brain occurs as an opportunistic infection in AIDS and other conditions associated with immunosuppression or in neonates.
- The acute infection leads to extensive brain necrosis surrounded by petechial hemorrhages.
- The infection most commonly affects the basal ganglia and brain stem.
- Microscopically there are areas of necrosis with *Toxoplasma* cysts, surrounded by infiltrates of macrophages.
- The chronic (treated) lesions are cystic and filled with necrotic material. Parasites are usually difficult to find in such lesions. Calcification may be prominent.

45. List the most important prion diseases.
- Creutzfeldt–Jakob disease (CJD), the most common prion disease, with an incidence of 1:1 million
- Gerstmann–Sträussler–Scheinker syndrome
- Fatal familial insomnia (FFI)
- Kuru
- Animal equivalents of the human disease: scrapie (sheep and goats), mink transmissible encephalopathy, and bovine spongiform encephalopathy (BSE; "mad cow disease")

46. What are prions?
Prions are abnormal proteins with a β-pleated sheet structure. The prion protein, PrPsc, is an isoform of the normal, ubiquitous, transmembrane protein PrPc that has an α-helical structure. The conformational change may occur spontaneously, but this process is rare and slow. It may also result from genetic mutations, but the infectious process is the consequence of protein–protein interactions—that is, the abnormal protein facilitates the structural change of the normal isoform. Thus the abnormal, exogenous, "infective" PrPsc transforms the normal PrPc protein, and the transformed, insoluble molecule causes the diseases. PrPc is encoded by the PRNP gene (chromosome 20); its point mutations cause familial CJD and FFI. Human consumption of meat from BSE-affected cows started a variant of CJD (vCJD) in Great Britain and France, with sporadic cases in other areas of Europe.

47. Describe the microscopic pathology of prion diseases.
The infected brain shows typically widespread spongiform degeneration and severe neuronal loss. In addition, many cases show plaques that are aggregates of PrPsc. The latter occur in various gray matter structures with a different distribution pattern in the various forms of prion disease: vCJD is characterized by a high number of "kuru plaques" in the extracellular space of the cerebral cortex as opposed to their predominance in the cerebellum in classic CJD. There is no inflammatory reaction; however, gliosis is common. The exact mechanism of vacuole formation (spongiform transformation) is unknown.

48. List the key facts about multiple sclerosis (MS).
- It is a demyelinating disease characterized by chronic relapsing and remitting course.
- Incidence is 1 or 2 per 1000, usually in the 25- to 45-year-old age group.
- Demyelinated plaques develop at random but are most often found along the central–medial, paraventricular axis, optic nerves, and the spinal cord.
- Clinical symptoms vary from case to case. The most common findings are limb weakness (40%); visual symptoms, such as diplopia or partial blindness and inability to focus (20%); paresthesia (20%); vertigo (5%); and bladder incontinence (5%).
- Infections are common, especially urinary infections.
- Motor disturbances predominate, leading to abnormal gait and joint deformities.

- Mental deterioration is noticed in long-lasting disease and may lead to dementia.
- Death results from widespread paralysis leading to respiratory failure.
- Peripheral nerves are usually spared.

49. **What is the pathogenesis of MS?**
    The exact pathogenesis and etiology of MS are not known. Current theories postulate that the disease is either infectious or caused by autoimmune mechanisms. The following are important epidemiologic data providing clues about the causation:
    - It is more common in moderate or cold climates distant from the equator than in the tropics.
    - If people move, they retain the same susceptibility as they would have had in the residence of their childhood.
    - Outbreaks and clustering of disease suggest an infection in some cases.
    - It is more common in whites than other races (90% of patients in the United States are white).
    - It is more common in females than in males (female:male ratio, 3:1).
    - Familial cases: 10 times higher risk if a sibling or parent is affected.
    - Genetic basis of the disease is suggested by a 30% concordance among monozygotic twins and 3% to 5% in dizygotic twins.

50. **Describe the morphology of the typical plaques of MS.**
    Acute/active MS plaques are relatively sharply outlined, slightly depressed, rather firm ("sclerosis"), oval or irregularly shaped, have the color of gray matter, and have variably sized lesions with edema. Microscopically, typical features are selective loss of myelin, lipid-rich debris within macrophages, perivascular lymphocytic cuffs, destruction of oligodendroglia, and preservation of axons.

    Inactive plaques are almost devoid of myelin, and the inflammation is replaced by astrocytosis and gliosis. A reduced number of axons are seen.

NEURODEGENERATIVE DISEASES

51. **What are the most common causes of dementia?**
    - Alzheimer's disease (AD; 60%)
    - Atherosclerosis and multiinfarct dementia (15%–20%)
    - Multifactorial dementia or a combination of Alzheimer and multiinfarct dementia (15%)
    - Various other less common forms of dementia

52. **List some less common forms of dementia.**
    - Parkinsonism (2%)
    - Chronic alcoholism (2%)
    - Pick disease (1%)
    - Huntington disease (1%)
    - AIDS (1%)
    - Syphilis (1%)
    - Creutzfeldt–Jakob disease (very rare, <1%)

KEY POINTS: NEURODEGENERATIVE DISEASES ✔

1. Neurodegenerative diseases are chronic brain diseases of unknown etiology.

2. Neurodegenerative diseases have unique pathologic features that correlate with diagnostic clinical symptoms of these diseases.

3. Alzheimer's disease is the most common neurodegenerative disease and the most common cause of dementia.

53. **List key facts about AD.**
   - It is a neurodegenerative disease of unknown etiology, clinically presenting as dementia.
   - In most instances, it is an old-age disease that occurs at random, but in 10% of cases, there is a family history of AD.
   - Familial forms of early-onset AD are linked to genetic markers (e.g., specific alleles of apoprotein E).
   - It is the most common cause of dementia, accounting for 60% of all cases in industrialized countries. In the United States, more than 4 million patients suffer from dementia of the AD type.
   - Pathologically characterized by atrophy of the brain and typical microscopic findings.

54. **What is the cause of AD?**
   The cause and the pathogenesis of AD are unknown. Clinical, laboratory, and epidemic findings suggest that several factors may play a pathogenetic role:
   - **Genetic factors:** Several potentially important genes have been identified in familial cases. This indicates that even the hereditary cases are multifactorial and polygenic. It is of interest that one of these candidate genes is located on chromosome 21, the same chromosome that is triploid in Down syndrome. The significance of this finding is not obvious, but it is worth noting that patients who have Down syndrome show early onset of histologic cerebral changes that are similar to those seen in AD.
   - **Apoprotein A:** Certain alleles of apoprotein A, especially ε-4 allele, are found in some cases of AD. Unfortunately, many others do not have this allele, and, conversely, some patients with the ε-4 allele do not have AD.
   - **β-Amyloid:** A unique form of amyloid is found in the brain of AD patients. This β-amyloid is derived from amyloid precursor protein (APP). Several mutations of the APP gene have been identified in familial cases, and the same genetic abnormalities are found in some sporadic cases. The exact pathogenetic role of amyloid deposition, however, has not been determined.
   - **Presenilin:** PS-1 and PS-2 genes encoding these transmembrane proteins are mutated in AD. Presenilins are thought to participate in the processing of β-amyloid. Mutations of PS-1 and PS-2 are found in half of all patients with early-onset AD.

55. **Describe the neuropathology of AD.**
   - There is atrophy of the brain with thin gyri, widened sulci, and dilatated ventricles. These changes can be documented during life by CT scanning.
   - Neurofibrillary tangles seen in the cytoplasm of pyramidal cells, especially in the hippocampus, amygdala, basal forebrain, and the raphe nuclei. These tangles consist of insoluble paired helical filaments composed of hyperphosphorylated forms of neurofilaments, tau-protein, ubiquitin, and β-amyloid. In advanced cases of AD, neurofibrillary tangles are found lying in the neuropil as "tombstones" of dead neurons, the nuclei and cytoplasm of which have disappeared.
   - Neuritic (senile) plaques appear as complex spherical structures. It is thought that they develop from damaged neurons, which form the core of the plaques. The core of typical mature plaques consists of paired helical filaments similar to those forming the intraneuronal neurofibrillary tangles. The core is heavily impregnated with β-amyloid. They can be seen in H&E-stained slides but are best visualized by silver impregnation or immunohistochemical stains (e.g., ubiquitin or β-amyloid). Most often these plaques are found in the hippocampus and cortex, but they may be found in other parts of the brain.
   - Granulovacuolar degeneration is primarily found in the hippocampus. Neurons of this area show an increased number of lysosomes in their cytoplasm. By light microscopy, these lysosomes appear as clear cytoplasmic vesicles with a central basophilic dot.
   - Hirano bodies appear as elongated bodies composed of actin filaments are also found in the hippocampus. They lie adjacent to neurons or, less often, within their cytoplasm.
   - Amyloid angiopathy presents as deposits of amyloid in the small cerebral arteries and arterioles. These deposits, however, are not specific for AD.
   See Fig. 22-4.

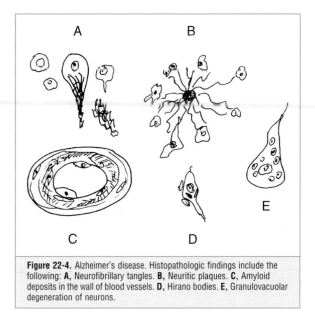

Figure 22-4. Alzheimer's disease. Histopathologic findings include the following: **A,** Neurofibrillary tangles. **B,** Neuritic plaques. **C,** Amyloid deposits in the wall of blood vessels. **D,** Hirano bodies. **E,** Granulovacuolar degeneration of neurons.

56. **Are neuritic plaques and neurofibrillary tangles diagnostic of AD?**
    No. A few plaques and neurofibrillary tangles can be found in the brain of most aging people. The diagnosis of AD is made by counting the plaques and neurofibrillary tangles or finding large numbers of these changes in the neocortex of a deceased person who had clinical evidence of dementia. Special stains such as silver impregnation to demonstrate neurofibrillary tangles or neuritic plaques are useful for counting these lesions in histologic sections.

57. **What are the symptoms of AD?**
    - Progressive loss of memory
    - Impairment of at least one of the following cognitive functions: judgment, abstract thinking, problem solving, language, visual–spatial function, and aphasia of the word-finding type
    - Impaired social functioning
    - Clear sensorium

58. **What is Pick disease?**
    It is a rare form of dementia that may be clinically indistinguishable from AD but occurs usually in younger people (40–60 years of age).
    There is selective atrophy of frontal and temporal lobes ("knife-edge" gyri and wide sulci, with hydrocephalus), but it also may involve the deeper gray matter structures (putamen and caudate nucleus).
    Histologic features include loss of neurons accompanied by gliosis. The remaining neurons become swollen (Pick cells), or their cytoplasm is filled with filamentous round inclusions (Pick bodies). These cytoplasmic inclusions consist of paired helical filaments and can be impregnated with silver stain. In contrast to AD, there are no neurofibrillary tangles and no neuritic plaques.

59. What is parkinsonism?

Parkinsonism (Parkinson syndrome) is a clinical syndrome characterized by any combination of the following symptoms:

- Tremor (it is involuntary, often of the "pill-rolling" type)
- Rigidity
- Bradykinesia (slowing of voluntary movements)
- Postural instability (stooped posture)
- Expressionless face and slurred speech
- Gait disturbances (festinating, shuffling, small steps, and frequent falling)
- Autonomic disturbances (constipation, hypotension, etc.)
- Depression and dementia develop in a significant number of cases over time

60. What are the causes of parkinsonism?

- Idiopathic Parkinson disease (paralysis agitans) is the most common cause
- Postencephalitic parkinsonism (rare today)
- Ischemia of basal ganglia (relatively common)
- Drugs (e.g., phenothiazine and haloperidol)
- Toxins (e.g., carbon monoxide poisoning and methanol)
- Head trauma, repetitive (e.g., boxers)
- Shy–Drager syndrome (idiopathic parkinsonism associated with hypotension and other autonomic symptoms)

61. What is idiopathic Parkinson disease?

- It is a common degenerative disease of basal ganglia. It affects more than 5% of all people older than the age of 70 years.
- The etiology is not known.
- Pathologically it presents with a loss of dopaminergic neurons in the pigmented nuclei of the brain stem and the disruption of the normal function of the nigrostriatal system (includes substantia nigra, caudate, putamen, globus pallidus, subthalamus, and thalamus).
- On gross examination of cross-sections of the brain, there is depigmentation of substantia nigra and locus ceruleus.
- Microscopically substantia nigra shows a loss of neurons and loss of pigment from the remaining neurons, which contain eosinophilic round Lewy bodies. Lewy bodies consist of neurofilaments, α-synuclein, and ubiquitin.

62. What is Huntington disease (HD)?

HD is an autosomal dominant disease involving the extrapyramidal motor system presenting with chorea, extrapyramidal signs, and progressive dementia. Symptoms begin appearing in the 35- to 45-year-old age group. The HD gene, known as ITI5, is located on the short arm of chromosome 4, contains 67 exons, and encodes for the protein huntingtin. The gene's CAG repeat is expanded in HD, which results in an abnormal huntingtin (expanded polyglutamine stretch), and this causes the disease. Pathologic findings include:

- Atrophy of caudate nucleus, putamen, and globus pallidus accompanied by "boxlike" dilatation of the lateral ventricles
- Loss of neurons in the atrophic basal ganglia, but also in parts of the cortex

63. What are the symptoms of HD?

The most typical finding is choreoathetosis (derived from Greek words for "dance" and "slow writhing movements") characterized by complex, jerky, usually rapid movements. These movements are hyperkinetic (excessive, abnormally increased muscular activity), dystonic (abnormal muscle tonicity), uncoordinated, and involuntary. Eventually, these movements are replaced by reduced activity, stiffness (rigidity), and slowness of movements (bradykinesia), which are characteristics of parkinsonism. Cognitive impairment often precedes choreoathetosis. Patients are unable to perform complex tasks, and both immediate and remote recall are lost. Hence, the dementia that develops is different from the type caused by cortical lesions and thus is classified as subcortical dementia.

64. **What is amyotrophic lateral sclerosis?**
    - It is a progressive, fatal motor neuron disease of unknown etiology, also known as Lou Gehrig disease.
    - Most cases are sporadic, but some cases are familial. Familial cases seem to be more common on some Pacific islands (e.g., Pacific Ocean islands—Guam and the Mariana Islands).
    - Both the upper and the lower motor neurons are affected. Neuronal death (apoptosis) is linked in some familial cases to mutation of the gene encoding the zinc/copper-binding superoxide dismutase.
    - Pathologically the spinal cord shows a loss of neurons from the anterior horn of the gray matter and the demyelination and loss of anterior corticospinal and lateral corticospinal tracts (Fig. 22-5).
    - Clinically the disease presents with fasciculation (due to loss of lower motor neurons and denervation of muscles) and progressive loss of muscle strength.
    - Spasticity, hyperactive tendon reflexes, and Babinski reflex are evident because of a loss of upper motor neurons.
    - Widespread paralysis develops over time. Median survival is 5 years. Death usually results from paralysis of respiratory muscles.

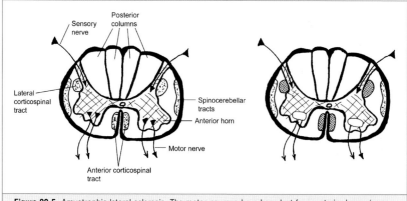

Figure 22-5. Amyotrophic lateral sclerosis. The motor neurons have been lost from anterior horns (*open circles* in anterior horns). Anterior and lateral corticospinal tracts *(shaded areas)* undergo degeneration due to a loss of upper motor neurons.

NUTRITIONAL, METABOLIC, AND TOXIC BRAIN DISEASES

65. **Which vitamin deficiencies affect the brain?**
    Brain lesions are most often found in deficiencies of the vitamin B complex:
    - B_1 (thiamine)—Wernicke–Korsakoff syndrome
    - B_6 (pyridoxine)—irritability and seizure in children
    - Nicotinic acid—pellagra with neurologic irritability, impaired memory, spastic weakness, delirium, and seizures
    - B_{12} (cyanocobalamin)—spinal cord and cortical lesions resulting in paresthesia, and motor symptoms progressing to paralysis and dementia ("megaloblastic madness")

66. **Describe the effects of vitamin B_1 deficiency on the nervous system.**
    Thiamine deficiency may present as either dry or wet beriberi. Wet beriberi involves the heart, but in dry beriberi, there are typical neurologic or psychiatric symptoms. Acute deficiency superimposed on chronic deficiency causes cerebral beriberi (Wernicke–Korsakoff syndrome).
    Dry beriberi is characterized by symmetric peripheral neuropathy. It presents with bilateral and symmetric sensorimotor neuropathy involving predominantly lower extremities, and with paresthesias of the toes, muscle cramps, and pain in the calves.
    Wernicke–Korsakoff syndrome includes delusions, confabulation, hallucinations, confusion, memory loss, ataxia, and nystagmus, often terminating in coma. The pathologic changes include hemorrhagic necrosis of the mammillary bodies and paraventricular regions of the brain stem and brain (e.g., hypothalamus, periaqueductal and tectal regions, cerebellum, pons, and optic chiasm). Usually there is dilatation of small capillaries with prominent endothelial cells, with eventual multifocal hemorrhages accompanied by siderophages, reactive gliosis, inflammation, and destruction—almost selectively—of serotoninergic neurons. The pathogenesis of these lesions is not understood, but most likely it is related to altered glycolysis caused by thiamine deficiency.

KEY POINTS: NUTRITIONAL, METABOLIC, AND TOXIC ✓ BRAIN DISEASES

1. Chronic alcohol abuse leads to direct brain injury and is also accompanied by vitamin B deficiencies that cause distinct neurologic lesions and symptoms.

2. Brain injury is encountered in many systemic metabolic diseases and in the course of major organ failure (e.g., liver failure and kidney failure).

67. **What are the most important neuropathologic consequences of vitamin B_{12} deficiency?**
    Vitamin B_{12} deficiency leads to subacute combined degeneration of the spinal cord. Axons in both the ascending tracts of the posterior column and the descending pyramidal tracts are affected. The initial signs include slight ataxia, then spastic weakness of the lower extremities and burning sensation in the feet, and lack of coordination of the musculature of the lower limbs due to altered postural sensibility. The disease may progress to paraplegia. In severe cases, the lesions may be found in the anterior horn and the cortical portions of the brain. See Fig. 22-6.

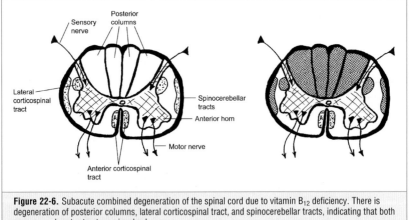

Figure 22-6. Subacute combined degeneration of the spinal cord due to vitamin B_{12} deficiency. There is degeneration of posterior columns, lateral corticospinal tract, and spinocerebellar tracts, indicating that both sensory and motor tracts are involved.

68. **What are the most significant neuropathologic consequences of alcohol abuse?**
Acute alcohol intoxication may be lethal or reversible. Chronic alcoholism may induce:
- **Cortical atrophy:** It is a result of the direct toxic effect of alcohol and malnutrition. Cerebral atrophy may be accompanied by nonobstructive hydrocephalus ex vacuo.
- **Atrophy of the cerebellum:** Histologically, the cerebellum shows a loss of granular cells of the cerebellar vermis and Purkinje cells of the cerebellar cortex, accompanied by proliferation of astrocytes. The cerebellar damage results in truncal ataxia, stumbling with or without intention, tremor, and nystagmus, and it is often accompanied by other alcohol-related conditions, such as delirium tremens, neuropathy, and encephalopathy.
- **Wernicke–Korsakoff syndrome:** It is a consequence of thiamine deficiency, a nutritional deficiency commonly found in chronic alcoholics.
- **Central pontine myelinolysis:** This is a rare complication characterized by focal areas of selective myelin loss within the pons. In mild forms, it may be asymptomatic, but sometimes it may cause quadriplegia and severe depression of consciousness. The exact pathogenesis of this lesion is not known, but it is thought that it represents a complication of too rapid correction of hyponatremia in chronic alcoholics.
- **Marchiafava–Bignami disease:** It is a rare complication characterized by coagulative necrosis of midline structures and commissures of the brain (e.g., corpus callosum).
- **Fetal alcohol syndrome (FAS):** It develops in infants born to mothers who drink alcohol. The features of FAS are low birth weight, slitlike eyes, birdlike flattened face, and slow psychomotor development.
- **Alcoholic neuropathy, myopathy, and myelopathy:** Peripheral sensory motor neuropathy is a complication of malnutrition combined with vitamin deficiencies.

69. **List the neuropathologic findings in drug addicts (substance abuse cases).**
- **Emboli:** Intravenous drug abuse is often complicated by endocarditis, which may serve as a source of septic emboli. These emboli may cause cerebral infarcts and abscesses.
- **Vasospasm:** Many recreational drugs, such as cocaine, amphetamine, and phencyclidine, cause vasospasm, which may lead to cerebral ischemia or hemorrhage.
- **Angiitis:** It may involve arteries of various sizes (hypersensitivity angiitis). This adverse reaction is poorly understood, but is seen at autopsy of people abusing amphetamine, cocaine, phenylpropanolamine, and several other drugs.

70. **What are the major characteristics of hepatic encephalopathy?**
Hepatic encephalopathy develops in severe liver failure. It may appear as acute hepatic encephalopathy characterized by rapidly developing coma. Portal-systemic shunting (in cirrhosis) or portacaval anastomosis (surgical due to portal hypertension in cirrhosis) cause chronic hepatic encephalopathy. The principal pathologic findings include diffuse cerebral edema that may cause herniations and the presence of Alzheimer type 2 astrocytes (astrocytes with swollen, vesicular, often lobulated nuclei and prominent nucleoli) in the cortex and basal ganglia. These cells are not pathognomonic of hepatic encephalopathy because they may be found in brains after hypoxemia and uremia and also in hyperammonemic states due to enzyme deficiencies of the urea cycle.

71. **Describe the CNS changes in Wilson disease.**
Wilson disease (hepatolenticular degeneration) is an autosomal recessive disease affecting copper metabolism. Copper-induced injury causes cirrhosis, Kayser–Fleischer ring of the cornea, and extensive loss of neurons from basal ganglia. Putamen is the most severely affected part of the brain, but basal ganglia such as globus pallidus and subthalamic and thalamic nuclei can be affected as well. Patients usually present with extrapyramidal symptoms (dysarthria, dysphagia, dystonia, and tremor), which may

progress to dementia. Other patients who predominantly have liver insufficiency may present with hepatic encephalopathy. The affected basal ganglia show neuronal loss and gliosis, which may be followed by spongy degeneration, cyst formation, or both.

NEOPLASMS

72. **How common are brain tumors?**
    - The incidence is low (10–17 per 100,00), but nevertheless there are 14,000 cases per year in the United States.
    - They occur in all age groups.
    - They account for 2% of all cancer deaths in adults and 20% of cancer deaths in children.
    - In children, brain tumors are the second most common type of malignancy.

73. **What are the risk factors for brain tumors?**
    Most brain tumors occur at random and are unrelated to any identifiable risk factor. The only known risk factor is therapeutic x-irradiation of children; such children are at higher than average risk for developing brain tumors. Some brain tumors develop in patients afflicted with certain hereditary syndromes.

74. **List the most important hereditary syndromes associated with an increased incidence of brain tumors.**
    - **Neurofibromatosis type 2:** Schwannomas of the eighth nerve
    - **Neurofibromatosis type 1:** Increased incidence of peripheral nerve neurofibromas and meningiomas
    - **von Hippel–Lindau syndrome:** Hemangioblastoma of the cerebellum and hemangioma of retina
    - **Li-Fraumeni syndrome:** Glioblastoma multiforme, in association with breast, ovarian, and colon cancer
    - **Tuberous sclerosis:** Subependymal giant cell astrocytoma

KEY POINTS: NEOPLASMS ✓

1. Most brain tumors are malignant and lethal because they directly destroy the brain and also increase intracranial pressure and cause many secondary changes in the brain.

2. Most brain tumors originate from glia cells.

3. Meningiomas and schwannomas are benign intracranial tumors.

75. **List the most common primary brain tumors.**
    - Gliomas (75% of tumors in adults; 60% of all gliomas are glioblastomas multiforme)
    - Meningiomas (15% of tumors in adults)
    - Undifferentiated composed of neuroectodermal precursor cells; common in children

76. **How are primary brain tumors classified histogenetically?**
    Histogenetic classification is based on the assumption that the histologic features of a given tumor betray its cell of origin. Using this principle, one can recognize a number of pathologic entities, listed in Table 22-2.

TABLE 22-2. HISTOGENETIC CLASSIFICATION OF TUMOR CELLS	
Cell of Origin	**Tumor**
Astrocyte	Astrocytoma Glioblastoma multiforme
Oligodendroglia cell	Oligodendroglioma
Ependymal cell	Ependymoma
Choroid plexus cell	Choroid papilloma
Neuronal precursor cell	Medulloblastoma
Meningeal arachnoid cell	Meningioma
Vascular cell	Hemangioblastoma
Lymphoid cell	Lymphoma
Schwann cells	Schwannoma
Embryonic remnants	Craniopharyngioma Germ cell tumor

77. How are tumors of the CNS classified topographically?
Three major groups are recognized (Fig. 22-7):
- Supratentorial tumors (i.e., cerebral tumors located above the tentorium cerebelli; most brain tumors found in adults [70%] are supratentorial.)
- Infratentorial tumors (i.e., tumors of the cerebellum and the brain stem located underneath the tentorium cerebelli; most brain tumors in children (70%) are found in this location.)
- Spinal cord tumors

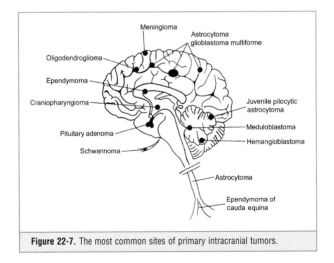

Figure 22-7. The most common sites of primary intracranial tumors.

78. List the pathogenesis of clinical signs and symptoms caused by brain tumors.
Brain tumors are space-occupying lesions that act on the adjacent brain, causing:
- **Compression:** The effects of compression depend on the location of the tumor. In general, the tumor may cause loss of motor functions (e.g., paralysis) or of sensory functions

(e.g., loss of sensation), or it may stimulate certain parts of the brain and cause epileptic fits or abnormal sensory stimuli.

- **Destruction:** Invasive tumors may destroy or stimulate nerve cells and produce the same symptoms as those tumors that are compressing the brain.
- **Infarction and hemorrhage:** The tumor may invade blood vessels or compress blood vessels and thus cause ischemic necrosis. Necrotic tumors tend to bleed.
- **Cerebral edema:** It is a typical response to all intracranial pathologic processes. Brain edema involves the peritumoral brain tissue but also parts of the brain at a distance from the tumor.
- **Obstruction of CSF flow:** This obstruction leads to formation of hydrocephalus.
- **Changes in the CSF composition:** CSF pressure is typically increased, and the CSF contains increased amounts of protein. Tumor cells may occasionally be seen, most often in tumors such as lymphoma and medulloblastoma.

79. **Why do brain tumors cause intracranial hypertension?**
The main reasons are:
- Mass effect of the tumor
- Brain edema
- Obstruction of the CSF and resulting hydrocephalus

80. **Do brain tumors metastasize?**
In general, brain tumors do not metastasize. Meningiomas and schwannomas are benign tumors, and one would not expect them to metastasize in any circumstances. Highly malignant tumors such as glioblastoma multiforme may theoretically metastasize, but in most instances, the patients die before such extracranial metastases develop.

81. **Can brain tumors metastasize?**
Yes. The best example is medulloblastoma, a highly malignant brain tumor of childhood. The tumor cells of these cerebellar tumors may enter the CSF, and such cells are then carried "downstream" into the spinal cord ("drop metastases"). Metastases have also been recorded following operations of brain tumor patients. It is thought that such tumors enter the blood during surgery or thereafter because the procedure has damaged the blood–brain barrier and made it more permeable.
   The third example of brain tumor metastases is tumors that have metastasized to the thoracic or abdominal cavity through the catheters and drainage tubes inserted by surgeons into the cranium to drain the CSF and thus reduce the intracranial pressure.

82. **Can benign brain tumors cause death?**
Yes. Benign tumors (e.g., meningioma) may cause death primarily because of their location. For example, a benign tumor may compress the vital centers of the brain stem. Some tumors are located such that they cannot be reached or resected by surgeons.

83. **What is the most common primary malignant brain tumor?**
- Glioblastoma multiforme is the most common primary brain tumor in adults, accounting for 40% of all brain tumors.
- Medulloblastoma is the most common tumor in children, accounting for 25% of all intracranial neoplasms in those younger than 10 years of age.

84. **How are astrocytic tumors classified?**
Astrocytic tumors are classified on the basis of the degree of their differentiation and by specific clinicopathologic parameters. Accordingly, these tumors were classified into four main categories, with astrocytoma Grade I being the best differentiated (low grade), and astrocytoma Grade IV, also known as glioblastoma multiforme, as the high-grade tumor. Subsequent

studies and discoveries have shown that this approach is too simplistic; therefore the current World Health Organization classification recognizes several more subtypes of astrocytic tumors, such as diffuse astrocytoma, anaplastic astrocytoma, glioblastoma multiforme, juvenile pilocytic astrocytoma, and pleomorphic xanthoastrocytoma.

85. **List key facts about diffuse astrocytoma.**
    - Also known simply as astrocytoma, it must be distinguished from circumscribed variants of astrocytic tumors (e.g., pilocytic astrocytoma and pleomorphic xanthoastrocytoma).
    - It accounts for 10% to 15% of all astrocytic tumors.
    - It occurs most often in young adults (peak age, 35 years). Approximately 60% of all tumors occur in the 20- to 45-year-old age group, but 30% are found in people older than 45 years.
    - Composed of well-differentiated neoplastic astrocytes infiltrating the surrounding brain.
    - The tumor has an intrinsic tendency to progress and transform into anaplastic astrocytoma or glioblastoma multiforme.
    - Mean survival with modern surgery and chemotherapy is 6–8 years.

86. **List key facts about glioblastoma multiforme.**
    - It is the most common glioma (60% of all gliomas), accounting for 15% of all intracranial tumors (including metastases).
    - The peak incidence in the 45- to 60-year-old age group, but it may occur in children, teenagers, and very old people as well.
    - It may begin as a highly malignant glioblastoma multiforme (primary glioblastoma multiforme), or it may develop from the progression of diffuse astrocytoma with early and frequent p53 mutations (secondary glioblastoma multiforme).
    - There is invasive growth; it may extend to the other side of the brain (bilateral "butterfly" lesions seen by CT scan or at autopsy). It may be multifocal.
    - Marked macroscopic and microscopic pleomorphism (note that it is called multiforme).
    - Gross examination shows areas of necrosis, hemorrhage, cystic change, and so on.
    - Microscopically, the diagnosis is made by recognizing the variegated pattern rather than a specific anaplastic cell. Typically tumors show anaplasia, pleomorphism, necrosis, numerous mitosis, and vascular-endothelial ("glomeruloid") proliferation.
    - It has an extremely bad prognosis. Mean survival is 1 year, and only 1% of all patients survive 3 years.

87. **What is a juvenile pilocytic astrocytoma?**
    - It is a slow-growing tumor of children and adolescents.
    - It accounts for 25% of all intracranial tumors in children younger than age 10 years.
    - It is most often located in the cerebellum.
    - It is cystic and well circumscribed on gross examination.
    - Histologically it is composed of fibrillar astrocytes, often showing Rosenthal fibers.
    - Most cerebellar tumors are curable and can be resected completely. Hypothalamic tumors cannot be removed completely and are lethal.

88. **What is oligodendroglioma?**
    - It is an uncommon cerebral tumor of adults (30–60 years), accounting for about 10% of all gliomas
    - It is most often found in the cerebral hemispheres
    - It is circumscribed and often calcified
    - Microscopically it is composed of uniform oligodendroglia cells, occasionally admixed to astrocytes; low mitotic rate
    - Tumors tend to recur after surgery.
    - The 5-year survival rate is 75%, and 10-year survival rate is 50%.

89. **List key facts about ependymoma.**
   - It is an uncommon tumor that occurs in all age groups but more often in children than adults. It accounts for 30% of all intracranial tumors in children younger than the age of 3 years.
   - It is derived from ependymal cells lining the ventricles and spinal canal, although may occur from ependymal remnants outside the CNS as well.
   - It is the most common neuroepithelial tumor of the spinal cord (60% gliomas).
   - In the brain, 60% of tumors originate in the fourth ventricle. In the spinal cord, the tumor can originate from the cauda equina (filum terminale).
   - Microscopically it is composed of ependymal cells forming perivascular pseudorosettes and tubules. Filum terminale tumors have a myxopapillary structure.
   - Prognosis depends on the location of the tumor, its resectability, and its histologic grade. It has a worse prognosis in children than in adults.

90. **What is medulloblastoma?**
   - It is a malignant tumor derived from primitive neuroectodermal cells.
   - It is a childhood tumor. More than 50% of all patients are younger than 20 years of age. Peak occurrence is at 7 years of age.
   - It accounts for 25% of all brain tumors in children younger than 10 years of age.
   - It may occur in young adults (20–30 years) but is extremely rare after age 40 years.
   - It involves vermis of cerebellum in children, but in older people it may involve the cerebellar hemispheres.
   - There are drop metastases through CSF to the spinal cord.
   - Histologically it is composed of densely packed small "blue" cells arranged into solid sheets. There are frequent mitoses and necrosis.
   - Prognosis has improved with modern chemotherapy, and the 5-year survival is 50% to 70%. Prognosis depends on the resectability of the tumor. The presence of metastasis is an unfavorable finding. Children younger than the age of 3 years have worse prognosis than adults.

91. **List key facts about meningioma.**
   - It is a benign tumor originating from the meningothelial (arachnoid cells) of the leptomeninges.
   - It accounts for 20% of intracranial tumors.
   - Peak age is 50 to 70 years, but it may occur at any age. It is more common in women.
   - It is attached to the dura, most often in the parasagittal region along the falx cerebri.
   - It is a well-circumscribed tumor compressing the brain from outside.
   - The overlying bone shows hyperostosis and infiltration by the tumor. Local invasion of bone does not mean that the tumor is malignant.
   - Histologically it is composed of meningothelial cells forming whorls, often with central calcifications (psammoma bodies). Several histologic subtypes are recognized, but histologic subtyping is of no clinical significance.
   - Prognosis is excellent but depends on the grade of the tumor. Three grades are recognized: Grade I tumors (93%) have excellent prognosis but may recur in 10% of cases; Grade II (atypical meningiomas) (5%) tend to recur in 30% of cases; and Grade III (malignant meningiomas) (2%) tend to invade the brain and may be lethal.

92. **What are intracranial nerve sheath tumors?**
   Nerve sheath tumors are classified as schwannomas or neurofibromas. These tumors most often develop from peripheral nerves and inside the cranium. They develop almost exclusively from the eighth nerve. Schwannomas of the eighth cranial nerve are benign tumors of the cerebellopontine angle found in neurofibromatosis type 2. Neurofibromas are the most common intradural extramedullary tumors of the nerve roots of the spinal cord.

93. What is cerebellar hemangioblastoma?
Hemangioblastoma of the cerebellum is a benign tumor composed of endothelial cells forming small blood vessels, surrounded by interstitial lipid-laden cells. With hemangiomas of the retina, cerebellar hemangioblastomas are part of the hereditary von Hippel–Lindau syndrome.

94. What is craniopharyngioma?
Craniopharyngioma is a benign tumor developing from the remnants of the Rathke pouch, the primordium of the pituitary. Typically it is located in the suprasellar region and tends to compress and destroy the hypothalamus. Panhypopituitarism is a common complication.

95. Which tumors tend to metastasize to the brain?
Up to 50% of all clinically diagnosed intracranial malignant tumors are metastases from other sites. The most common tumors that metastasize to the brain are:
- Lung cancer
- Breast cancer
- Kidney cancer
- Gastrointestinal cancer
- Melanoma
- Thyroid cancer
  Mnemonic to remember these tumors is *breast*:
  Breast
  Renal
  Enteric (colon)
  Aerorespiratory tract
  Skin (melanoma)
  Thyroid

PERIPHERAL NERVES

96. How do peripheral nerves react to injury?
Peripheral nerves consist of myelinated and nonmyelinated fibers. Injury of the perikaryon leads to irreversible degeneration of both myelinated and nonmyelinated axons. Transection of the axon, however, can be repaired, and the axon can regenerate as long as the perikaryon is viable.
In myelinated nerves, three types of axonal injury are recognized:
- **Distal axonal degeneration:** Injury of the perikaryon leads to "dying back" injury of the axon, which starts most distally and spreads proximally toward the perinuclear portion of the cytoplasm. Degeneration of the axon is accompanied by a breakdown of the myelin enveloping the damaged axon (secondary demyelination). This form of injury is typically seen in toxic and drug-related neuropathies (e.g., isoniazid neuropathy) and vitamin deficiency (e.g., vitamin B_1 deficiency).
- **Wallerian degeneration:** This type of injury typically occurs in transected axons. Distal to the site of transection, the axon degenerates together with its myelin sheath. Proximally, the axon dies back to the next node of Ranvier, but the stump can regenerate, and the new axon is formed. It is remyelinated by the adjacent Schwann cell.
- **Segmental demyelination:** Axonal injury is secondary, and it follows an injury of Schwann cells, leading to a loss of myelin sheath (primary demyelination). Fragmented myelin is phagocytized by macrophages. This type of injury typically occurs following ischemia, due to immune injury of myelin sheaths, or toxic neuropathies. Hereditary neuropathies also involve injury of myelin sheaths, which is sometimes accompanied by concentric regeneration of Schwann cells in the form of hypertrophic "onion bulbs."

KEY POINTS: PERIPHERAL NERVES ✔

1. Peripheral nerve injuries are caused by metabolic, toxic, nutritional, circulatory, and immunologic diseases, but they may also be hereditary.

2. Diabetic neuropathy is the most common peripheral nerve disease.

97. How are neuropathies classified clinically?
Peripheral neuropathies can be classified according to their etiology (e.g., toxic and metabolic), duration (e.g., acute and chronic), or distribution of lesions:
- **Mononeuropathy:** This form of disease presents with symptoms pertaining to a single nerve, such as the radial or ulnar nerve in carpal syndrome.
- **Mononeuritis multiplex:** This form of disease presents with symptoms pertaining to several isolated nerves usually affected in an unpredictable manner, as in polyarteritis nodosa.
- **Polyneuropathy:** Numerous, sometimes all, nerves are involved, as in various toxic neuropathies, alcoholic neuropathy, Guillain–Barré syndrome, carcinomatous neuropathy, and so forth.

98. How does polyneuropathy present clinically?
Three forms are recognized:
- Predominantly motor neuropathy (e.g., Guillain–Barré syndrome)
- Predominantly sensory neuropathy (e.g., carcinomatous neuropathy)
- Combined sensorimotor (e.g., alcoholic or diabetic neuropathy)
Peripheral neuropathy is most often of the sensorimotor type.

99. List principal peripheral neuropathies.
- Hereditary
  - Charcot–Marie–Tooth disease
  - Dejerine–Sottas syndrome
  - Neuropathy in various hereditary metabolic diseases (e.g., porphyria and hereditary amyloidosis) and neurologic diseases (e.g., Friedreich ataxia)
- Autoimmune
  - Inflammatory demyelinating neuropathy (Guillain–Barré syndrome)
- Metabolic
  - Diabetic
  - Uremic
  - Hypothyroid
  - Porphyric
- Nutritional/toxic
  - Alcoholic
  - Beriberi (vitamin B_1 deficiency)
  - Vitamin B_{12} deficiency
- Ischemic
  - Peripheral vascular (atherosclerotic) disease
  - Diabetic microangiopathy
  - Polyarteritis nodosa
- Infectious
  - Herpes zoster
  - Leprosy (rare in the United States, more common in tropics)
  - AIDS
  - Diphtheria toxin (rare today!)
  - Lyme disease

100. What is inflammatory demyelinating neuropathy (IDN)?
IDN (also known as Guillain–Barré syndrome) is a peripheral nerve disease presenting with an acute onset of motor symptoms, such as muscle weakness or paralysis. Resolution of symptoms begins 2 to 4 weeks after onset, with complete recovery in most patients. In some patients, it may have a protracted course. The disease may occur in several settings:
- Sporadic form without any obvious precipitating event
- Following immunization or surgery
- Following a viral or mycoplasmal infection
- As a paraneoplastic syndrome in patients with cancer

101. Describe the pathologic findings in inflammatory demyelinating neuropathy.
- It can affect any part of the peripheral nervous system: peripheral nerves, spinal roots, cranial nerves, autonomic nerves, and peripheral ganglia.
- Affected nerves are infiltrated with lymphocytes and macrophages.
- Demyelination is prominent, but the axons are spared.
- Onion bulbs resulting from recurrent demyelination and remyelination are seen in chronic stages of the disease.
- Complete recovery is the norm.

102. What is the most common peripheral neuropathy encountered in clinical practice?
It is diabetic neuropathy.

103. What is the most common infectious neuropathy in the United States?
It is HIV infection and AIDS polyneuropathy. This may be related directly to HIV infection but may also be a complication of the body's immune response or toxicity of drugs used in the treatment. It occurs in several forms:
- **Chronic axonal polyneuropathy:** This is the most common form of AIDS peripheral neuropathy. Axonal degeneration is typically associated with sensory symptoms (paresthesias, tingling, and loss of touch and pain).
- **Inflammatory demyelinating neuropathy:** Typical Guillain–Barré syndrome may develop in the course of the HIV infection before the onset of full-blown AIDS, but it may also present in a chronic form.
- **Infectious polyneuropathy:** It is most often caused by CMV infection or herpes zoster.
- **Toxic neuropathy:** It is related to drugs used in the treatment of HIV infection.

104. How does amyloid affect peripheral nerves?
Deposits of amyloid may be found in the wall of small blood vessels providing blood to the peripheral nerves or in the extracellular matrix of the endoneurium surrounding the axons. These deposits may cause axonal and myelin sheath injuries. Deposits of amyloid in ganglia are typically associated with autonomic symptoms.

105. Which diseases cause amyloid deposits in the peripheral nerves?
Amyloid may be found in the nerves in several settings:
- AL amyloid is deposited in multiple myeloma.
- AA is deposited in systemic (secondary) amyloidosis, complicating chronic infectious diseases.
- Transthyretin-derived amyloid is found in familial hereditary amyloid polyneuropathy.

106. What is the most common form of chronic peripheral neuropathy in children?
Hereditary neuropathy such as Charcot–Marie–Tooth disease, an autosomal dominant disease, is the most common form of chronic polyneuropathy in children. It is characterized by

demyelination and axonal degeneration. Subsequent remyelination leads to the formation of onion bulbs and remarkable thickening of peripheral nerves.

107. **List the most important peripheral nerve tumors.**
Most peripheral nerve sheath tumors are benign:
- Neurofibroma
- Schwannoma (neurilemmoma)

Malignant tumors are uncommon and may develop from benign tumors. The most important is malignant peripheral nerve sheath tumor (also known as neurofibrosarcoma).

WEBSITES

1. http://www.ncbi.nlm.nih.gov/entrez/query.fcgi?db=PubMed
2. http://www-medlib.med.utah.edu/WebPath/webpath.html#MENU
3. http://virtualtrials.com/btlinks/index.cfm?catid=11&catname=Pathology

BIBLIOGRAPHY

1. Ellison D, Love S, Chimelli L, et al: Neuropathology, 2nd ed., London, Mosby, 2005.
2. Lee JM, Grabb MC, Zipfel GJ, Choi DW: Brain tissue responses to ischemia. J Clin Invest 106:723–731, 2000.
3. Louis DN. Molecular pathology of malignant gliomas. Annu Rev Pathol 1:97–117, 2006.
4. Prusiner SB: Shattuck lecture—neurodegenerative diseases and prions. N Engl J Med 344:1516–1526, 2001.
5. Rowland LP, Shneider NA: Amyotrophic lateral sclerosis. N Engl J Med 344:1688–1700, 2001.
6. Saperstein DS, Katz JS, Amato AA, Barohn RJ: Clinical spectrum of chronic acquired demyelinating polyneuropathies. Muscle Nerve 24:311–324, 2001.
7. Sul J, Posner JB: Brain metastases: epidemiology and pathophysiology. Cancer Treat Res 136:1–21, 2007.
8. Townsend GC, Scheld WM: Infections of the central nervous system. Adv Int Med 43:403–448, 1998.

INDEX

Page numbers in **boldface type** indicate complete chapters. Page numbers followed by *t* indicate tables; *f*, figures.

Ascites, 40
  cirrhosis-related, 270, 270f
  hemorrhagic, 293
  hemorrhagic pancreatitis-related, 294
Aspartate aminotransferase
  as acute viral hepatitis indicator, 272
  as cell injury indicator, 11
  as liver function/injury indicator, 264, 293–294
  as pancreatitis indicator, 293–294
Aspirin
  as gastritis cause, 241
  as prolonged bleeding time cause, 179–180
Asthma, 61, 206t, 209
  atopic, 209
  bronchial, 208–210
  extrinsic, differentiated from intrinsic, 209
  as pneumothorax cause, 223
Astler-Coller staging system, for colorectal cancer, 260t
Astrocytic tumors, 470–471
Astrocytoma
  diffuse, 471
  juvenile pilocytic, 471
Ataxia, Friedreich, 107
Ataxia telangiectasia, 85, 92, 103
Atelectasis, 203, 203f
  compression, 204
  contraction, 204
  obstructive, 204
  patchy, 204
Atheroma, 122
  aortic, 122–123
  as infarct cause, 123
  ulcerated, 127–128
Atherosclerosis, 111, 121–122
  clinical manifestations of, 127–128
  coronary, 69, 125–126, 137
  diabetes mellitus-related, 299
  differentiated from arteriosclerosis, 121
  as ischemic heart disease cause, 139
  lesions of, 122
  pathogenesis of, 127f
    theories of, 122, 126, 128
  risk factors for, 123, 125
Athlete's foot, 395
Atresia, 99
  definition of, 235
  esophageal, 236
Atrophy, 15, 15f
  cerebellar, alcohol abuse-related, 467
  cortical, alcohol abuse-related, 467
  definition of, 16
  neurogenic muscle, 436, 436t, 437–438, 438f
  pathologic, 16
  physiologic, 16
Auspitz sign, 399
Autocrine stimulation, 365, 365f
Autoimmune disease, 67
  cutaneous, 396, 398
  definition of, 67

Autoimmunity, development of, 67
Autosomal dominant diseases, 108t, 109
  of muscle/musculoskeletal system, 109t, 443
Autosomal dominant inheritance/traits, 105, 106,
    107–108, 108f
Autosomal dominant polycystic kidney disease, 304,
    304f, 305t
Autosomal recessive diseases, 111, 111f, 111f, 112f
  as cancer risk factor, 86
Autosomal recessive inheritance/traits, 99, 106, 111
Autosomal recessive polycystic kidney disease, 304,
    304f, 305t
Axons
  distal degeneration of, 473
  injury reaction in, 448
  injury to, 451, 455
Azotemia, 301–302

B
Babinski reflex, 465
Bacteremia, pneumonia-related, 212
Bacteria. *See also specific bacteria*
  eosinophil-mediated killing of, 31
  leukocyte-mediated killing of, 23, 23f, 24
    congenital defects in, 24–25
  neutrophil-mediated killing of, 24
  opsonization of, 26
Bacterial infections. *See also specific bacterial
    infections*
  cutaneous, 393
  as diarrhea cause, 250, 250t
  as esophagitis cause, 239
  hepatic, 271, 276–277, 277f
  as myositis cause, 445
Bacteriuria, 303
Balanitis, 331
Baritosis, 215
Barr bodies, 104
Basal cell carcinoma, 389f, 401–402, 402f
B cells. *See* B lymphocytes
bcl-2 gene
  chronic lymphocytic leukemia/lymphoma-
    associated, 92
  follicular lymphoma-associated, 191
Bcl-2 protein, in B-cell lymphoma, 15
Beck triad, 154
Bence Jones proteins, 193f, 194, 320
"Bends," 52
Benign prostatic hyperplasia (BPH), 17, 335–336, 336f,
    338
Benzene, carcinogenicity of, 88
Berger disease (immunoglobulin A nephropathy), 311,
    312, 314–315, 314f
Beriberi, wet or dry, 466, 474
Berylliosis, 215, 217
Bile ducts, common, carcinoma of, 289
Biliary excretion, measurement of, 264
Biliary obstruction
  extrahepatic, 268

Hereditary diseases/syndromes
  brain tumor-associated, 468
  as cancer risk factor, 85
  definition of, 98
Hermaphroditism, 105
Hernia/herniations
  cerebral or cerebellar, 449, 450f
  congenital diaphragmatic, 238
  hiatal, 237–238, 237f, 239
  inguinal scrotal, 330
  as intestinal obstruction cause, 247, 248f
  scrotal, 331
Herpangina, 228
Herpes genitalis, 393
Herpes labialis (cold sores), 227, 393
Herpes simplex virus infections, 389f, 457
  cutaneous, 393
  as esophagitis cause, 239
  oral, 227
Herpes simplex virus-2 infections, 342
  in females, 339–340
  in males, 331
Herpes virus 8, carcinogenicity of, 89
Herpes virus infections, 101, 451
Herpes zoster virus infections, 389f, 475
High-density lipoprotein (HDL), 124–125
Hilar cell tumors, 354
Hirschsprung disease, 103, 247
Hirsutism, 408
Histamine, 26
  as bronchospasm cause, 209–210
Histiocytoma, malignant fibrous, 446
Histiocytosis
  Langerhans cell, 400, 407
  sinus, 187
Histocompatibility antigens (HLA), characteristics
  of, 59
Histoplasmosis, 30, 383, 396
Hives, 396
Hodgkin disease (lymphoma), 80, 196
  age factors in, 87
  definition of, 195
  differentiated from non-Hodgkin lymphoma, 196,
    196t
  staging of, 188, 196
  subtypes of, 195
Homocysteine, as neural tube defect risk factor,
    100
Hormones. See also specific hormones
  definition of, 365
  main types of, 366
Horner syndrome, lung cancer-related, 221
Human chorionic gonadotropin, as ovarian cancer
  marker, 354
Human immunodeficiency virus (HIV) infection,
    73, 101
  complications of
    adrenal insufficiency, 383
    central nervous system effects, 459

Human immunodeficiency virus (HIV) infection
    (Continued)
    central nervous system malformations, 451
    glomerulonephritis, 309
    neoplasms, 74
    nephropathy, 313
    neurologic consequences, 74
    polyneuropathy, 176
    renal complications, 313–314
  transmission of, 73
Human papillomavirus, 85, 335, 339, 341–343,
    393–394, 394f
  carcinogenicity of, 89
Human T-cell leukemia virus-1 (HTLV-1), 195
Huntington disease, 107, 461, 464–465
Hydatidiform mole, 355–356, 356f
Hydradenitis suppurativa, 395
Hydrocele, 330–331
Hydrocephalus
  intracranial, brain tumor-related, 470
  meningitis-related, 456, 459–460
  Pick disease-related, 463
Hydrochloric acid, as esophagitis cause, 239
Hydronephrosis, 322
Hydrops fetalis, 173
Hydrothorax, 222–223
21-Hydroxylase deficiency, 383
Hyperaldosteronism, 270. See also Conn syndrome
  primary, 382–383
  secondary, 382
Hyperbilirubinemia, 265
  benign isolated conjugated, 267
  mixed, 267
  unconjugated, 267
Hypercalcemia
  hyperparathyroidism-related, 379, 379f
  as pancreatitis cause, 292
  as paraneoplastic syndrome, 96
  as renal calculi cause, 322
  renal cell carcinoma-related, 324
Hypercholesterolemia, 124
  familial, 108t, 111
Hypercoagulable states, 47
Hypercortisolism, 368. See also Cushing syndrome
Hyperemia, 40–41
  active, 40
  passive, 40
Hyperemic tissues, color of, 40–41
Hyperestrinism, 271
Hyperextension injury, to the spinal cord, 451
Hyperflexion injury, to the spinal cord, 451
Hyperglycemia, diabetes mellitus-related,
    297–299
Hyper-immunoglobulin G syndrome, X-linked, 72
Hyperlipidemia
  as atherosclerosis cause, 123–124
  as gout cause, 432
  nephritic and nephrotic syndromes-related,
    302, 312t